Current Issues
in Nursing

Current Issues in Nursing

Edited by

Joanne Comi McCloskey

Professor and Director of Doctoral Program
University of Iowa, College of Nursing

Helen Kennedy Grace

Program Director
W.K. Kellogg Foundation

Third Edition

The C. V. Mosby Company

St. Louis • Baltimore • Toronto   1990

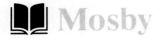

Editor: Linda L. Duncan
Production and editing: Editing, Design & Production, Inc.
Book design: Rey Umali
Cover design: Elise Stimac

Third Edition

Copyright © 1990 by The C.V. Mosby Company

Previous editions copyrighted 1981, 1985

Printed in the United States of America

The C.V. Mosby Company
11830 Westline Industrial Drive, St. Louis, Missouri 63146

Library of Congress Cataloging-in-Publication Data

Current issues in nursing/edited by Joanne Comi McCloskey, Helen
  Kennedy Grace.—3rd ed.
    p.   cm.
  Includes bibiliographical references.
  ISBN 0-8016-5525-0
  1. Nursing. 2. Nursing—United States. I. McCloskey, Joanne
Comi. II. Grace, Helen K.
  [DNLM: 1. Ethics, Nursing. 2. Nursing. 3. Philosophy, Nursing.
WY 16 C976]
RT63.C87   1990
610.73—dc20
DNLM/DLC
for Library of Congress   89-13080
                                     CIP

CONTRIBUTORS

Fadwa A. Affara, MA, MSC, RGN, SCM, RNT
Director, Regulation of Nursing Project
Florence Nightingale International Foundation
International Council of Nurses
Geneva, Switzerland

Genrose J. Alfano, RN, MA, FAAN
Editor, *Geriatric Nursing*
Editor, *Journal of Care for the Aging*
Freeport, New York

Linda K. Amos, RN, EdD, FAAN
Dean and Professor
College of Nursing
University of Utah
Salt Lake City, Utah

Gail Ardery, RN, PhD
Patient Care Coordinator
Iowa City Hospice
Iowa City, Iowa

Susan M. Awbrey, PhD
Assistant Professor
Coordinator of Learning Resources
College of Nursing
Michigan State University
East Lansing, Michigan

Myrtle K. Aydelotte, RN, PhD, FAAN
Professor and Dean Emeritus
College of Nursing
University of Iowa
Iowa City, Iowa

Judy Baigis-Smith, RN, PhD
Director, Long-Term Care and Health Promotion
Johns Hopkins University School of Nursing
Baltimore, Maryland

Ruth M. Barnard, RN, PhD
Associate Professor of Nursing
School of Nursing
University of Michigan
Ann Arbor, Michigan

Marjorie Beyers, RN, PhD, FAAN
Associate Vice President
Nursing and Allied Health Services
Sisters of Mercy Corporation
Farmington Hills, Michigan

Gillian Biscoe, RNG
Consultant, Human Resource Management and
Organizational Change
Department of Health
Lambton Quay, New Zealand

Judith L. Brett, RN, PhD
Director, Nursing Systems
Robert Wood Johnson University Hospital
New Brunswick, New Jersey

Pamela J. Brink, RN, PhD, FAAN
Professor and Associate Dean, Research
Faculty of Nursing
University of Alberta
Edmonton, Alberta, Canada

Kathleen Coen Buckwalter, RN, PhD
Professor
College of Nursing
University of Iowa
Iowa City, Iowa

Gloria M. Bulechek, RN, PhD
Assistant Professor
College of Nursing
University of Iowa
Iowa City, Iowa

Betty L. Chang, RN, DNS, FAAN
Professor
University of California
Los Angeles, California

Grace H. Chickadonz, RN, PhD, FAAN
Professor and Dean
College of Nursing
Syracuse University
Syracuse, New York

Olga Maranjian Church, RN, PhD, FAAN
Professor and Chair, Graduate Program
School of Nursing
University of Connecticut
Storrs, Connecticut

Trevor Clay, RGN, RMN, FRCN
General Secretary
The Royal College of Nursing of the United Kingdom
London, England

Joyce Colling, RN, PhD, FAAN
Associate Professor
School of Nursing
The Oregon Health Sciences University
Portland, Oregon

Colleen Conway-Welch, RN, PhD, FAAN
Professor and Dean
School of Nursing
Vanderbilt University
Nashville, Tennessee

Connie R. Curran, RN EdD, FAAN
President, Curran Group
Chicago, Illinois

Carolyne Kahle Davis, RN, PhD
National and International Health Care Advisor
Ernst and Whinney
Cleveland, Ohio

Vivien M. DeBack, RN, PhD
Project Director, NCNIP
Alverno College
Milwaukee, Wisconsin

Georgina de Carrillo, RN, PhD
Directora del Instituto de Pedagogia
Fac. de Ciene. Medicas
Quito, Ecuador

Connie Delaney, RN, PhD
Assistant Professor
College of Nursing
University of Iowa
Iowa City, Iowa

Elizabeth C. Devine, RN, PhD
Assistant Professor
School of Nursing
University of Wisconsin-Milwaukee
Milwaukee, Wisconsin

Barbara A. Donaho, RN, MA, FAAN
Vice President, Nursing and Patient Services
Shands Hospital at the University of Florida
Gainesville, Florida

M. Patricia Donahue, RN, PhD, FAAN
Associate Professor
College of Nursing
University of Iowa
Iowa City, Iowa

Rosemary Donley, RN, PhD, FAAN
Executive Vice President
The Catholic University of America
Washington, District of Columbia

Dorothy J. Douglas, RN, PhD
Professor
School of Nursing
University of Wisconsin-Madison
Madison, Wisconsin

Eileen McQuaid Dvorak, RN, PhD
Visiting Professor
The Marcella Niehoff School of Nursing
Loyola University of Chicago
Chicago, Illinois

Sharon A. Eck, RN, MA
Nursing Operations Manager
Le Bonheur Children's Medical Center
Memphis, Tennessee

Eunice K.M. Ernst, RN, MPH

Director, National Association of Childbearing
Centers, Inc.
Perkiomenville, Pennsylvania

Sharon L. Firlit, RN, PhD

Assistant Professor
Rush Medical Center
Chicago, Illinois

Mary Jean Flaherty, RN, PhD, FAAN

Associate Professor
The Catholic University of America
Washington, District of Columbia

David Anthony Forrester, RN, PhD

Associate Professor
University of Medicine and Dentistry of New Jersey
Newark, New Jersey

Stephen S. Fox, PhD

Professor
Department of Psychology
University of Iowa
Iowa City, Iowa

Maryann F. Fralic, RN, PhD

Senior Vice President for Nursing
Robert Wood Johnson University Hospital
New Brunswick, New Jersey

Mildred I. Freel, RN, MEd

Associate Professor
College of Nursing
University of Iowa
Iowa City, Iowa

Sara T. Fry, RN, PhD

Associate Professor
School of Nursing
University of Maryland
Baltimore, Maryland

Betty S. Furuta, RN, MS

Assistant Dean
Student Academic Service
School of Nursing
University of California, San Francisco

Lucia Gamroth, RN, MS

Associate Administrator
Benedictine Nursing Center
Mt. Angel, Oregon

Julia Fry Gibson, RN, JD

Director
Center for Labor Relations, Economic and Social Policy
American Nurses' Association
Kansas City, Missouri

Helen Kennedy Grace, RN, PhD, FAAN

Program Director in Health
W. K. Kellogg Foundation
Battle Creek, Michigan

Judith R. Graves, RN, PhD

Associate Professor
College of Nursing
University of Utah
Salt Lake City, Utah

Edward J. Halloran, RN, PhD, FAAN

Associate Professor
School of Nursing
University of North Carolina
Chapel Hill, North Carolina

Sally Brosz Hardin, RN, PhD

Professor
College of Nursing
University of South Carolina
Columbia, South Carolina

Sue Thomas Hegyvary, RN, PhD, FAAN

Professor and Dean
School of Nursing
University of Washington
Bellevue, Washington

Ada Sue Hinshaw, RN, PhD, FAAN

Director, National Center for Nursing Research
National Institutes of Health
University of North Carolina at Greensboro
Greensboro, North Carolina

Linda C. Hodges, RN, PhD

Associate Dean and Professor
School of Nursing
University of North Carolina at Greensboro
Greensboro, North Carolina

Constance A. Holleran, RN, MSN, FAAN

Executive Director, International Council of Nurses
Geneva, Switzerland

Mary Louise Icenhour, RN, PhD

Assistant Professor
School of Nursing
Duke University
Durham, North Carolina

Lucille A. Joel, RN, PhD, FAAN

Professor and Chair, Department of Adults & the Aged
College of Nursing
Rutgers University
Newark, New Jersey

Marion Johnson, RN, PhD

Assistant Professor
College of Nursing
University of Iowa
Iowa City, Iowa

Karlene M. Kerfoot, RN, PhD, FAAN

Senior Vice President, Nursing
St. Luke's Episcopal Hospital
Houston, Texas

Karen Kauffman Knibbe, RN, MSN

Gerontological Nurse Practitioner
Doctoral Candidate at the School of Nursing
University of Pennsylvania
Philadelphia, Pennsylvania

Robert J. Kus, RN, PhD

Associate Professor
College of Nursing
University of Iowa
Iowa City, Iowa

Anita M. Langford, RN, MS

Director of Nursing
The Mason F. Lord Chronic Hospital and Nursing
Facility
Baltimore, Maryland

Madeline M. Leininger, RN, PhD, FAAN

Professor of Nursing and Anthropology
College of Nursing
Wayne State University
Detroit, Michigan

Juliene G. Lipson, RN, PhD, FAAN

Associate Professor
School of Nursing
University of California, San Fransisco

Maxine E. Loomis, RN, PhD, FAAN

Professor and Director, PhD Program
College of Nursing
University of South Carolina
Columbia, South Carolina

Sally Peck Lundeen, RN, PhD

Assistant Professor/Director Nursing Center
School of Nursing
University of Wisconsin-Milwaukee
Milwaukee, Wisconsin

Joan E. Lynaugh, RN, PhD, FAAN

Associate Professor and Director
Center for the Study of the History of Nursing
School of Nursing
University of Pennsylvania
Philadelphia, Pennsylvania

Meridean L. Maas, RN, PhD

Associate Professor and Chairperson
College of Nursing
University of Iowa
Iowa City, Iowa

Catherine Malloy, RN, PhD

Professor and Associate Dean for Academic Programs
George Nathan University
Fairfax, Virginia

Pamela J. Maraldo, RN, PhD, FAAN

Chief Executive Officer
National League for Nursing
New York, New York

Hans O. Mauksch, PhD

Professor Emeritus—University of Missouri at Columbia
Lecturer—University of Georgia
Athens, Georgia

Joanne Comi McCloskey, RN, PhD, FAAN

Professor and Director of Doctoral Program
College of Nursing
University of Iowa
Iowa City, Iowa

Kathleen M. McKeehan, RN, PhD
Director, Himalayan Institute
School of Nursing
University of Pennsylvania
Philadelphia, Pennsylvania

Catherine P. Murphy, RN, PhD
Associate Professor and Chairperson of the Graduate
Program
School of Nursing
Boston College
Chestnut Hill, Massachusetts

Ellen K. Murphy, RN, MS, JD
Assistant Professor
School of Nursing
University of Wisconsin-Milwaukee
Milwaukee, Wisconsin

Mary D. Naylor, RN, PhD, FAAN
Associate Professor and Director of Undergraduate
Studies
School of Nursing
University of Pennsylvania
Philadelphia, Pennsylvania

Roseann Netzer, RN, MS
Certified Psychiatric Clinical Specialist
Dedham, Massachusetts

Vuyelwa Ndiki Ngcongco, RN, PhD
Undersecretary for Manpower Development
Ministry of Health
Gaborone, Botswana

Philda Nomusa Nzimande, RN, PhD
Chair of Nursing Administration
Director of Nursing Research
University of Zululand
Republic of South Africa

Karen S. O'Connor, RN, MA
Director, Division of Nursing Practice and Economics
American Nurses' Association
Kansas City, Missouri

Karen A. O'Heath, RN, MA
Clinical Manager, Department of Nursing
The University of Chicago Hospitals
Chicago, Illinois

Virginia M. Ohlson, RN, PhD, FAAN
Professor, College of Nursing
University of Illinois at Chicago
Chicago, Illinois

Ellen Frances Olshansky, RNC, DNS
Assistant Professor
School of Nursing
University of Washington
Seattle, Washington

Patricia M. Ostmoe, RN, PhD
Professor and Acting Vice Chancellor for Academic
Affairs
School of Nursing
University of Wisconsin-Eau Claire
Eau Claire, Wisconsin

Rebecca Partridge, RN, PhD
Coordinator, Education and Quality Assurance Division
Kaiser-Permanente Medical Center
Oakland, California

Geeta Lawot Pfau, RN, PhD
Gaborone, Botswana

Timothy Porter-O'Grady, RN, PhD
Senior Health Consultant
Affiliated Dynamics, Inc.
Avondale Estates, Georgia

Gaye W. Poteet, RN, EdD
Professor
East Carolina University
Greenville, North Carolina

Marilyn L. Rothert, RN, PhD
Associate Professor
Director, Lifelong Education
College of Nursing
Michigan State University
East Lansing, Michigan

Nancy Hanley Ryan, RN, MS
Staff Specialist, Pediatric Nursing Service
Massachusetts General Hospital
Boston, Massachusetts

Marla E. Salmon, RN, ScD, FAAN

Chairman & Associate Professor, Public Health Nursing
School of Public Health
University of North Carolina-Chapel Hill
Chapel Hill, North Carolina

Janet C. Scherubel, RN, PhD

Research Coordinator
Rush University College of Nursing
Chicago, Illinois

Joyce M. Schowalter, RN, MEd

Executive Secretary
Minnesota Board of Nursing
Minneapolis, Minnesota

Carole A. Shea, RN, PhD

Graduate Director and Associate Professor
Northeastern University
College of Nursing
Boston, Massachusetts

Maxine K. Sliefert, RN, PhD

Associate Professor and Department Head
Department of Nursing
Cardinal Stritch College
Milwaukee, Wisconsin

Gloria R. Smith, RN, PhD, FAAN

Professor and Dean
College of Nursing
Wayne State University
Detroit, Michigan

Joy Smith, RN, BSN

Director of Nursing
Benedictine Nursing Center
Mt. Angel, Oregon

Alina A. Souza, RN, PhD

Associate Professor
Universidade de Brasilia
Campus Universitario, Asa Norte
Brazilia, Brazil

Rita Kisting Sparks, RN, PhD

Professor
Assistant Dean, Continuing Education
University of Wisconsin-Eau Claire
Eau Claire, Wisconsin

Maureen Beirne Streff, RN, MS, CS

Certified Psychiatric Clinical Specialist
Streff Associates
Acton, Massachusetts

Neville E. Strumpf, RNC, PhD, FAAN

Assistant Professor
Director, Gerontological Nurse Clinician Program
School of Nursing
University of Pennsylvania
Philadelphia, Pennsylvania

Elizabeth A. Swanson, RN, PhD

Associate Professor and Chairperson
College of Nursing
Iowa City, Iowa

Sandra S. Sweeney, RN, PhD

Professor
School of Nursing
University of Wisconsin-Eau Claire
Eau Claire, Wisconsin

Geraldine J. Talarczyk, RN, EdD

Associate Professor
Director of Undergraduate Program
College of Nursing
Michigan State University
East Lansing, Michigan

Rosalie A.E. Thompson, RN, RM, DNE

Professor and Chair
Department of Nursing
Faculty of Medicine
University of Capetown
Republic of South Africa

Toni Tripp-Reimer, RN, PhD, FAAN

Professor
College of Nursing
University of Iowa
Iowa City, Iowa

Patience Vanderbush, MA

School of Public Health
University of North Carolina
Chapel Hill, North Carolina

Glenn A. Webster, PhD
Associate Professor of Philosophy
Associate Professor of Nursing
University of Colorado
Denver, Colorado

Kay Weiler, RN, JD
Assistant Professor
College of Nursing
University of Iowa
Iowa City, Iowa

Harriet H. Werley, RN, PhD, FAAN
Distinguised Professor
School of Nursing
University of Wisconsin-Milwaukee
Milwaukee, Wisconsin

Karen E. Witt, RN, MSN
Assistant Professor
School of Nursing
University of Wisconsin-Eau Claire
Eau Claire, Wisconsin

Karen Zander, RN, MS
Organizational Development Specialist, Department of Nursing
Director of Consultation, Center for Nursing Case Management
New England Medical Center
Boston, Massachusetts

CeCelia R. Zorn, RN, MSN
Doctoral Candidate
School of Nursing
University of Wisconsin-Milwaukee
Milwaukee, Wisconsin

PREFACE

Nursing, worldwide, is a profession undergoing rapid change. The changes in nursing are related to the changes in society: in the wake of the women's movement, nurses have become more personally and politically assertive; more flexible education patterns and government's increasing financial support for education have led to acceptance of university education for nurses, advanced degrees, and the generation of new nursing knowledge; automation and increasing technology have caused specialization. Nursing is also influenced greatly by the changes in health care: an aging society with more chronic health care problems has promoted the nursing specialty of gerontology with more attention to the problems of long-term care and nursing homes; prospective payment and cost-containment efforts in health care have created concerns in nursing about cost of services and about adequate education of managers; AIDS and the care of these patients raised issues related to ethics, nursing knowledge, and practice. And more than ever, amid all the change, nurses are practicing independently, expanding their roles, and requesting equal participation in the important decisions affecting patient care and health care policy.

In periods of rapid change, decisions must often be made quickly. With many issues confronting such a large and diverse profession, there is danger that decisions will be made without full knowledge or without sufficient opportunity to discuss and debate. Worse yet, issues may be ignored and decisions not made. The purpose of this book is to provide a forum for knowledgeable debate on the important issues that concern all of today's nurses so that intelligent decision making can occur.

As in the previous two editions, the issues are identified and addressed in 12 sections: definitions of nursing, nursing knowledge, changing education, changing practice, quality assurance, governance, government intervention, cost effectiveness, personal and professional assertiveness, role conflict, cultural diversity, and ethics. As in previous editions, each section includes an overview of the section, a debate chapter, and several viewpoint chapters. Of the 89 chapters in this third edition, 3 are reprints from the second edition, 20 are updates from the second edition, and 66 are totally new. None have been published elsewhere. New to this edition and in keeping with the rapidly developing international flavor of nursing is the inclusion of chapters from other countries; all but one section concludes with a chapter written from an international perspective.

In each overview we briefly introduce the section and the chapters in that section. The overview, which highlights some of the important points in each chapter and raises some related issues, will assist readers to select chapters to read. Each debate chapter is a debate of one of the problematic issues in nursing. A listing of the titles of debate chapters in the edition gives some idea of the scope of the issues:

- Nursing theory and nursing practice: Do they connect?
- Is nursing research used in practice?
- Entry into practice: Will the 1985 proposal ever happen?
- Is there anything new about this nursing shortage?
- Quality control: Professional or institutional responsibility?
- Does nursing have the power to change the health care system?
- Controlling health care expenditures: Strategies for cost containment in long-term care
- Can health care costs be contained?
- Career development: Its status in nursing
- Can there be one nursing organization?
- Cultural diversity in nursing: How much can we tolerate?
- Truth telling

In the first edition, the debate chapters were a result of master's students' participation in an issues course at the University of Illinois College of Nursing. The chapters were based on actual oral debates that took place in class. For each debate a small group of students (anywhere from two to five) were asked to choose a topic, make up a reading list for advance distribution, and present all sides of the issue in a debate format to the rest of the class. Each group was instructed to stress the facts and research findings and to be as creative in presentation as they could. The approach was intellectual but the mood was fun. Several groups conducted their own surveys of class knowledge and opinions prior to class. Others dressed for and acted out parts. For example, in one class there was a physician's assistant and nurse practitioner who dressed exactly alike in their lab coats and stethoscopes, and in another the students played the parts of nursing deans to argue out the merits of a Ph.D. or a D.N. program.

Each group was required to state their debate topic in a debate form; the same topic could lead to several debates. For example, the topic of the expanded role for nurses resulted in one group in a debate entitled, "Should Nurses Practice Dependently, Independently or Interdependently?" and in another group resulted in a debate entitled "Nurse Practitioners or Physicians' Assistants?" In a two-hour course, one hour was allocated for the debate presentation and one hour for questions and debate with the rest of the class.

Some of the class debates were written up and published in the first edition. In the second and third editions we have kept the same format, because we think debates are an excellent medium for teaching this content. Student debaters as well as their audience are involved in sorting out the complicated issues surrounding the debate. Many times just knowing all the facts leads to effective decision making; other times, it leads to the knowledge of what further research is needed before effective decision making can occur.

In the viewpoint chapters, each author gives her or his own view and critical analysis of one particular aspect of the section's general topic. Viewpoints are those of the individual authors and may involve their taking a controversial stand, presenting a case study or results of some research, reviewing the past and current status of a topic, or outlining problems and future directions. The viewpoint chapters differ from the debate chapters as the words viewpoint and debate differ: the viewpoint chapters, for the most part, offer only one side or a piece of an issue. It is hoped that the viewpoint chapters provide material and ideas for other debates, that readers will agree or take issue, that after reading a viewpoint they will be stimulated to think and seek out more information. It is impossible to list all the many viewpoints here but a sample list of titles will, we hope, get you thirsting to read these and more.

- Nursing intervention taxonomy development
- Potential and pitfalls of expert systems in nursing
- How to choose a graduate program
- Case management: A golden opportunity for whom?
- Standards of regulatory agencies: Blueprint for quality or bureaucratic morass?
- Why are we seeing more unionization?
- The aftermath of DRGs: The politics of transformation
- Women and the empowerment of leaders: Lessons from the Geraldine Ferraro case
- Has the front-line nurse been abandoned?
- Rationing of health care services: Ethical issues for nursing

As we stated before, this edition includes for the first time some international chapters. Reading of these chapters will expand the horizons of all nurses. Their titles are:

- Theoretical underpinnings of community based primary care in developing countries
- The development of nursing service administration as a subdiscipline of nursing and administration in South Africa
- Models of nursing education for developing countries: The Bahrain model
- Nursing practice in developing countries: The Latin American experience
- International nursing: The role of the International Council of Nurses and the World Health Organization

- Government intervention in a developing country: The Botswana experience
- Who pays for the costs of care in other countries?
- Imagery issues in international nursing
- Traditional roles of women and nurses in the developing countries
- Cultural diversity: The international student
- What are the ethical issues from a worldwide viewpoint?

As the size of the book attests, it is a fairly complete source of all of today's important nursing issues. Careful reading, thought, and debate today can result in correct decisions, actions, and achievements tomorrow.

Joanne Comi McCloskey
Helen Kennedy Grace

WHO IS THIS BOOK FOR?

This book is appropriate for several audiences. First, it is an ideal book to use in a senior-level undergraduate or graduate level issues course. A teacher using this book could easily have her class orally present the debates written here or could structure a whole new set of debates using the readings here as source material.

Second, it is a good book to use as a core text for a graduate curriculum. There is something here that will fit with most nursing courses. For example, the sections on definitions of nursing and nursing knowledge are appropriate for nursing theory courses, the section on education for education courses, the sections on practice and cost effectiveness for nursing administration courses, the section on personal and professional assertiveness for leadership classes, and so on. By picking and choosing from the numerous viewpoints, every class in the graduate curriculum can benefit from the use of this book. By using one text throughout the curriculum, the department can help to achieve financial savings for the individual student and consistency in expectations from the faculty. Attesting to its comprehensive approach is the fact that the book is frequently used by graduate students to help prepare for comprehensive exams.

Third, the book is of interest to all nurses or nonnurses interested about the profession of nursing. The book is an excellent source of information about the nursing profession and about the issues confronting the profession. It is a stimulating and envigorating book that revitalizes one as it is read. It would make a good gift for a new RN or for a nurse going back to graduate school.

ACKNOWLEDGMENTS

Every book, especially one of this size that involves so many authors, takes many people to finish the job. For help with the third edition, we wish to thank:

Richard Zorab, former editor-in-chief at Blackwell Scientific Publications, who initiated the third edition, worked with us on the new outline, helped to establish the process, and, as always, was enthusiastic about the book and our work.

James Krosschell, who replaced Richard at Blackwell, and his assistants, Denise Gilpin and Cindy Kogut, who provided assistance with early correspondence to authors.

Alison Miller, Vice President of the Nursing Division at The C.V. Mosby Company, and, especially, Linda Duncan, our editor at Mosby who helped us finish the book and ensure that it was published in a timely manner. Just as we had chapters ready to be copy edited, Blackwell sold its nursing books to Mosby. The transaction took longer than we expected and caused us some tense moments but we successfully changed horses in the middle of the stream.

Gail Ardery, who worked for us for a year and a half as an Administrative Assistant. She made it possible for two busy people to add a book to their workloads.

At both of our work places, there were others who also helped with typing, phone calls, photocopying, etc. Joanne wishes to thank Hien Ong, Nancy Goldsmith, Debra Carlson and Rose Weldon for their help. Helen thanks Anita Clifton, and Norma Larsen Pugh.

The authors also deserve credit. As the results demonstrate, each of them took seriously the task. Yes, there were a few who needed several reminders to respond, but as their chapters demonstrate they are a very responsible and knowledgeable group of people.

Finally, we are grateful for the continued support and enthusiasm for this book from the nursing community. We hope that this edition continues to meet your needs.

CONTENTS

FIVE   **QUALITY ASSURANCE**

SIX   **GOVERNANCE**

VIEWPOINTS

PART ONE

DEFINITIONS OF NURSING

Nursing theory and related considerations

JOANNE COMI McCLOSKEY
HELEN KENNEDY GRACE

Throughout its history, nursing has struggled with definitions. Embedded firmly in traditional mothering roles, nursing has found it difficult to make transitions into the professional and scientific realms. The recent advances in nursing research and the growing number of doctoral programs in nursing are beginning to have an impact on nursing theory. What are the current issues in defining nursing?

In the debate chapter to this section, Firlit begins by examining the relationship of nursing theory and nursing practice to the philosophical foundations of the discipline. She says that the metaparadigm of nursing is continuing to evolve with emerging specificity of the concepts of person and nursing. Current thinking is supportive of multiple perspectives and diverse viewpoints. According to Firlit, this has stimulated theory development but has also perpetuated a degree of dissonance between theory and practice. Her debate is a presentation of arguments that support and refute the contention that there is a connection between theory and practice. For example, supporting the contention is the fact that in the past only the scientific mode was valued in nursing theory development, but now there is growing acceptance of the aesthetic, ethical, and personal knowledge modes. Also, nursing literature is replete with examples of how practicing nurses are applying theory. Evidence that there is little connection between nursing theory and nursing practice is that nursing theories are too abstract for practice and only a small percentage of graduate students who learn about theories in school use a model in practice. Firlit's review and critique of the theory development literature will be of help to many; her arguments for a stronger theory-practice connection should make sense to all.

In the next chapter, Webster questions the widely held assumption that nursing is or should become a science. He examines the distinctions between a science and a profession and concludes that nursing is not a science and should not try to become one because science is too limiting for nursing. He says that a nurse's education should be in those disciplines and sciences that are useful for understanding the particular (humanities, history, philosophy) rather than the general: "The nurse should be trained to recognize and respect each person in his or her uniqueness." He argues that nursing should use philosophies of science that "illuminate the differences and relations among the various branches of science, rather than fostering the illusion that the only sciences are the physical sciences." Those who have found Webster and Jacox's discussions of the Received View in earlier editions helpful and stimulating will also appreciate this chapter.

The development of classification systems is an approach used to clarify a domain. According to Douglas and Murphy, these have been appearing with increasing frequency in the nursing literature since the early 1970s. The best known, most widely used, and perhaps most controversial classification in nursing is that of nursing diagnosis. Douglas and Murphy examine the evolution of the concepts of nursing process and nursing diagnosis. That nursing can benefit from this taxonomic approach is clear, but the authors worry that the expectations for nursing diagnosis and other nursing taxonomies are far too high. They warn that the concept of nursing diagnosis has become so popular that unrealistic accomplishments are expected of it. They also point out that the imprecise use of the term *taxonomy* in nursing may compromise its potential as a tool. Douglas and Murphy urge continued efforts to refine and categorize nursing diagnoses but warn that it is dangerous to pin all hopes on nursing diagnosis alone. They believe that a single taxonomy is undesirable in that it focuses energies on reaching premature closure, thereby limiting further growth.

Although the nursing diagnosis movement has pointed to the need for standardized language for treatments, no classification or taxonomy of nursing interventions exists at present. Bulechek and McCloskey discuss the need for such a taxonomy and also conceptual issues related to the development. Such a classification is needed to standardize nomenclature about nursing treatments; to expand nursing knowledge about the links between diagnoses, treatments, and outcomes; to facilitate development of nursing information systems; to assist in the planning for resource use in practice settings; and to provide a language to communicate the unique function of nursing. The chapter discusses two conceptual issues: whether an inductive or deductive approach should be used in the development and what type of nursing activities should be included. The authors are leaders of a research team that is working to develop such a taxonomy.

Another way to look at the structuring of nursing knowledge is to examine the continuing debate on specialization versus generalization. According to Chickadonz, the debate continues because "we have not defined and structured the body of knowledge" and therefore we are not sure whether it belongs at an undergraduate or graduate level. Chickadonz compares and contrasts positions on this issue from two well-known nurse leaders, Donna Diers and Rosella Schlotfeldt. Because these authors have "different views of nursing's social mission, they have different conceptualizations of the body of knowledge required." Chickadonz presents some history of nursing practice and nursing education, including the diversity of master's programs, the credentialing of nurses, and the knowledge needed by clinical specialists and administrators. She proposes two criteria for specialists: that they have mastery of knowledge more specialized than what is obtained at the undergraduate level and that they have knowledge and skills different from other specialists. She outlines a future in which both generalist and specialist knowledge is needed by all types of nurses.

In the last chapter of this section, the discussion concerns theory development and the issues confronting nursing in South Africa. Thompson says that South Africa is both a developing and a developed country that reflects in microcosm the challenges facing the First World and Third World countries. In many developing countries, the major focus and practice area of nursing is in the community. There are three facets to Thompson's chapter. First, she addresses the concept of community-based primary care, which has received renewed attention since the 1978 conference held in Alma-Ata (USSR). According to Thompson, nurses have been practicing a form of community-based primary care for decades as community health or district nurses, but they have lacked the theoretical underpinnings that the study of epidemiology provides. Thompson then discusses health care and nursing in South Africa. She concludes with some recommendations for change. She proposes that the sickness and illness model of nursing be exchanged for a wellness one and that the home and family be the pivotal unit in nursing programs rather than the hospital. She concludes with a list of seven ingredients of a wellness service that would enable and empower people to care for their own health.

The authors in Part One have pointed out several considerations in the efforts to define nursing and to develop nursing theory. These include the structuring of knowledge through taxonomies, the issue of generalist versus specialist knowledge, the focus on illness or wellness, and the setting of the hospital versus the home. The authors in Part Two concentrate on issues related to knowledge development. The authors in Part One provide a beginning for a discussion about nursing, but in a sense the entire book continues their efforts.

CHAPTER 1

Debate

Nursing theory and nursing practice
Do they connect?

SHARON L. FIRLIT

The premise that nursing theory and nursing practice are mutually interdependent has been established.[17,29,32] However, the degree to which this relationship is perceived as congruent varies. Within the profession, divergent views exist regarding the *connectedness* of nursing theory and nursing practice. Before presenting arguments to support each outlook, I will review the relationship of nursing theory and nursing practice to the philosophical foundation of the discipline of nursing.

PHILOSOPHICAL BASIS
Nursing's metaparadigm

The metaparadigm of any discipline is its identification of overall areas of interest. A metaparadigm reflects the philosophical orientation or worldview espoused by members of a discipline. This gestalt forms the foundation and boundaries for inquiry and knowledge (theory) development within the profession.

The metaparadigm of nursing continues to evolve. In 1980 Flaskerud and Halloran[18] documented consensus within the nursing profession for the central concepts of person, environment, health, and nursing. In 1984 Fawcett[15] formalized these concepts along with three recurring themes originally identified by Donaldson and Crowley[14] as the metaparadigm of nursing. However, alternative metaparadigms have been proposed. In 1983 Kim[23] specified three conceptual domains of nursing: client, environment, and nursing action. Further work[24] led her to revise these to a typology of four domains: client, environment, client-nurse, and practice. In 1985 Meleis[29,30] identified seven central nursing phenomena: nursing client, health, en-

vironment, interaction, nursing process, transition, and nursing therapeutics. Most recently (1988), in an analysis of the philosophical roots of four contemporary nursing theories, Sarter[38] identified seven shared themes to contribute to the development of a metaparadigm for nursing. They are process, evolution of consciousness, self-transcendence, open systems, harmony, relativity of space-time, pattern, and holism. What appears to be emerging is greater specificity of the concepts person and nursing. Sarter expands the phenomena of person, and Kim and Meleis further differentiate nursing practice: process, interaction, and actions (therapeutics).

Within a discipline, several paradigms may coexist. Each paradigm represents a distinctive view of reality within which the metaparadigm phenomena are explicated. Furthermore, each paradigm reflects a research tradition in which methods of investigation or ways of knowing are specified. Therefore each paradigm contains metaphysical and epistemological beliefs that guide inquiry related to the metaparadigm phenomena.

Fawcett[15] identifies current conceptual models in nursing as paradigms, because they each represent a distinctive frame of reference. Examples include King's open system model, Levine's conservation model, Orem's self-care model, Rogers' life process model, and Roy's adaptation model. Parse[34] pools conceptual frameworks into two paradigms. One is the totality paradigm, which is the traditional and most widely held view. Theorists within this paradigm include Roy, King, and Orem. The newer paradigm is the simultaneity paradigm represented by Rogers and

Parse. The paradigms differ in their assumptions about humans and health, the goals of nursing, and methodology for research and practice. At one time many people argued for a single, unified model of nursing. However, current thinking is supportive of multiple perspectives in mapping the domain of nursing.[15,22,26,45,47]

Nursing theory

A theory is a statement about the relationship(s) of specifically defined concepts that describe, explain, or predict some phenomenon and, in professional disciplines, prescribe action.[3,12,29] Theories are generally developed within a research tradition, that is, they are based on a particular view of reality and method of inquiry. Nursing theories specify relations among variables derived from the central concepts of nursing's metaparadigm. The way the variables are defined is dependent on the paradigm or conceptual framework used by the theorist.

Conceptual models of nursing have generated nursing theories.[25,28,37] Each of these theories has addressed one or more concepts within the model. An example is King's theory of goal attainment,[25] which was derived from the concept of interpersonal systems in her conceptual framework. The nurse-client dyad is one type of interpersonal system. The theory describes the nature of nurse-client interactions that lead to the achievement of goals. Characteristics of the interaction that are specifically defined are perception, communication, transaction, self, role, stress, growth and development, and time and space. A list of propositions, some dealing with process, others with outcome, indicates the predictive value of the concepts in the theory.

Models and theories from other disciplines have also contributed to the development of nursing theory. Walker and Avant[49] identify this approach to theory building as derivation. With derivation the terminology or structure from one field shifts to another. When derivation is used in nursing theory development, concepts or other components of the original theory or model are redefined or adapted to the nursing metaparadigm. Using this approach, Roy[37] derived the concept of adaptation from Helson's adaptation level theory, and Benner[5] described the stages of nursing practice based on a model of skill acquisition developed by Dreyfus and Dreyfus.

Nursing theories have also been based on broad paradigms or worldviews shared by a variety of disciplines. For example, theories of psychotherapy, education, and other social sciences have been founded on the phenomenological tradition that seeks to understand meanings of human experiences.[11] Paterson and Zderad[35] used this approach exclusively in developing their humanistic nursing practice theory. The focus of this theory is the meaningfulness derived from the nursing situation in which "interhuman relating is purposely directed toward nurturing the well-being or more-being of a person with perceived needs related to the health-illness quality of living."[35] Benner[5] also used this approach in interpreting skilled nursing practice. As an outcome of her work, seven domains of nursing practice were identified and described. Beliefs and methods of the phenomenological tradition and also naturalistic inquiry comprise the human science paradigm discussed by Watson.[50]

In summary, nursing theories continue to evolve from a variety of inter- and intradisciplinary paradigms. This diversity allows for theory development based on observation of extant practice as well as ideas about what nursing ought to be. Nursing theories describe and prescribe different aspects of nursing care. Because practice situations vary, nursing theories with multiple perspectives need to be developed.

Nursing practice

Nursing practice is something more than the application of theoretical knowledge. Donaldson and Crowley[14] state that "clinical practice is always to some extent empirical, pragmatic, intuitive, and artistic."[14] Carper[7] identifies four fundamental patterns of knowing in nursing and concludes that nursing practice "depends on the scientific knowledge of human behavior in health and in illness, the aesthetic perception of significant human experiences, a personal understanding of the unique individuality of the self and the capacity to make choices within concrete situations involving particular moral judgments."[7] Elaborating on Carper's work, Chinn and Jacobs[8] propose that aesthetics, the art of nursing, is the foundation for the integration of all patterns of knowing.

Frameworks have been identified to guide practitioners in integrating various ways of knowing within clinical situations. The model for situation-producing nursing theories proposed by Dickoff, James, and Wiedenbach[13] constitutes "conceptualization of the *relations* that must exist between, on the one hand, whatever predictive theories are required and, on the other hand, other things and theories necessary to produce situations of the kind deemed professionally good by the practice discipline in question."[13] So, in addition to the consideration of empirical or scientific theories, aesthetic, existential, and moral knowledge is used in situation-producing theory. Because the purpose of situation-producing theory is to achieve a desired goal, values are included as a moral component, and aesthetic and personal knowledge components are included in descriptions of survey list activities, such as internal resources of the agent and procedures.

Other frameworks cited include Shotter's theory of personal action discussed by Clarke[10] and Kuypers' metatheory for practice.[26] In essence, the argument is that nurses use some model, often unconsciously, to choose, adapt theories, and integrate them with other knowledge derived from the clinical situation in providing nursing care (goal-directed action). The explication of this underlying framework is in itself a theory that can be used to guide further nursing practice.

Although these theories can explain how nurses use knowledge in their practice, controversy over the unique nature of nursing practice continues. The American Nurses' Association's (ANA) Social Policy Statement[2] defines nursing as "the diagnosis and treatment of human responses to actual and potential health problems."[2] Schlotfeldt[39] contends that this definition is in conflict with nursing's traditional goal "to assist human beings attain, retain, or regain the highest possible levels of physical, physiological, social and emotional function and comfort of which each is capable."[39] Orlando[33] criticizes the ANA definition as being too general and incapable of distinguishing the function of nursing practice from that of other health care professions. She defines the distinct function of nursing as "attending to individuals when in distress because they can't find their own encouragement; they can't look after themselves; they can't nourish, nurture or protect themselves; they can't give themselves curative care when they are ailing."[33] Smith[43] reports a panel discussion by six nursing leaders on major issues in nursing. There was no consensus on what makes nursing unique. Smith[43] concludes: "that there is disagreement is heartening."[43] Others would differ with this view, holding that a fundamental, philosophical agreement about the nature of nursing is paramount for the viability of the profession.

To summarize, nursing theory and nursing practice are based on philosophical beliefs related to reality and knowing. However, diverse viewpoints coexist within the profession. Although this has stimulated theory development, it has also perpetuated a degree of dissonance between nursing theory and nursing practice. Based on this overview, the debate that follows presents arguments from nursing literature that either refute or support the connection between nursing theory and nursing practice. The term *theory* is used here in a broad sense, as a way of looking at and interpreting the world. Therefore, reference to conceptual models as well as theories will be made.

THE NURSING THEORY–NURSING PRACTICE CONNECTION

Arguments supportive of an interaction between nursing theory and nursing practice can be categorized into those that view nursing practice as necessary for theory development and theory validation and those that reflect application of theory in practice.

Practice as a basis for nursing theory development

"Theory is born in practice, is refined in research, and must and can return to practice."[12] Dickoff, James, and Wiedenbach made this contention about the interdependence of nursing theory, nursing practice, and nursing research in 1968. At that time only "embryos of nursing theory" existed.[12] Over the past 20 years, however, numerous theories have been developed. Furthermore, resources contributing to theory development are expanding. These include the recognition and integration of different patterns of knowing, the acceptance of multiple philosophical and methodological perspectives, and the increase in doctorally prepared nurses who can facilitate theory advancement.[22]

Carper[7] demonstrated that the body of knowledge that serves as the rationale for nursing practice includes empirical, aesthetic, ethical, and personal knowledge patterns. In the past, only the empirical (scientific) mode has been valued in nursing theory development. However, growing acceptance of each of the patterns as necessary for full knowledge development holds promise for a stronger nursing practice–nursing theory development bond. Nurse scientists have already begun to look more openly at the type of knowledge that can be derived from the study of clinical practice. In Benner's study[5] of nursing practice, all four patterns of knowing were documented as components of expert nursing care. Agan[1] studied holistic nursing practice and described the use of intuitive knowing, an aspect of personal knowledge. Clarke[10] proposed that if nursing theory is anchored within the reality of nursing practice, nursing actions become central and ethical issues assume importance. Thus using nursing practice as a basis for theory development promotes not only a broader view of reality but also an increased relevance of theory to practice. As Benner[5] contends:

> Adequate description of practical knowledge is essential to the development and extension of nursing theory. . . . There is much to learn and appreciate as practicing nurses uncover common meanings acquired as a result of helping, coaching, and intervening in the significantly human events that comprise the art and science of nursing.[5]

Validation of nursing theory in practice

Although it is arduous and complex, to Chinn and Jacobs[8] the theory validation process is the essence of the theory-practice relationship. This activity involves the empirical testing of theoretical propositions in the practice setting. If repeated results provide evidence of a theory's accuracy, the theory is valid. Theory testing also provides feedback to refine the theory so that it better represents reality.

The number of research studies based on conceptual models of nursing has increased substantially.[28,42,51] However, Silva[41] contends that little progress has been made in the actual testing of these models. In an assessment of 62 research studies based on 5 nursing models, only 9 met all of the criteria for the explicit testing of nursing theory. Silva[41] attributes this low figure in part to a lack of commitment of theorists and investigators to follow through with a systematic program of theory testing. She recommends that nurse theorists make explicit key assumptions, propositions, and hypotheses that need to be tested. Such specification would focus and streamline the process of theory building. Examples of theorists who have done so are King[25,51] and Roy.[37] Furthermore, Silva recommends that criteria for research-based theory testing be clarified in nursing theory and nursing research courses.

Dickoff, James, and Wiedenbach[13] discuss testing theory in terms of its coherency, palatability, and feasibility claims. In arguing for the importance of theory testing, they maintain that

> Unless within his limits man makes such an attempt he is forever compelled to act without the light of theory and so to remain at the level of inarticulate art—a position having grave consequences for educating an adequate number of able practitioners, as well as for the quality of practice. Or else he must dumbly follow a theory of dubious validity.

Numerous nursing models and theories are in the process of being tested. The practical validation of a theory is a process that requires concerted effort over a period of time. Because validation of nursing theories takes place within clinical settings, practicing nurses are involved with testing and collection of the data used to verify the theory in question. Thus, practitioners have input into the process of confirming or refining a theory. They provide a vital link in the nursing theory–nursing practice connection.

Application of nursing theory in practice

Although nursing theories may not be fully validated, they serve as a guide to practice for many nurses. In justifying the application of a theory in practice, Chinn and Jacobs[8] advise that the following prerequisites be considered:

1. The goals of the theory should be examined and compared with the outcomes or goals that are judged to be of value in nursing practice.
2. The circumstances under which the theory is expected to apply should be congruent with the situation in which the theory actually will be applied.
3. Comparison should be made between the variables important in the construction of the theory and variables recognized to be directly influencing the practice situation.
4. The relationships within the theory should provide sufficient explanation to provide a basis for planning and implementing nursing actions.
5. There should be evidence from actual research that supports the validity of the theory.
6. The potential for observing and recording factors that are relevant to the theory's application should be assessed.

Ideally each of these prerequisites should be met before proceeding with application. However, Chinn and Jacobs propose that the practitioner is justified in applying the theory if most of the prerequisites are met. If not all the prerequisites are met, they recommend that a research approach be used to document the results of the application.

Nursing literature is replete with examples of practicing nurses applying nursing theory. Nurses from the University of Michigan hospitals developed and use an assessment tool derived from the modeling and role-modeling nursing theory.[6] Graduates of the McGill University School of Nursing have applied the McGill model of nursing (a practice-derived model) in various practice settings, such as ambulatory care, intensive care, and communities.[19] In Winstead-Fry's compendium,[51] various nurses relay how they have applied one of eight different nursing theories. Uys[46] contends that conceptual models of nursing are more like philosophies than theories. They each provide a particular perspective or view of nursing that often becomes an unconscious approach to practice. This is reflected in one nurse's comment: "I don't consciously decide to use Orlando's theory. Rather it is a way of thinking, a way of responding that is integrated into my total practice."[40] Thus in serving as a guide to practice, nursing theory connects with nursing practice.

NURSING THEORY SEPARATE FROM PRACTICE

Arguments that question a nursing theory–nursing practice interaction may be categorized into those that refute the presence of practice theory in nursing and those that maintain that current nursing theory is not congruent with nursing practice. These views have implications for both the practicing nurse and the profession.

Nursing practice theory does not exist

Walker[48] appears to have been the first to query the nature and necessity of a practice theory in nursing. Based on the definition of practice theory as sets of principles or directives for practice, Walker holds that this view represents an "odd use of the term 'theory' for 'theory' is typically employed in the context of systematic description and explanation." Walker further argues that principles of practice constitute a part of the practical aspects of nursing knowledge rather than the theoretical component of a domain.

Christman[9] extends discussion of the distinction between theories as abstract concepts used to describe, explain, and predict phenomena and theories as constructive actions used to modify events in a desirable

direction. Christman equates constructive actions to applied science and maintains that there is no one theory of applied science. Applied scientists use a mixture of scientific theories that allow the best management of their work effort. Nursing is an applied science, and "everything that nurses do for patients arises from some element in the fundamental sciences, either behavioral or biophysical or both."[9] Christman further cautions against the adherence to conceptual frameworks that may lead to locked-in thinking and thus limit the application of science in nursing.

Beckstrand[4] argues that what is meant by practice theory is vague. She discusses the application of the methods of science, ethics, and philosophy to the problems nurses experience in practice. She maintains that none of these ways of theorizing is unique to practice. They are methods available to all who seek to comprehend some aspect of the world. When these theories arise within the purview of a particular discipline, such as nursing, "they can be called the scientific and philosophical knowledge of the discipline."[4]

Walker, Christman, and Beckstrand disclaim the need for nursing theory to be practice theory. They caution against confusing the thought with the act. They see the practice of nursing as the application of basic scientific and other forms of abstract knowledge. The implication this view has for the profession can be summed up in Christman's warning: "If nurses stray from the orderly process of the methods of science, they may be accused of dilettantism and/or pseudoscience and risk losing credibility with the universe of scientists."[9]

Nursing theory is not congruent with nursing practice

Findings from a national survey of graduate nursing students and faculty[21] revealed that although all in the sample ($n = 676$) indicated they were familiar with at least one conceptual model of nursing, only 35% reported that they used a nursing model in their practice outside of the educational program. Other authors have attributed the divergence of nursing theory from nursing practice to either the abstractness, irrelevance, or insufficiency of nursing theory for practice.

Smith[44] and Lundh, Soder, and Waerness[27] articulate the stance that nursing theories are too abstract for application in practice. Smith, a practitioner, asks why nurses must be "afflicted with baroque nursing theories couched in stilted pseudo-intellectual jargon."[44] She accuses theoreticians of obscuring the obvious by their use of vague phrases and grand verbiage. After giving several examples, Smith queries: "Who, besides academic luminaries, benefits from this blizzard of inflated words?"[44] She concludes that the obscure language of theorists limits efforts by practitioners to discuss nursing in a realistic, relevant, constructive way and thereby presents a professional loss that nurses should not accept. She recommends to theorists: "If what you really want to do is provide nurses with guidelines and a direction to follow, how about saying things in plain English?"[44]

Lundh, Soder, and Waerness[27] question the usefulness of theories as guides to practice because of their abstract character: "The rules of action that they lead to are seldom more concrete than the theories themselves. They therefore appear trivial and largely a matter of common sense."[27] Furthermore, "they fail to say anything of interest about the social reality in which nursing takes place. . . . The classless and genderless participants have been abstracted out of their social context."[27]

Miller[31] contends that theories of nursing bear little relationship to the reality of nursing practice and are perceived as idealized and irrelevant by many nursing practitioners. This discrepancy is due to the incongruity of values and attitudes held by practitioners and theorists. Practitioners often are employed in settings in which cure rather than care is the dominant perspective. In addition, although theorists may advocate the active involvement of patients in their own care, patients are often viewed as passive recipients of health care. Perry[36] holds a similar view—that little consensus exists between theorists and practitioners regarding professional values and attitudes. This lack of consensus, she believes, is made evident by the discrepancy between the conceptual orientations of theory and practice.

Others argue that nursing models and theories do not provide a sufficient base of knowledge for nursing practice. Hoon[20] points out that death and dying are not addressed in conceptual models. Field[16] agrees that nursing models are incomplete. She contends that knowledge from the biological and behavioral sciences, in addition to intuition, is needed to make nursing practice judgments. Lundh, Soder, and Waerness[27] argue that nursing actions "often occur on premises other than those of instrumental 'scientific' rationality." This does not mean that they are irrational but that they are based on a different type of rationality: a "rationality of caring" that "focuses on the unique rather than on the general and emphasizes flexibility and adaptiveness to the situation."

What these arguments imply is that if nursing theory is to be useful to nursing practitioners and to facilitate communication within the profession, nursing theory needs to be concrete, to address the reality of the practice situation, and to reflect the values and attitudes of practicing nurses. Until this is done, the theory-practice gap will continue.

SUMMARY

The views presented here exemplify the diversity of opinion that exists regarding the connection of nursing theory with nursing practice. Arguments may be summarized as those addressing the nature, relevance, and validity of the nursing theory—nursing practice interaction.

A theory is a statement that specifically describes, explains, or predicts some phenomenon. In nursing, theories have developed inductively as a result of describing extant practice[5] and deductively by extrapolating propositions from conceptual models of nursing.[25,37] Considerable support is given to the notion of incorporating knowledge other than scientific into nursing theories.[8,12] In addition, some have advocated the development of prescriptive theories for nursing.[12,29] Others argue that the prescriptive view of theory development does not fit the acceptable methods of scientific theory development.[4,9,48] They admit that nurses apply scientific theories and other knowledge in practice but contend that how this is done cannot be explained by a scientific theory. Therefore, they disclaim a nursing theory—nursing practice interaction.

That nursing theories are relevant for nursing practice is demonstrated by numerous examples in which nursing theories or models have been used as guides or organizing frameworks for nursing practice.[6,51] Yet there are those who dispute this premise because of the abstractness of nursing theories and their failure to give concrete direction in specific clinical situations[27] and because of the incongruence of values and attitudes between idealized nursing theories and realistic nursing practice.[31,36]

Theory development is a process that includes articulation and validation of descriptions and/or explanations of phenomenon. In nursing, validation of theories is taking place,[42,51] but few if any theories are considered valid at present. Therefore, one could argue, to advocate that nursing practice be based on nursing theories may be inappropriate because the evidence for theoretical validity is insufficient. Furthermore, even if used, current nursing theories do not always provide adequate guidance for many nursing care situations.[16,20]

Most arguments address current weaknesses in the connection between nursing theory and nursing practice rather than question the premise that there is an interdependence between nursing theory and nursing practice. Within this postulate, nursing theory arises out of nursing practice, either inductively through the observation of practice or deductively from the conceptualizations of nurses. Nursing theory is verified in practice and then can be used to explain or direct practice. Nursing practice under the guidance of nursing theory leads to theory refinement and expansion. Thus nursing theory and nursing practice operate in both directions, each improving and developing the other.

From the perspective of the individual nurse, a nursing theory–nursing practice interaction may or may not exist. Factors that determine whether such an interaction exists include familiarity with nursing theories, congruity of personal and organizational values with those of a theory, and the effectiveness of using a theory in one's practice. With the inclusion of nursing theory content within most professional nursing educational programs and the increase in theory testing and application activities in clinical settings, one can forecast a continued increase in the number of practitioners who perceive and put into practice a nursing theory–nursing practice connection.

From the perspective of the profession, recent nursing theory development has broadened in scope by recognizing various patterns of knowing in nursing practice. In addition, theorists and investigators are depending more on the collaboration of practicing nurses in the initial development, testing, and refining of nursing theory. If continued, these activities will strengthen the nursing theory–nursing practice connection. Furthermore, as Visintainer[47] contends: "As nursing strives to understand itself both as a user-applier and discoverer-inventor of knowledge and theory, it provides a model for other practice professions and academic disciplines."

REFERENCES

1. Agan RD: Intuitive knowing as a dimension of nursing, Adv Nurs Sci 10(1):63, 1987.
2. American Nurses' Association: Nursing: a social policy statement, Kansas City, Mo, 1980, American Nurses' Association.
3. Argyris C and Schon DA: Theory and practice: increasing professional effectiveness, San Francisco, 1974, Jossey-Bass.
4. Beckstrand J: A critique of several conceptions of practice theory in nursing, Res Nurs Health 3(2):69, 1980.
5. Benner P: From novice to expert: excellence and power in clinical nursing practice, Menlo Park, Calif, 1984, Addison-Wesley Publishing Co.
6. Campbell J and others: A theoretical approach to nursing assessement, J Adv Nurs 10:111, 1985.
7. Carper BA: Fundamental patterns of knowing in nursing, Adv Nurs Sci 1(1):13, 1978.
8. Chinn PL and Jacobs MK: Theory and nursing: a systematic approach, ed 2, St Louis, 1987, The CV Mosby Co.
9. Christman L: There is no theory of nursing. Paper presented at Chautaugua '82, Vail, Colo, August 1982, Colorado Nurses' Association.
10. Clarke M: Action and reflection: practice and theory in nursing, J Adv Nurs 11:3, 1986.
11. Cohen MZ: A historical overview of the phenomenological movement, Image 19(1):31, 1987.
12. Dickoff J, James P, and Wiedenbach E: Theory in a practice discipline part 1: practice oriented theory, Nurs Res 17(5):415, 1968.
13. Dickoff J, James P, and Wiedenbach E: Theory in a practice discipline part 2: practice oriented research, Nurs Res 17(6):545, 1968.
14. Donaldson SK and Crowley DM: The discipline of nursing, Nurs Outlook 26(2):113, 1978.
15. Fawcett J: The metaparadigm of nursing: present status and future refinements, Image 16(3):84, 1984.
16. Field PA: The impact of nursing theory on the clinical decision making process, J Adv Nurs 12:563, 1987.
17. Firlit SL: Nursing theory and nursing practice: separate or linked? In McCloskey JC and Grace HK, editors: Current issues in nursing, ed 2, Boston, 1985, Blackwell Scientific Publications, Inc.
18. Flaskerud JH and Halloran EJ: Areas of agreement in nursing theory development, Adv Nurs Sci 3(1):1, 1980.
19. Gottlieb L and Rowat K: The McGill model of nursing: a practice-derived model, Adv Nurs Sci 9(4):51, 1987.
20. Hoon E: Game playing: a way to look at nursing models, J Adv Nurs 11:421, 1986.
21. Jacobson SF: Studying and using conceptual models of nursing, Image 19(2):78, 1987.
22. Jennings BM: Nursing theory development: successes and challenges, J Adv Nurs 12:63, 1987.
23. Kim HS: The nature of theoretical thinking in nursing, Norwalk, Conn, 1983, Appleton-Century-Crofts.
24. Kim HS: Structuring the nursing knowledge system: a typology of four domains, Scholar Inq Nurs Pract 1:99, 1987.
25. King IM: A theory for nursing: systems, concepts, process, New York, 1981, John Wiley & Sons.
26. Kristjanson LJ, Tamblyn R, and Kuypers JA: A model of guide development and application of multiple nursing theories, J Adv Nurs 12:523, 1987.

27. Lundh U, Soder M, and Waerness K: Nursing theories: a critical view, Image 20(1):36, 1988.

28. Malinski VM, editor: Explorations on Martha Rogers' science of unitary human beings, Norwalk, Conn, 1986, Appleton-Century-Crofts.

29. Meleis AI: Theoretical nursing: development and progress, Philadelphia, 1985, JB Lippincott Co.

30. Meleis AI: Theory development and domain concepts. In Moccia P, editor: New approaches to theory development, New York, 1986, National League for Nursing.

31. Miller A: The relationship between nursing theory and nursing practice, J Adv Nurs 10:417, 1985.

32. Moccia P: Theory development and nursing practice: a synopsis of a study of the theory-practice dialectic. In Moccia P, editor: New appraoches to theory development, New York, 1986, National League for Nursing.

33. Orlando IJ: Nursing in the 21st century: alternative paths, J Adv Nurs (12)405, 1987.

34. Parse RR: Nursing science: major paradigms, theories, and critiques, Philadelphia, 1987, WB Saunders Co.

35. Paterson JG and Zderad LT: Humanistic nursing, New York, 1976, John Wiley & Sons.

36. Perry J: Has the discipline of nursing developed to the stage where nurses do 'think nursing'? J Adv Nurs 10:31, 1985.

37. Roy C and Roberts SL: Theory construction in nursing: an adaptation model, Englewood Cliffs, NJ, 1981, Prentice-Hall.

38. Sarter B: Philosophical sources of nursing theory, Nurs Sci Q 1(2):52, 1988.

39. Schlotfeldt R: Defining nursing: a historic controversy, Nurs Res 36(1)64, 1987.

40. Schmiedling NJ: Orlando's theory. In Winstead-Fry P, editor: Case studies in nursing theory, New York, 1986, National League for Nursing.

41. Silva MC: Research testing nursing theory: state of the art, Adv Nurs Sci 9(1):1, 1986.

42. Silva MC: Conceptual models of nursing. In Fitzpatrick JJ and Taunton RL, editors: Annual review of nursing research, vol 5, New York, 1987, Springer.

43. Smith MJ: Perspectives on nursing science, Nurs Sci Q 1(2):80, 1988.

44. Smith SR: "Oremization," the curse of nursing, RN 44(10):83, 1981.

45. Stevens BJ: Nursing theories: one or many? In McCloskey JC and Grace HK, editors: Current issues in nursing, ed 2, Boston, 1985, Blackwell Scientific Publications, Inc.

46. Uys LR: Foundational studies in nursing, J Adv Nurs 12:275, 1987.

47. Visintainer MA: The nature of knowledge and theory in nursing, Image 18(2):32, 1986.

48. Walker LO: Toward a clearer understanding of the concept of nursing theory, Nurs Res 20(5):428, 1974.

49. Walker LO and Avant KC: Strategies for theory construction in nursing, Norwalk, Conn, 1983, Appleton-Century-Crofts.

50. Watson J: Nursing: human science and human care, Norwalk, Conn, 1985, Appleton-Century-Crofts.

51. Winstead-Fry P, editor: Case studies in nursing theory, New York, 1986, National League for Nursing.

CHAPTER 2

Viewpoints

Nursing and the philosophy of science

GLENN A. WEBSTER

In addition to the tenets of the received view of the nature of science, the logical positivistic philosophy of science passed on to nursing an assumption concerning the desirability of disciplines becoming sciences that is traceable at least back to the eleventh and twelfth centuries in European and Middle Eastern thought. The purpose of this chapter is to question the value of this assumption, especially for nursing, by examining critically the distinctions among science, profession, and discipline. These distinctions will make it easier to answer often-asked questions about the relation of nursing to the sciences and the relevance of philosophy and the philosophy of science to nursing.

THE NATURE OF SCIENCE

Science per se is a systematic body of knowledge for knowledge's sake. It is theoretical rather than practical, and it is concerned with truth rather than action. It is not necessarily concerned with the general, as Aristotle claimed,[1] but may be concerned with the particular. The best example of a science of the particular is history.* The various sciences may not be unified by reduction to one basic science, as the 1930 Vienna Circle logical positivists believed would be the case.[8] But in order for a body of knowledge to be a

science, it must be systematic and cohere with the rest of the sciences.

There are two theses here: (1) A body of knowledge must be systematic to be a science, and (2) each science must cohere with all of the other sciences. There is no need for nursing to accept the narrow definition of system offered by logical positivism: axiomatization and formalization by translation into the grammar of the first order predicate calculus. This leaves incomplete the task of defining the sense in which a body of knowledge must be systematic. Perhaps the truth in Paul Feyerabend's methodological anarchism is the rejection of any a priori conception of the nature of systematization needed for a discipline to be a science.[5] We may be rightly suspicious of closure on the issue of the nature of systematization while avoiding Feyerabend's apparent relativism and skepticism.

It is easier to be clear about the second thesis: there are no independent sciences. For example, astrology is a pseudoscience rather than a science because, although it is systematic, it does not cohere with the rest of the sciences in the late twentieth century. Astrology's view of the causal influences of the stars and planets on human affairs is incoherent with physics, astronomy, astrophysics, and both macro- and microbiology. Further, the worldview that is coherent with astrology is a minority worldview of the early Middle Ages and not the worldview of the late twentieth century. It is no accident that the science fantasy novels in which astrology plays a major role have settings reminiscent of the early Middle Ages.[7] Why is the late twentieth century preferable to the

---

*The position that history is concerned with the unique and non-repeatable is a natural consequence of the sweep of Western philosophy over 2600 years. Whitehead[13] articulates the *reasons* for this belief well enough to allow for a confident claim: History is non-repeatable, as is the individual.

early Middle Ages in our approach to knowledge and truth? Again, the hint from art is helpful: the sciences and theories that cohere in the late twentieth century are much more complex and achieve coherence in spite of their greatly heightened complexity.* In addition, the sciences and theories of the late twentieth century are in general much more precise in their descriptions of the various domains constituting the world. Precision brings cognitive risk. Karl Popper is correct: theories that successfully run higher cognitive risks are preferable to theories that avoid risk through vagueness or other means.[10] Even if positive empirical verification of such theories is impossible, theories that survive high empirical risks may be considered empirically justified, at least provisionally.

Coherence is a philosophical concept that cannot be succinctly defined. It is more than logical consistency; that is, it is more than lack of contradiction. The best way to explain coherence is by analogy to art. Classical aesthetics from Aristotle to Whitehead holds that beauty is the result of organic unity within a work.[2] The beautiful work must be reasonably complex. Each part of such a work must be so related to the other parts of the same work that they all mutually enhance the meaning and significance of one another. In the ideally perfect work of art, no part may be added, subtracted, or changed without diminution of the value of all parts and of the whole. By analogy, within the sciences, each theory within a science and each science within the body of human knowledge as a whole should enhance the plausibility and significance of all other theories and sciences. Coherence in science is the analog of beauty in art. Hence it is no accident that aesthetic beauty has played a major role in the development of the theories of the established sciences. Incoherence is ugly.

The analogy is truer than it seems because the coherence among the sciences is conceptual coherence, better understood in terms of aesthetics than formal logic. This is because scientific coherence at least strives for concrete particularity rather than abstract form. Concrete particularity is the hallmark of art and aesthetics;[4] abstract form is the concern of symbolic logic.† This is appropriate because the corpus of science at any one time is a particular, and the actuality that it is trying to know—the world—is another particular. There is a paradox here, because scientists are part of the world that they are attempting to know by means of science. This paradox is illustrated nicely by the painting by Maurice Escher in which a man is holding a mirrored sphere containing himself and the world.[6]

Logical consistency is comprehensible, and so is aesthetic coherence. But "logical coherence" is either meaningless or indistinguishable from "aesthetic coherence." "Conceptual coherence" seems more abstract and general than aesthetic coherence; but a clarification of conceptual coherence leads to the same notions of concrete particularity and nonrepeatability characteristic of aesthetic coherence. Hence, it was no accident that Truth and Beauty were two of the five syncategorematic concepts (terms or concepts transcending the ordinary metaphysical categories) of medieval philosophy. Truth is to be achieved through an organic unity similar, if not identical, to the organic unity that grounds Beauty. The other syncategorematic concepts were Unity, Reality, and the Good. Unity and Reality tie the other three together. (This is a bit of Neoplatonism inherited from Plotinus in the second century and developed by early medieval Western philosophy.)

Hence, those who contend that nursing is both a science and an independent body of knowledge would seem to be mistaken about at least one of these two points—mistaken about the first and confused about the second.

PROFESSIONS, DISCIPLINES, AND SCIENCES

Nursing is primarily a profession. It has developed an academic discipline to support the profession and facilitate the education and training of nurses. The truth in the view that nursing should develop its own independent body of knowledge is that each such discipline develops a body of literature special to itself. The problems of training new nurses are different from the problems of training new physicians. Hence, the disciplines of nursing and medicine are independent,

---

*See A.N. Whitehead, *Adventures of Ideas* (New York, 1933, Macmillan); and Larry Laudan, *Progress and Its Problems* (Berkeley, 1977, University of California Press). Laudan emphasizes the importance of coherence among theories and, implicitly, among extant viable research traditions in various sciences. Whitehead provides an aesthetic/metaphysical exposition of the nature of coherence.

†Symbolic logic is only able to analyze propositions and theories in accordance with repeatable forms. If it deals with the particular, it is only via the general or repeatable.

with separate texts and guides for the training of new professionals. But, as has been argued above, there are no independent sciences. In the sense in which nursing and medicine are independent disciplines, neither is a science.

Both nursing and medicine use the sciences, and both contribute to the sciences. There are good reasons, however, for denying that there is either a science of nursing or a science of medicine; the goal of the two disciplines is practical rather than theoretical. The word *science* is loaded with positive value connotations. Every discipline wants to be called a science for reasons of politics and self-esteem, with the interesting exception of law, which has enough self-esteem and political power not to need added support from the label "science."

Can there be sciences that are primarily practical, that are concerned with the development of theory and the guidance of research, the goal of which is improvement of the practice of a profession? How are such putative practical sciences related to the theoretical sciences? Is technology practical science or to be distinguished from science? Again, the word *science* is being fought over because it is positively valued. Setting such value issues aside, it is useful to distinguish knowing from doing, knowledge from action. Our best technology makes extensive use of our best science and vice versa, but technology should be distinguished from science. Canons of wise practice are canons of technology rather than science. Nursing, medicine, and law all augment our ability to act (or at least the ability of the professional to act); hence, they are comparable to engineering or architecture rather than physics or biology. Just as engineering needs solid-state physics, among other sciences, nursing and medicine need anatomy and physiology, and nursing may have a greater need for the social sciences and human sciences than does medicine.

The relations between professions and supporting sciences are rich and two way: specific sciences are financed and promoted because of their relevance and importance to one or more professions. Much work in contemporary microbiology has this kind of support; health science campuses support such work because of its importance to research on many of the more intractable diseases, such as cancer. Genetic engineering is a branch of technology in symbiotic relationship to the science of microbiology. There is a similar symbiotic relationship between the technology that produces dense, integrated chips and solid-state physics.

SCIENCES OF SPECIAL RELEVANCE TO NURSING

Are there sciences or will there be sciences primarily supported by nursing?

Science presupposes an existing domain; the scientist is trying to understand what is already there. But the goal of the nursing profession as a profession is to create something new, not merely to understand something already in existence. What distinguishes nursing from other professions is the nature of that which it wishes to create: the enhancement of the health of the individual and community. Many sciences are relevant to the accomplishment of this goal, and nursing as a profession is learning to make better use of these independent and largely preexisting tools. But certain sciences, especially the human sciences, have not received the attention, funding, and encouragement that they need to flourish. Unfortunately for nursing, these are exactly the sciences for which nursing has the most need. Nursing is not a human science; it is a profession. However, nursing needs to foster and make use of the human sciences.

The nurse is the health professional whose focus of professional expertise is the needs of the patient as a person, usually in the context of some health deficit. The nurse must have a foundation in the biological sciences and in psychology in order to handle the health deficits. But the primary focus in the education of a nurse should be on those disciplines and sciences that are useful for understanding the particular rather than the general; for persons as such are unique individuals. Humanities and history should be in every nursing curriculum. Philosophy is indispensable for ethics and theories of human nature and for understanding the difference between the repeatable and the nonrepeatable.

Hence, the nurse is the health professional who should be trained to recognize and respect each person in his or her uniqueness. For the nurse, training in human relations (Buber[3]) is more important than training in epidemiology, although some knowledge of the latter is also useful and expected.

NURSING AND THE PHILOSOPHY OF SCIENCE

Which traditions in philosophy and philosophy of science are most useful for supporting nursing as a discipline and profession? Will there be any differences in the traditions that are most useful for supporting the sciences of special relevance to nursing? Should nursing be supporting sciences in the traditional sense, or would it be more helpful to the discipline and profession of nursing for nursing to support certain types of history and case studies, perhaps certain new branches of philosophy? The caring literature is a case in point. Nursing needs much richer sources in literature and philosophy than presently exist. Should the research effort and funds of nursing support such endeavors as the writing of a new genre of short story and novel focusing on the experience of individuals and their families with health problems? Would it not be useful to nursing to have new work in philosophy expounding and developing the concept of caring? The concept of person?

I see my role as a philosopher of science concerned with nursing to be largely therapeutic (hence the series of articles with Ada Jacox in which we tried to exorcise the ghost of the received view[11]). Nursing per se is not a science, so the relevance of philosophy of science is largely that of putting science in perspective so that nursing can develop without the onus of trying to become a science following one model or another. Part of the legacy of the received view was the pressure to transform disciplines into sciences, even when such a transformation was inappropriate.

But philosophy of science can be helpful in understanding the relationship of nursing to the sciences. The most helpful traditions are not the received view but the more pragmatic and idealistic alternatives to the received view. I personally find Whitehead more helpful than straight phenomenology, because Whitehead provides a philosophical basis for integrating the physical sciences with the metaphysics of experience. Phenomenology, as is the case with any developed philosophical system, is also able to handle the physical world and the physical sciences. But this is not phenomenology's strength.

A strong case can be made for the relevance of both existentialism and phenomenology as useful for the conceptual enlargement of the professional nurse. These traditions in philosophy are far more useful for heightening one's moral sensitivity than British empiricism. And if one's interest is in the development of the social sciences rather than the physical sciences, one should read the work of such contemporary Continental philosophers as Jürgen Habermas.* Other work of potential value is that of the contemporary neo-Whiteheadians such as Robert C. Neville.[9]

Nursing has a special problem in understanding the sciences and its relation to the sciences because of nursing's need to balance experience and physical reality. People act. Action involves both physical reality and understanding, intention, interests, and goals, among others. The latter are mental phenomena. But the former also can be described by those sciences that have added time and motion to the description of static structure. However, no matter how complete and sophisticated the physical science, human action eludes it. The physiologist has something to say about the relationships among bone, muscle, and tendons as a human arm is raised. The neurologist makes a contribution to the picture. But the two together are unable to bridge the gap between events involving muscles, tendons, bones, and nerves, and intentional actions. Somehow the latter involves the former and is impossible without it; but the physical sciences are at present unable not only to explain the relationship, but also to do so *in theory*.

This is a version of the famous mind-body problem. The distinction between inquiries into the reasonableness and nature of human actions and inquiries into the functioning of the body, inclusive of the nerves and the brain, is a particularly troublesome distinction philosophically, whether or not one is a mind-body dualist. An inquiry into the body is not going to reveal the intentionality of actions; an inquiry into actions cannot possibly separate out physical events alone. Whitehead's analysis of reality—physical and mental—into experient occasions is tempting but does not finally resolve all of the puzzles about the relationships between the "two worlds." We want to view reality as one, but we are left with two.

Returning to an earlier question, the philosophies of sciences that are relevant to nursing include those that enable us to make sense of the human sciences. A narrow philosophy of science that illuminates only certain physical sciences is largely a waste of time for nursing. Nursing needs broader philosophies of science that reveal the differences and relations among the various branches of science rather than those that foster the illusion that the physical sciences are the only sciences. If nursing prospers as a profession, it may play an important role in the reintegration of

---

*For instance, *The Theory of Communicative Action*, Volume 1, *Reason and the Rationalization of Society* (Boston, 1984, Beacon Press). The work of the Frankfort School of Philosophy may prove to be quite valuable to philosophy in general and nursing in particular, but it is difficult work, not for beginners.

science and human knowledge, because it is exactly integrated science and knowledge that nursing needs. Medical specializations find scientific specialization useful and foster it. Nursing needs a gestalt or holistic understanding of person and society. Overspecialization is an obstacle to such understanding. In brief, the nurse needs the Renaissance approach to philosophy and science rather than late nineteenth-century German departmentalization and specialization.

CONCLUSION

Nursing theory and research is handicapped at the present time by the misconception, fostered by economic and political pressures, that such theory and research should be viewed as science or developing science. Here the distinction among science, profession, and discipline may be liberating. Much nursing theory and research is directed to the production of literature designed to inspire the profession and provide direction to the discipline. It is visionary and hortatory. In contrast, science is cautious, objective, and nonjudgmental. The scientist wants to know and does not care, as a scientist, whether the knowledge will be useful, beneficial, or dangerous. Fortunately most scientists are also persons. The key to these distinctions is the contrast between preparation for wise and humane action and the testing and extension of human knowledge. Knowledge is needed for wise and humane action, but it is not enough.[1,6] Vision and ethical commitment are at least as important to the viability of professions such as nursing—a helping and caring profession.

REFERENCES

1. Aristotle: Nichomachean ethics, Bk VI, Ch. 3. In McKeon R, editor: The basic works of Aristotle, New York, 1942, Random House.
2. Aristotle: Poetics. In McKeon R, editor: The basic works of Aristotle, New York, 1942, Random House.
3. Buber M: The knowledge of man: a philosophy of the inter-human, New York, 1966, Harper & Row.
4. Collingwood RG: The principles of art, New York, 1958, Oxford Univ Press.
5. Feyerabend P: Against method, London, 1978, Verso.
6. Hofstadter DR: Gödel, Escher, Bach: an eternal golden braid, New York, 1980, Random House.
7. Kurtz K: The chronicles of the Deryni, Garden City, NY, 1973, Nelson Doubleday, Inc. Zelazny, R: Sign of chaos, New York, 1987, Arbor House. Donaldson, SR: The mirror of her dreams, New York, 1986, Ballantine Books.
8. Neurath O, Carnap R, and Morris C: Foundations of the unity of science, vols 1 & 2, Chicago, 1955, 1970, The Univ of Chicago Press.
9. Neville RC: Reconstruction of thinking, Albany, 1981, State Univ of New York Press.
10. Popper K: The logic of scientific discovery, New York, 1959, Basic Books.
11. Webster GA, Jacox A, and Baldwin B: Nursing theory and the ghost of the received view. In McCloskey JC and Grace HK, editors: Current issues in nursing, Boston, 1981, Blackwell Scientific Publications.
12. Whitehead AN: Process and reality, corr ed, New York, 1978, Free Press.

CHAPTER 3

Nursing process, nursing diagnosis, and emerging taxonomies

DOROTHY J. DOUGLAS
ELLEN K. MURPHY

INTRODUCTION

Classification systems, often called taxonomies or taxonomic approaches, have appeared with increasing frequency in nursing literature since the early 1970s. In 1974, influenced in part by the publication of Sokal's article on classification,[52] many nurse authors began to describe and develop classification systems for nursing with renewed enthusiasm.

According to the literature cited below, comprehensive taxonomies for nursing will facilitate the clear, concise, comprehensive, predictive, and continued growth of the discipline. This approach seems particularly attractive, because nursing as a discipline is grounded in the natural and social or behavioral sciences basic to the health care field. In fact, to the degree that we emulate the medical model, we are tempted to believe that the development of adequate classification systems unique to the practice of nursing will differentiate us from other health professionals, assure our recognition as scientists in our own right, aid us in achieving a high level of practice, and further other goals important not only to the individual nurse but to the nursing profession as a discipline.

That nursing can benefit to some degree from a taxonomic approach is clear. Such an approach is especially useful in a rapidly developing profession. It aids the processes of evolution, growth, change, adaptation, and interaction with cognate professions. As Sokal notes,[52] classification systems facilitate communication, assist in the development of research hypotheses, point toward future trends, and identify, simplify, and give structure to hitherto undiscovered characteristics of classes of objects or behaviors. (Note that Sokal does not include identification of the profession that develops the taxonomy among the purposes of taxonomy.) Such systems also serve the profession and the professional in efforts to avoid false, misleading, or transitory concepts. As is true of any good tool, a taxonomy (whether or not it is yet fully developed) should be carefully honed and used only for the purpose for which it was designed.

In *nursing process* and *nursing diagnosis* we have two excellent examples of long-term attempts to develop concepts that would accomplish goals similar to those outlined for taxonomies. It is useful to examine the evolution of these concepts. By so doing, we may be able to avoid some of the problems and pitfalls inherent in classification systems, and thereby maximize their potential utility.

NURSING PROCESS AND NURSING DIAGNOSIS
Evolution of concepts

The terms *nursing process* and *nursing diagnosis* first surfaced in the early 1950s. These concepts began to occur with increasing frequency in the nursing literature of the 1960s, although they were often used inconsistently. Their continued evolution through the 1980s included attempts not only to refine definitions but also to identify the cognitive processes inherent in their operationalization. Despite significant advances in definition and operationalization, concern regarding these concepts and their uses and functions pervades the literature today.

A review of the nursing process–nursing diagnosis literature reveals an interplay of concepts that serves to both obscure and elucidate their respective definitions and functions. Since *process* and *diagnosis* first appeared in the literature, each term has been used to define the other without having an intrinsic definition of its own. This is symptomatic of the difficulty inherent in investing intangible concepts with concise and unambiguous meaning. The process of defining and operationalizing a new concept may begin with labels that are essentially devoid of meaning or have meaning only through prior associations. As the concept develops, the meaning gradually accrues and is modified. (The development of the concept *primary nursing* is a case in point.)

Although the first recognized use of the term *nursing diagnosis* predated the first recognized use of *nursing process*,[16,38,58] nursing diagnosis was generally subsumed under the assessment component of nursing process.[20] In 1960 Abdellah[1] referred to nursing diagnosis as a process in identifying "five basic elements of nursing." In 1962 Chambers[10] defined nursing diagnosis as an investigation of facts to determine the nature of a nursing problem, during which the nurse would systematically collect facts, interpret facts in view of the particular patient, identify nursing problems, decide the course of action, and evaluate the results. These elements are remarkably similar to what we now label nursing process. In 1963 Komorita[34] defined nursing diagnosis as a process that provides systematic assessment of problems and needs.

By the late 1960s the concept of nursing process as we know it had evolved, apparently without much controversy, under a variety of rubrics including the definition and philosophy of nursing, clinical inference, and even nursing diagnosis.[58] A faculty group at the Catholic University School of Nursing in Washington, D.C. summarized the phases of nursing process in 1967 as assessing, planning, implementing, and evaluation.[58] In 1971 Carrieri and Sitzman[9] stated that the unique elements of the nursing process had been identified as observation, inference, validation, assessment, action, and evaluation. By the second half of the 1970s, nursing process was usually described as an initial stage in which data are collected, assessment is made, and one or more nursing diagnoses are formulated. This stage is typically followed by planning, implementing, and evaluating phases. This formulation has persisted to the present.

From the many references to it in nursing literature, there would appear to be wide acceptance of the concept *nursing process*. In fact, we were unable to locate an article published before 1982 that challenged the received opinion. In that year, Henderson[27] questioned

whether "problem solving is all there is to nursing (so that it can be called *the* nursing process) and whether problem solving is peculiar to nursing (or whether it can be called the *nursing* process)."

The interrelationship of nursing diagnosis and nursing process is obscured by the apparent need to proceed through the steps of data collection, assessment and evaluation, and problem-solving to arrive at the diagnosis—which is, in turn, recognized as a piece of the larger nursing process.[14,26] Although most authors seem to agree that nursing diagnosis is a piece of nursing process, it has received separate (and more controversial) treatment in the literature.

Early definitions of nursing diagnosis were similar to what we now recognize as nursing process. Initially the label alone was used, leaving the reader to intuit its meaning,[16] while the bulk of the article dealt with the function and utility of a particular diagnostic label or the process of nursing diagnosis in general. Komorita[34] noted in 1963 that although the term was frequently used, there was little agreement among nurses as to its meaning. In 1974 Bloch[5] included nursing diagnosis among frequently used concepts in nursing in need of clarity and common understanding. Authors began to use the term *diagnosis* as an end product of a preceding process such as assessment,[18,48] or as a chronological step in a larger process. For example, nursing diagnosis must be preceded by validation of data and followed by a care plan.[42] The definition of the term underwent further refinement as a result of attempts to describe the cognitive steps necessary to develop diagnostic models and paradigms[4,19,31] and to assist the practitioner in their use.[22,23,25,40] Gordon stated in 1979 that defining nursing diagnosis is a major conceptual issue confronting researchers,[19] and, in 1982, noted the dearth of such research.[22] More recently, the literature contains discussion of diagnosis implementation.[44] Aydelotte and Peterson note that multiple definitions remain.[2]

Need for critique

Attempts to differentiate nursing diagnosis from medical diagnosis date from the 1950s. Early authors found it necessary to justify nursing's use of the term *diagnosis*.[29,33] One author proposed the term *trophicognosis* as an alternative, to avoid the inevitable confusion with medical diagnosis.[39] In the late 1970s through the 1980s, authors included in their discussions of nursing diagnosis comments about its similarity to[3,19,24,28] or difference from medical diagnosis.[3,4,19,28,53]

Did the furor over the legitimate use of the term *diagnosis* mask the need for a critical analysis of this concept? We found literature to avoid this issue prior to Williams' article in 1980,[57] which was followed by that of Shamansky and Yanni in 1983.[50] Shamansky and Yanni felt the need to call theirs a minority opinion, as they suggested that nursing diagnosis may actually limit practice, create obstacles to clear communication, and constrain inference and intuition. Although this view was strongly attacked by Kritek,[37] these authors precipatated debate over a problematic concept. In 1988 Jenny[30] questioned whether the accepted diagnostic label *knowing deficit* is really a diagnosis at all, since it does not meet the criteria for a nursing diagnosis. As such, she suggested, it is theoretically invalid and has limited utility. In general, however, the support for nursing diagnosis remains overwhelming among nurse authors.

TAXONOMIES

The descriptive label *taxonomy* has been frequently associated with nursing diagnosis.[17,18,24,28] Less frequently, nursing process has been called taxonomic approach, or has been thought to encompass taxonomies.[49] Nurse educators have referred to Campbell's textbook as a useful taxonomy, despite the author's disavowal.[8] In fact, *taxonomy* as used in nursing is already dangerously close to becoming jargon. Its imprecise use ultimately may compromise its potential as an aid in articulating and analyzing the processes of nursing.

According to *Webster's Third Unabridged Dictionary*, *taxonomy* refers both to the "study of the general principles of scientific classification" and to the systematic distinguishing, ordering, and naming of type groups within a subject field. *Roget's Fourth International Thesaurus* lists taxonomy as a synonym for classification, analysis, categorization, ranking, partitioning, pigeonholing, rating, and organization.[46] Classic examples of taxonomies are chemistry's periodic table and biology's classifications of plants and animals.

Sokal[52] added to this definition of taxonomy by noting that such classification systems arrange or order objects into groups or sets on the basis of their relationships. He listed several purposes of classification, including economy of memory and ease of manipulation, and stated that the paramount purpose of a classification system is to describe the structure and relationships of constituent objects to one another and

to similar objects, simplifying these relationships in such a way that general statements can be made about classes or objects. Because classifications based on many different properties of the classified objects are necessarily general, they are unlikely to serve specific purposes, although they might be useful for a variety of purposes. For example, in the 1980s, classification systems other than nursing diagnoses are being utilized for specific administrative purposes. The nursing administration literature has dealt extensively with patient classification systems that are not based solely on nursing diagnosis. The U.S. government has chosen to use (medical) diagnosis-related groupings (DRGs) as the basis for the prospective federal payment system.

Nursing taxonomies

Abdellah's classification of 21 nursing problems[1] or McCain's assessment paradigm of 13 functional areas[32] may be considered precursors of the attempt to systematize knowledge through a taxonomic approach. The ongoing attempts to classify nursing diagnoses are the best-known use of the taxonomic approach.[2,18,41,47] Through the efforts of individual nurses who convened at seven national conferences, nursing diagnoses have been identified and categorized using principles of classification. These categories have been further classified into a systematic format labelled Taxonomy I by the North American Nursing Diagnosis Association (NANDA).

Functionally, then, nursing diagnosis has been viewed by the profession as a part of the nursing process. However, it has also been viewed as furnishing a classifiable quantum of data, thus evolving a taxonomy with which to define our profession. That is, if the premise is accepted that nursing diagnosis is a part of a process unique to nursing, then a taxonomy of nursing diagnoses will define the nursing profession by telling what it does. Nurse authors take this a step further by characterizing the development of taxonomies as theory development activity.[26,32,35,36,41] Their position appears to be that theory is like natural law: it is something that is there all the time, and we need only to identify and describe it. Some of these authors have recognized taxonomy development as the first step of theory development.[26,35] Suppe and Jacox[54] caution that characterizing theory development as a stepwise process, with one level requiring completion before higher level theories can be developed, ignores the intertwining of concept and theory development.

And, as Porter[43] reminds us, promoting the unique identity of the nursing profession may be commendable, but it is quite different from the traditional purpose of taxonomic development to categorize an object and thereby explain why it possesses the properties it does.

UTILITY

The expectations for nursing process, nursing diagnosis, and taxonomies are monumental. Nursing process has been hailed as the foundation of nursing practice,[2] a model for uniform nursing practice,[38] and the core and essence of nursing.[58] Others hold that nursing diagnosis will allow us to define a body of unique nursing knowledge[15] and to further quality assurance programs;[6] it will clarify the role of the nurse and make individual nurses more accountable, thus increasing our stature as members of an autonomous profession.[15,38] Nursing diagnosis will delineate the components of health care for which nursing is responsible, and will enhance our professional identity.[6,15] It will facilitate intraprofessional and interprofessional communication, consultation, continuity of care, and third-party reimbursement.[55] It will provide a focus for the content of our clinical education and research.[21] All these potential accomplishments and goals rest on a concept that is not yet 35 years old. Any obstacles to attaining these goals will presumably be removed by further classification efforts. Proponents of NANDA Nursing Diagnosis Taxonomy I now project remarkably similar purposes for its development.[43]

The Third National Conference on Classification of Nursing Diagnosis developed this definition: Nursing diagnosis is a concise phrase or term summarizing a cluster of empirical indicators describing characteristics of unitary man.[33] This definition seems a bit too expansive if it is to accomplish all the specific goals previously enumerated. We are concerned that the profession is pinning too much hope on nursing diagnosis and what it can do for us. Certainly nursing diagnosis is becoming an important part of nursing practice, and it has accomplished much in its quest to articulate what nursing is. Viewed in the context of the history of health care, nursing has made great strides in developing the nursing diagnosis concept. Unfortunately, the concept is so popular that it has elevated expectations beyond a realistic level. If the literature can be believed, we are to rely on one concept to define a profession that is rapidly changing, developing, and being shaped, in part, by events outside the profession.

Will the development of classification systems allow us to define the profession of nursing in terms of what uniquely belongs to it? The question as it stands is unanswerable, but if we were to assume such a result, we can readily see some difficulties. We would be defining the profession as it is today rather than shaping it to meet tomorrow's needs and expectations. Although it is valuable to describe and differentiate existing classes of objects or behavior with an eye to predicting objects or behavior not yet discovered (analogous to the development of the periodic table in chemistry), it is something else to rely on a single classification system, such as nursing diagnosis, to define the profession of nursing. Suppe and Jacox[54] question the premature adoption of Rogers' conceptual framework for organizing nursing diagnoses, and suggest that additional frameworks should be considered and developed.

Yura and Walsh's review of the professional literature[58] revealed that there have been no new initiatives relating to the development of theoretical-conceptual frameworks proposed, presented, or published from 1980 through 1986. The energies of researchers, practitioners, and educators instead have been directed to the application of theoretical-conceptual structures proposed in the 1960s and 1970s. Similarly, only one revised definition of nursing has appeared since 1980, whereas the 1960s produced seven published definitions and the 1970s, five.[59]

The question occurs as to whether this pattern indicates consensus, directed creative energies, or numbing of critical challenge. Porter's suggestion that human-environment interactions can be recognized as the primary phenomena of nursing and the subject matter of a taxonomy is encouraging continued debate and creativity.[43] So too is Rasch's assertion[45] that the true nature of what nurses diagnose has yet to be elaborated and that until this is done, the logic of inductively developing a taxonomy based on the essential characteristics of nursing diagnoses is at best questionable. Also laudable are NANDA's continuing efforts in providing the profession with a developing taxonomy to serve as an imperfect model. These efforts should not be abandoned nor should they be impervious to challenges.

Another caveat applicable to nursing should be mentioned. Cultural and personal bias affect the categories selected, so that once taxonomists become convinced a particular trait is of great importance they will more readily use categories that support this view and will fail to recognize others. This tendency could have a limiting effect on the development of nursing and would assuredly limit its utility to the North American culture that dominated its development.

Of what use is all this effort, and where can we go from here? Any in-depth thinking about these questions is useful for the profession and practice of nursing by demonstrating the dynamic interaction between the clinical practice of a professional and the theoretical bases undergirding that practice. Of course, an effort in one specific direction cannot bear the freight of all the questions we would like answered about the theory and practice of nursing. Such efforts shed light on the interaction between clinical practice and its underlying theoretical bases. At their best they foster salutary discussions, critiques, and the exchange of views. Thus a taxonomic approach has practical value in addressing both professional and theoretical questions in nursing. That the results from this approach can be misused, misapplied, and misinterpreted in no way lessens their value.

However, this emphasis on classification of nursing diagnosis may be counterproductive. A single taxonomy for nursing may be undesirable. We do not share Weidmann and North's forecast[56] that one system will emerge as best for all fields of nursing. A single taxonomy may be an impossibility, and focusing nursing energies on such a task not only could be frustrating and wasteful but could unduly narrow our vision. The American Nurses' Association committee established to monitor developments in classification systems was originally assigned to develop a taxonomy for nursing practice. After some deliberation the committee realized that nursing is "too rich in data to settle on a single classification system of taxonomy at this time."[11]

We by no means suggest abandoning efforts to refine and categorize nursing diagnoses. In 1985 we suggested that the profession should not feel compelled to "finish" work on nursing diagnoses before proceeding to other critical investigations, such as those into nursing interventions and their impact.[13] Nurses are indeed proceeding with the development of individual diagnoses and the interventions associated with them.[2] There are now entire textbooks devoted to interventions.[7,51] Also encouraging is the continued development and utilization of alternative classification systems in nursing such as the Omaha Classification System.[56]

One of the difficulties faced in efforts to advance knowledge in our profession is that we are dependent to a greater or lesser degree on advances in other areas of the basic and applied sciences. The health care professions are so interdependent that a great advance in one can be effectively canceled by a relatively small advance in the other. Similarly, our profession can be substantively changed by advances in technology and fundamental changes in society (for example, the women's movement, the graying of America, the restructuring of health care financing).

How shall we proceed? We can use emerging taxonomies in a Hegelian manner to synthesize a new direction. We do not need ideal classification systems to make progress. As systems develop and are widely discussed the profession and the individual nurse should feel free to proceed in whatever direction(s) seem useful. For example, it may be useful to consider whether nursing diagnosis has been misplaced in the care continuum. Doesn't it make more sense to classify after all data are in, all treatment given, all outcomes evaluated, and definitive conclusions reached?

Sokal's notion of using taxonomies to generate hypotheses is a useful one. For example, the assessment category of nursing process can now be thought of as raising questions about, as well as adding categories to, nursing diagnoses. Nursing diagnoses, in turn, raise questions and encourage hypotheses about the process of nursing as it exists today.

Advances in any field are made with one creative insight or formulation building on another. Even if the building blocks are redesigned or discarded, the work that has preceded assists us toward our goals. Closure is not necessary, but continued growth is.

REFERENCES

1. Abdellah FG and others: Patient centered approaches to nursing, New York, 1960, Macmillan.
2. Aydelotte MK and Peterson KH: Keynote address: nursing taxonomies—state of the art. In McLane AM, editor: Classification of nursing diagnoses: proceedings of the seventh conference, St Louis, 1987, The CV Mosby Co.
3. Aspinall MH: Nursing diagnosis: the weak link, Nurs Outlook 24:433, 1976.
4. Avant K: Nursing diagnosis: maternal attachment, Advances in Nursing Science 2:45, 1979.
5. Bloch D: Some crucial terms in nursing: what do they really mean? Nurs Outlook 22:689, 1974.
6. Bruce JA: Implementation of nursing diagnosis, Nurs Clin North Am 14:509, 1979.

7. Bulechek GM and McCloskey JC: Nursing interventions: treatments for nursing diagnoses, Philadelphia, 1985, WB Saunders Co.

8. Campbell C: Nursing diagnosis and intervention in nursing practice, New York, 1978, John Wiley & Sons.

9. Carrieri VK and Sitzman J: Components of the nursing process, Nurs Clin North Am 6:115, 1971.

10. Chambers W: Nursing diagnosis, Am J Nurs 62:102, 1962.

11. Committee monitors development of classifications for practice, American Nurse 15(7):3, 1983.

12. Dickoff J and others: Theory in a practice discipline, Nurs Res 17:543, 1968.

13. Douglas DJ and Murphy EK: Nursing process, nursing diagnosis and emerging taxonomies. In McCloskey JC and Grace HK, editors: Current issues in nursing, ed 2, New York, 1985, Blackwell Scientific.

14. Durand M and Prince R: Nursing diagnosis: process and decision, Nurs Forum 5:50, 1966.

15. Field LL: The implementation of nursing diagnosis in clinical practice, Nurs Clin North Am 14:497, 1979.

16. Fry VS: The creative approach to nursing, Am J Nurs 53:301, 1953.

17. Gebbie K and Lavin MA: Classifying nursing diagnoses, Am J Nurs 74:250, 1974.

18. Gebbie K and Lavin MA: Classification of nursing diagnoses, St Louis, 1975, The CV Mosby Co.

19. Gordon M: Nursing diagnoses and the diagnostic process, Am J Nurs 76:1298, 1976.

20. Gordon M: The concept of nursing diagnosis, Nurs Clin North Am 14:487, 1979.

21. Gordon M and Sweeney MA: Methodological problems and issues in identifying and standardizing nursing diagnoses, Advances in Nursing Science 2:1, 1979.

22. Gordon M, Sweeney MA and McKeehan K: Nursing diagnosis: looking at its use in the clinical area, Am J Nurs 80:672, 1980.

23. Gordon M and others: Development of nursing diagnosis, Am J Nurs 80:669, 1980.

24. Gordon M: Nursing diagnosis, New York, 1982, McGraw-Hill Book Co.

25. Guzzetta CE and Forsyth GL: Nursing diagnostic pilot study: psychophysiologic stress, Advances in Nursing Science 2:27, 1979.

26. Henderson B: Nursing diagnosis: theory and practice, Advances in Nursing Science 1:75, 1978.

27. Henderson V: The nursing process: is the title right? J Adv Nurs 7:103, 1982.

28. Hickey M: Nursing diagnosis in the critical care unit, Critical Care Nursing 3:91, 1984.

29. Hornung G: Nursing diagnosis: an exercise in judgment, Nurs Outlook 4:29, 1956.

30. Jenny JL: Knowledge deficit: not a nursing diagnosis, Image 19:184, 1987.

31. Jones JA: Clinical reasoning in nursing, J Adv Nurs 13:185, 1988.

32. Jones PE: A terminology for nursing diagnosis, Advances in Nursing Science 2:65, 1979.

33. Kim MJ and Moritz DA: Classification of nursing diagnoses. Proceedings of the third and fourth national conferences, New York, 1982, McGraw-Hill Book Co.

34. Komorita NI: Nursing diagnosis, Am J Nurs 63:83, 1963.

35. Kritek PB: The generation and classification of nursing diagnoses: toward a theory of nursing, Image 10:33, 1978.

36. Kritek PB: Commentary: the development of nursing diagnosis and theory, Advances in Nursing Science 2:73, 1979.

37. Kritek PB: Nursing diagnosis in perspective: response to a critique, Image 17:3, 1985.

38. Lash AA: A re-examination of nursing diagnosis, Nurs Forum 17:332, 1978.

39. Levine ME: Trophicognosis: an alternative to nursing diagnosis. In ANA Regional Clinical Conference Proceedings, Kansas City, Mo, 1965, American Nurses' Association.

40. Matthews CA and Gaul AL: Nursing diagnosis from the perspective of concept attainment and critical thinking, Advances in Nursing Science 2:17, 1979.

41. McKay RP: What is the relationship between the development and utilization of a taxonomy and nursing theory? Nursing Researcher 26:222, 1977.

42. Mundinger MO and Jauron GD: Developing a nursing diagnosis, Nurs Outlook 23:94, 1975.

43. Porter EJ: Critical analysis of NANDA nursing diagnosis taxonomy I, Image 18:136, 1986.

44. Rantz MJ and Mass M, editors: Nursing diagnosis: implementation, Nurs Clin North Am 22:873, Dec 1987.

45. Rasch RFR: The nature of taxonomy, Image 19:147, 1987.

46. Roget's International Thesaurus, Fourth Edition, New York, 1977, Thomas Crowell & Sons.

47. Roy C: A diagnostic classification system for nursing, Nurs Outlook 23:90, 1975.

48. Roy C: The impact of nursing diagnosis, AORN J 21:1023, 1975.

49. Sculco CD: Development of a taxonomy for the nursing process, J Nurs Educ 17:40, June 1978.

50. Shamansky S and Yanni C: In opposition to nursing diagnosis: a minority opinion, Image 15:2:47, 1983.

51. Snyder M: Independent nursing interventions, New York, 1985, John Wiley and Sons.

52. Sokal RR: Classification: purposes, principles, progress, prospects, Science 185(27):1115, 1974.

53. Stein M: Nursing diagnosis: use in neonatal ICU, Dimensions of Critical Care Nursing, 7:104.

54. Suppe F and Jacox AK: Philosophy of science and the development of nursing theory, Ann Rev Nurs Res 3:251, 1985.

55. Weber S: Nursing diagnosis in private practice, Nurs Clin North Am 14:533, 1979.

56. Weismann J and North H: Implementing the Omaha classification system in a public health agency, Nurs Clin North Am 22:971, 1987.

57. Williams AB: Rethinking nursing diagnosis, Nurs Forum 19:357, 1980.

58. Yura H and Walsh MB: The nursing process, ed 3, New York, 1978, Appleton-Century-Crofts.

59. Yura H and Walsh MB: The nursing process, ed 5, New York, 1988, Appleton-Century-Crofts.

CHAPTER 4

Nursing intervention taxonomy development

GLORIA M. BULECHEK
JOANNE COMI McCLOSKEY

The development of nursing knowledge has been facilitated by use of the nursing process, which has a 25-year history in American nursing. The major emphasis during this time has been on the assessment phase of the process. The underlying assumption was that if nurses had a consistent data base they would automatically know what and how to treat. The nursing diagnosis movement is altering this assumption. Clinical decision making is seen as vital to a valid nursing diagnosis, in deciding both the data needed and how to analyze them. The profession is quickly realizing that if a nursing diagnosis is made there is an ethical and legal obligation to treat the patient. Attention is focusing on nursing treatments and outcomes, in addition to nursing diagnoses. The growth of knowledge about phases of the nursing process is reciprocal; as more is learned about nursing interventions and nursing outcomes, refinement and refocusing of the assessment and diagnosis will occur. The development of diagnostic and intervention labels is formulating a unique body of nursing knowledge, the factor isolating level of theory generation. This chapter discusses the need for a taxonomy of nursing interventions and describes two conceptual issues related to its achievement.

BACKGROUND

The phenomenon of concern in nursing interventions is nurse behavior, those things nurses do to assist clients in moving toward a desired outcome. This differs from nursing diagnoses, where the phenomenon of concern is client behavior. Previous research about nurse behavior has focused on two areas, job performance and patient classification.

Job performance studies have attempted to provide valid and reliable criteria for the appraisal of nursing care. Examples include the Phaneuf Nursing Audit,[33] the Slater Nursing Competencies Rating Scale,[34] the Quality Patient Care Scale,[32] the Rush Medicus Methodology for Monitoring the Quality of Nursing Care,[12] and Schwirian's Six Dimension Scale of Nursing Performance.[24,25] These tools have been used both in studies of quality assurance and job performance and as examples for the design of performance appraisal programs. They have been shadowed by interrater reliability issues and problems in construct validity.[16,30]

Patient classification research has attempted to quantify the amount of nursing care required by a client. Two types of patient classification tools exist: prototype tools and factor evaluation tools.[1] Such tools are in widespread use in the allocation of nursing resources. The factor type features a list of critical indicators of direct care given. These were developed to predict staffing needs but have been used recently in defining the cost of nursing care. Examples of the factor type of patient classification include the Rush-Medicus Classification Instrument,[14] the Grace-Reynolds Application and Study of PETO (GRASP) system,[20] and the patient classification system at Abbott Northwestern Hospital (Minneapolis, Minn.).[2] Many hospitals have developed their own classification systems or have modified previously purchased systems subsequent to the 1980 mandate by the Joint Commission on Accreditation of Hospitals, which required that a systematic methodology for determining nursing requirements be in place in hospitals.[23] Giovannetti and Mayer[9] list 16 problems faced by nursing departments in planning and implementing a patient classification system. The problems, relating to predictive validity and interrater reliability, can be overcome only through staff development and continued monitoring.

The classic tools listed above are inadequate as a taxonomy of nursing interventions. Those tools were developed for specific purposes, namely, quality assurance, allocation of resources, and productivity measurement. The nursing activity items they include are only a sample of all the activities that nurses perform. The items include a mixture of concrete tasks and more abstract actions. They include a variety of assessments, needs, diagnoses, and treatments. For the most part, they overlook the conceptual issue of how to define the independent and collaborative aspects of nursing practice. Using these tools, it is not possible to identify appropriate nurse action for a specific nursing diagnosis. Indeed, the description of nurse behavior has evolved from job performance and patient classification issues to the need for a logical classification of nursing treatments.

SIGNIFICANCE

At a conference on nursing information systems in 1983, a study group pointed out that although nurses spend much of their time documenting care provided, this documentation has not been systematically organized to advance nursing knowledge, to develop nursing practice, or to improve patient care.[28] In 1984 Zielstroff[38] asserted that the major impediment to the development of computerized nursing information systems is deficiencies in nursing's knowledge base:

Those who work in the design and development of nursing information systems constantly bemoan the fact that there are so few clinical problems in nursing for which the etiology, symptoms, treatment, and expected outcomes are known. There are no known probability estimates for prevalence or incidence of common nursing problems; or for relating symptoms to diagnosis, or treatment to outcome. Indeed, there is neither a standard terminology nor a widely accepted format for data gathering. It is impossible to derive hard and fast rules for computer assistance in decision making with such an ill-defined data base.

Recently there have been numerous efforts reported in the literature to "cost out" nursing. For the most part these studies had small sample sizes, were conducted in one institution, and used patient classification systems without much regard to their validity and reliability.[18] The wide variety of and lack of standardization in patient classification systems is, in fact, a key reason that it is difficult to obtain large data sets

for the comparison of nursing costs. McCloskey[17] has proposed a model of determining nursing costs using nursing diagnoses and interventions. To implement such a model, a list of standardized interventions is needed.

Thus it appears that the essential first step in organizing and standardizing nursing information is to develop meaningful categories of data and establish a uniform terminology. Werley[37] has emphasized the importance of this work by establishing the Nursing Minimum Data Set. Six content areas—assessment, diagnoses, interventions, outcomes, acuity or intensity, and demographics—were developed at a national invitation conference. Eighteen variables were accepted for the initial pilot study. As expected, the variables describing nursing practice proved troublesome. Taxonomy I developed by the North American Nursing Diagnosis Association (NANDA) was accepted as the classification for nursing diagnoses. A 7-category system and a 16-category system of nursing interventions were pilot-tested. Werley[35] reported at the International Nursing Conference on Clinical Judgment and Decision Making (May 1987, Calgary) that the pilot study findings indicated that neither intervention classification system was satisfactory, because the categories did not prove to be mutually exclusive.

In 1986 the board of directors of the American Nurses' Association (ANA) adopted a policy statement urging the uniform classification of four areas of nursing practice: assessment, diagnosis, intervention, and outcome.[3] NANDA was acknowledged as the organization developing the diagnosis taxonomy.[10,22] Definitive plans for developing the other three classification systems are yet to be formulated. At the January 1988 Conference on Research Priorities in Nursing Science, the National Center for Nursing Research (NCNR) identified as a high priority the development of nursing information systems.[21] To achieve this goal, standardized data sets are needed that document nursing care across settings, and a taxonomy is needed to classify nursing phenomena in a standard language.

In summary, a classification of nursing interventions is needed for the following reasons: (1) to standardize the nomenclature of nursing treatment; (2) to expand nursing knowledge about the links between diagnoses, treatments, and outcomes; (3) to facilitate the development of nursing information systems; (4) to assist in planning for resources needed in nursing practice settings; and (5) to provide a language to communicate to others the unique function of nursing.

CONCEPTUAL ISSUES

One of the major methodological issues in the development of an intervention taxonomy is whether to use a deductive or an inductive approach. A deductive approach, whereby interventions are identified and placed in an existing conceptual framework, does not appear a good choice at this time. Although there are several intervention classification schemes—Benner's eight domains of nursing,[4] the minimum data set intervention lists,[36,37] the Omaha classification scheme for interventions,[31] the 17 categories of nurse activities in the study by the National Council of State Boards of Nursing,[15] Henderson's and Nite's list of therapeutic measures,[13] Sigma Theta Tau's International Classification of Nursing Knowledge,[26] and Bulechek and McCloskey's beginning taxonomy of nursing interventions[5]—none are ready for the task at hand. All of these represent very preliminary attempts at identifying and classifying nursing interventions; most are the efforts of a single individual; few are empirically derived; and none are complete and validated. Other conceptual frameworks that relate to nursing diagnosis, such as NANDA's Taxonomy I,[19] Gordon's functional health patterns,[11] and the Omaha classification of nursing diagnoses,[27] are not appropriate for use in a deductive attempt to construct a taxonomy of nursing interventions.

Because there are few conceptual frameworks of nursing interventions and those that do exist are tentative and incomplete, and because there are numerous data sources containing thousands of concrete nursing activities, an inductive approach is a more logical choice. For several decades nurse educators and theorists have written about nursing actions or activities or those things a nurse should do as part of the intervention or implementation step of the nursing process. These writings are available in nursing textbooks and, more recently, in nursing care planning books and information systems. In all of these sources interventions are viewed as discrete actions; there is little conceptualization of how these actions fit together. For example, the following are typical of interventions listed in current nursing textbooks: "position the limb with sandbags," "raise the head of the bed 30 degrees," "encourage the patient to take deep breaths," and "explore the need for attention with the patient." Textbooks frequently include several hundred of these interventions, with the list for any one patient or for treatment of any one diagnosis numbering several dozen. Campbell's list of nursing interventions[8] features more than 2500! Thus it seems more logical to use an inductive approach in which these concrete actions can be grouped and categorized.

A second major conceptual issue is deciding what types of nursing activities (concrete actions) should be included in an intervention taxonomy. This issue focuses on the definition of a nursing intervention. In 1985 we defined a nursing intervention as an "autonomous action based on scientific rationale that is executed to benefit the client in a predicted way related to the nursing diagnosis and the stated goals."[6] This definition captured the independent role of the nurse in the treatment step of the nursing process. However, it does not encompass all of the treatment activities performed by the nurse. To be useful for multiple purposes a taxonomy of nursing interventions must include all types of treatments that nurses perform.

In a presentation at NANDA's Eighth Conference on the Classification of Nursing Diagnoses,[7] we described seven groups of nursing activities:

1. Assessment activities to make a nursing diagnosis
2. Assessment activities to gather information for a physician to make a medical diagnosis
3. Nurse-initiated treatments in response to nursing diagnoses
4. Physician-initiated treatments in response to medical diagnoses
5. Daily essential function activities that may not relate to either medical or nursing diagnoses but are done by the nurse for the client
6. Activities to evaluate the effects of nursing and medical treatments (these are also assessment activities but they are done for purposes of evaluation, not diagnosis)
7. Administrative and indirect care activities that support the delivery of nursing care.

Some of these categories require some elaboration. Category 3, "nurse-initiated treatments in response to nursing diagnoses," includes those nursing treatments resulting from the client's response to medical interventions. If a medical intervention caused a problem amenable to nursing treatment, then the nurse would make a diagnosis and treat it.

Categories 3 and 4 include monitoring or surveillance actions of nurses when these are done as treatments. Unfortunately, the words *monitoring* and *assessment* are used in many ways to mean different things in nursing. In categories 1, 2, and 6 they are used to refer only to data-gathering activities.

The daily essential functions referred to in category 5 differ from what are called activities of daily living (ADLs). If a client is unable to perform ADLs (e.g., bathing, hair combing) he or she would be diagnosed as having a self-care deficit and these activities would be carried out as nursing treatments under category 3. The activities included in category 5 are those that nurses often spend a great deal of time doing because others are not available to do them. A survey[29] listed among these such activities as answering the phone, finding supplies, obtaining prescribed drugs, cleaning equipment, picking up meal trays, and moving furniture. These are important to the patient and are often done by the nurse. If nurses are better able to conceptualize and articulate these issues we will be better equipped to seek ancillary help.

Category 7, administrative and indirect care activities, includes activities related to staff development, recordkeeping, staffing and scheduling, and so on.

These are all activities performed by the nurse to benefit the client—but are they all nursing interventions? Our 1985 definition[6] refers to category 3 above, the nurse-initiated treatments. Many nurses, authors of nursing texts, and nursing information systems, however, do not distinguish among these categories. An activity in any of these categories is often labeled a nursing action, intervention, or treatment.

We have expanded our previous definition of a nursing intervention as follows to include three of the seven types of nursing activities.[7]

A nursing intervention is any direct care treatment that a nurse performs on behalf of a client. These treatments include nurse-initiated treatments resulting from nursing diagnoses, physician-initiated treatments resulting from medical diagnoses, and performance of the daily essential functions for the client who cannot do these.[7]

We believe that the core of nursing interventions should be the nurse-initiated treatments (category 3), but any listing of nursing interventions (say, for a computerized care planning system) must also include physician-initiated treatments and the daily essential function activities (categories 4 and 5). At this time we believe the activities in categories 1 and 2 to be assessment (prediagnosis) and not intervention (post-diagnosis) functions. Category 6 focuses on evaluation and is best identified when a classification of patient outcomes is articulated. Category 7, administrative ac-

---

DEFINITIONS OF TERMS RELATED TO NURSING INTERVENTION TAXONOMY DEVELOPMENT

Nursing activities

Those actions that nurses do to assist clients to move toward a desired outcome; these activities include seven types: two types of assessment activities, three types of intervention activities, evaluation activities, and administrative activities. Nursing activities are at the concrete level of action and examples include: "raise the head of the bed 30 degrees," "explore the need for attention with the patient," and "observe for coughing."

Nursing intervention

Any direct care treatment that a nurse performs on behalf of a client which includes nurse-initiated treatments, physician-initiated treatments, and performance of daily essential functions. These are at the conceptual level and require a series of actions or activities to carry them out.

(1) Nurse-initiated treatments—interventions initiated by the nurse in response to a nursing diagnosis: "an autonomous action based on scientific rationale that is executed to benefit the client in a predicted way related to the nursing diagnosis and the stated goals."[6] Examples include patient contracting, counseling, reminiscence therapy, preparatory sensory information, bathing, oral hygiene, and positioning.

(2) Physician-initiated treatments—interventions initiated by a physician in response to a medical diagnosis but carried out by a nurse in response to a doctor's order. Examples include medication administration, electrolyte restoration, and intervenous fluid administration.

(3) Daily essential function activities—interventions that are not related to either nursing or medical diagnoses but are often done by the nurse for the client who cannot do them. Examples include bedmaking, equipment management, and a setup and disposal.

---

tivities, involves supporting (or indirect or overhead) activities and would not be included in a listing of nursing interventions because these are not direct care activities (see the box above for a summary of terminology related to nursing intervention taxonomy development).

We lead a research team at the University of Iowa

that is developing a taxonomy of nursing interventions. A qualitative approach is being taken to develop a classification of intervention labels with accompanying definitions and practice activities. Further work will be needed to organize the intervention labels into a taxonomic structure with accompanying rules for placement.

CONCLUSION

There is a need for a taxonomy of nursing intervention labels that includes all direct care treatment activities that nurses do on behalf of clients. This classification will parallel NANDA's taxonomy of nursing diagnoses. It will create a standardized language for the treatment portion of the nursing process. The explication of interventions and their defining activities (conceptual labels with examples) will be a major step forward in describing nursing practice. The standardized language can be computerized and linkages between diagnoses, interventions, and outcomes can be discovered through documentation and study of actual patient care.

Acknowledgement

Members of the research team include: Joanne C. McCloskey, Ph.D., R.N.; Gloria M. Bulechek, Ph.D., R.N.; Martha J. Craft, Ph.D., R.N.; Janice A. Denehy, Ph.D., R.N.; Marlene Z. Cohen, Ph.D., R.N.; John D. Crossley, M.A., R.N.; Orpha J. Glick, Ph.D., R.N.; Meridean Maas, Ph.D., R.N.; Colleen M. Prophet, M.A. candidate, R.N.; and Toni Tripp-Reimer, Ph.D., R.N.

REFERENCES

1. Abdellah F and Levine E: Better patient care through nursing research, New York, 1965, Macmillan.
2. American Hospital Association: Nursing patient classification systems. Unpublished manual accompanying live satellite teleconference, Chicago, 1985.
3. American Nurses' Association: Minutes of board of directors meeting, Kansas City, December 1986.
4. Benner P: From novice to expert, Menlo Park, Calif, 1984, Addison-Wesley.
5. Bulechek GM and McCloskey JC: Nursing interventions: what they are and how to choose them, Holistic Nursing Practice 1(3):36, 1987.
6. Bulechek GM and McCloskey JC: Nursing interventions: treatments for nursing diagnoses, Philadelphia, 1985, WB Saunders Co.
7. Bulechek GM and McCloskey JC: Nursing interventions: treatments for potential nursing diagnoses. In Carroll-Johnson RM,

editor: Classification of nursing diagnoses: proceedings of the eighth conference, Philadelphia, 1989, JB Lippincott.
8. Campbell C: Nursing diagnosis and intervention in nursing practice, ed 2, New York, 1984, John Wiley & Sons.
9. Giovannetti P and Mayer G: Building confidence in patient classification systems, Nursing Management 15(8):31,1984.
10. Gordon M: Report of the president: book of reports from the NANDA biennial business meeting, St. Louis, Mo., March 15, 1988.
11. Gordon M: Manual of nursing diagnosis, New York, 1982, McGraw-Hill Book Co.
12. Haussmann R and others: Monitoring quality of nursing care, Health Serv Res 9:135, 1974.
13. Henderson V and Nite G: Principles and practice of nursing, ed 6, New York, 1967, Macmillan Publishing Co.
14. Jelinek RC and others: A methodology for monitoring quality of nursing care, US Department of Health, Education and Welfare Pub No HRA 76-25, Washington, DC, 1974, US Government Printing Office.
15. Kane M and others: A study of nursing practice and role delineation and job analysis of entry-level performance of registered nurses, Chicago, 1986, National Council of State Boards of Nursing, Inc.
16. Lang N and Clinton J: Assessment of quality of nursing care. In Werley H and Fitzpatrick J, editors: Annual review of nursing research, vol 2, New York, 1984, Springer Publishing Co.
17. McCloskey JC: Implications of costing out nursing for reimbursement, Nursing Management 20(1):44, 1989.
18. McCloskey JC, Gardner DL, and Johnson MR: Costing out nursing services: an annotated bibliography, Nursing Economics 5(5):245, 1987.
19. McLane AM: Classification of nursing diagnoses: proceedings of the seventh conference, St Louis, 1987, The CV Mosby Co.
20. Meyer D: GRASP: Grace-Reynolds Application and Study of PETO, Morgantown, NC, 1978, MCS.
21. National Center for Nursing Research: Report on the national nursing research agenda. Paper presented at the Conference on Research Priorities in Nursing Science, Washington, DC, January 1988.
22. North American Nursing Diagnosis Association: Developments in taxonomy, Nursing Diagnosis Newsletter 14(2):5, 1987.
23. Riccolo D: Institutional approaches to costing out nursing. In: Johnson M, editor: Series on nursing administration, vol 1, Menlo Park, Calif, 1988, Addison-Wesley.
24. Schwirian PM: Prediction of successful nursing performance, parts III and IV, US Department of Health, Education, and Welfare Pub No HRA 79-15, Washington, DC, 1979, US Government Printing Office.
25. Schwirian PM: Evaluating the performance of nurses: a multidimensional approach, Nurs Res 27:347, 1978.
26. Sigma Theta Tau International Honor Society of Nursing: Introduction to the international classification of nursing knowledge, Indianapolis, 1987, Sigma Theta Tau.
27. Simmons DA: Nurse planning information systems: a classification scheme for client problems in community health nursing, US Department of Health and Human Services Pub No HPA 80-16, Washington, DC, 1980, US Government Printing Office.
28. Study Group on Nursing Information Systems: Computerized

nursing information systems: an urgent need. Res Nurs Health 6(2):101, 1983.

29. Survey of nonnursing functions spots time wasters, Am J Nurs 88(4):429, 1988.

30. Ventura M and others: Interrater reliability for two measures of nursing care quality, Res Nurs Health 3:25, 1980.

31. Visiting Nurse Association of Omaha: Client management information system for community health nursing agencies, US Department of Health and Human Services Pub No HRP-0907023, Washington, DC, 1986, National Technical Information Service.

32. Wandelt M and Ager J: Quality patient care scale, New York, 1974, Appleton-Century-Crofts.

33. Wandelt M and Phaneuf M: Three instruments for measuring the quality of nursing care, Hospital Topics 50(8):20, 1972.

34. Wandelt M and Stewart D: Slater nursing competencies rating scale, New York, 1975, Appleton-Century-Crofts.

35. Werley HH and Devine EC: The nursing minimum data set: status and implications. In Hannah KJ and others, editors: Clinical judgment and decision making: the future with nursing diagnosis, New York, 1987, John Wiley & Sons.

36. Werley HH and Lang NM: Proceedings of the postconference task force meeting on the nursing minimum data set, Chicago, 1985.

37. Werley HH, Lang NM, and Westlake SK: The nursing minimum data set conference: executive summary, J Prof Nurs 2(4):217, 1986.

38. Zielstorff RD: Why aren't there more significant automated nursing information systems? J Nurs Adm 14(1):7, 1984.

CHAPTER 5

Clinical specialization versus generalization

New perspectives on an old issue

GRACE H. CHICKADONZ

The debate on clinical specialization versus generalization ought to be declared a nonissue in its current form. Two divergent views are presented here to provide perspectives on what this debate is about. In the first Diers discusses the preparation of practitioners, clinical specialists, and clinicians and argues persuasively that all of nursing is specialized practice.[7]

There is no longer any such thing as "generalized" nursing practice. While undergraduate programs must prepare generic (meaning "of a [same] kind") nurses, once nurses have graduated, all become specialized. In institutional settings, nurses work with children or adults, with patients being treated surgically or medically. Their patients have diseases or disorders of the lungs, legs, or lymph. Community health nursing, once thought to be the most "generalized" has increasingly recognized its special knowledge as health planning, epidemiology, and the study of the family and/or community. Brand new BSN graduates express a preference for their first work assignments, and if they are lucky enough to get it, become specialists from that point on.*

Diers believes that all of nursing is specialized practice because of the explosion of nursing knowledge.[7]

The shape of nursing's educational, administrative, and practice patterns has been determined not by politics or organizational positions but by the growth of knowledge both in nursing and in related fields. When nursing's repertoire of knowledge rested on comfort measures, hygiene, and diet, it was possible to train and place nurses as generalists because there was not enough knowledge to warrant specialization. Now, the territory of each nurse is huge. It is impossible for every nurse to know everything necessary to practice even safely, not to say elegantly, in every special field, whether the fields are defined by disease, organ system, medical care organization, severity of patient condition, or institutional base. . . . What characterizes specialization is specialized knowledge, not job description or title. Inevitably, specialization forces depth over breadth, specific over general. That being the case, advanced education is not and cannot be just more of the same.

Despite her argument that specialization is inevitable because of the growth of knowledge in different subject areas, Diers fails to address the issue that not all advanced knowledge is unique to each separate specialty.

The debate about clinical specialization versus generalization will not die because it encompasses a tangled web of issues that are at the core of nursing's history and evolution toward the future. These disagreements sometimes involve only definitions of terms, but usually they involve substantive issues and often become quite heated. The issues include roles in nursing practice, education for different roles and levels of responsibility, the nature of nursing as a profession, nursing's knowledge base and the educational process itself, the needs of society, and the changing nature of health care in America. At present the ways these issues are connected is not always clear, either in theory or practice environments, where there is usually a shortage of appropriately educated and utilized people. Always the ideal is compromised by the realities. Schlotfeldt[20] addresses the situation and acknowledges the need for nursing to identify and resolve some major issues within the field:

Those issues derive from conflicting views of the profession's essential mission or goal, its practice domain, and jurisdiction; the system of education through which some lay persons are transformed into professionals known as

---

*Through preceptorships and electives, some undergraduate programs now help students gain experiences that match their specialty interests, thus increasing the likelihood that they will be selected for their preferred first assignments.

nurses, and others into nurses' assistants; and the regulation and control of nursing education and nursing practice.

Acknowledging the increasing amount of scholarship about nursing and its system of knowledge, Schlotfeldt notes nonetheless the paucity of nursing theories, which may be due to the conflicting views of nursing's world of work and inquiry. In discussing these conflicting views, she elaborates on the concept of health and the nature of human beings.[20]

Whereas physicians who fulfill their mission logically view human subjects as being vulnerable to ills, nurses who fulfill their professional role logically conceive the persons they serve to be, by nature, health-seeking beings. It is thus incumbent upon nursing's scholars to identify and classify the human health assets—the health-seeking mechanisms and health-seeking behaviors with which they are naturally endowed and subsequently acquire, frequently with assistance of nurses. It is also their responsibility to learn more than is currently known about them and about the factors that influence health-seeking mechanisms and behaviors, both favorably and adversely. Newly discovered and substantiated knowledge of those mechanisms, behaviors and influencing factors can then be incorporated into nursing's scientific knowledge and made available to practitioners for their use in preserving, protecting, and enhancing the health of all to whom they give care and help to achieve independence and self-fulfillment.

Herein lies the generalist knowledge base that forms the basis for professional practice.

The health-seeking behaviors of individuals, families, and communities, as well as strategies for enhancing or augmenting them, are not dependent on an individual's state of health at any given time. Neither are these health-seeking behaviors and strategies totally dependent on a person's age or type of infirmity. It is unlikely that all the factors involved in understanding and enhancing health-seeking behaviors can be learned at an undergraduate level. Neither the scope and depth of knowledge nor the emotional and developmental maturity of the typical undergraduate student make that realistic. But the debate continues because we have not defined and structured the body of knowledge and therefore cannot place the knowledge at appropriate undergraduate and graduate levels. Nor do we have clearly delineated practice roles for nurses with different levels of knowledge. Schlotfeld[20] writes:

There can be no question that a crucial ingredient for preparing professionals is identification of a body of knowledge that is fundamental to professional practice and about

which there is agreement by a cadre of qualified professionals. However, as yet there is no consensus among qualified professionals in nursing concerning the *subject matter* that should represent the intellectual armamentarium of professionals called nurses.

If the issue of generalist knowledge were settled, Schlotfeldt believes, it would be possible to identify specialist knowledge. She notes, however, that there is little agreement about nursing specialties, the preparation necessary for each specialty, or the knowledge and skills expected of such specialists.

Schlotfeldt[20] begins by defining nursing's social mission and on that basis develops a plan for identifying generalist and specialist knowledge. She suggests that nursing should claim its long heritage and declare that nursing provides a professional service from which all members of society can benefit when they are well as well as when they are ill.

Diers[7] approaches the task differently:

The problems that patients present define the knowledge base. Labeling specialties by patient problem, . . . is as good a way as any other of defining knowledge. Patients present differently according to disease or dysfunction, . . . by setting, . . . by organ system. . . . For the present, the narrowness of specialty does not matter. . . . The fact that nursing is creating specialty definitions that seem now to be at different levels of abstraction or to come from different concepts reflects, more than anything else, the evolution of knowledge. What is important . . . is only that such specialties *are* being created and labeled, for nursing increasingly is specialist practice.

One crucial distinction between the approach of Diers and that of Schlotfeldt is the conceptualization of the person as client. Diers[7] defines the knowledge base in relation to patients, thus implying that they are already "in" the health care system. Schlotfeldt[20] defines the recipient of nursing as all human beings (including patients), thus leaving open the question of how nurses create contact with the specific persons to be served.

There is, however, much similarity in their views of the professional practitioner. Their writings, in fact, do not represent different positions in the generalization versus specialization debate. They reflect, rather, different views or aspects of nursing's social mission, and they therefore present different conceptualizations of the body of knowledge required to support nursing practice. How did nursing arrive at such divergent views?

THE EMERGENCE OF NURSING TODAY

Two forces have created the interplay of ideas that define nursing in the 1980s. The first is the role of nursing in the system of health care, primarily in hospitals, in which nursing is both a provider of its own professional service and a facilitator for the provision of other professional services, primarily medical. The advent of nurse-practitioners has blurred the boundaries further, because the services they perform are sometimes a substitute for medical services. The second force is the process by which nursing has developed an educational system that prepares nurses for the world of work.

The emergence of clinical specialization occurred because nurses needed and wanted to know more about how to take care of people in many different kinds of health situations, most of which they encountered in hospitals organized to support medical practice. The advances in medical technology have had a profound influence on this escalating demand for nursing knowledge in clinical practice. Several authors have reviewed the emergence of this emphasis on clinical knowledge, which has increased from the early 1940s to the present.[5,16,18] Over the same period of time, a significant shift in focus in graduate programs occurred to match the clinical focus that was advocated by nurse leaders. The emphasis in the 1940s on the functional roles of teacher, administrator, researcher, or consultant was gradually replaced by an almost universal focus on the expert nurse clinician with a specialized body of knowledge and practice.[4,16] The focus on nursing content shifted correspondingly from knowledge of teaching, supervision, administration, and consultation to consistent efforts to define and structure nursing's body of clinical knowledge.[12,16,19]

One of the significant debates that emerged out of this shift to a clinical focus is the issue of clinical specialization or generalization. In exploring the evolution of this issue, Reed and Hoffman[18] note the shift to clinical nursing but also point out that this shift was not accompanied by any agreement about the meaning of the terms *specialization* or *generalization* or the nursing content specific to either focus.[1,5,6,13]

More recently Starck[24] and Williamson[25,26] have described the diversity of master's programs and outlined the impact of that diversity on the opportunities in the marketplace for nurses with master's degrees. Starck[24] noted that the 1986 National League for Nursing Directory of Graduate Nursing Programs[14] listed 143 programs offering 257 different titles of programs; 20 different titles were used to describe programs related to the care of children alone. Also 21 titles were used to describe curricula in nursing administration. Stark[24] noted that in none of the titles is there evidence of consensus about the body of knowledge related to the title of a program. Williamson[26] further called attention to the importance of choosing names for program titles that would given an accurate indication of the program's curriculum.

Similar confusion exists in relation to the problem of certifying competency in a particular specialty. Efforts to test nurses in specialty areas for the purpose of granting credentials have resulted in some identification of knowledge relevant for different areas of specialization. However, a major difficulty is the number of clinical specialty titles, many of which overlap, and the lack of clear definitions of specialized content relating to those titles. The American Nurses' Association (ANA) certification plan[3] currently lists 17 different categories for clinical certification and an additional 2 for nursing administration. (At least 10 other organizations also certify specialty status.[2]) To complicate matters further, two levels of certification exist for some categories in the ANA plan; only one level requires graduate preparation.[3]

During the same time that the pendulum was swinging toward a clinical focus, issues were being raised about roles in nursing administration and the preparation available for these roles.[15] Originally the need for advanced knowledge in education and administration led to the first graduate courses in nursing.[15] But as the emphasis on clinical practice increased, not enough nurse leaders were prepared for the administrative roles. These roles were vital for creating the systems in institutions that support the delivery of expert clinical nursing services and the delivery of medical services. Blair[1] outlined the situation: "As the emphasis on clinical nursing increased, the emphasis on administration in nursing decreased. Concern and research related to the setting, systems, outcomes, costs and resources needed for the delivery of nursing care became devalued."

Research has clarified the role of the nurse executive[1,10,15,17] as a person functioning at the executive level of an organization, managing 10- to 15-million-dollar budgets in major teaching hospitals, and developing effective systems for delivery of care. Similarly, the head nurse in the role of midlevel manager is emerging as the key to facilitating the system of care.[5,9] Clearly, nursing education must respond to the need for expert managerial knowledge as well as clinical knowledge. But what is the appropriate response? The clinical specialization versus generalization issue relates to both the clinical specialist role and head nurse or midlevel manager role in institutional settings and also to roles of nurse-practitioners and community health nurses in ambulatory and community settings.

The generalist-specialist issue raises multiple questions. What are the outcomes of nursing care? What knowledge is required to achieve those outcomes in a variety of health care settings? Is clinical knowledge by itself enough? Is managerial knowledge enough? Does nursing benefit only those who are ill, or does it benefit everyone, including those who are ill? Is the goal to attain, maintain, or regain health or to diagnose and treat the disease?

The value to our society of having a healthy population cannot be overestimated. An empowered society whose members are able to take responsibility for their own lives and health is a goal we must begin to explore, given the exploding cost of medical care in this country. What we are currently achieving with our resources focused on illness is not enough. Furthermore, the changing political and health care systems have placed limitations on those resources. In some cases new modes of care are being created, such as home care. In others, increasing numbers of people are becoming disenfranchised by the exploding costs of medical care and medical insurance. Nursing must position itself to discover new answers.

The conceptualization of nursing proposed by Schlotfeldt[20] is based on a philosophical orientation that recognizes and respects the inherent capabilities of human beings, who are by nature health seeking. She identifies the intellectual work to be done based on this orientation.

A major task for nursing's scholars is to identify and classify the human health assets (health-seeking mechanisms and behaviors) with which people typically are naturally endowed and subsequently acquire, and that provide focus for nurses' work. A second, major task for nursing scholars is to identify and structure the system of knowledge that is fundamental to general and specialized nursing practice. . . .

Resolution of issues concerning nursing's specialties could be a simple matter once agreement is reached concerning the professional's body of basic knowledge. Based upon the assumption that newly developed specialties are legitimate when specialists must have command of knowledge and skills that surpass those had by generalists, two criteria are proposed: 1) each specialty must be demonstrated to require mastery of knowledge that is more extensive and more narrowly focused than is general nursing knowledge and require skills that are more complex; and 2) each specialty must be demonstrated to require mastery of knowledge and skills that are different from those required for all other nursing specialties.

SOME HOPEFUL PREDICTIONS FOR THE FUTURE

Nursing's leadership for the future will be provided by those with graduate preparation and advanced knowledge in the discipline of nursing.[11] A significant part of that leadership will come from scholarly nurse-practitioners who are expert in areas of generalized and specialized nursing practice, and some of those expert practitioners will be doctorally prepared for autonomous nursing practice.[21] Their expertise will be based on clinical knowledge and judgment that assesses the needs of persons and the interventions that lead predictably to desired outcomes, along with the cost-effective utilization of resources and design of care systems that ensure accountability for professional services. Professional nursing services available in society will be for those who are well and those who are ill and will focus on enhancing the health-seeking assets of everyone and on teaching people to protect their own health status and quality of life.

Nursing knowledge will be structured, and consensus will be achieved while knowledge continues to evolve through scholarly inquiry.[22] Knowledge for clinical practice will be both generalized and specialized and will be reflected in graduate curricula, about which there will be consensus across similar programs with similar titles. Areas of generalized knowledge will also be structured and agreed on and will transcend different specialty programs as appropriate to each specialty focus. Clinical research will provide a basis for guiding practice in areas of both generalized and specialized knowledge.

Faculty who teach clinical nursing will be educated at the doctoral level. They will be expert in nursing knowledge and practice in their area of specialization and will engage in clinical practice and research relevant to their areas of specialized knowledge.

Head nurses and midlevel managers will have master's degrees based on specialized clinical knowledge coinciding with their areas of work and also knowledge in the management of clinical nursing and systems of care. The clinical knowledge will form the basis for managing clinical care, the management knowledge for managing staff and resources to provide clinical care.

Nurse executives in major institutions will have doctoral degrees and will function with generalized nursing knowledge and specialized management knowledge. They will build on a base of specialized nursing knowledge and practice from their master's preparation; that is, they will be expert in some aspect of specialized nursing knowledge and practice before becoming nurse executives.

New models for education and practice will prepare nurses for roles as scholarly nurse-practitioners and will provide social and institutional support for autonomous professional nursing practice.[21] Nursing will be recognized by society as playing a major role in meeting the health needs of a diverse population and as doing so within reasonable boundaries, given the financial resources of the society.[8,23]

REFERENCES

1. Blair EM: Needed: nursing administration leaders, Nurs Outlook 24:550, 1976.
2. Bulechek GM and Maas ML: Nursing certification: a matter for the professional organization. In McCloskey JC and Grace HK editor: Current issues in nursing, ed 2, Boston, 1985, Blackwell Scientific Publications, Inc.
3. The career credential: professional certification, St. Louis, 1988, American Nurses' Association.
4. Characteristics of master's education in nursing, Pub No 15-1759, New York, 1987, National League for Nursing.
5. Chickadonz GH and Perry AM: Clinical specialization versus generalization: perspectives for the future. In McCloskey JC and Grace HK, editor: Current issues in nursing, ed 2, Boston, 1985, Blackwell Scientific Publication, Inc.
6. Defining clinical content, graduate nursing programs. Four monographs: Community health nursing, Maternal child health nursing, Medical-surgical nursing, and Psychiatric nursing. Boulder, Colo, 1967, Western Interstate Commission for Higher Education.
7. Diers D: Preparation of practitioners, clinical specialists and clinicians, J Prof Nurs 1(1):41, 1985.
8. Donley R: Nursing: 2000, an essay, Image 16(1):4, 1984.
9. Fralic MF: Developing the head nurse role: a key to survival. In Chaska N, editor: The nursing profession: a time to speak, New York, 1983, McGraw-Hill.
10. Goodrich NM: A profile of the competent nursing administrator, Ann Arbor, Mich, 1982, UMI Research Press.
11. Hart SE, editor: Introduction. In Issues in graduate nursing education, New York, 1987, National League for Nursing.
12. Kohnke MF: Curriculum design for the master's candidate in nursing. In The case for consultation in nursing: designs for professional practice, New York, 1978, Wiley Publications.
13. McLane AM: Core competencies of masters-prepared nurses, Nurs Res 27:48, 1978.
14. Master's education in nursing: route to opportunities in contemporary nursing, New York, 1986-1987, National League for Nursing.
15. Molen MT, Blyth JJ, and McCloskey JC: The preparation of nurse administrators. In McCloskey JC and Grace HK, editor: Current issues in nursing, ed 2, Boston, 1985, Blackwell Scientific Publications, Inc.
16. Nahm H: Graduate education of the nurse. In Abdellah FG and others, editors: New directions in patient-centered nursing: guidelines for systems of service, education and research, New York, 1973, Macmillan Co.
17. Poulin MA: Study of the structure and functions of the position of nursing service administrator, doctoral dissertation, New York, 1972, Columbia University.
18. Reed SB and Hoffman SE: The enigma of graduate nursing education: advanced generalist? specialist? Nurs Health Care 7(1):43, 1986.
19. Rogers ME: Emerging patterns in nursing education. In Williamson J, editor: Current perspectives in nursing education: the changing scene, St. Louis, 1978, The CV Mosby Co.
20. Schlotfeldt RM: Resolution of issues: an imperative for creating nursing's future, J Prof Nurs 3(3):136, 1987.
21. Schlotfeldt RM: The scholarly nursing practitioner. In Lindeman CA, editor: Alternate conceptions of work and society: implications for professional nursing, Washington, DC, 1988, American Association of Colleges of Nursing.
22. Schlotfeldt RM: Structuring nursing knowledge: a priority for creating nursing's future, Nurs Sci Quarterly 1(1):35, 1988.
23. Slavinsky AT: Psychiatric nursing in the year 2000: from a nonsystem of caring to a caring system, Image 16(1):17, 1984.
24. Stark PL: The master's prepared nurse in the marketplace: what should they do? In Hart SE, editor: Issues in graduate nursing education, Pub No 18-2196, New York, 1987, National League for Nursing.
25. Williamson JA: Crisis in academic nursing. In Chaska NL, editor: The nursing profession: a time to speak, New York, 1983, McGraw-Hill.
26. Williamson JA: Masters education: a need for nomenclature, Image 16:99, 1983.

CHAPTER 6

Theoretical underpinnings of community-based primary care in developing countries

ROSALIE A.E. THOMPSON

At a recent annual meeting and scientific session of the American Academy of Nursing, Dr. Rhetaugh Dumas observed:

In the light of the changing world around us, it is imperative that in this last decade of the century we continue to raise fundamental questions about the nature of nursing and nursing education.

Sociopolitical, economic, and environmental changes must influence our thinking and planning in nursing education. We have many options open to us, but we need to make the right choices now for the profession to continue to have relevance in the future and to be effective in meeting the health challenges of the new economic era.

I have chosen to approach the subject primarily from the perspective of my own country, South Africa, and to focus on the challenges of community-based primary care for the nurse and for nursing education in a developing country.

South Africa is both a developing and a developed country; it reflects in microcosm the challenges that face the countries of the First World and Third World. Before discussing the fundamental issues for nurses providing effective community-based primary care in a developing country, and some of the implications of these for nursing education, this chapter will address the concept of community-based primary care and its challenges in a developing country.

DEFINITION OF COMMUNITY-BASED PRIMARY CARE

The term *community-based primary care* is relatively new in the nursing literature. Community care has, in nursing, generally been seen as an alternative to hospital care. This is unfortunate because hospitals are themselves communities (in fact a community within a community) serving a particular group of people. Hospital staff who send patients home without adequate preparation seem in so doing to assume that the community is a functioning social unit outside the hospital that can be depended on to provide the continuing care needed by a recovering patient.[5] This is certainly not so, as O'Neill suggests: "The greatest self-inflicted loss of all is the loss of a caring community, the loss of the once widely held belief that looking after yourself and your own was the first role of the individual, the family and the community."[10]

What, in fact, do we mean by community? Definitions are varied; some imply homogeneity, others heterogeneity, as the following examples illustrate.

Communities are characterized by people's engagement in activities that demand interrelationship of efforts, they give rise to shared culture, and they are often sited in a particular geographic locale. Community is then an aspect of the way men relate to one another . . . which goes far and beyond the coerced and the necessary.[9]

The term [community] should not refer to a cohesive, homeostatic association of people but to a stratified arrangement of groups, interests and resources, some of them having more power and status than others. Considerable competition and even conflict is likely to be present in any given community and some change in the internal structure of communities may occur over time.[22]

The community is a social space in which the concept of meeting the needs of this group and its internal power will be incorporated for making decisions regarding the solution of its problem.[11]

These definitions illustrate different ways to understand the term *community*. Now consider what is meant by primary health care.

Although as a branch of health care it has been relatively neglected for generations, primary health care is the oldest form of care. As long as nursing has existed there has been a health practitioner acting as first contact for care. Irrespective of the term used to describe this form of practice, it is an essential level of care in every health care system.

A milestone in the rebirth of interest in primary health care was the 1978 International Conference on Primary Health Care held in Alma-Ata (USSR), which defined primary health care as

. . . essential health care based on practical, scientifically sound and socially acceptable methods and technology made universally accessible to individuals and families in the community through their full participation and at a cost that the community and country can afford to maintain at every stage of their development in the spirit of self-reliance and self-determination. It forms an integral part of the country's health system, of which it is the central function and main focus, and of the overall social and economic development of the community. It is the first level of contact of individuals, the family and community with the national health system bringing health care as close as possible to where people live and work, and constitutes the first element of a continuing health care process.[20]

Community-based primary care is, then, the practice of primary care within a defined population using programs based on epidemiological analyses that address the major health needs of the community, plan services, and evaluate the effects of care. It is important that the needs of all those in the defined population are assessed, not only the needs of those who come to the service. These programs may include the promotion of health, the prevention of disease, curative and rehabilitative care for individual patients and families, as well as a special focus on the community and its subgroups. At all levels, the participation of the community is essential. Primary health care should be not only geographically and financially accessible to the patient population, but also culturally accessible—a consideration all too frequently overlooked.

Once information on the precise health status of the community is available, the practice can decide which problems—for example, hypertension, motor vehicle accidents, the need for immunization, teenage pregnancy—are the most common. On the basis of this information, decisions can be made that will affect the health education and disease prevention activities of the practice as a whole as well as those of the clinician (whether doctor or nurse) in the examination room.

Community-based primary care may be found in a variety of settings in the public sector, but it can also be found in the private sector. A team approach to meeting the health needs of the specific community is essential. Even though the level of training of the professional members of the team will vary in different community contexts, the basic premise of community-based primary care remains the same.

Nurses have been practicing a form of community-based primary care for decades as community or district nurses, but without the scientific framework provided by epidemiology, notably in relation to the identification of community health problems and in the monitoring of program outcomes. At best, nurses have been dependent on the extrapolation from secondary data sources where these exist.

Individual, family, and community health care are closely interrelated but require different, although parallel, strategies in addressing the needs of each. In the past they have been unnecessarily separate, which may not have been a deliberate policy, but this separation cannot be maintained now. The health needs of all peoples require otherwise.

Having discussed what is meant by *community* and *primary health care,* it is useful to consider the concept of development. "Development is one of the most compelling concepts of our time. It provokes painful questions about values, techniques, and choices."[4] The term *development* is frequently used with reference to Third World countries; however it should also be seen as a process in industrialized nations. Industrial nations fall far short of realizing their human potential.

Additionally they are part of the reason why the third world finds development so difficult. . . . relations with the third world cannot be improved simply by exporting technology and increasing trade. Development means increasing the capacity of people to influence their future. . . . It means that projects and programmes not only need to accomplish physical and concrete changes, but to do so in such a way that people have a greater capacity to choose and to respond to these changes. It means that planned change has to be concerned with the potential of individuals and with the inviolability of their persons.[4]

HEALTH CARE IN SOUTH AFRICA

Like many countries, South Africa is developing in the First World as well as in the Third World sense. The unique needs and challenges of such a country need to be addressed. In order to do so, the major characteristics of a developing country require some consideration.

South Africa is a young country of 27.7 million

people.* Settlers from western Europe first arrived in 1652. It is a country of great diversity geographically, climatically, culturally, economically, and sociopolitically. Approximately one quarter of the population enjoys a First World lifestyle, and the lifestyle of the remaining three quarters is that of the Third World. The profile of disease and mortality is directly related to the distinctive socioeconomic stratification; there are diseases of affluence and diseases of poverty. With increasing wealth and urbanization, diseases of poverty are exchanged for those of affluence. South Africa is not a poor country and has a relatively high gross national product (GNP), but for all its economic potential, the life expectancy of its people is typical of that of a developing country.[7]

The age distribution in South Africa shows the characteristics of a developing country, with a large percentage of the population under 14 years of age (almost 40% among the Black, Asian, and Colored population), and also the characteristics of a developed country, with 4.1% of the people older than 65 years. A high birth rate and a predominantly young population will remain the norm for decades to come and will impose great and growing demands on the provision of health care services and indeed affect all aspects of development.[6] Population projections for 1980 to 2000 predict a 35% increase for Whites but a 73% increase for Blacks. The geographical distribution of the population is wide. In 1980 approximately 47% of the population lived in rural areas,[12] but a dramatic shift in this distribution among Blacks is taking place. In the year 2000 between 75% and 79% of the Blacks are expected to be living in urban areas.[3]

This trend towards urbanization has important implications for the demand for, and the provision of Health Services. Urban communities are more easily brought within reach of organised health services. Remote rural populations however, present significant problems as adequate health care is hampered by natural barriers, poor roads, inadequate transport services and, as populations are often sparse, the doctor/population ratio is not economically viable.

The effect of this on the practice of nurses in particular, as well as on other health care professionals, is significant.[17]

The stress produced by massive urbanization and rapid cultural change is of particular significance. The adjustment required in one generation to move from a rural and often traditional tribal setting to the mushrooming "cities within cities" is phenomenal. Most deaths among young adults are from nonnatural causes: motor vehicle accidents (in all population groups) and homicides (among Black and Colored adults).[3] The psychosocial stress associated with change and urbanization and the need for an understanding of culturally conditioned psychiatric illness present major challenges to the mental-health practitioner and the community at large. Information about the mental health of the population is grossly lacking—a not uncommon situation in a developing country.

Although South Africa currently spends 5.9% of the gross national product on health (the World Health Organization [WHO] recommends at least 5%), expenditures among geographic, social, and economic groups and between preventive and curative services vary widely.[3] The major portion is spent on curative services in urban areas, but it is estimated that only 4.5% to 4.7% is spent on preventive and health-promotion services.[7] Information on private and public expenditures on health is lacking, but it is estimated that approximately one half of the total health expenditure is from the private sector. The move toward privatization to alleviate the problems of financing health care may produce more problems than solutions.

Nurses form the largest health care profession (47%) in South Africa,† and their geographic distribution is also far more favorable than that of any other category of health care professionals. There is currently (1985) one registered nurse for every 435 people.[17] The WHO considers a nurse to population ratio of 1:500 necessary to deliver basic comprehensive health care in a Third World country. Although the ratio of practicing nurses to population is not quite as good, there is nonetheless a very high percentage of nurses who are practicing. When the ratio for racial categories is considered, the situation is not as good. There is currently (1985) one registered Black nurse per 721 Black people, so the number of Black nurses admitted to the profession needs to increase markedly if the WHO ratio (1:500) is to be attained by the year 2000.

The ratio of medical practitioners and interns to total population was 1:1490 in 1983.[17] Of these approximately 78% (in 1980) resided in urban areas;

---

*Including the National States but not the Independent States. The population of the latter is estimated at 5.5 million.

†In 1987 there were 65,000 registered nurses in South Africa.

25% (1983) were specialists and thus not involved in primary care. The 1983 ratio of nonspecialist medical practitioners to population in urban areas of the provinces was 1:900, as compared to 1:4100 in the rural areas of the provinces.[23] However, in the self-governing (national) states, the ratios are 1:9784 and 1:22,360, respectively.[2]

THE FUTURE OF PRIMARY CARE IN DEVELOPING COUNTRIES

Because nurses, of all the health professionals, are closest to people and closest to the largest number of people, they hold "the key to an acceptance and expansion of primary health care" and, I believe, to community-based primary care as well.[8]

The focus of nursing must change from the sickness model to a health model. At present most nurse education programs are firmly tied to the perspectives of curative medicine and are connected to hospitals. The traditional assumption of the hospital as the appropriate place for preparation for a career in nursing indicates a "sickness concept of nursing." Concern about this concept was reported by Smith in 1979 when he wrote "the acute hospital-medical-surgical model of care which presently dominates basic programmes will be a totally inappropriate model for future nursing practitioners."[16] Ten years later, I believe this model of care is indeed inappropriate.

Many education programs will require reorientation if nurses are to develop the skills for planning and providing the kind of nursing that is necessary for meeting current and future health needs.[14] The nurse of the future must be more than a hospital nurse. We will always need nurses to give direct care to the sick in institutional settings, but we must redress the balance in orientation and not allow the sickness concept to dominate our entire view of what nursing is about.

In looking at the education of the professional nurse, it seems to me that to contemplate improvements in curriculum design is to contemplate only the lesser problem. My concern is much more with the nature of the academic and clinical experience, its meaning, and its value for the students attempting to develop their potential as human beings and as professional persons. We need to develop concepts of education so that students can gain carefully timed and graduated experience in exploring and exercizing their own humanness in the series of human encounters that constitutes their professional program. I believe the education of a nurse should shift toward a person- and health-centered approach. This shift requires an emphasis on individual, family, and community health.

Because the family unit is a microcosm of society, it reflects the needs of society at large. The family is the primary social unit and therefore the basic unit for determining health progress. Social values, health behaviors, and health perceptions are family oriented and transmitted, and therefore any significant change in individual and group or community behavior must also have a family orientation. The family, as the nuclear unit in society, should be a key area of experience for young nurses at the beginning and throughout their programs. Because the hospital has been the pivotal unit for nursing activity, everything else has been seen as peripheral. If the home (family) is presented as the pivotal unit, then the hospital will be seen as a means of returning the person to that unit rather than as an end in itself.

If nursing is to meet today's and tomorrow's health needs, students must, from the outset, be in close and committed contact with people in their everyday world. Family attachments[14] provide opportunities for learning what is really important to people. Students come to see the health needs of the family and the health care services provided through the eyes of the public, not only through those of the professional. When this happens, students see from the beginning the importance of the public's perspective on health care and specifically nursing care. Family attachments emphasize the broader issues of health and its maintenance and the importance of understanding how health needs are met in the community and as part of everyday life. These attachments also provide excellent opportunities to work with and to learn from the community—to form an active partnership and to appreciate the impact of culture on lifestyle and health behavior. All these are essential prerequisites for an effective professional practice and, specifically, a community-based practice. I believe that professional attitudes (rather than knowledge and skills per se) are the key to bringing about the necessary changes in the provision of health care. I also believe that the content and bias of basic education are major determinants of professional attitudes. For this reason I have focused considerable attention on some key aspects of nursing education.

Before the practice of nursing can realize its potential contribution to community health, not only in the provision of effective care but also in the deeper understanding of health and the etiology of disease, basic changes in family and community nursing practice must be subjected to rigorous scientific research. Long-held assumptions need to be challenged, hypotheses tested, and new methods developed.[13]

Within the total philosophy of community care, a satisfactory community-based primary care team will have to be organized to meet each country's unique needs—a health team that responds and is responsible to the local community, serves its needs, and actively promotes good health. "Resources can then be channelled towards preventing illness in the first place and to managing rather than trying to cure some of the new diseases."[13]

In preparing for a community-based primary care practice in a developing country, the professional nurse needs a balanced basic education as a generalist nurse. In South Africa all professional nurses are trained* to practice within four spheres: general, community, and psychiatric nursing, and midwifery—in order to provide a comprehensive, community-based health service.

Today's health problems require a nursing service that will work to:

1. Change public and corporate policies to make them conducive to health. A question that needs to be addressed is "How can nursing contribute to the development of a nation's health care strategy?" Events can be influenced by those who understand not only the factors that bear directly on health and illness, but also the social and political context in which they occur. "The pressure is on for a shift by nurses from their traditional roles to the assumption of greater responsibility in a much wider arena."[21] "Nurses should be able to use effective strategies . . . to present their particular point of view. Techniques such as networking, creating alliances, negotiation and management of conflict and confrontation should become part of the armoury of every nurse in a leadership position."[21]

2. Reorient service and education to the maintenance and promotion of health in the population and ensure that the necessary range of services is provided in the context of community needs.

This will require nurses who are innovative and competent and able to participate meaningfully in the planning and evaluation of health programs, to initiate services where necessary, and to be leaders and managers of primary health care teams.[19] "Nurses will need to participate more actively in interprofessional and intersectoral teams for health development."[8]

In terms of priorities, a society may value the care of sickness over the promotion of health. Indeed in many countries the pinnacle of civilization is the local hospital. No doubt much of the blame can be laid at the door of health care professionals, because they usually wait for people to be sick before offering help. A shift in the attitudes of the public as well as in those of the health professionals will need to be encouraged, and this includes the need to change perceptions of the role of the nurse.

Nurses will need to act as agents for change—as motivators, negotiators, facilitators, teachers, and communicators in the field of health. These skills are generally underestimated and underdeveloped in most spheres of nursing. To do this nurses themselves need to be healthy role models. "It's not enough to teach and encourage people how to be healthy, they must want to be healthy."[15]

The role of the nurse will change as more nurses move from the hospital into the community. In some countries it may be necessary to change the regulatory mechanisms governing the scope of nursing practice and nursing education in order to ensure an optimal community-based primary care nursing service.

3. Monitor and assess demographic, political, technological, cultural, ethical, and economic trends. All these affect the health needs and health status of the community. In addition, the availability of adequate health-status data is essential. At all levels of the health care service, computer assistance is necessary.

4. Enable and encourage individuals and groups to be their own advocates in health issues and to be involved in the maintenance and protection of their own health and in their community's development. Nurses have unique opportunities to provide health education, to promote healthy living, and to organize groups of patients to help each other (the self-care and self-help concept).

---

*Professional nurses follow a 4-year program, receiving either a bachelor's degree or a diploma offered at a nursing college in association with a university department of nursing.

Yet few perceive these opportunities and take up the challenge.

5. Recognize the importance of social forces and social relationships as determinants of values and behavior relevant to health and as significant resources for coping with stress and maintaining health.[13] Unless the social nature of health and illness is understood, nurses will not be able to function competently. Ensuring an environment that is socially and emotionally appropriate for each community is the key in the maintenance of health.

6. Recognize the safe traditional beliefs and practices relating to health and sickness. This is of particular importance in a multicultural society such as South Africa.

7. Use the mass media and other new information technologies to increase knowledge and to disseminate information relating to the improvement of health.

The challenge is to provide a true health service—a wellness service—to enable and to empower people to care for their own health. But in this challenge nurses have identified a dilemma that has been well described by Nita Barrow. She poses the following questions:[1]

1. Can nurses admit that persons or communities can be involved in their own health care and perform measures independently of nurses without considering those persons or communities threats to their professional standing?

2. Can knowledge be passed on to enable others to perform such tasks without this being seen as weakening the nurse's status?

3. How best can nursing continue to grow as a caring, sharing profession, concerned with people and their needs, and at the same time realize that this growth will actually be promoted by giving away some of the knowledge, skills, and prerogatives of the profession to people with little training and also to the wider community itself?

Perhaps this last is the essential question for nurses to answer.

REFERENCES

1. Barrow N: Nursing: the art, science and vocation in evolution, Contact 59:142, 1980.

2. Botha JL, Bradshaw D, and Gowan R: How many doctors are needed in South Africa by 1990? S Afr Med J 69:252, 1986.

3. Bradshaw D, Yach D, and Fellingham S, editors: Community based essential health care services in Southern Africa, Parow, 1988, Medical Research Council.

4. Bryant C and White LG: Managing development in the third world, Boulder, Colo., 1982, Westview Press.

5. Clark J and Henderson J, editors: Community health, London, 1983, Churchill Livingstone.

6. Department of National Health and Population Development: The 1985 census, Epidemiological Comments 14(1):12, 1987.

7. Klopper J: The role of community health in South Africa, Cape Town University, 1986.

8. Mahler H: Nurses lead the way, Geneva: WHO Features, No 97, June 1985.

9. Minar DW and Greer S: The concept of community. In Clark J and Henderson J, editors: Community health, London, 1983, Churchill Livingstone.

10. O'Neill P: Health crises 2000. London, 1983, Heinemann.

11. Ordonez C: quoted in WHO Study Group Community-based education of health personnel, Geneva, 1987, WHO.

12. Report of the Science Committee of the President's Council: Demographic trends in South Africa, Cape Town, 1983, Government Printer.

13. Skeet M: Unpublished, 1988.

14. Skeet M. Thompson R. Creative Nursing. Processive care and more? J Adv Nurs 10:15-24, 1985. World Health Organization: WHO. A guide to curriculum review for basic nursing education. Orientation to primary health care and community health. Geneva: WHO, 1985. United Kingdom Central Council for Nursing, Midwifery and Health Visiting. Project 2000. London: UKCC, 1986.

15. Smith J: Janforum. The relationship between rights and responsibilities in health care: a dilemma for nurses, J Adv Nurs 8(5):438, 1983.

16. Smith J: Editorial, J Adv Nurs 4:589, 1979.

17. Thompson R: The development of nursing in South Africa. In White R, editor: Nursing politics past, present and future. London, 1988, Wiley.

18. Thompson R: Today's nursing for tomorrow's health, Curationis 9(4):1, 1986.

19. United Kingdom Central Council for Nursing Midwifery and Health Visiting: Project 2000, London, 1986, UKCC.

20. World Health Organization: Alma-Ata 1978. Primary health care. Report of International Conference on Primary Health Care, Alma-Ata USSR, September 6-12, 1978, Geneva, 1978, WHO.

21. World Health Organization: Leadership in nursing for health for all: a challenge and strategy for action, Geneva, 1987, WHO.

22. World Health Organization: Regional office for South East Asia. Team work for primary health care: report of WHO expert group. New Delhi, 1981. In WHO Study Group: Community-based education of health personnel, Tech Rep Ser 746, Geneva, 1987, WHO.

23. Zwarenstein M: Estimating the distribution of health care services in South Africa, master's thesis, London, 1987, London School of Tropical Health and Hygiene.

PART TWO

NURSING KNOWLEDGE

Defining and refining nursing knowledge

JOANNE COMI McCLOSKEY
HELEN KENNEDY GRACE

Any discussion of nursing soon leads to a discussion of what knowledge is unique to nursing. Nursing has long been criticized for not having a unique, defined body of knowledge. In recent decades nursing has made considerable strides to change this situation. More nurses are doing nursing research, producing nursing knowledge, and using this knowledge in practice. Yet as the numbers of nursing researchers increase and the volume of nursing research grows, troublesome issues develop. One of these relates to the use of research in the practice setting.

Is nursing research used in practice? This is the title of the debate chapter in Part Two, by Weiler and Buckwalter. Examining the pro arguments, they list three factors that have positively influenced the use of nursing research in practice: (1) changes in the conceptualization of nursing and the value of research, (2) advances in the preparation of nurses to use research, and (3) removal of barriers to research dissemination and use. Examining the con arguments, they list three factors as current barriers to research use: (1) values and qualifications of practicing nurses, (2) the process of implementation, and (3) institutional factors. The authors conclude the chapter with a discussion of strategies for increasing the use of nursing research in practice. The strategies are predicated on the notion of planned change and the asumption that the quantity and quality of nursing research will continue to grow.

The next three chapters outline strategies for the development of nursing knowledge. One strategy for assisting the science of nursing to grow is mentorship. In the first of the section's viewpoint chapters, Ardery takes a refreshing look at mentoring and proposes that it be used as a strategy for knowledge generation. She advocates a shift in the goals for mentoring relationships from career enhancement of individuals toward the development of the body of nursing knowledge.

Although nursing has promoted mentoring as a key to personal growth, Ardery points out that the concept has never been operationally defined and that much of the literature is based on unexamined assumptions. In a very interesting approach to the topic, she calls for a reformulation of the goals of mentoring and an examination of the content of the relationship. She proposes Daloz's constructs of support, challenge, and vision as the basis of future mentoring relationships. Mentoring relationships, she says, should be evaluated, not by the extent of career enhancement, but by the amount of knowledge generated.

Another strategy that will assist the science of nursing to grow is the proposed Nursing Minimum Data Set (NMDS). Werley, Devine, and Zorn outline the efforts toward and the purposes of establishing a uniform standard for the collection of comparable essential nursing data. The proposal is that all health care agencies collect and report key elements of nursing data about clients in a uniform way. The standardization of nursing data would allow research on multiple questions related to nursing care. The proposed data set has 16 elements including the four nursing elements of diagnosis, intervention, outcome, and intensity of nursing care. The authors discuss implementation of the data set in relation to four issues: documentation, computerization, cost, and acceptance. Although barriers to implementation exist, the NMDS rates as perhaps the most important development in nursing in the past decade. All nurses should be aware of the concept and work toward its implementation.

Computer use can be listed as yet another strategy in the defining and refining of nursing knowledge. In her chapter Chang explains the potentials and pitfalls of intelligent computers or expert systems. An expert system is a computer program that uses artificial intelligence technology to represent human knowledge, experience, and judgment. Potential uses include providing consultation, clarifying decision making, preserving and expanding knowledge, and unifying nursing language. Only recently have expert systems been used in nursing. Chang describes her work on one that will help nurses make nursing diagnoses in the self-care deficit area. One difficulty in developing expert systems in nursing is the lack of knowledge about the decision-making processes that nurses use. Although several hurdles need to be surmounted, the use of expert systems in nursing offers much potential for the development and testing of nursing knowledge.

As more nursing knowledge is accumulated, the question of how it should be classified arises. In a very thoughtful and comprehensive chapter, Loomis discusses the organization of nursing knowledge and the impact that category systems have on the science and practice of nursing. Loomis reviews many classification systems and demonstrates that there has been little similarity in approach. On the one point of agreement, the distinction between clinical and nonclinical research, Loomis takes issue. She presents her own recent work on knowledge classification. In her proposed model of nursing science she defines nursing as the science of health and healing. She subdivides nursing science into the study of clinical nursing therapeutics and the study of social issues in relation to nursing. Loomis says it is possible to develop one classification system that can be used to classify both nursing research and the practice of nursing.

In another chapter related to the difficult task of classification, Barnard discusses previous efforts to classify nursing research and then presents an overview of the work of Sigma Theta Tau (STT) in this area. As chairperson of STT's Research Committee, Barnard has headed the organization's effort to establish a classification system that could be used for a research depository. The plan for a depository was put on a back burner in order to develop the system of classification, which has been published in two editions entitled the *Directory of Nurse Researchers*. It is important to have a system to help organize the expanding body of research and to facilitate retrieval and sharing. Barnard's review of STT's system and many others including *Index Medicus* and the *Cumulative Index to Nursing and Allied Health Literature (CINAHL)* is very informative and gives an excellent picture of the challenges involved in such an endeavor.

However it is classified, current nursing knowledge is understood better when it is put in historical per-spective. In her chapter Church discusses the lessons that are learned from historical inquiry. Until recently nursing's history was undiscovered or ignored. Currently there is a resurgence of interest in nursing history, which Church says bodes well for the profession. The truths about nursing's past should serve to define its future. Although "historical awareness should be viewed as a prerequisite to a professional mentality and identity," nurse historians must demonstrate the relevance of their efforts to nursing care today.

O'Heath, Swanson, and McCloskey return in the next chapter to the theme of research dissemination and use, which was begun in Chapter 7. A key mechanism in the dissemination of knowledge to the nursing community is publication of research findings in nursing journals. The 1970s and 1980s were years in which nursing journals proliferated, reflecting the rapid development of the knowledge base of nursing. In an effort to better understand this proliferation, the authors compare 60 nursing journals established before 1981 with 25 nursing journals established between 1981 and 1986. The more recently established journals share many characteristics with the older journals; they differ, however, in having smaller readerships, being more specialized, reporting more research, and taking less time to publish a manuscript once it is accepted. The authors report actual statistics of individual journals, because features vary a good deal from one journal to another. Readers who find this information helpful in learning about the journal publishing process in nursing will want to refer to previous work by some of the same authors. Dissemination of nursing knowledge through journal publication is an important link between knowledge generation and knowledge utilization. The debate chapter in Part 2 raised the question of whether nurses use research is their practice. How much responsibility should nursing journals assume to promote research use in practice?

In the last chapter, Nzimande gives us a concrete illustration of many of the issues raised by previous authors as she addresses knowledge development and education in the developing subdiscipline of nursing service administration in South Africa. Readers who are interested in international nursing, nursing service administration, and the process of knowledge development and use will find this chapter useful. In South Africa nurses have some very particular needs, such as the need to begin a nursing journal. Other needs, such as development and the sorting out of relationships with physicians, echo those in other countries, including the United States. Nzimande's chapter demonstrates that nurses worldwide are involved in the process of nursing knowledge development and dissemination.

The development of nursing knowledge occurs in the context of other professional developments. For example, the defining of nursing knowledge received a major boost with the formation of the National Center for Nursing Research in 1986 within the Institutes of Health. Hinshaw writes about this important development in Chapter 49. The center has improved nursing's image as a scientific profession, but some troublesome issues are beginning to emerge. For example, what type of nursing research can and will the center fund? How does funding of research affect the development of the knowledge base?

The last decade in nursing has been a time of rapid gains in the development of nursing knowledge. But another recent development in nursing is the widespread and severe nursing shortage. Lynaugh writes in Chapter 23 about how this shortage is different from previous shortages. Will the development of nursing knowledge be able to continue at its current pace as the profession now must pay more attention to problems of recruitment and retention? As the forces that shape nursing change, the defining and refining of nursing knowledge continues. The direction or pace may change somewhat, but the process will continue.

CHAPTER 7

Debate

Is nursing research used in practice?

KAY WEILER
KATHLEEN COEN BUCKWALTER

The use of nursing research in practice continues to be an issue of vital concern to the profession. Position papers and editorials have been written describing the importance of research to practice. However, the key concerns remain: Is nursing research being encouraged? Is it being professionally supported? Are we achieving improved patient care? The establishment of the National Center for Nursing Research (NCNR), the commitment of the American Nurses' Association (ANA), and the international vision of Sigma Theta Tau all demonstrate the profession's pledge to define areas of research and translate the findings into improved patient care. However, this collective effort does not assure us that we have significantly advanced the profession's application of research to practice, nor does it persuade us that yesterday's research findings are being implemented today.

Florence Nightingale set an early example in combining dedicated patient care with vigorous research. She used systematic documentation of her interventions in combination with precise morbidity and mortality statistics to guide her evaluation of nursing outcomes and her determination of nursing practice.[16,40,56] Unfortunately, the nursing profession did not continue this groundwork of documentation, classification, and verification. Nursing focused on other ways of learning (e.g., tradition, reference to authority, experience, trial and error). Meanwhile, other professions addressed questions that were considered appropriate topics of nursing research and inquiry.[14]

In the 1950s the first nursing journal dedicated to the promotion and dissemination of nursing research was founded. *Nursing Research* was established with two main purposes, "to give members of the nursing profession the benefits of new knowledge resulting from research and to keep them informed about research which is under way."[75] It is significant that until 1976 the journal could not claim that more than 50% of the yearly published research articles were applicable to clinical practice.[5,15]

The debate presented in this chapter concerns whether nursing research is used in practice. A basic premise of this debate is the need to mesh nursing research, teaching, and practice. All three require that the nursing profession be vigilant so that there is a "a periodic review of ground already covered; a recognition of current needs and gaps; and a clarification of emerging problems, possibilities, and challenges."[2]

This chapter is also based on the premise that it is appropriate and beneficial for nursing research to be used in nursing practice because nurses observe specific phenomena and provide care that is different from what other health care personnel observe and provide. Further, the authors believe that validated behaviors and interventions should be incorporated into nursing practice in order to provide patients with optimum care.

This chapter examines issues related to the transfer of knowledge generated by nursing research and addresses the question, "Are research findings influencing the quality of patient care?" The authors believe that this topic lends itself to discussion and debate but that resolution of the issue is perhaps premature and inappropriate. Rather than attempting to resolve the question, we focus on strategies for increasing the use of research in nursing practice.

In this chapter we also consider other questions

stimulated by this issue and urge the reader to examine these related questions as well:[47] "Who is responsible for the complex set of activities involved in using research in practice—the individual nurse, the organization, or both? What factors influence the use of research in practice? What constitutes successful utilization of research in practice? Does nursing research make a difference in practice, and if so, what difference does it make?"

NURSING RESEARCH IS USED IN PRACTICE

The three factors that have contributed to the use of nursing research in practice are (1) changes in the conceptualization of nursing and the value of research, (2) advances in the preparation of nurses to use research, and (3) removal of barriers to research dissemination and use.

Changes in the conceptualization of nursing and the value of research

Changes in the conceptualization of nursing and the importance of research to nursing practice have occurred in two predominant areas: (1) professional direction, support, and nurturance; and (2) the identification of theoretical frameworks and models on which to base scientific inquiry and methodology.

The ANA's professional commitment to the importance of nursing research has remained steadfast for more than 3 decades. However, the suggested application of research directives to patient care, nursing interventions, and general public health policy has changed with an expanded vision of the application of nursing research. For example, the 1962 ANA Blueprint for Research[2] suggested six major areas of nursing research. The document especially stressed the importance of comparing cost assessment for nursing interventions but did not emphasize clinical research.[88]

By 1985 the ANA Priorities for Nursing Research in the Twenty-first Century[22] had evolved to include research goals, strategies for goal attainment, and minimum criteria to be achieved by the 1990s:

- to ensure an increased supply of nurse-scientists by the year 2000
- to generate knowledge about the well-being and optimum functioning of human beings, the effective delivery of nursing services, excellence in nursing education, and the impact of the profession on health policy
- to develop environments that support nursing in-

quiry, including opportunities to initiate and implement nursing investigations and access to subjects, personnel, research facilities, and equipment
- to disseminate the results of nursing research to clinicians, the scientific community, the general public, and health policymakers and to increase use of the results

Thus the profession has strengthened its commitment to the strategies necessary for the development and dissemination of research findings and has expanded its efforts in the direction of national health care policy. Nursing has demonstrated that it is no longer willing to react and respond to enacted legislation; rather, nurses are interested in applying research to the formation of health care policy.

To be able to influence national health care policy, nursing must explain and demonstrate the applicability of nursing research to the proposed policy. Nursing must be able to (1) conceptualize the nursing research from macro- and microperspectives, (2) demonstrate a systematic assessment of major concerns and health care needs of society, (3) articulate the discipline's particular perspective on those concerns and needs, and (4) demonstrate contributions that can be made from research programs of nurse-scientists.[45,46]

As the professional honorary society, Sigma Theta Tau has taken a leadership role in supporting nursing research philosophically and financially. This organization has been outspoken in its belief that the scope of nursing research must not be limited to individual patients, client groups, or even national concerns but must have international implications.[21]

In tandem with professional commitments to research, nursing has also made advances in the development of theoretical bases for nursing practice. These frameworks have provided the foundation for research development and model testing. "Within the profession and from external sources, there are demands for nursing to demonstrate the scientific basis for its practice."[38]

Increasingly, nursing interventions and protocols are based on systematic data collection and analysis. Watson and colleagues assert that quality assurance research assists in the development of a research-based practice and leads to the utilization of research findings in nursing practice.[89] Although in its infancy, nursing diagnosis research is facilitating the establishment of a more scientific basis for practice and may contribute to the theory base in nursing as well.

The Western Interstate Commission for Higher Education in Nursing (WICHEN) conducted a nation-wide Delphi survey to determine in part whether research was being used in practice. In response to the question, "What items are the most important areas of research value for the profession?" three of the top four answers were related to the use of research and included:[65]

- determine means for greater use of research in practice
- determine effective means of communicating, evaluation, and implementing change in practice
- establish relationship between clinical nursing research and quality care

Projects that have been developed and funded recently deal explicitly with the translation of research findings into practice.[7,43,63] Perhaps the best example of this type of endeavor is the CURN project undertaken at the University of Michigan. The primary objective of this project was to develop and test a model to facilitate the use of scientific nursing knowledge in clinical practice settings.[72]

Barnard[6] further suggests that nurse researchers are now feeling more of a responsibility to go beyond the mere reporting of their findings. The research process can be viewed as extending through to the actual implementation phase.[58] The burden for implementation is no longer borne by the staff nurse alone. Nurse researchers are sharing the responsibility for transmitting their results into practice.

Advances in the preparation of nurses to use research

The National League for Nursing (NLN)[74] has taken the position that the preparation of nurses to conduct research generally belongs at the doctoral level. In 1987 the NLN[23] reported 45 nursing education programs that offered a doctoral program in nursing. The mission of these programs is to develop curricula with a strong emphasis on research to train nurse-scientists.[50]

To form the foundation for conducting research, students in baccalaureate programs should acquire an understanding of the research process and its contribution to nursing practice as well as the ability to evaluate research findings for applicability to nursing practice. Similarly, the ANA Resolution on Priorities in Nursing Research[1] stresses development of information relevant for the practice of nursing. The majority of baccalaureate nursing programs now include content related to nursing research in their curricula.[25,85] There is an increasing emphasis on acquiring

the skills to read research reports critically and to critique them. Teaching methods and tools have been developed recently to help students evaluate research results and apply research findings.[3] Nursing students are also being taught to use research findings as a basis for nursing interventions. Along with this curricular shift toward the understanding and use of research has been an increase in the number of research-based texts. This fact is significant because nursing education textbooks are still the primary source of knowledge for practice.

O'Connell[77] analyzed 145 studies published in *Nursing Research* in the 1970s. She found increases in the number of investigators, nonnurse investigators, authors with Ph.D.'s, collaborative research with nonnurses, and studies funded by federal research grants. She concluded that there had been an upgrading of the quality of research in the last half of the decade.

Brown, Tanner, and Padrick[12] identified the characteristics of nursing research in the 1980s and noted positive changes and trends in the past three decades. They reported that (1) the amount of nursing research has increased considerably; (2) the focus of the research has shifted to clinical problems, (3) the research has become more theoretically oriented, and (4) the research has become more methodologically sophisticated.

Jacox[50] has identified additional factors that point to the increasing competence of nurses to design, conduct, and use nursing research. These factors include: an increase in the expectation that nursing faculty members will conduct research and publish their findings, the number of nurse researchers in clinical agencies, the number of nurses belonging to the ANA Council of Nurse Researchers, the level of federal funding for nursing research and training, the number of research proposals submitted to the Division of Nursing and the NCNR, and the proportion of current nursing research that is related to clinical practice.

Removal of barriers to research dissemination and use

Horsley[72] has stated that research results are ready for dissemination and use when they (1) are consistent with prior research findings, (2) hold true when examined from different perspectives, (3) interpret only findings that meet significance and magnitude criteria, (4) interpret trends and hunches that need further testing, and (5) do not interpret unsupported or insignificant data unless evident in prior research.

Similarly, Haller, Reynold, and Horsley's criteria[41]

to determine whether research is ready for use in practice include (1) the need for replication to provide greater confidence in the reliability and validity of findings, which usually means more than one study in a research base; (2) examination of each study's scientific merit, especially validity, reliability, generality, and statistical significance; and (3) determination of any potential risks to patients.

Once these criteria have been met, the information must be transmitted to nurses who need it and can use it in their daily practice. This hurdle is not an easy one to overcome, but the recent development of nursing models for research utilization and the increased avenues for publication and dissemination of nursing research have helped to solve the problem.

Nursing models for research utilization

Several studies have tested the utilization of nursing research in practice. For example, the Regional Program for Nursing Research Development was designed to be a demonstration project to develop models to overcome barriers to research utilization.[60]

Nursing Child Assessment Satellite Training (NCAST), another utilization program, was actually a series of three training projects carried out over a 10-year period.[7] "All of these projects have emphasized translating and disseminating research findings for the practicing nurse,"[17] and activities were designed to increase nurses' awareness of new research and to persuade them that research was valuable for practice.

The Conduct and Utilization of Research in Nursing (CURN) project was undertaken at the University of Michigan.[72] The primary objective of the project was to develop and test a model to facilitate the use of scientific nursing knowledge in clinical practice settings. (This model is discussed in more detail later under strategies for increasing the use of research in practice.)

Brett[9] reported on a study of 14 nursing research findings and the extent to which nurses used them in practice. Nine of the findings were developed from the research literature, and five were gathered from the CURN Project.

Brett[9] found that "The majority of nurses were aware of the average innovation, were persuaded about it, and used the average innovation at least sometimes." It was reassuring to note that none of the innovations ranked in the "unaware" stage; however, only one innovation fell in the "always use" stage. Brett[9] expressed caution that the "diffusion of these selected research findings might provide optimism about the state of research dissemination and use, but few studies exist against which to compare these findings."

In Brett's study[9] there was a statistically significant relationship between a nurse's willingness to adopt a nursing innovation and hours per week the nurse devoted to reading professional literature (specifically *Nursing Research* and *RN*) and the nurse's attendance at a nursing research conference. This suggests that nursing journals convey information that is being integrated into clinical practice. However, it was frustrating to note that Brett found no statistically significant relationship between the adoption of nursing practice innovations and the years of education, type of education, number of degrees, or level of education of the nurses in her sample. Perhaps the effectiveness of our educational system in teaching the continued application of research to practice needs further examination.

Continuing education programs may be one effective alternative. There has been a dramatic increase in recent years in the number of research utilization projects developed by and for nurses to help bridge the gap between research and practice. One popular format for these projects has been a long-term (i.e., 2- or 3-year) continuing education model, featuring several 2- to 3-day conferences held within a discrete geographic region. These projects offer a combination of formal presentations of theories, models, and methods of research utilization along with expert consultation or guidance for participants, who are expected to apply the knowledge and skills acquired in a research utilization project in their home setting. Eligible participants include those nurses with master's or doctoral degrees who are in a position to implement research-based change in practice and management, integrate research-based knowledge in curricula, and teach research utilization content.[78]

Use of journals for dissemination of research

The "central function of journals is to provide current information related to practice, trends, and issues affecting a discipline."[87] The breadth and diversity of nursing make dissemination of research difficult. However, the increased number of specialty journals presenting research reports,[84] the publication of research-based articles in the nonrefereed journals traditionally subscribed to by clinicians,[67] and the development of a computerized nursing index for research[90] should make targeting and retrieval of research much easier.

Innovative publications are appearing that assist in the dissemination of research information to practitioners. The *Annual Review of Nursing Research*[34] is approaching its seventh year and dramatically demonstrates the scope and amount of nursing research. *The Research Review: Studies for Nursing Practice*,[18] a bimonthly publication newsletter, provides abstracts of recent research reports, scientific updates, and new and noteworthy research projects. A regular section in the *Western Journal of Nursing Research*, "Using Research in Practice," presents practical applications of reported research.[10]

In May 1988 the inaugural issue of *Applied Nursing Research (ANR)*,[33] a journal devoted to the advancement of nursing as a research-based profession, appeared. *ANR* focuses on the clinical implications of nursing research and integrates scientifically documented information in a readable manner for nurses in a variety of settings—practice, education, research, and management. Rather than emphasizing methodological or analytical strategies, this journal highlights the clinical applications of research. In keeping with this purpose, every manuscript submitted is jointly reviewed by a clinician and a researcher. In addition to original manuscripts, *ANR* features research briefs, columns devoted to clinical problems and methods, and an "ask an expert" section in which practicing nurses can discuss clinical problems or potential innovations they would like to see studied by nurse researchers. The advent of journals such as *ANR*, designed as a forum for all professional nurses, should help to bridge the gap between research and practice and enhance research utilization in practice settings.

Other evidence that barriers to the conduct and use of research are gradually eroding include more positive attitudes toward research by clinicians, increasing institutional and administrative support for nursing research, and the establishment of more nursing research positions in clinical settings.[86] This latter change provides practitioners with a person who can (1) facilitate the identification of scientific knowledge useful in practice, (2) develop research-focused meetings and discussion groups to promote the implementation of findings, and (3) identify current and potentially researchable problems relevant to nursing practice, administration, and education.[19,59,86]

In summary, there is evidence that research is used in practice. Nursing has made a good beginning and

has laid the foundation that will eventually lead to a scientific basis for practice. However, at present not enough research is being used in practice settings. What is being used is taking too long in the translation process, a problem that will be discussed below.

NURSING RESEARCH IS NOT USED IN PRACTICE

Nursing has suffered from the idea that nurses are technical caregivers, not scientists, and further that there are not many researchable problems in nursing. Three factors that have inhibited or delayed the transmission of nursing research into practice are (1) values and qualifications of practicing nurses, (2) the process of research implementation, and (3) institutional factors.[53]

Values and qualifications of practicing nurses

Most nurses lack the preparation necessary to evaluate and implement research in their own environments.[30,51,73] Although many baccalaureate programs now include some orientation to research, more preparation is needed. Most practicing nurses have not had courses in nursing research, and in fact the majority of current practitioners have either diplomas or associate degrees and may not be able to understand, critically evaluate, and implement research findings.[53,55] Furthermore, these nurses tend to read clinical journals that do not present research findings.[55,68,84,87] Circulation statistics show that most nurses depend on one of four journals: *American Journal of Nursing, RN, Nursing '85,* or *Nursing Life.*[84] These journals contain relatively few research reports, which limits opportunities for communication between clinicians and researchers, as Ketefian has shown.[52] The small percentage of nurses with graduate-level preparation suggests it is unrealistic to depend solely on them to translate research into practice. As noted earlier, Brett[9] has demonstrated that even advanced graduate education may not guarantee the implementation of nursing research into practice.

Beyond consideration of the educational preparation of nurses are other factors related to their socialization, attitudes toward research, and orientation to nursing. Most nurses are regarded as having a "doer" orientation rather than a view of themselves as scholars and creative thinkers.[30,55,69,76] This orientation has lead to a devaluation of nursing knowledge and diminished accountability for data-based practice.

Hunt[48] concluded that relevant research findings are not put into practice because practitioners (1) do not know about them, (2) do not understand them, (3) do not believe them, (4) do not know how to apply them, or (5) are not allowed to use them. Dracup and Weinberg[24] identified yet another reason for the gap between nursing practice and research: many nurse researchers are *not* practicing clinicians and therefore frequently identify research problems with little relevance for practice. This view is supported by McBride, Diers, and Schmidt,[67] who conclude, "No matter how good the nursing research, it will affect practice only when it deals with phenomena that are seen as problems by practitioners." They further caution researchers from going "back into the ivory tower" to congratulate themselves on their nursing practice research.

Greenwood[39] was more emphatic in describing the crux of the problem: "*Clinical nurses do not perceive research findings as relevant to their practice.* And further, they do not perceive them as relevant to their practice because frequently they *are not* relevant to their practice."

The process of research implementation

Integrating research into practice is not an easy task. The process requires not only education and intellectual capacity but also judgment, discipline, and perseverance.[30] The CURN project[72] suggests that in order to incorporate research-based knowledge into the delivery of patient care, nurses must be able to (1) identify and synthesize results from many studies in a common research base, (2) transform knowledge into clinical protocols, (3) create specific nursing actions from the protocols, and (4) evaluate the innovations. Translating knowledge into practice also requires a planned social change effort.[53] Nurses need specific instructions on the implementation of findings.[20] However, at the present time practitioners have few guidelines on how to use research or how to critique the literature for application of research in their own clinical settings.[81] Regrettably, the isolation of research from practice documented by Ketefian[52] in 1975 continues today, and nurses still have difficulty locating, reviewing, and analyzing research findings useful in their practice.[42] More studies need to include concrete suggestions for use of the findings in the practice setting.

Nursing research reports also contribute to the barriers encountered in the implementation of their results. A review of the reports indicates that methodological investigations are scarce and that data sources are limited and need to encompass a wider variety of forms (e.g., records, archives, observational techniques, unobtrusive measures, longitudinal studies). Nursing needs to change the pervasive attitude that all research must be experimental or quasi-experimental to be meaningful. Case study methods and qualitative investigations are equally valuable to the profession. The results need to indicate replications, multivariate analyses, relationships to the results of other studies, and uses in future research. Most important, the research activities need to indicate a systematic building of a science for nursing practice.[12]

Other barriers to the implementation of research include (1) research jargon, which is perceived as foreign and unusable by many clinicians;[66,80] (2) research reports that are unclear or disorganized;[71] (3) a substantial time lag in publication of research findings, which may be as long as several years;[71] and (4) a tremendous lack of replication studies necessary to validate clinical findings.[31,42] Similarly Haller and colleagues[41] suggest that replication and construct validity are important criteria for the use of research findings in practice. Rather than building discrete knowledge bases through systematic study of various content areas, current research efforts tend to be diffuse and unfocused.[77]

Even when these barriers are absent or have been overcome, not all research findings are ready to be implemented clinically.[31] Theoretical development in nursing is not yet at a level to stimulate research[29] that in turn would guide and be influenced by practice. Ideally, the relationship between theory, research, and practice is a dynamic reciprocal interchange, as depicted in Figure 7-1. The nursing profession is still striving toward this ideal, and it is no accident that the link between research and practice forms the base of this ideal triangle. Fawcett[31] decries the lack of a clear theoretical base for many studies and suggests that such studies contribute little to nursing knowledge.

Institutional factors

Other impediments to the use of research in nursing practice are related to organizational factors. Many staff nurses lack authority and control over their practice. They may feel powerless to effect changes in their clinical setting.[53] Jacox[51] suggests that role conflict and lack of support for new graduates who question established procedures may further contribute to the problem. Insufficient time and money can also prohibit involvement in nursing research.[30,69]

Institutional support is a critical factor in the conduct and use of research, and the nurse administrator is in a particularly influential role.* For successful implementation of research findings, nursing service administrators must demonstrate a genuine commitment to research, which entails development of self, staff, and resources.[42]

Other modifications in organizational expectations eed to be considered. The addition of research as an item in the position description for nurses at all levels and specifically for the position of clinical nurse specialists is necessary.[61] Informational mechanisms need to be established to provide clinicians with opportunities to discuss research findings, new ideas, and views regarding possible testing protocols.[6,61] In particular, employment of nurse researchers by clinical facilities might promote the conduct and use of research. Unfortunately, only a few institutions have established this role.[70] Although many positive changes are under way, to date institutional support for nursing research is not widespread, and scientific knowledge has not yet become the basis for nursing practice.

STRATEGIES FOR INCREASING USE OF RESEARCH IN PRACTICE

The nursing profession is acutely aware of the problems discussed above, and a number of ways to facilitate the translation of nursing research into practice have been advanced. A number of authors have discussed the value of disseminating the results of nursing research and offer suggestions to achieve this goal. Recommendations for bringing research findings to the attention of practicing nurses include the use of satellite communication modes,[54] marketing strategies,[11,32] and organizational mechanisms.[19] The consortium approach is also effective in facilities that are low in library and financial resources but that wish to share information.[91]

Davis[19] addressed issues surrounding the incorporation of research findings into practice and cited the need to recognize the organizational and cultural aspects of nursing practice that influence the research environment. She further described organizational

*References 4, 19, 26, 38, 42, 51.

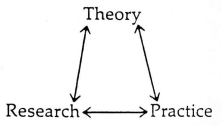

Fig. 7-1 Reciprocal relationship between theory, research, and practice.

mechanisms in one practice setting that legitimize research activity, such as released clinical time for research and recognition through the formal reward system. Fugleberg[35] asserted that there should be a specific performance criteria for all nursing managers in order to encourage research in the practice setting. She also maintained that if all nursing staff were encouraged to assist graduate student research, general staff interest in nursing would increase. Networking has been cited as a method of sharing resources and providing educational offerings that would stimulate staff interest in nursing research.[49] Analysis of quality assurance programs has been another method of providing research in a practical, applicable way.[62] Most of these strategies have been predicated on the notion of planned change.

Planned change

Hersey and Blanchard[44] present two models for change—directive and participative. With one modification, the authors have found the latter approach (Figure 7-2) more appropriate for implementing change in nursing research in clinical settings. Rather than concentrating initially on making new knowledge available to clinicians it is more effective to first begin changing attitudes. Developing a positive attitude and a commitment among clinicians in the direction of the desired change promotes the use of research findings in their particular setting. Involvement of an individual nurse or group of nurses in helping to determine the methods by which research will be reviewed and translated into practiice is particularly effective and is analogous to group participation in problem solving. Translating commitment into behavior is not an easy task. It is helpful to identify respected clinicians who may already be familiar with and value research and to attempt to gain their support for using more research in practice. If this can be done, organizational

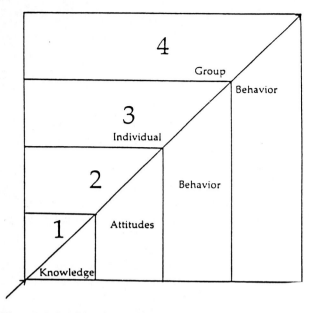

Fig. 7-2 Participative change cycle. *(From Hersey P and Blanchard K: Management of organizational behavior, ed 4, 1982, Englewood Cliffs, NJ, Prentice-Hall.)*

change may be facilitated by getting other nurses to pattern their behavior after the clinicians they admire and perceive to be in leadership roles.[44]

In examining the change process, Kurt Lewin[64] identified three phases: unfreezing, changing, and refreezing. Stevenson[83] has recommended Lewin's framework as one that is effective in developing staff research potential and overcoming resistance to research. Briefly, Lewin's three phases are as follows:

1. Unfreezing involves breaking down the old traditions and customs to make way for new alternatives. Nurses might be motivated to abandon their usual approach to practice based on intuition and to substitute a desire to provide patient care based on tested theories and knowledge about human responses to health and illness.
2. Changing requires new patterns of behavior acquired through the mechanisms of identification and internalization. For example, nurse researchers who serve as models of the desired behaviors may be introduced to the clinical setting (identification), or the staff nurses could be placed in situations in which they had to use research findings in their practice in order to function successfully (internalization).

3. Refreezing is the process by which the newly acquired behaviors become integrated into the nurse's personality and work role. Even when new behaviors such as the use of research findings are adopted, the behaviors must be reinforced and sustained or they will be extinguished.[6]

The CURN project,[72] which focused on transferring research-based knowledge into protocols for nursing practice, has identified seven specific steps in the research use process that must be incorporated into any planned change effort:

- systematically identifying patient care problems
- identifying and assessing research-based knowledge to solve identified patient care problems
- designing a nurse practice innovation to meet the needs of the clinical problem
- conducting clinical trials and evaluating the innovation
- deciding whether to adopt, alter, or reject the innovation
- developing means to extend the new practice to other units
- developing mechanisms to maintain the innovation over time

Thus far, ten protocols have been developed that provide a synthesis of the research literature and transform findings into clinically relevant knowledge. The work of the CURN project is most noteworthy because it provides guidelines for the identification, implementation, and evaluation of data-based answers to patient care problems.

OTHER MODELS FOR USE OF RESEARCH FINDINGS

Stetler and Marram[81] developed a three-phase model for evaluation of research findings for application in clinical settings that provides another useful framework. Theory stages are (1) validation—critical examination of research to determine strengths and weaknesses, (2) comparative evaluations—assessing the desirability and feasibility of research for a particular setting, and (3) decision making—defining the most appropriate type of application of the research finding. Hefferin, Horsley, and Ventura[42] proposed the addition of a fourth phase to this model. This step entails evaluation of the proposed practice change using pretest and posttest strategies. A significant feature of their recommendation is relating "both the degree

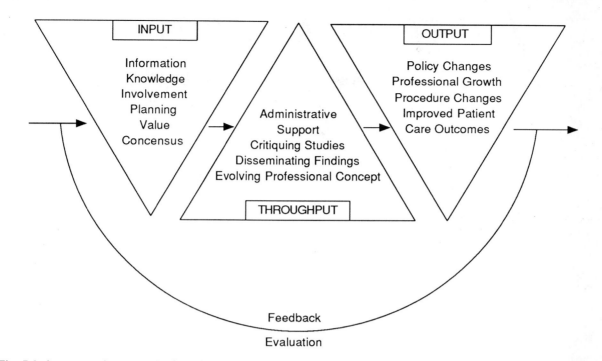

INPUT

Information
Knowledge
Involvement
Planning
Value
Concensus

Administrative
Support
Critiquing Studies
Disseminating Findings
Evolving Professional Concept

THROUGHPUT

OUTPUT

Policy Changes
Professional Growth
Procedure Changes
Improved Patient
Care Outcomes

Feedback

Evaluation

Fig. 7-3 A systems theory model for using new research-based knowledge. (*From Goode CJ and others: J Nurs Admin 17:11, 1987.*)

and direction of this effect to the appropriate theoretical bases for change."[42]

Krone and Loomis[57] reported on the work of Glaser and others,[36] who maintain that the use of research findings can be encouraged by getting nurses involved in various aspects of the research process. For this involvement to be most effective, they recommend that it be related to problems of personal interest and concern to the clinician.

An excellent example of personal interest and commitment to research-based practice was reported by Goode, Lovett, Hayes, and Butcher.[38] Goode and her colleagues reported three nursing protocols that were developed from identified patient care needs, based on professional research, implemented to meet the needs of their specific patient population, and evaluated to determine if they were achieving the desired results (Figure 7-3). These demonstrate the potential patient benefits and personal rewards that may result when nurses are committed to improved patient care. In an effort to increase the use of research findings in nursing clinical practice, Goode[37] has developed a videotape that depicts a step-by-step method for implementing research-based practice in a health care facility. These endeavors demonstrate the potential patient benefits

and personal rewards that may result when nurses are committed to improved patient care.

Davis[19] effectively argued that organizational and cultural factors play a significant role in the introduction of nursing research into clinical settings. Rewards for using and conducting research must be built into the system—pay increases, promotions, paid leaves, and funded travel to attend research conferences. Again, administrative support for research-related activities cannot be underrated.

In analyzing the interaction of nursing research utilization, Horsley[47] has noted that research may be used in the development of new studies, the testing of presented theories, the generation of new theories, or the verification or documentation of changes in practice (Figure 7-4). Horsley has identified two target audiences—practicing nurses and nursing students—that have different mechanisms available for the transmission of information and the modification of nursing practices. Horsley has further defined the research utilization model to identify research components and research products for each of the target audiences. The model identifies potential areas of investigation and calls for innovative instructional strategies for nursing students and an extension of the projects directed to-

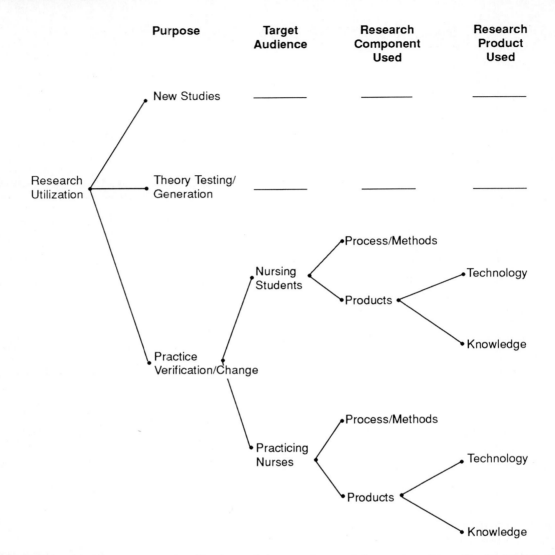

Fig. 7-4 Relationship between research utilization and the use of research in practice. *(From Horsley JA: West J Nur Res 7:135, 1985.)*

ward practicing nurses. Although the list of issues regarding research utilization in practice is long, Horsley concludes, "the list of validated solutions is essentially blank."[47]

Barnard[6] proposed consideration of a conceptual model developed by Rogers[79] for the adaptation of new nursing knowledge. The Rogers model has four stages: (1) awareness, (2) persuasion, (3) decision making, and (4) adoption. Even within this framework, however, there will necessarily be a time lag between awareness of a new idea and its implementation.

Finally, Watson and associates have identified a two-track model that includes research utilization and research conduct. The model involves staff nurses at the unit level as a key component and provides a framework for linking nursing practice and education through nursing research. The outcome of both tracks of the model is the dissemination of information by publication.

All the strategies discussed share common elements and have value in terms of helping nurses use research in their practice. As nurses become more aware of these approaches and adopt a strategy that is comfortable for them and relevant to their practice setting, the profession will move toward its goal of practice that is research based, with theoretical underpinnings from nursing and other professions. There is hope that Bloch's model[8] for conceptualizing nursing research and science, in which the dissemination and use of findings in education and practice is the outcome, may indeed become a reality.

CONCLUSION

In summary, there is general agreement that the conduct of clinical research and the translation of relevant research findings into clinical practice are important professional objectives. The degree to which these objectives are being addressed is evident in part by the amount of current literature devoted to topics related to nursing research, the strong endorsement of research by professional organizations, the number of nursing research conferences, and federal funding available for the conduct and utilization of research. Research values and activities appear well accepted in some professional arenas, but there is limited evidence of the presence of such activities and values in the hospital practice setting. Although reports of individual efforts to promote a positive research environment can be found in the literature,[8,19] it is also evident that research values and activities have not generally been translated into practice.[13,19,82]

Communication of the results of nursing research to the practicing nurse and the need for continued efforts to build a theory-based practice have been encouraged, supported, and accepted by the nursing profession for more than two decades.[19,28,54,82,88] However, only limited knowledge about the specific mechanisms available to facilitate the conduct and implementation of nursing research is apparent in the nursing literature.[27,42] The implementation of research findings in clinical practice with the subsequent goal of maintaining a research-based practice is promoted as one of the major movements toward the achievement of full professional status for nursing.[82]

REFERENCES

1. American Nurses' Association Commission on Nursing Research: Resolution on priorities in nursing research, 1974 convention, Am Nurs 6:9, 1974.
2. American Nurses' Association Committee on Research and Studies: ANA blueprint for research in nursing, Am J Nurs 62:69, 1962.
3. Aslakson MA and Heermann J: Evaluating research findings for application to nursing practice. In Evaluating research preparation in baccalaureate nursing programs. Proceedings of the National Conferences for Nurse Educators, Iowa City, 1982.
4. Aydelotte MK: Nursing research in clinical settings: problems and issues, Reflections 2:3, 1976.
5. Baer ED: "A cooperative venture" in pursuit of professional status: a research journal for nursing, Nurs Res 36:18, 1987.
6. Barnard KE: The research cycle: nursing, the profession, the discipline, West J Nurs Res 4:1, 1982.
7. Barnard KE and Eyres SJ, editors: Child health assessment: part 2. The first year of life, DHEW Pub No HRA 79-25, Washington, DC, 1979, US Government Printing Office.
8. Bloch DA: Conceptualization of nursing research and nursing science. In McCloskey JC and Grace HK, editors: Current issues in nursing, Oxford 1981, Blackwell Scientific Publications, Inc.
9. Brett JLL: Use of nursing practice research findings, Nurs Res 36:344, 1987.
10. Brink PJ and others: Western journal of nursing research, Newbury Park, Calif, 1988, Sage Publishing Co.
11. Brooten DA: Is soft sell enough? Nurs Res 31:195, 1982.
12. Brown JS, Tanner CA, and Padrick KP: Nursing's search for scientific knowledge, Nurs Res 33:26, 1984.
13. Buckwalter KC: Is nursing research used in practice? In McCloskey JC and Grace HK, editors: Current issues in nursing, Oxford, 1981, Blackwell Scientific Publications, Inc.
14. Carnegie ME: The shifting of research emphasis and investigators, Nurs Res 23:195, 1974.
15. Carnegie ME: The editor's report—1976, Nurs Res 25:3, 1976 (editorial).
16. Cohen IB: Florence Nightingale. Sci Am 250:128, 1984.
17. Crane J: Using research in practice: research utilization—nursing models, West J Nurs Res 7:494, 1985.
18. Cronenwett L, editor: Research review: studies for nursing practice, Baltimore, 1987, Williams & Wilkins.
19. Davis MZ: Promoting research in the clinical setting, J Nurs Adm 20:22, 1981.
20. Dickoff J, James P, and Semradek J: 8-4 research: part 1, Nurs Res 24:84, 1975.
21. Diers D: On going international, Image 19:166, 1987 (editorial).
22. Directions for nursing research: toward the twenty-first century, ANA Cabinet on Nursing Research, Kansas City, Mo, 1985.
23. Doctoral programs in nursing 1986-87, NLN Council of Baccalaureate and Higher Degree Programs. NLN Pub No 15-1448, New York, 1987.
24. Dracup K and Weinberg SL: Another case for nursing research, Heart Lung 12:3, 1983.
25. Duffy ME: The research process in baccalaureate nursing education: a ten-year review, Image 19:87, 1987.
26. Egan EC, McElmury BJ, and Jameson HM: Practice-based research: assessing your department's readiness, J Nurs Adm 20:26, 1991.
27. Elliot JE, Krueger JC, and Kearns JM: Update on nursing research in the west, Nurs Res 29:184, 1980.
28. Fagin CM: The economic value of nursing research, Am J Nurs 82:1844, 1982.

29. Fawcett J: The relationship between theory and research: a double helix, Adv Nurs Sci 1:49, 1978.

30. Fawcett J: Integrating research into the faculty workload, Nurs Outlook 27:259, 1979.

31. Fawcett J: Contemporary nursing research: its relevance for nursing practice. In Chaska NL, editor: The nursing profession: a time to speak, New York, 1983, McGraw-Hill.

32. Fine RB: Marketing nursing research, J Nurs Adm 10:21, 1980.

33. Fitzpatrick JJ, editor: Applied nursing research, Philadelphia, 1988, Saunders Co.

34. Fitzpatrick JJ and Taunton RL, editors: Annual review of nursing research, New York, 1987, Springer Publishing Co.

35. Fugleberg BB: Nursing research in the practice setting, Nurs Adm Q 11:38, 1986.

36. Glaser E and others: Putting knowledge to use: a distillation of the literature regarding knowledge transfer and change, Rockvill, Md, 1976, NIMH.

37. Goode CJ: Using research in clinical nursing practice, Horn Video Productions, Ida Grove, Iowa.

38. Goode CJ and others: Use of research based knowledge in clinical practice, J Nurs Adm 17:11, 1987.

39. Greenwood J: Nursing research: a position paper, J Adv Nurs 9:77, 1984.

40. Grier B and Grier M: Contributions of the passionate statistician, Res Nurs Health 1:103, 1978.

41. Haller KB, Reynolds MA, and Horsley JA: Developing research based innovation protocols: process, criteria and issues, Res Nurs Health 2:45, 1979.

42. Hefferin EA, Horsley JA, and Ventura MR: Promoting research-based nursing: the nurse administrator's role, J Nurs Adm 12:34, 1982.

43. Henry B and others: Delineation of nursing administration research priorities, Nurs Res 36:309, 1987.

44. Hersey P and Blanchard K: Management of organizational behavior, ed 4, Englewood Cliffs, NJ, 1982, Prentice-Hall.

45. Hinshaw AS: Using research to shape health policy, Nurs Outlook 36:21, 1988.

46. Hinshaw AS: The national center for nursing research: challenges and initiatives, Nurs Outlook 36:54, 1988.

47. Horsley JA: Using research in practice: the current context, West J Nur Res 7:135, 1985.

48. Hunt J: Indicators for nursing practice: the use of research findings, J Adv Nursing 6:189, 1981.

49. Hunt V and others: Networking: a managerial strategy for research development in a service setting, J Nur Adm 13:27, 1983.

50. Jacox A: The coming of age of nursing research, Nurs Outlook 34:276, 1986.

51. Jacox AK: Nursing research and the clinician, Nurs Outlook 22:382, 1974.

52. Ketefian S: Application of selected nursing research findings into nursing practice, Nurs Res 24:89, 1975.

53. Ketefian S: Selected issues in the translation of research to nursing practice, West J Nurs Res 2:249, 1980.

54. King D, Barnard KE, and Hoehn R: Disseminating the results of nursing research, Nurs Outlook 29:164, 1981.

55. Kirchhoff KT: Should staff nurses be expected to use research? West J Nurs Res 5:245, 1983.

56. Kopf EW: Florence Nightingale as statistician, Res Nurs Health 1:93, 1978.

57. Krone KP and Loomis ME: Developing practice relevant research: a model that worked, J Nurs Adm 21:38, 1982.

58. Krueger JC: A vital link in the nursing research cycle, West J Nurs Res 1:148, 1979.

59. Krueger JC: A survey of research utilization in community health nursing, West J Nurs Res 4:244, 1982.

60. Krueger JC, Nelson AH, and Wolanin MO: Nursing research: development, collaboration, and utilization, Germantown, Md, 1978, Aspen Systems Corp.,

61. Kruse LC and others: Nursing research in Iowa Hospitals, unpublished manuscript, 1988.

62. Larson E: Combining nursing quality assurance and research programs, J Nurs Adm 13:32, 1983.

63. Lewandowski LA and Kositsky AM: Research priorities for critical care nursing: a study by the American Association of Critical Care Nurses, Heart Lung 12:35, 1983.

64. Lewin K: Field theory in social sciences, New York, 1951, Harper & Row,

65. Lindeman CA: Priorities in clinical nursing research, Nurs Outlook 23:693, 1975.

66. Ludeman R: The language and importance of nursing research, West J Nurs Res 2: 432, 1980.

67. McBride MA, Diers D, and Schmidt RC: Nurse-researcher: the crucial hyphen, Am J Nurs 70:1256, 1970.

68. McCloskey JC and Buckwalter KC: Publishing in non-refereed journals is not only o.k. it's necessary, West J Nurs Res 4:255, 1982.

69. Martinson IM: Nursing research: obstacles and challenges, Image 8:3, 1976.

70. Mayer GG: The clinical nurse-researcher: role-taking and role making. In Chaska NL, editor: The nursing profession: a time to speak, New York, 1983, McGraw-Hill.

71. Mercer RT: Nursing research: the bridge to excellence in practice, Image 16:47, 1984.

72. Michigan Nurses Association: Using research to improve nursing practice: a guide, New York, 1983, Grune & Stratton.

73. Murdough C, Kramer M, and Schmalenberg CE: The teaching of nursing research: a survey report, Nurs Educ 6:28, 1981.

74. National League for Nursing: Perspectives for nursing and goals of the National League for Nursing, 1979-1981, Pub No 11-1782, 1979:

75. A new magazine for nurses, Am J Nurs 52:664, 1952 (editorial).

76. Notter LE: The case for nursing research, Nurs Outlook 23:760, 1975.

77. O'Connell KA: Nursing practice: a decade of research. In Chaska NL, editor: The nursing profession: a time to speak, New York, 1983, McGraw-Hill.

78. Proposal submitted to Division of Nursing, USPHS, by Linda R Cronenwett and Cheryl Stetler, Special Projects Grants, 1986.

79. Rogers EM and Showmaker FF: Communication of innovations, New York, 1971, Free Press.

80. Schrader ES: Gobbledygook as a barrier to research, AORN J 30:13, 1979.

81. Stetler CB and Marram G: Evaluating research findings for applicability iin practice, Nurs Outlook 24:559, 1976.

82. Stevens B: Nursing theory, analysis, application, evaluation, Boston, 1984, Little, Brown & Co.

83. Stevenson JS: Developing staff research potential: overcoming

nurse resistance to research. In Machan L, editor: The practitioner-teacher role: practice what you teach, Wakefield, Mass, 1980, Nursing Resources.
84. Swanson E and McCloskey J: Publishing opportunities for nurses, Nurs Outlook 34:227, 1986.
85. Thomas B and Priice M: Research preparation in baccalaureate nursing education, Nurs Res 29:259, 1980.
86. Todd A and Gortner S: Researchmanship: removing obstacles to research in the clinical setting, West J Nurs Res 4:329, 1982.
87. Vaz D: An investigation of the usage of the periodical literature of nursing by staff nurses and nursing administrators, J Contin Educ Nurs 17:22, 1986.
88. Wald FS and Leonard RC: Towards a development of nursing practice theory, Nurs Res 13:309, 1964.
89. Watson CA, Bulechek GM, and McCloskey JD: QAMUR: A quality assurance model using research, Journal of Nursing Quality Assurance 2:21, 1987.
90. Werley HH and Westlake SK: Impact of nursing research on public policy: an examination of ANA research priority statements, J Prof Nurs 1:148, 1985.
91. Zalar MK, Welches LJ, and Walker DD: Nursing consortium approach to increase research in service setting, J Nurs Adm 15:36, 1985.

CHAPTER 8

Viewpoints

Mentors and protégés

From ideology to knowledge

GAIL ARDERY

All ideologies must be seen in perspective. One must not take them too seriously. One must read them like fairytales which have lots of interesting things to say but also contain wicked lies, or like ethical prescriptions which may be useful rules of thumb but which are deadly when followed to the letter.

P. FEYERBEND[15]

The term *mentor* has been adopted from Greek mythology to denote an experienced guide, adviser, or advocate who assumes responsibility for promoting the growth and professional advancement of a less experienced individual—the *protégé*. Mentoring, the process by which a mentor promotes a protégé, can take a variety of forms, each with its own distinctive label. In the business community, for example, the term *mentoring* connotes a long-term, personal dyadic relationship, in which the mentor commits large amounts of time, energy, and caring to help the protégé achieve success. Nurses have tended to adopt less intense and more short-term relationships with their less experienced coworkers, serving as preceptors, coaches, peer pals, and clinical colleagues. Although these varying types of relationships can differ widely in both their structure and their goals, all are intended to enhance the effectiveness of relatively inexperienced workers. In this sense they all are manifestations of mentoring.

Nurses have viewed mentoring, in all its varied forms, as a panacea for the reality shock experienced by new nurses and as a key to professional growth.[17,22,34] Indeed, mentoring has become a new ideology for personal career advancement in nursing. Like any other budding ideology, however, mentoring's value to the nursing profession warrants careful examination. In this chapter, I propose that mentoring relationships be examined, not in terms of the structure of the relationships themselves, but rather in terms of the pieces of knowledge content generated through those relationships,[13] as well as the specific techniques or processes with which mentors foster learning. Moreover, I propose a shift in goals for mentoring relationships, away from the career enhancement of individual protégés and toward the development of a professional body of nursing knowledge.

MENTORING RELATIONSHIPS

In the business community it has been common for successful, well-established professionals to assume voluntarily long-term responsibility for the career development of younger colleagues. The goal of these relationships typically is to promote the success of the younger colleague. Although the mentor and protégé initially hold unequal amounts of influence and expertise, their relationship can evolve into a peer relationship as the protégé matures.[33] This form of mentoring has been seen as necessary for advancement of young businessmen. Benefits accrued by protégés have included career advice and support, skills and knowledge, opportunities and resources, exposure and visibility, and maturation. Mentors, in return, have developed a sense of generativity, gained a dependable coworker, and been rewarded for promoting new talent.[8,30]

Women in the business world also have been involved in this form of mentoring relationship. Established men are frequently eager to sponsor a younger female colleague, although sexual and paternalistic tensions often plague these dyads. In addition, because women are socialized differently from men, they frequently have difficulty fitting into a mentoring system rooted in male culture.[8] Despite these problems, mentoring is still viewed as a way for women to gain confidence in their abilities and develop into successful professionals.[11]

Mentoring relationships have been well utilized by nurses in administrative and academic positions. Of the 71 nurse influentials studied by Vance,[38] 83% reported having had mentors at some point in their careers. Seventy-nine percent of their mentors were female, and only 21% were male. Mentors helped these nurses through "(1) career promotion, door opening, and creating opportunities; (2) professional career role modeling; (3) intellectual and scholarly stimulation; and (4) inspiration."[38] More important, a full 93% of the nurse influentials had served as mentors to others.

In recent years nurses have advocated the spread of mentoring beyond administrative and academic settings. Mentoring in clinical practice has usually involved a short-term arrangement to facilitate staff orientation and socializatioin. Preceptors, for example, tend to function as short-term, intense educators and role models for students, new graduates, and staff orienting to a new specialty area.[27] Coaches help less experienced coworkers determine specific needs for growth, set clear and challenging tasks to facilitate growth, and provide feedback on performance and goal attainment.[4] Peer pals, on the other hand, serve more as support persons, sharing information and strategies, providing advice, and serving as a sounding board.[14] None of these varied forms of mentoring has

been widely adopted by nurses. Failure to form mentoring relationships more widely may be due to any of a number of factors: lack of exposure to the concept, minimal participation in team sports as children, lack of self-esteem, socialization toward affiliation, or absence of a career orientation.[14,19] Campbell-Heider[8] has claimed that because nurses practicing in clinical settings are not career oriented, the type of mentoring prevalent in the business world fails to meet their needs. Rather, Campbell-Heider argued, nurses who function as preceptors, peer pals, and career guides can best help their inexperienced colleagues. Benner and Benner,[3] however, have attributed the general absence of any form of mentoring in nursing to differences in values and expectations in the educational and service arenas, to stereotyping of new graduates by nursing service personnel, to distrust of the novice's technical competence, and to resentment by established practitioners of newcomers' attempts to institute change.

Nurse authors have attributed numerous potential benefits to varying forms of mentoring: rapid socialization of workers to differing roles and work environments,[12,17,36] increased commitment to professional values,[25] effective education of nurses for leadership and administrative positions,[7,14,19,22,38] enhanced recruitment and decreased turnover rates, greater valuation of self,[9] more effective utilization of collective power,[38] and better opportunities for achieving personal success.[7,25]

Most discussions of mentoring that have cited learning as a postive outcome focused on the basic or entry-level knowledge of individual nurses. Various mentoring strategies have been viewed as tools for ensuring safe and effective functioning of new graduates or nurses new to a specialty area.[9,34] Particular emphasis has been given to the individualized instruction made possible through mentoring arrangements.[36,37] The mentoring role, when compared to other roles such as team leader, also might enable clinicians to share their knowledge more broadly.[1] Clinical preceptors have been used to provide baccalaureate students with hands-on experiences in clinical nursing research. Such programs promote the view that research and the development of research-based knowledge is an integral and essential aspect of nursing practice.[6] Blackburn, Chapman, and Cameron[5] cited increased scholarly productivity as an individual outcome for academicians who had mentors in graduate school. But only infrequently has mentoring been praised as a way to increase the general body of nursing knowledge.[35]

BEYOND THE IDEOLOGY

In recent years beliefs about the value—even the desirability—of mentoring relationships have increasingly been questioned. Mentoring has not solved all individual and corporate ills. Some mentors or individuals who could serve as mentors have inhibited less experienced colleagues and students, stifling their innovativeness and discouraging them from taking calculated risks.[28] Most mentors have selectively denied some employees access to the system.[24]

Hagerty,[18] in a thoughtful commentary on mentoring, listed several additional criticisms that warrant repeating. First, the concept of mentoring has never been conceptually defined, nor has its validity as a construct been demonstrated. Different authors have discussed the persons, the process, the purposes, and the activities involved in the same terms—as if they were all the same thing. These weaknesses render testing of the concept impossible. Accordingly, research on mentoring has had to rely on anecdotal, retrospective descriptions of mentoring relationships, most typically obtained through self-designed questionnaires whose validity and reliability have not been demonstrated. Qualitative studies[21] have accumulated large amounts of data regarding nurses' responses to specific mentoring programs, but these data lack generalizability.

In addition, much of the literature on mentoring is based on one or more of the following unexamined assumptions: (1) having a mentor is necessary for success; (2) succeess, particularly upward movement in an organization, is a desirable goal for everyone; (3) mentoring can occur in the same form and with equal effectiveness across widely varying professions and organizations; (4) lack of mentoring has hampered career advancement among women; and (5) nursing has a shortage of mentors.[2] As Hagerty correctly noted, each of these claims should be treated as hypotheses, rather than as assumptions, and should be subjected to empirical testing. Finally, Hagerty questioned whether the rush to embrace mentoring represents another attempt by nurses, most of whom are female, to imitate an institution developed by males that might not even be worth imitating!

Also untested is the assumption that female socialization patterns impede the development of mentoring relationships among women. According to one version of this belief, women are socialized toward affiliation, and men are socialized toward competition. Further, achievement is somehow inherently linked to competition, whereas affiliation is inherently linked to powerlessness.[19] In contrast, the same socialization patterns also have been claimed to make women competitive with one another.[25] The relationship between socialization patterns and professional interactions remains at best undefined. Moreover, it remains unclear why achievement cannot be enhanced through both affiliation and competition. Mentoring itself, even in its most elitist, "male" form, represents a type of affiliation—a relationship often described as very personal and dependent on the right mix of chemistry.[31] Using this line of reasoning, women should be even better at mentoring than men. The unclarity and inconsistency in these discussions signals the need for more serious investigations of mentoring.

Data collected on mentoring relationships have not always demonstrated beneficial effects. A study of role conceptualization and role deprivation did not find significant differences among student who were involved in preceptorships and those who were not.[20] And research data strongly supporting relationships between mentoring and career success have not yet been provided.[8]

Williams and Blackburn[39] found that junior faculty with and without mentors did not differ in overall research productivity. Faculty with mentors had significantly more often served as a coprincipal grant investigator, edited a book within the past 2-year period, served as a consultant, and participated in a refereed forum. Of the various mentoring activities analyzed in this study, only role-specific modeling/teaching emerged as a predictor of productivity, and then only of research activities. Role-specific activities for mentors included helping the protégé plan a research project, write a grant proposal, and also coauthoring. Serving as the protégé's advocate, socializing the protégé to the organization, and encouraging protégés' dreams had little effect on output. This study suggests that mentoring relationships might have subtle interactions with work and learning outcomes and illustrates the need to apply rigor in mentoring research.

The focus on personal achievement and advancement so frequent in the mentoring literature creates further concerns. Nursing's tradition has long been rooted in the ethic of caring for others. Our approach to clients still assumes a philosophy of caring, and we still measure our effectiveness (at least in clinical areas) in terms of the outcomes our patients attain. Being part of a relationship whose goal is personal advancement may not be congruent with our profession's emphasis on improving the health and well-being of others.

NEW APPROACHES TO MENTORING

Mentoring relationships are not inherently good or bad. What we make of them and what we accomplish with them will determine their value. I believe that mentoring can serve as a vehicle for increasing nursing's body of knowledge. However, mentoring's effectiveness in this area will be facilitated if nurses make two shifts in their thinking.

The first shift is to reformulate our goals within mentoring relationships. We all tend to invest energy discriminately, to maximize our chances of goal attainment. If our primary goal is personal success, our efforts will be directed at endeavors that promote personal success. If, on the other hand, our primary goal is increasing our profession's body of knowledge, we will concentrate on activities that help us reach that goal. If individuals participating in mentoring relationships were to view their goals as increasing knowledge—both their individual knowledge and the larger body of nursing knowledge being accumulated by the profession—the amount of knowledge transacted or attained through that relationship would be expanded. Faculty at top-ranked schools of nursing have demonstrated this type of commitment, both to the development of a knowledge base for nursing and to the sharing of that knowledge with their colleagues. At these institutions, mentoring relationships among faculty, between faculty and students, and between faculty and clinicians have been widely utilized to facilitate research endeavors.[32]

The second shift is to change the way we examine and evaluate mentoring as a construct. As noted earlier, most discussions of mentoring have focused on the structure of the relationship, describing its personal or emotional nature, or delineating specific characteristics seen as desirable for mentors and protégés. However, the benefits of mentoring might become more apparent if we were to examine the content of the relationship—that is, the knowledge that is shared or mutually generated—and the particular techniques mentors use to effect growth in knowledge. We might ask, for example, whether particular types of knowledge are especially appropriate to this type of instruction. We might wish to determine what teaching strategies mentors find effective. And evaluation can be focused primarily on measuring learning outcomes rather than on describing the nature of the relationship itself.

Daloz[10] has proposed a model of mentoring that is compatible with both these shifts. Daloz's model characterizes mentoring as three distinct types of activities performed by mentors: supporting, challenging, and providing vision. Support "refers to those acts through which the mentor affirms the validity [of the protégé's] present experience" and creates trust.[10] Support is provided by listening, giving structure, expressing positive expectations, serving as an advocate, sharing oneself, and making the relationship special. In contrast to support, challenge divides the mentor and protégé, creating a gap that is tension producing for the protégé. Challenging entails setting tasks, engaging in discussion, constructing hypotheses, and setting high standards.

Support and challenge have distinct individual effects as well as combined effects on a protégé's development. Protégés are expected to fall within four developmental categories, with the attained developmental level depending on the amount of support and challenge activities undertaken by influential others.

In the category called "confirmation," in which support is high but challenge is low, protégés feel good about themselves but lack the necessary skills to function productively in their work world. The category called "stasis," in which both support and challenge are low, is characterized by an absence of any action and maintenance of the status quo. Challenge without support causes the protégé to enter the category of "retreat" and develop a rigid worldview in which some semblance of security can be maintained. True "growth" is possible only with an appropriate mix of challenge and support.

Challenge and support are not sufficient. Mentors also provide vision to their protégés, illuminating long-range goals and sketching dreams of what the future can hold. Mentors provide vision by modeling, explaining traditions, offering new mental maps, suggesting new languages, and providing mirrors. Vision creates a context in which both support and challenge function to effect transformation. Vision thus provides both a "climate of expectations" and a "sense of continuity" that persist even in the mentor's absence.[10]

Daloz's model provides a beginning for more meaningful examinations of mentoring relationships. The support and challenge constructs could be used to test hypotheses about specific teaching processes involved in these relationships. Perhaps more important, the construct of vision could be adopted to describe the transmission of knowledge between mentors and protégés. Conceptualizing the transmission of knowledge as a sharing of vision might also help us examine how mentors approach information, perceive it in novel ways, and mold it into new meanings. Sharing of those visions can only accelerate the development of a comprehensive body of nursing knowledge.

For all this to be possible, large amounts of work must be done. The concepts described by Daloz, or alternative parallel constructs, will have to be conceptually and operationally defined. Learning or knowledge outcomes must similarly be specified and defined. Then the constructs can be subjected to empirical testing to obtain research-based data regarding the effectiveness of mentoring as a teaching and learning form.

Finally, I suggest that we not limit our examinations to traditional, dyadic mentoring relationships. The constructs of support, challenge, and vision are sufficiently abstract to be useful in a variety of teaching and learning situations, including classroom instruction, clinical and laboratory instruction, seminar discussions, graduate research assistantships, thesis and dissertation supervision, work orientation programs, and ongoing staff development and education. Moreover, these same constructs might be appropriate for examining how knowledge is acquired and shared through collaborative research projects, particularly in those instances in which project participants do not have equal levels of experience and expertise. In collaborative research projects the expertise of a number of researchers is focused on a single topic, making complex projects more manageable and providing project members with opportunities to learn from one another and increase their competencies. Collaboration can also enhance personal growth and self-awareness.[29]

CONCLUSIONS

Mentoring, though not widely practiced, appears to be an increasingly popular teaching and learning form. The National League for Nursing's most recent directory of internship programs for nursing students lists 118 separate programs within the United States.[26] A few graduate nursing programs have incorporated extended practicum experiences into their administration role components. Various forms of mentoring also are being advocated in nursing literature from other countries.[2,23] We do not know, however, whether mentoring indeed constitutes an effective teaching and learning form, which mentoring activities most enhance learning, and precisely how mentoring can aid in the development of a comprehensive body of nursing knowledge.

Fortunately, we are beginning to accumulate a small amount of research-based evidence on the value of mentoring. For instance, we know that the existence of faculty research interest groups has been a characteristic of top-ranked schools of nursing.[32] In addition, role-specific modeling and teaching activities appear to have a positive effect on the research productivity of junior faculty members.[39] We simply need to know much more.

Mentoring continues to hold great promise as a type of coworker or teacher-learner relationship that can foster the generation of nursing knowledge. Increased participation by nurses in varying types of mentoring relationships will enable researchers to better examine its usefulness and describe its essential components. The time has come to take this concept seriously, to define it rigorously, and to evaluate empirically its effectiveness in various teaching and learning situations. Without rigorous evaluation, the value of mentoring to nursing can only be considered potential.

REFERENCES

1. Atwood AH: The mentor in clinical practice, Nurs Outlook 27(11):714, 1979.
2. Bajnok I and Gitterman G: Nurses as colleagues and mentors, Canadian Nurse 84(2):16, 1988.
3. Benner P and Benner RV; The new nurse's work entry: a troubled sponsorship, New York, 1979, The Tiresian Press.
4. Binger JL and Huntsman AJ: Coaching: a technique to increase employee performance, AORN J 47(1):229, 1988.
5. Blackburn RT, Chapman DW, and Cameron SM: "Cloning" in academe: mentorship and academic careers, Research in Higher Education 15(4):314, 1981.
6. Brand KP: Options for clinical nursing research experiences, Nurse Educataor 12(2):35, 1987.
7. Cameron RK: Wanted: mentor relationships within nursing administration, Nursing Leadership 5(1):18, 1982.
8. Campbell-Heider N: Do nurses need mentors? Image 18(3):110, 1986.
9. Chinn PL and Wheeler CE: Feminism and nursing: can nursing afford to remain aloof from the women's movement? Nurs Outlook 33(2):74, 1985.
10. Daloz LA: Effective teaching and mentoring, San Francisco, 1987, Jossey-Bass Publishers.
11. Diamond H: Patterns of leadership, Image 11(2):42, 1979.

12. Dobbs KK: The senior preceptorship as a method for anticipatory socialization of baccalaureate nursing students, J Nurs Educ 27(4):167, 1988.

13. Down FS: Doctoral education: our claim to the future, Nurs Outlook 36(1):18, 1988.

14. Duncan J and Partridge R: Peer pals: overcoming the obstacles to leadership development, Nursing Leadership 3(2): 18, 1980.

15. Feyerbend P: How to defend society against science. In Hacking I, editor: Scientific revolutions, New York, 1981, Oxford Univ Press.

16. Gibbons LK and Lewison D: Nursing internships: a tri-state survey and model for evaluation, J Nursing Administration 10(2):31, 1980.

17. Glass B and others: A nurse colleague program: one solution to nurse turnover, Neonatal Network 5(6):16, 1985.

18. Hagerty B: A second look at mentors: do you really need one to succeed in nursing? Nurs Outlook 34(1):16, 1986.

19. Hamilton MS: Mentorhood: a key to nursing leadership, Nursing Leadership 4(1):4, 1981.

20. Itano JK, Warren JJ, and Ishida DN: A comparison of role conceptions and role deprivation of baccalaureate students in nursing participating in a preceptorship or a traditional clinical program, J Nurs Educ 26(2):69, 1987.

21. McGrath BJ and Princeton JC: Evaluation of a clinical rpeceptor program for new graduates—eight years later, Journal of Continuing Education in Nursing 18(4):133, 1987.

22. McLean PH: Reducing staff turnover: the preceptor connection, Journal of Nursing Staff Development 3(1):20, 1987.

23. McMurray A; Preceptoring: a link between theory and practice, Australian Nurses Journal 16(3):42, 1986.

24. Megel ME: New faculty in nursing: the role of the mentor, J Nurs Educ 24(7):303, 1985.

25. Meisenhelder JB: Networking and nursing, Image 14(3):77, 1982.

26. National League for Nursing: Directory of nurse internship programs. Reprinted in Imprint 34(5):24, 1987/88.

27. O'Brien A: Choosing the role in staff development that's best for you, AORN J 35(7):1262, 1982.

28. O'Connor KT: For want of a mentor, Nurs Outlook 36(1):38, 1988.

29. Pender NJ and others: Collaboration in developing a research program grant, Image 19(2):75, 1987.

30. Phillips-Jones L: Mentors and Proteges, New York, 1982, Arbor House.

31. Pilette PC: Mentoring: an encounter of the leadership kind, Nursing Leadership 3(2):22, 1980.

32. Pollock SE: Top ranked schools of nursing: network of scholars, Image 18(2):58, 1986.

33. Roche GR: Much ado about mentors, Harvard Business Review 57(1):14, 1979.

34. Schempp CM and Rompre TM: Transition programs for new graduates: how effective are they? Journal of Nursing Staff Development 2(4):150, 1986.

35. Schlotfeldt RM: Mentorship: a means to a desirable ends. In McCloskey JC and Grace HK, editors: Current issues in nursing, ed 2, Boston, 1985, Blackwell Scientific Publications Inc.

36. Shamian J and Inhaber R: The concept and practice of preceptorship in contemporary nursing: a review of pertiinent literature, International Journal of Nursing Studies 22(2):79, 1985.

37. Talarczyk G and Milbrandt D: A collaborative effort to facilitate role transition from student to registered nurse practitioner, Nursing Management 19(2):30, 1988.

38. Vance C: Women leaders: modern day heroines or societal deviants? Image 11(2):37, 1979.

39. Williams R and Blackburn RT: Mentoring and junior faculty productivity, J Nurs Educ 27(5):204, 1988.

CHAPTER 9

The nursing minimum data set (NMDS)

Issues for the profession

HARRIET H. WERLEY
ELIZABETH C. DEVINE
CECELIA R. ZORN

The development of the Nursing Minimum Data Set (NMDS) is an initial effort to establish uniform standards for the collection of comparable, minimum, essential nursing data. There are a variety of issues surrounding the testing and implementation of the NMDS that are identified in this chapter. These can be categorized into issues related to nursing as a practice profession and issues related to health policy. Before the issues are discussed, background information is provided about the NMDS concept, development, purposes, and elements. Future directions for the NMDS are presented in the final section.

NMDS CONCEPT, DEVELOPMENT, PURPOSE, AND ELEMENTS
Concept

The NMDS is based on the concept of the Uniform Minimum Health Data Sets (UMHDSs). A UMHDS has been defined as "a minimum set of items of information with uniform definitions and categories, concerning a specific aspect or dimension of the health care system which meets the essential needs of multiple data users."[4] The concept was developed in 1969 out of efforts to identify national health data standards and guidelines.[9,10,11] Several different UMHDSs have been developed in the areas of long-term care, hospital discharge, and ambulatory care.[12,13,14] However, the Uniform Hospital Discharge Data Set (UHDDS) is the only minimum health data set in widespread use today.[4,5,6]

At the 1969 Conference on Hospital Discharge Abstract Systems[8,11] several criteria were set forth for the development of minimum health data sets. These were as follows: (1) data items included in the set must be useful to most if not all potential users, such as health care professionals and administrators; planning, regulatory, and legislative bodies at local, state, and federal levels; insurance agencies; and the research community; (2) items selected must be those that can be collected readily with reasonable accuracy; (3) items should not duplicate data available from other sources; and (4) confidentiality of health care information should be protected.

Built on the concept of the UMHDSs, the NMDS represents nursing's first attempt to standardize the collection of essential nursing data. By adapting the definition given for a UMHDS, the NMDS can be defined as a minimum set of items of information with uniform definitions and categories concerning the specific dimension of nursing that meets the information needs of multiple data users in the health care system. The NMDS includes those specific items of information that are used on a regular basis by the majority of nurses across all types of settings in the delivery of care.

Development

Work on the NMDS began in the late 1970s. A Nursing Information Systems Conference was held in 1977 at the University of Illinois College of Nursing, Chicago, to assess the state of the art of nursing information systems (NISs) and to provide stimuli that might encourage nurses to move in this direction. Initial conceptualization of a basic nursing data set was done through the small group work at that conference and was explicated in the Newcomb[15] chapter of the Werley and Grier volume.

In 1985 the NMDS was developed by consensus

ELEMENTS OF THE NURSING MINIMUM DATA SET

Nursing care elements
1. Nursing diagnosis
2. Nursing intervention
3. Nursing outcome
4. Intensity of nursing care

Patient or client demographic elements
*5. Personal identification
*6. Date of birth
*7. Sex
*8. Race and ethnicity
*9. Residence

Service elements
*10. Unique facility or service agency number
11. Unique health record number of patient or client
12. Unique number of principal registered nurse provider
*13. Episode admission or encounter date
*14. Discharge or termination date
*15. Disposition of patient or client
*16. Expected payer for most of this bill (anticipated financial guarantor for services)

---

*Elements comparable to those in the Uniform Hospital Discharge Data Set.

through the efforts of a national group of 64 experts, who participated in the 3-day invitational NMDS Conference. It was sponsored by the University of Wisconsin-Milwaukee School of Nursing and funded largely by the Hospital Corporation of America (HCA) Foundation. The NMDS Conference was modeled after other conferences that had been conducted to identify the earlier UMHDSs. The participants at the conference included nurse experts in practice, administration, research, and education; health policy spokespersons; information systems, health data, and health record specialists; and persons knowledgeable about the development of the UMHDSs.[23,24,25]

Purposes

The purposes of the NMDS are to (1) establish comparability of nursing data across clinical populations, settings, geographic areas, and time; (2) describe the nursing care of patients or clients and their families in a variety of settings, both institutional and noninstitutional; (3) demonstrate or project trends regarding nursing care provided and allocation of nursing resources to patients or clients according to their health problems or nursing diagnoses; and (4) stimulate nursing research through links to the detailed data existing in NISs and other health care information systems (HCISs).

Elements

The NMDS includes three broad categories of elements: (1) nursing care, (2) patient or client demographics, and (3) service elements. Ten of the sixteen elements also are included in the previously mentioned UHDDS.[6,12] Those elements presumably would not need to be re-collected in hospitals, where they should be available through existing relational data-base management systems. The NMDS elements are listed in the box on this page.

ISSUES RELATED TO NURSING AS A PRACTICE PROFESSION

There are four major issues concerning the NMDS that relate to nursing as a practice profession. These include (1) the need for consistent documentation of nursing data, (2) nursing's role in developing and using computerized data and NISs, (3) the cost of data collection and use of the NMDS, and (4) acceptance of the NMDS by the profession.

Need for documentation

A practice issue related to testing and implementing the NMDS is the need for consistent documentation of nursing data. Because the NMDS is an abstraction tool for data in the health care record, the data must be documented consistently so that they can be abstracted later. The NMDS draws on the documentation of the nursing process that is used when nurses provide care to people in any setting. It can be effective only if nurses in practice and administration document fully both the care provided and the nurse resources used to provide that care.

The tremendous demands on clinicians' time often limit their ability to document nursing care and nurse resource consumption data consistently. However, unless mechanisms are developed to ensure accurate and complete documentation, health records will be an inadequate source of the nursing data needed by clinicians, administrators, researchers, educators, and health policymakers. Any efforts to increase the quality of documentation must minimize the additional demands made on clinicians, who already are experiencing considerable stress in providing care under growing cost-containment measures.

Computerization of nursing data

In addition to documentation, the computerization of data is an issue related to the testing and implementation of the NMDS. In certain areas computerization of nursing information is becoming more common. However, in the past many nurses have not been involved either in philosophical discussions preceding adoption of an information management system or in the day-to-day decision making about NISs. In addition, nurses often have not taken action to ensure that the available information technology served the profession, assuming that because the technology existed, it would advance the discipline. Computerized nursing data are not always retrievable; the data must be saved so that they will be available for later abstraction and use. The entry of nursing information must be done in such a way that the data are keyed and can be retrieved as needed.[28] In the future these NISs will be computerized and operational at the institutional or agency level where, through relational data-base management systems, the nursing data can be related to other HCISs. The goal is to include the NMDS elements in the NISs as these systems are being developed and refined, so that the data set can be incorporated into ongoing data collection systems.

Cost considerations

Related closely to computerization of data are several other issues associated with cost considerations. Nurse clinicians and administrators must develop strategies to obtain funding for NIS computerization from both internal and external sources. Research and development monies frequently are available internally, but nurses often do not request or demand these resources. Hence, they do not recieve nursing's proportionate share of the total support available in facilities for the development of computerized information systems. Similarly, external funding sources, such as the National Center for Health Services Research, are not used by nursing administrators and practitioners for the support of information system research, development, and management.

There has been far too much delay in nurses taking advantage of the technology related to the information management and computerization age. Groups and individuals outside of nursing also recognize the need for NISs. For example, Randall,[16] Director of Marketing Health Services of McDonnell Douglas Automation Company, commented that the emphasis on computerization in the health care delivery systems has been largely on financial aspects of billing and collecting. He noted that more recently hospital communication systems have received attention, patient care systems have emerged, and there is a growing subindustry targeted to special purpose functions such as radiology, laboratory, and pharmacy. He stated: "In all that activity there appears to be a forgotten element. One which, for whatever reason, rarely receives the attention it deserves, considering its importance in the totality of the health care delivery process."[16] Randall was referring to nursing; he identified nurses' contributions and commented that the decade of the 1980s will belong to them. The decade of the 1980s is now over, and what have nursing leaders done to bring nursing into the information management and computerization age? Have they made sure that nursing receives its fair share of the total dollars invested for facility computerization, so that nursing, the largest service unit, is not lagging behind?

The cost of implementing the NMDS is also an issue that must be addressed. Because the NMDS is built on the UHDDS, which currently is required for clients under Medicare coverage in hospitals, the cost of implementation may be considerably less for this particular patient group. This is an advantage, both financially and practically in implementation of the NMDS. Only 4 nursing care elements and 2 of the service elements are additional; the other 10 elements are comparable to those already being collected in the UHDDS. Nurses should recognize the merits of having built the NMDS on the UHDDS and capitalize on this fact in justifying that the data set elements be included in NISs and other HCISs.

Acceptance by the profession

Acceptance of the NMDS for implementation by nurses is the final professional issue to be identified. Such acceptance can be encouraged best by emphasizing the benefits of the NMDS, as identified and described briefly below.

1. Access to comparable, minimum nursing care and resources data at local, regional, national, and international levels
2. Enhanced documentation of nursing care provided

3. Identification of trends related to client problems (nursing diagnoses) and nursing care provided
4. Impetus to improved costing of nursing services
5. Improved data for quality assurance evaluations
6. Impetus to development and refinement of nursing information systems
7. Comparative research on nursing care, including research on nursing diagnoses, nursing interventions, nursing outcomes (resolution status of nursing diagnoses), and referral for further nursing services
8. Contributions toward advancing nursing as a research-based discipline

There is obvious value in having a minimum data set usable by the entire profession. It must be understood that the NMDS is not a series of minimum data sets for current clinical decision making in the various areas of nursing, which would result in a proliferation of data sets having questionable comparability. Instead it is a set for retrospective collection of comparable, minimum, essential, common-core data across all settings, a set that describes the nursing care provided and the nurse resources used.

Use of the NMDS also would facilitate the evaluation component of the nursing process. As nurses assume more autonomy for their practice, the ability to evaluate adequately and demonstrate their contribution becomes even more crucial. In addition, increased accountability is required for the resources used and the client outcomes achieved. Access to comparable data across settings and populations related to patient outcomes, or the resolution status of the nursing diagnoses, would enhance greatly the evaluation of nursing care provided. For example, nursing outcome and intensity of nursing care (hours of nursing care and staff mix), as two elements of the data set, could contribute substantially toward the evaluation of nursing care.

Two crucial ongoing efforts in nursing, the development and testing of the NMDS and the development of nursing diagnosis and intervention classification systems for nursing practice,[26] are closely related. The early work on the NMDS spurred further development of intervention classification schemes and highlighted the importance of the nursing diagnosis taxonomy movement.[19,22] Testing and implementation of the NMDS will be facilitated by the continuing development and refinement of classification systems for nurs-

ing practice. One important example of such work is the intervention classification project of Bulechek, McCloskey, and colleagues at the University of Iowa College of Nursing. Additionally, testing of the NMDS will provide considerable data for the continual refinement of classification systems for nursing diagnoses, interventions, and outcomes.[26]

The knowledge that nurses possess and the information they generate are essential for theory building in nursing. Implementing the NMDS can result in readily retrievable data for research focused on a variety of nursing concerns. This research then can serve as a link to develop theories that are based on nursing practice.

ISSUES RELATED TO HEALTH POLICY

A variety of changes within nursing and the health care industry may influence testing and implementation of the NMDS. Nurses are practicing in settings more diverse than ever before. The move in health care from acute-care settings to community settings is changing the employment and practices of many nurses. The elderly population is increasing dramatically. Health care expenditures in this country are rising rapidly, and cost containment is a crucial national concern. With all of these changes, the need for retrievable, essential, core nursing data is essential for health policy decision making.

Nursing data: the missing component

With increased data on the description of nursing care, as well as the identification of trends in nursing care practices and allocation of nurse resources, health policy decisions can be made considering issues pertinent to nursing. Up to now these decisions frequently were made without regard to nursing concerns, because nursing's data simply were not available or were not comparable. Recently Trevino[18] noted that ". . . all too often the utility of potential information resources is significantly diminished because of a lack of comparability in the definitions, codes, classifications, terminology, and sampling frames used by different agencies at the federal, state, and local levels." He identified several consequences of this lack of comparability, which included (1) difficulty in making meaningful comparisons, (2) increased cost in collecting new data in an attempt to make up for inconsistencies, and (3) major gaps in data where much information still is lacking.

An example of the inconsistencies in data documentation and collection for a specific client population was described recently by Westermeyer[27] in the *American Journal of Public Health*. A strategy for an alcoholism social indicator system using information already collected by various institutions was developed. A major difficulty in using this method was the variation in agency coding schemes. Westermeyer found that the only demographic variables routinely collected by all nine agencies in the study were age and gender, and these were the only two that could be compared readily. Significant differences were found in the coding schemes of the agencies for race, county of residence, marital status, education, occupation, employment status, and religion, so that none of these could be compared across agencies. These differences were found despite the fact that five of the agencies were state and two were federal, and some consistency in coding of these common demographic variables could be expected. Because of this inconsistency, Westermeyer found the ability to assess needs of alcoholic individuals, present an epidemiological portrayal of this population, and evaluate treatment programs was diminished greatly.

Westermeyer's[27] description of inconsistencies in data documentation and collection has implications for nursing. Nurses must ensure that nursing data are documented more consistently within and among health care institutions. However, this does not always happen. For example, in the initial test of the NMDS, nursing diagnoses were not documented consistently according to the classification scheme endorsed by the institution, such as the North American Nursing Diagnosis Association system.[7] In addition, nursing outcomes (resolution status of the nursing diagnosis) also were documented inconsistently across health care records. See Devine and Werley[3] for further report of the pilot study findings.

Expanded opportunities

A significant change in the health care delivery system is the growth and development of additional organizations for nursing care delivery. For example, the number of nursing centers in the United States is increasing rapidly; 51 academic centers were identified in a survey of all National League for Nursing accredited baccalaureate programs,[2] and 30 additional nonacademic centers have been identifed.[17] As new centers are established and as personnel in existing nursing centers become more sophisticated in their

data management, it is crucial that essential, minimum nursing data from this type of health care setting be readily retrievable. Health care policy making will become acutely focused on cost containment in the ambulatory health care setting, following the recent constraints in the hospital setting. If nursing centers can provide readily retrievable data (computerized) supporting the effectiveness of care in these settings, both in terms of cost and outcome, an important contribution will be made to the profession, health care industry, and consumers. There is an established Council for Nursing Centers within the National League for Nursing to assist in the organization, planning, and operation of nursing centers and in the computerization of their nursing services data, which it is hoped will include the NMDS elements.

Similar opportunities to enhance the contribution of nursing data to health care policymaking exist in other settings. Nurses may experience considerable difficulty in developing or installing NISs in the acute care setting, where they often must compete with many others for information management resources. In home health care and long-term care settings, however, nurses frequently are the chief executive officers and may be in a more powerful position to influence the allocation of information management and computerization resources. In these settings nurses could incorporate the NMDS in their initial NIS development. The data then would be available in an ongoing data collection system to influence policymakers concerned with health care in these settings.

FUTURE DIRECTIONS

In consideration of the NMDS issues related to nursing as a practice profession and to health policy, the following essential efforts in the continuing development of the NMDS must be carried forward.

1. Expand the NMDS testing effort (regionally, nationally, and internationally), with refinement of the NMDS definitions and data collection procedures as indicated.
2. Demonstrate the types of research that can be done, using the NMDS elements alone and with additional data through the use of audit trails to NISs and other HCISs.
3. Demonstrate through research the administrative and programmatic value of the NMDS.
4. Promote inclusion of the NMDS elements in

existing and developing NISs to facilitate the ongoing collection of uniform, comparable nursing data that may be aggregated and/or used for purposes of comparative research.

5. Promote national and international sessions on nursing documentation using the nursing process and the NMDS definitions.
6. Encourage computerization of NISs nationally and internationally.
7. Facilitate implementation of the 1986 American Nurses' Association resolution on computerization of nursing services data.[1]

As these efforts in the continuing development of the NMDS are accomplished, methods for improving health care for specific client groups may be revealed, more efficient and effective use of resources may be identified, and new methodologies for costing nursing services may be explicated. The effort of many individuals will be needed to accomplish the continuing development of the NMDS. There are a variety of implications of the NMDS for nurses in clinical practice, administration, research, and education. These are enumerated by Werley and Devine[20] and Werley, Devine, and Zorn.[21] Specific activities may be focused on facilitating, participating in, and organizing conferences and continuing education offerings to enhance documentation and involvement in computerization. And more concerted efforts must be made by nurses in clinical and administrative positions to see that both nursing care and management data are computerized.

The NMDS project team makes a continual effort to disseminate information about the NMDS. At both national and international meetings, the benefits and implications for nurses and nursing are discussed; in addition, benefits for health policymakers and for the health care industry are highlighted. Responses also are given to requests for guidance on what NMDS elements to include in computerized NISs, as health care personnel are progressing with development of their information systems.

SUMMARY

The development of the NMDS is an initial effort to establish uniform standards for the collection of minimum, essential nursing data. Within this chapter, the concept of the NMDS was presented, and selected issues related to professional practice and health policy were discussed. Testing and implementation of the

NMDS are dependent on consistent documentation of the data set elements by practitioners. Computer systems must be developed to facilitate both the management of nursing data and the relationship between the nursing data management system and the general data management system. Therefore nursing leadership is essential to the design and use of data management systems. The cost of implementing the NMDS can be minimized in certain instances, because many of the data set elements are already part of the data base required for hospitalized Medicare patients. The information obtained through use of the NMDS will facilitate evaluation of nursing practice and the continued development of classification systems for nursing diagnoses, interventions, and outcomes. The NMDS also will provide documentation of the relationships among such factors as nursing diagnoses, interventions, outcomes, and the use of nursing resources. Enhanced specification and understanding of these crucial relationships undoubtedly will contribute to nursing practice, the ability of nurses to influence health policy decisions, and health care for the consumers.

REFERENCES

1. American Nurses' Association: Development of computerized nursing information systems in nursing services (resolution no 24), Kansas City, Mo, 1986, American Nurses' Association.
2. Barger SE: Academic nursing centers: a demographic profile, J Prof Nurs 2:246, 1986.
3. Devine EC and Werley HH: Test of the nursing minimum data set: availability of data and reliability, Res Nurs Health 11:97, 1988.
4. Health Information Policy Council: Background paper: uniform minimum health data sets (unpublished), Washington, DC, 1983, Department of Health and Human Services.
5. Health Information Policy Council: 1984 revision of the uniform hospital discharge data set (unpublished), Washington, DC, 1984, Department of Health and Human Services.
6. Health Information Policy Council: 1984 revision of the uniform hospital discharge data set, Federal Register 50(147):31038, 1985.
7. McLane AM, editor: NANDA nursing diagnosis Taxonomy I. In Classification of nursing diagnoses: proceedings of the seventh conference, St Louis, 1987, The CV Mosby Co.
8. Murnaghan JH: Uniform basic data sets for health statistical systems, Int J Epidemiol 7:263, 1978.
9. Murnaghan JH, editor: Ambulatory care data: report of the conference on ambulatory medical care records, Med Care 11(2, suppl):1, 1973.
10. Murnaghan JH, editor: Long term care data: report of the conference on long-term health care data, Med Care 14(5, suppl):1, 1976.
11. Murnaghan JH and White KL, editors: Hospital discharge

data: report of conference on hospital discharge abstract system, Med Care 8(4, suppl):1, 1970.

12. National Committee on Vital and Health Statistics: Uniform hospital discharge data: minimum data set, Pub No (PHS) 80-1157, Hyattsville, Md, 1980, US Department of Health, Education, and Welfare.

13. National Committee on Vital and Health Statistics: Long-term health care: minimum data set, Pub No (PHS) 80-1158, Hyattsville, Md, 1980, US Department of Health and Human Services.

14. National Committee on Vital and Health Statistics: Uniform ambulatory medical care: minimum data set, Pub No (PHS) 81-1161, Hyattsville, Md, 1981, US Department of Health and Human Services.

15. Newcomb JB: Issues related to identifying and systemizing data—group discussion. In Werley HH and Grier MR, editors: Nursing information systems, New York, 1981, Springer Publishing.

16. Randall AM: The nursing system—a computer challenge for the 80s! Computers in Hospitals 3(3):50, 1982.

17. Riesch SK: Personal communication, June 8, 1988.

18. Trevino FM: Uniform minimum data sets: in search of demographic comparability, Am J Public Health 78:126, 1988 (editorial).

19. Werley HH: Nursing diagnosis and the nursing minimum data set. In McLane AM, editor: Classification of nursing diagnoses: proceedings of the seventh conference, St Louis, 1987, The CV Mosby Co.

20. Werley HH and Devine EC: The nursing minimum data set: status and implications. In Hannah KJ and others, editors: Clinical judgment and decision making: the future with nursing diagnosis, New York, 1987, Wiley.

21. Werley HH, Devine EC, and Zorn CR: The nursing minimum data set: effort to standardize collection of essential data. In Ball J and others, editors: Nursing informatics, New York, 1988, Springer-Verlag.

22. Werley HH, Devine EC, and Zorn CR: Status of the nursing minimum data sets (NMDS) and its relationship to nursing diagnosis. In Carroll-Johnson RM, editor: Classification of nursing diagnoses: proceedings of the eighth conference, Philadelphia, JB Lippincott Co (in press).

23. Werley HH and Lang NM, editors: Identification of the nursing minimum data set, New York, 1988, Springer Publishing.

24. Werley HH, Lang NM, and Westlake SK: Brief summary of the nursing minimum data set conference, Nursing Management 17(7):42, 1986.

25. Werley HH, Lang NM, and Westlake SK: The nursing minimum data set conference—executive summary, J Prof Nurs 2:117, 1986.

26. Werley HH and Zorn CR: The nursing minimum data set and its relationship to classification for nursing practice. In Classifications for nursing practice, Kansas City, Mo, American Nurses' Association (in press).

27. Westermeyer J: Problems with surveillance for alcoholism: differences in coding systems among federal, state, and private agencies, Am J Public Health 78:130, 1988.

28. Zielstorff RD, McHugh ML, and Clinton J: Computer design criteria for systems that support the nursing process, Kansas City, Mo, 1988, American Nurses' Association.

CHAPTER 10

Potential and pitfalls of expert systems in nursing

BETTY L. CHANG

Will expert systems replace nurses? Is an expert system the same as artificial intelligence (AI)? These are some of the questions asked about nursing systems and computers. This chapter discusses AI and one of its applications, expert systems. Expert systems in medicine are reviewed, followed by a review of existing expert systems in nursing. A visionary approach is taken to the potential of expert systems in nursing, followed by a description of common pitfalls. Finally, ongoing work on one expert system, Computer Aided Research in Nursing (CARIN), is briefly described.

What is artificial intelligence?

Artificial intelligence is a branch of computer science concerned with designing intelligent computer systems, that is, systems exhibiting the characteristics we associate with human intelligence.[2] These include the abilities (1) to respond to situations with flexibility, (b) to make sense of ambiguous or contradictory messages, (c) to recognize the relative importance of elements of a situation, and (d) to find similarities and differences among situations. Areas of research in AI include the following: expert system design of computer software to provide consultation or advice; intelligent computer-assisted instruction, a special application of expert systems to individualize learning; speech recognition, the recognition of human speech by computers, vision, the ability of computers to sense the environment; robotics, the designing of devices to perform specific tasks; and neural networks, the attempt to emulate the brain's complex patterning. Areas of research for computer programmers include the improvement of natural language processing and automated programming. Natural language processing is divided into two types, generational and understanding. Natural language generation is a method of having the computer produce English so that the user can use the system more readily. Natural language understanding provides a method for the computer to understand instructions in English (rather than programming only in numbers).

EXPERT SYSTEMS
What can expert systems do?

An expert system is a computer program that uses AI technology to represent human knowledge, experience, and judgment in a particular domain. Expert systems are also known as knowledge-based systems, because they involve knowledge bases consisting of facts and heuristics for applying those facts. Expert systems allow users to analyze complex data, diagnose problems, or suggest the best way to deal with a situation. They can only serve as aids to nurses, not as replacements for them. An expert system differs from a database system in that it is designed for reasoning rather than computation. Although both types of programs allow for storage and retrieval of data, an expert system may serve as a consultant in diagnosing a patient or suggesting a treatment, while a database system enumerates facts about patients. Databases contain factual or declarative knowledge that allows users to draw their own conclusions; expert systems contain both factual and procedural knowledge, or knowledge of rules for decision making. The combination of factual and procedural knowledge allows the expert system to simulate to a limited extent the reasoning processes of human experts.

Are expert systems restricted to specialized computers?

Expert systems have been developed that run on computers of various sizes and types. Very large computers can be used for highly complex research prototypes; however, minicomputers and desktop com-

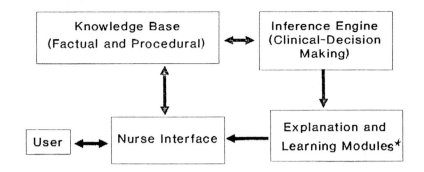

★ Additional Modules that may be optional.

Fig. 10-1 Components of an expert system.

puters are now used for expert systems in education, business, and industry. Remote terminals or stand-alone personal computers can be used for expert systems in a variety of settings where expert consultation and assistance are relied on to save time and reduce errors. Most computers are able to accommodate some type of expert system program.

Furthermore, there are few restrictions on the programming languages that can be used. Although many research systems use LISP (an AI programming language), a number of natural programming languages have been used in the development of expert systems. A wide selection of language and utilities programs and expert shells also are available to the expert system developer. An expert shell is a programming structure used in building an expert system.

Components of an expert system

The development of software modules varies depending on conceptual approach, programming language selected, and the specific domain for development. The most simplified modules include the three systems (knowledge base, inference engine, and user interface) diagrammed in Figure 10-1. The knowledge base contains both factual knowledge about patients and procedural knowledge or rules governing how decisions are made. However, the database alone will not provide the nurse with expert consultation; inferences must be made about nursing diagnoses.

The inference engine controls the expert system by deciding what rules are to be used, accessing the appropriate rules in the knowledge base, exercising those rules, and determining when an acceptable solution has been reached.

The user interface is that part of the program that allows a nurse to communicate with the expert system. The interface is generally written to facilitate ease of use by avoiding unnatural syntax and language and unnecessary keypunching.

Additional modules included in some systems are the explanatory module and the learning module. An explanatory module explains the reasons for a decision proposed by the program. A learning module accumulates information as individual cases are processed. Through this accumulation of data the system notes corrections that need to be made in its knowledge base. The system is thus said to be able to learn from experience.

APPLICATIONS OF EXPERT SYSTEMS
Applications in medicine

Expert systems have been developed in manufacturing, mining, space projects, and business, as well as in health care. One of the earliest developments of expert systems for scientific research was Stanford University's DENDRAL, a program for determining the chemical structure of compounds.[6] Perhaps the best-known program in medicine is MYCIN, started in 1976 by Shortliffe to help diagnose infectious diseases.[6] Many programs have since been developed, including TEIRESIAS, which may be used with expert systems to create a body of metaknowledge (knowledge about knowledge) and to allow users to communicate with an expert system without using a computer programmer.

Other well-known programs include INTERNIST, developed by Myers and Pople at the University of Pittsburgh in the early 1970s for the diagnosis of about 500 diseases.[23] CADUCEUS is an extension of INTERNIST and includes several improvements. Other programs in medicine include ONCOCIN, developed to give advice regarding the treatment of cancer[25]; DIGITALIS ADVISER, for determining digitalis dosages[26]; WHEEZE and PUFF, for respiratory diseases; and CASNET, for glaucoma.[6] It is interesting to note that expert systems in medicine have been confined to the research laboratory. This fact has led to serious questions about the professional acceptance of expert systems.[16] Thus, although the potential of expert systems may be great, their actual use as clinical advisors in medicine is minimal.

Nursing applications

To date only a few expert systems exist in nursing. The COMMES (Creighton On-Line Multiple Medical Expert System), developed at Creighton University and using a semantic net to link key concepts, has been widely reported.[10,11,23] The system was designed to serve as a resource and consultant to three major nursing groups: undergraduate students, in-service educators, and practicing nurses. The system provides objectives for patient care and identifies various medical diagnoses or nursing problem areas. It can also suggest nursing problem areas corresponding to particular signs and symptoms and can provide resources and suggested reading material for in-service educators concerned with the nursing care of patients with specific problems.[24] More recent work focuses on the useful information provided by COMMES, compared with that of nursing experts.[9] Ozbolt[22] has noted that COMMES contains knowledge at the beginning generalist level that is limited to usual care for common problems.

Other prototypes have been reported by Ozbolt and colleagues over a period of years.[12,20,21] These systems are based on McCain's and Orem's nursing models, and have been developed using Bayesian* theory and Apple computers.[19] However, Ozbolt and colleagues have chosen not to extend the present prototypes. Further work on expert systems for diagnosis, treatment planning, and evaluation are in progress at Case Western Reserve University.[22] Bloom, Leitner, and Solano[3] describe an expert system prototype that can generate nursing care plans based on nursing diagnosis. This system, too, is in the prototype stage. Still another system is in the process of development at the University of California at Los Angeles (UCLA) by Chang

and colleagues; it will be described in greater detail later in this chapter.

Several hospital-oriented nursing programs for the documentation of nursing care are in use. Although they may not provide clinical consultation, as expert systems do, the hospital systems do generate written care plans and are often mentioned in conjunction with nursing diagnosis.[4,5,17]

POTENTIAL OF EXPERT SYSTEMS FOR NURSING

The potential of expert systems in nursing may be envisioned as follows: (a) serving as aids or consultants in nursing, (b) clarifying or encoding the reasoning or decision-making processes of experts, (c) preserving knowledge and expanding the expert knowledge base, and (d) unifying nursing language and diagnostic nomenclature.

Serving as an aid or consultant

Expert systems, by their very definition, are designed to make inferences and serve as consultants in selected domains. The consultation function will be useful to practicing nurses if the system is readily available and easily accessible. If availability and program or information accessibility are limited, the usefulness of the system is diminished (in comparison to that of a library, for example).

Potential applications include the use of expert systems for in-service nursing or nurse orientation. Also, continuing education units can be offered for isolated modules. The potential long-term savings of using expert systems to supplement classes for nurses are clear.

If the program is designed for easy entry and quick information display, the system also can serve as a consultant to staff nurses. This function would be especially useful to nurses who are caring for patients with unfamiliar conditions. For example, a nurse from an orthopedic unit may be temporarily assigned to an oncology unit and may quickly obtain consultation regarding a patient's treatment and nursing care, such as chemotherapy.

Encoding the decision-making process

The development of expert systems can lead to contributions in testing clinical decision-making processes. Only if this process is explicated and encoded can a truly functional expert system be developed. As computer information nurse specialists—called

---

*Bayesian theory is a system of predicting outcomes by assigning probabilities to individual events and applying mathematical formulas to them.

nurse informatists—and expert clinicians work on the problem the process increasingly will become clarified.

Preserving and expanding expert knowledge

Knowledge derived from human experts is preserved in the expert system's program and can be updated as new knowledge or information is obtained. In most present systems, the knowledge base is programmed by knowledge engineers. However, in some systems, such as TEIRESIAS, users may change parts of the program themselves. (TEIRESIAS is an expert system designed to be used in building or revising other expert systems.) In the future it may be possible for a program to update itself. The expert system will be built including a learning system, so that the expert system automatically makes corrections or changes based on new data from patients.

Unifying nursing language

The computerization of nursing information has been a great impetus for unifying terminology and nomenclature in nursing. The effort to computerize nursing information has led nurses to seek universally acceptable nomenclature. Computerization may significantly contribute to the codification of nursing terminology and even the clarification of nursing science.

The potential of expert systems in nursing is not without pitfalls. A system is as good as it has been built. A few broad areas of difficulty are described below.

PITFALLS IN THE DEVELOPMENT OF EXPERT SYSTEMS

Certain problematic areas have been identified in the nursing literature and as a result of personal experience. These issues include (a) identification of a problem appropriate to the capabilities of an expert system, (b) methods of acquiring knowledge and representing what is known and the rules governing the decision-making process, and (c) selecting the conceptual framework.

Appropriate identification of a problem

Problem identification is important[25] as the first stage in the development of an expert system. The exact nature of the problem and the system's goals need to be stated. First, the problem selected must be narrow but not trivial in scope.[1,15] Second, the problem

should require judgment and cognitive skills that can be replicated. If the problem is extremely broad and requires much complex reasoning, it will be difficult to program. Third, the problem should be widely acknowledged by experts in the field, in this case professional nurses.

Questions to be asked include: Is the problem well defined? Are we expecting a computer to resolve ambiguity? Problem identification is an iterative process in which the domain experts state a problem and the programmers describe the problem as they understand it.

Knowledge acquisition and knowledge representation

Knowledge acquisition involves explicating the facts and procedures necessary for arriving at an inference or decision so that the knowledge can be understood by an expert systems programmer or knowledge engineer. Knowledge representation is the symbolic abstracting and programming of the knowledge. These tasks are two of the most difficult in the development of expert systems.

The difficulties involved in knowledge acquisition are increasingly acknowledged in the literature.[14,16,21] It has been hypothesized that one of the pitfalls of systems developed in the last decade may be the incorporation of inappropriate models of decision making.[16] A number of attempts to explicate the clinical nursing decision-making process are found in the literature, but there is no agreement regarding the nature of this process. This lack of agreement has been seen as one of the more serious hurdles to be surmounted in expert system development.

The hypothetical-deductive model of decision making has been proposed.[7] However, other cognitive models have been proposed that attempt to emulate the descriptive knowledge and the processing knowledge of nurses.[16] Abraham and Fitzpatrick[1] have suggested that Carper's structure of ways of knowing[8] be considered by nursing informatists. They point out that nurses use not only empirical, verifiable knowledge but also aesthetic knowledge involving affect and appreciation; ethical knowledge, focusing on the determination of moral judgments and values; and personal knowledge, derived from one's relationships with others.[1]

Methods of knowledge representation receive considerable attention in computer science research.[22] The selection of programming languages and methods of symbolic representation is hotly debated among programmers and nurse informatists. Examples of representational schemes in current systems are semantic networks* and production rules. Some people believe that expert systems are incapable of serving as intelligent consultants and place more hope in the newer neural networks technology. This technology, a method of pattern recognition, is based on the model of the human brain, in which individual cells, whose functions are governed by complex formulas, are connected by dendrites into neural networks. The network is programmed in certain patterns, and new patterns can be entered into the network to see if there is a match. This technology is used for aspects of decision making.

Selection of a conceptual framework

A dilemma encountered by domain experts (for example, clinical nurse specialists) in developing a system for nursing diagnoses is the nursing framework within which the diagnoses will be labeled. Some may decide to use the taxonomy adopted by the North American Nursing Diagnosis Association (NANDA) and the American Nurses' Association.[18] Others have chosen Orem's framework[19] or Gordon's functional health patterns.[13] The incompleteness of certain frameworks has been cited as an impediment to expert system development.[21]

These difficulties notwithstanding, my UCLA colleagues and I view the potential of expert systems for nursing as great, and we are involved in developing an expert system for nursing diagnosis research, discussed below.

AN EXAMPLE OF A SYSTEM IN PROGRESS
Problem and framework selection

At UCLA our team of several clinical nurse specialists and computer scientists has begun the development of an expert system for nursing diagnosis in the area of self-care deficit. We selected NANDA's Taxonomy I framework as the nursing assessment framework and self-care deficit as the alteration in human response. Self-care deficit was selected as the problem based on these criteria: it is well accepted in nursing, it is not trivial in nature, and many of its elements can be named and cognitively processed.

*Semantic networks represent facts as nodes and then interrelationships as links. A production rule is a heuristic (problem solving method) written in the form of "IF—THEN" statements.

Automation of assessment guide

The system is called CARIN, Computer-Assisted Research in Nursing, because it was developed to retrieve patient data in a statistically meaningful manner to facilitate nursing research. It is being designed in two phases. Phase I serves as an automated assessment guide, using Taxonomy I as a framework. The 9 categories of patterns of human responses are used, as well as 27 alterations in function. Phase II will offer diagnoses based on patient data. In this phase clusters of defining characteristics of the patient will be matched to a diagnosis already programmed into the computer.

We have programmed the automated assessment guide and are testing it at patients' bedsides prior to proceeding to phase II. We have decided to program the software using programming language C and Borland's expert system shell, PROLOG.[27] It has been designed to run on an IBM-compatible laptop computer, which is taken to the patient's bedside.

Field-testing the system

The automated assessment guide is currently being tested in a hospital setting. The automated guide without its expert system components may be of interim value to nurses in documenting signs and symptoms. We may eliminate worksheets used for jotting down patient assessments. At its simplest level the computerized printout provides an orderly record of patient data. Presently we are correcting errors in the program and adjusting to many of the practical aspects of using computers at the bedside. The clinical nurse specialist explained the assessment procedure to the patients who agreed to participate. The patients did not react negatively to the use of the computer.

Phase II will be a challenge to the UCLA team, as the process has been to other developers of expert systems. We are mindful of the limitations of AI technology, yet hopeful that most of the rules and heuristics can be captured.

SUMMARY

In this chapter I have discussed the role of expert systems within the larger field of AI technology. I have differentiated the capabilities of expert systems and data-base systems. Although expert systems have been developed in medicine, their acceptance by professionals in the field has been limited. The potential of expert systems includes nursing consultation, assisting in the clarification and encoding of the decision-making process, preserving and expanding the knowledge base, and unifying nursing language and nomenclature. Areas of difficulty in the development of nursing expert systems include identification of an appropriate problem, knowledge acquisition and the representation of rules in clinical decision-making, and the selection of a conceptual framework.

I have also described a research system, CARIN, in the process of development at UCLA. Some of the developmental tasks to be surmounted may require a great deal of research into the science of nursing and AI technology, as well as a measure of compromise.

Expert systems using AI techniques may not be globally applicable to nursing diagnoses in general, but specific applications certainly may help us examine selected nursing problems more critically.

REFERENCES

1. Abraham IL and Fitzpatrick JJ: Knowing for nursing practice: patterns of knowledge and their emulation in expert systems. In Stead W, editor: Proceedings the eleventh annual symposium on computer applications in medical care, Los Angeles, 1987, IEEE Computer Society Press.
2. Barr A and Feigenbaum EA: The artificial intelligence handbook, vol 2, Los Altos, Calif, 1982, William Kaufmann.
3. Bloom KC and others: Development of an expert system prototype to generate nursing care plans based on nursing diagnoses, Computers in Nursing 5(4):140, 1987.
4. Brooks CA: Computerized nursing care planning: utilizing nursing diagnosis. In Proceedings of nursing and computers, third international symposium on nursing use of computers and information science, St Louis, 1988, The CV Mosby Co.
5. Brooks CA and others: Computerized nursing care planning utilizing nursing diagnosis, Washington, DC, 1984, Oryn Publications, Inc.
6. Buchanan BG and Shortliffe EH: Rule based expert systems, Reading, Mass, 1984, Addison-Wesley Publishing Co, Inc.
7. Carnevali D: Nursing care planning: diagnosis and management, ed 3, Philadelphia, 1983, JB Lippincott Co.
8. Carper BA: Fundamental patterns of knowing in nursing, Advances in Nursing Science 1:13, 1978.
9. Cuddigan J and others: Evaluation of an artificial intelligence based on nursing decision support system in a clinical setting. In Proceedings of nursing and computers, third international symposium on nursing use of computers and information science, St Louis, 1988, The CV Mosby Co.
10. Evans S: Implementation of a computer-based test generation to evaluate health professions continuing education. In Proceedings of the first annual conference of the American Association for Medical Systems and Information, Los Angeles, 1982, IEEE Computer Society Press.
11. Evans S: The COMMES nursing consultant system: a practical clinical tool for patient care. In Proceedings of nursing and computers, third international symposium on nursing use of computers and information science, St. Louis, 1988, The CV Mosby Co.
12. Goodwin J, Ozbolt JG, and Edwards B: Developing a computer program to assist the nursing process: Phase I—from systems analysis to an expendable program, Nurs Res 24:299, 1975.
13. Gordon M: Manual of nursing diagnosis, New York, 1982, McGraw-Hill Book Co.
14. Grosso C: Knowledge and knowledge acquisition for the development of expert systems for nursing. In Proceedings of nursing and computers, third international symposium on computers and information science, St. Louis, 1988, The CV Mosby Co.
15. Hayes-Roth F, Waterman DA, and Lenat DB: Building expert systems, Reading, Mass, 1983, Addison-Wesley Publishing Co, Inc.
16. Hyslop A and Jones BA: A cognitive model as a nursing expert system: potential for decision support and training in patient assessment. In Proceedings of nursing and computers, third international symposium on nursing use of computers and information science, St Louis, 1988, The CV Mosby Co.
17. Korpman RA: Patient care information systems: looking to the future. In Software in healthcare, San Bernardino, Calif, 1984, Health Data Sciences Corporation.
18. McLane AM: Section IV, NANDA Taxonomy I, patterns of human response. In Classification of nursing diagnosis: proceedings of the seventh conference, North American Nursing Diagnosis Association, St Louis, 1987, The CV Mosby Co.
19. Orem DE: Nursing: concepts of practice, New York, 1985, McGraw-Hill Book Co.
20. Ozbolt JG: A prototype information system to aid nursing decisions. In Proceedings of the sixth annual symposium on computer applications in medical care, Los Angeles, 1982, IEEE Computer Society Press.
21. Ozbolt JG and others: Developing expert systems for nursing practice. In Proceedings of the eighth annual symposium on computer applications in medical care, Los Angeles, 1984, IEEE Computer Society Press.
22. Ozbolt JG Developing decision support systems for nursing: issues of knowledge representation, Medinfo, North Holland, Amsterdam 1986, Elsevier Science Publishers BV.
23. Pople H: The formation of composite hypotheses in diagnostic problem solving: an exercise in synthetic reasoning, International Joint Conference on Artificial Intelligence 5:1030, 1977.
24. Ryan S: Applications of a nursing knowledge-based system for nursing practice, inservice, continuing education and standards of care. In Dayhoff RE, editor: Proceedings of the Seventh Annual Symposium on Computer Applications in Medical Care, Los Angeles, 1983, IEEE Computer Society Press.
25. Shortliffe EH: Update on oncocin: a chemotherapy advisor for clinical oncology. In Computer applications in medical care, Los Angeles, 1984, IEEE Computer Society Press.
26. Swartout WR: A digitalis therapy advisor with explanations, Report No TR-176, MAC Project, Computer Science Department, Massachusetts Institute of Technology, 1977.
27. TurboProlog, Borland International, Scotts Valley, Calif (computer program).

CHAPTER 11

The organization of nursing knowledge

MAXINE E. LOOMIS

In his introduction to *The Mismeasure of Man*, Stephen Jay Gould[9] warns of "the myth that science itself is an objective enterprise, done properly only when scientists can shuck the constraints of their culture and view the world as it really is." He goes on to say:

Science must be understood as a social phenomenon, a gutsy human enterprise, not the work of robots programmed to collect pure information. Science, since people must do it, is a socially imbedded activity. It progresses by hunch, vision, and intuition. Much of its change through time does not record a closer approach to absolute truth, but the alteration of cultural contexts that influence it so strongly.

Gould's insight provides an appropriate introduction to this chapter on the organization of nursing knowledge, for any attempt to categorize the collected information of a discipline must be viewed in its social context. Nursing leaders provide the initial structure within which students learn and nurses practice. This structure must resemble current reality enough to be credible, yet must challenge that reality so as to further and improve the practice of nursing.

The purpose of this chapter is to stimulate thinking and discussion about the organization of nursing knowledge and the impact various category systems have had on the science and practice of nursing. An initial review of the various systems used to categorize nursing research will be followed by a brief discussion of the structure of the discipline of nursing. Finally, several recent models that I have developed are presented in an attempt to explore the similarities and differences between the science and practice of nursing.

CLASSIFICATION OF NURSING RESEARCH

Research means to search or investigate thoroughly. It is a process of investigation or experimentation aimed at the discovery and interpretation of facts, the revision of accepted theories or laws in the light of new facts, or the practical application of such new or revised theories or laws. Research provides the bridge between the academic discipline of nursing science and the professional practice of nursing therapeutics. Research should be either theory testing or theory generating in nature, and this union of research and theory should provide the foundation for nursing practice. Research is therefore a logical place to begin the search for a system by which to organize nursing knowledge.

Major trends in nursing research were documented by Roberts[18]; Brown[4]; Simons and Henderson[23]; Abdellah[1]; Notter[16]; Gortner, Bloch, and Phillips[7]; and Gortner and Nahm[8]. These reviews produced a clear lineage of the progress of nursing research over the past decades. Each contributed to the development of categories by which nursing research can be classified.

Despite the relative paucity of nursing research at that time, Simmons and Henderson[23] developed a comprehensive list of categories that included historical, philosophical, and cultural studies; issues related to the conduct of research (facilities, personnel, support, and method); and categories that can be grouped into the broad areas of nursing practice, education, and administration.

As nursing research progressed, Abdellah[1] developed a comprehensive classification of research projects in nursing from 1955 to 1968 supported by the United States Public Health Service (USPHS). The 167 grants actually cited in that report (see box on p. 78) were distributed across the following categories: health care personnel in nursing (22.1%); measurement of patient care systems (15.6%); the nurse role and its impact on patient care systems (15.5%); organizations of patient care systems and their impact on the delivery of health services (15.5%); faculty research development grants (11.3%); clinical research

CLASSIFICATION OF USPHS-SUPPORTED RESEARCH PROJECTS IN NURSING, 1955-1968

	No.	%
1. **Clinical research of problems related to nursing practice** (cardiac nursing, nursing in chronic illness, intensive care nursing, mental health and psychiatric nursing, parent-child health nursing, rehabilitation nursing, cancer nursing, medical-surgical nursing)	12	7
2. **Model and theory development** (application of models and theories, appliances and devices)	10	6
3. **Measurement of patient care systems** (methodologies used to measure quality patient care, quality of nursing care—criteria of nursing practice)	26	15.6
4. **Organizations of patient care systems and their impact on the delivery of health services** (hospital-based studies, outpatient and extra-hospital-based studies)	25	15.5
5. **The nurse role and its impact on patient care systems** (role behaviors, clinical nurse specialist role)	26	15.5
6. **Health economic systems affecting patient care**	2	1
7. **Health care personnel in nursing** (recruitment, selection, and evaluation; research in nursing education programs—teaching methods and curricula; the professionalization process in nursing; historical research)	37	22.1
8. **Health communications systems** (research conferences, tools for research)	10	6
9. **Faculty research development grants**	19	11.3
TOTAL	167	100%

From Abdellah FG: Nurs Res 19:6-17; 151-162; 239-252, 1970.

CONTRIBUTIONS OF NURSING RESEARCH TO PATIENT CARE

1. Building a science of practice
2. Refining the artistry of practice (clinical therapeutics)
3. Establishing structures for optimal patient care
4. Developing methodology
5. Application of research findings

From Gortner SR, Bloch D, and Phillips TR: J Nurs Adm 23, March-April 1976.

of problems related to nursing practice (7%); health communications systems affecting patient care (6%); model and theory development (6%); and health economic systems affecting patient care (1%).

Gortner, Bloch, and Phillips[7] elaborated the subcategories of building a science of practice, artistry of practice, establishing structures for optimal delivery of care, developing methodology, and application of research findings in their review of the contributions of nursing research to patient care (see box above). Gortner and Nahm[8] presented a historical overview of nursing research in the United States that included developments in nursing education and nursing practice research as well as the development of research resources.

In its 25th anniversary year *Nursing Research* published 5 articles reviewing the history of clinical nursing research from 1952 through 1975 by specialty areas. Barnard and Neal[3] reviewed 78 manuscripts from *Nursing Research* from 1952 to 1976, the *ANA Clinical Conference Series* from 1965 to 1973, and the *WICHE Communicating Nursing Research* series from 1968 to 1973 that related to maternal-child health (see box on p. 79). They reported studies in the following categories: care of the sick or hospitalized child (23%), childrearing (18%), special populations (12.8%), childbearing (11.5%), nurse's role (10.3%), and breast care and breast-feeding (6.4%). Their approach was based on human growth and development, recognizing deviations from the norm and the role of the nurse.

Highriter[12] reviewed 115 community health nursing articles obtained through a MEDLARS worldwide search and published from 1972 through 1976 (see box on p. 79). Her report included review and methodology studies (31.3%), service evaluation studies (24.4%), client need assessment (13%), service description studies (13%), community health nursing ed-

---

THE HISTORY OF CLINICAL NURSING RESEARCH, 1952-1975

Maternal-child nursing research	*No.*	%
1. Care of the sick or hospitalized child	18	23
2. Childrearing	14	18
3. Newborn, term, and premature infants	13	18
4. Special populations	10	12.8
5. Childbearing	9	11.5
6. Nurse's role	8	10.3
7. Breast care and breast-feeding	5	6.4
TOTAL	77	100

From Barnard KE and Neal MV: Nurs Res 26: 193, 1977.

THE HISTORY OF CLINICAL NURSING RESEARCH, 1952-1975

Community health nursing research	*No.*	%
1. Service evaluation	28	24.4
2. Client need assessment	15	13
3. Service description studies	15	13
4. Community health nursing education	13	11.3
5. Attitude studies	8	7
6. Study reviews and methodology	36	31.3
TOTAL	115	100

From Highriter ME: Nurs Res 26:183, 1977.

THE HISTORY OF CLINICAL NURSING RESEARCH, 1952-1975

Medical-surgical nursing research

1. Most prevalent
   A. Preoperative or postoperative nursing care
   B. Patients with cardiac disease
   C. Patients with diabetes mellitus

2. Next most frequently studied
   A. Patients with tuberculosis
   B. Patients with neurologic or orthopedic problems
   C. Patients with pulmonary disorders
   D. Patients with gastrointestinal disorders

From Ellis R: Nurs Res 26:177, 1977.

THE HISTORY OF CLINICAL NURSING RESEARCH, 1952-1975

Gerontological Nursing Research
1. Psychosocial characteristics and nursing needs of the elderly
2. Attitudes of nursing personnel toward the elderly
3. Psychosocial nursing interventions to meet needs of the elderly

From Gunter LM and Miller JC: Nurs Res 26:208, 1977.

THE HISTORY OF CLINICAL NURSING RESEARCH, 1952-1975

Psychiatric nursing research
1. Studies of the person
2. Studies of interpersonal relationships
3. Studies of the social system

From Sills GM: Nurs Res 26:201, 1977.

---

ucation (11.3%), and attitude studies (7%). These categories reflect an emphasis on delivery systems and client aggregates. Ellis[6] summarized the most prevalent medical-surgical nursing studies (see box on this page). These included over 200 such studies published in *Nursing Research* from 1952 through 1975. These involved preoperative and postoperative teaching, patients with cardiac disease, and patients with diabetes mellitus. A secondary set of studies of patients with tuberculosis, neurologic or orthopedic problems, or pulmonary or gastrointestinal disorders was also cited. Emphasis in this body of research was on patient condition.

Gunter and Miller[10] organized their review of nursing gerontology research by critical conceptual issues in what was then an emerging field of study (see box above). Sills' review of research in psychiatric nursing[22] included 310 research endeavors (see box on this page). The research was analyzed according to historical and theoretical trends in psychotherapy: the person (a trend occurring prior to World War II), the relationship (a trend dominant from 1945 to 1955), and the social system (from 1955 through 1977). Finally, O'Connell, and Duffey[17] conducted an analysis of the research in nursing practice published in *Nursing Research* from 1970 through 1975 (see box on p. 80). Their sample of 88 studies was classified along a num-

---

RESEARCH IN NURSING PRACTICE, 1970-1975

Procedure or technique
1. Monitoring techniques
2. Physical care techniques
3. Psychiatric treatments
4. Teaching techniques
5. Assessment techniques
6. Organization of staff

Specific needs of patients
Physical needs
1. Food and nutrition
2. Rest and sleep
3. Cleanliness
4. Exercise
5. Elimination
6. Respiration
7. Relief of pain
8. Protection
9. Medication

Nonphysical needs
1. Emotional support
2. Communication
3. Recreation
4. Religious
5. Family

Status
1. Inpatients
2. Outpatients
3. Healthy client

Age
1. Neonates
2. Children
3. 18 through 64 years
4. 65 and over

Specific patient states
1. Anorexia
2. Anxiety and fear
3. Bedridden
4. Dying
5. Fever
6. Healthy
7. Hyperactivity or hypoactivity
8. Incontinence or constipation
9. Infection, inflammation
10. Insomnia
11. Malnutrition
12. Nausea
13. Pain or distress
14. Prematurity
15. Preoperative or postoperative states
16. Reactions to nursing
17. Psychological maladaptation
18. Shock
19. Unconsciousness

From O'Connell KA and Duffey M. In Chaska NC, editor: The nursing profession: views through the mist, New York, 1978, McGraw-Hill Book Co.

---

ber of dimensions including investigator characteristics, study content, and research methods. Study content was specifically classified according to the general diagnostic category of the subjects (primarily reflecting traditional medical specialty areas), the procedure or technique investigated, the specific needs of patients addressed in the research (including physical and nonphysical needs), and the state of condition of the subject.

Sigma Theta Tau International recently revised the research topic category system used in compiling its Directory of Nurse Researchers.[21] The box on p. 81 contains descriptive information about the Sigma Theta Tau members research as well as the current research topics . The timeliness of this topic was also emphasized by the inclusion of a well-attended symposium, "The development of a taxonomy for nursing research," sponsored by the American Nurses' Association's Cabinet on Nursing Research, at the 1987 International Nursing Research Conference in Arlington, Virginia.

STRUCTURE OF THE DISCIPLINE OF NURSING

To date there has been little similarity in the systems used to classify general or specialized areas of nursing research. The only distinction that has endured for the last 25 years is that between clinical and nonclinical research, or, stated another way, between research related to nurses and nursing and research related to clinical practice. My concern about these

---

SIGMA THETA TAU INTERNATIONAL: DIRECTORY OF NURSE RESEARCHERS, 1987

1. **Descriptive information**
   Nursing model usage
   Ages of human subjects
   Categories of human subjects
   Species of animal subjects
   Sites of current research activities
   Funding source for current research activities
   Methodology

2. **Current research topics**
   A. Environment and health
   B. Clinical topics
      1. Development stages and events
      2. Emotional states and feelings
      3. Mental states
      4. Physiological states
      5. Functional ability and restoration
      6. Health problems, pathological states, and disease categories
      7. Health problems and unhealthy behaviors
      8. Health promotion and wellness behaviors
      9. Parent-infant health and parenting
      10. Family health
      11. Women's health
   C. Nursing care
      1. Nursing care and assessment
      2. Nursing care and interventions
   D. Cultural research
   E. Historical studies
   F. Methodologic research
   G. Nursing education
   H. Nursing philosophy
   I. Professional issues
   J. Systems research
      1. Multisystem issues
      2. Patterns of care

From Sigma Theta Tau International, Directory of nurse researchers, Indianapolis, 1987.

---

distinctions is that they set up unnecessary polarities that tend to divide rather than unify our scientific efforts.

A more recent distinction with little practical utility is that between basic and applied research. Part of the problem is that the parameters of applied research often are so narrowly constructed as to include only the direct practice of nursing in the clinical setting. It is inappropriate and divisive to exclude philosophical, ethical, historical, economic, political, social, and cultural concerns from the study of clinical nursing. My own definition of clinical or applied research is any investigation in which clients or client analogues are among the dependent or descriptive variables.

There is general agreement within the discipline regarding the components of nursing's metaparadigm: person, environment, health, and nursing. These concepts were used by Ozbolt and others in developing a classification system of nursing-related dissertations for University Microfilms International (see box on page 82). The major categories are age-related client groupings (including family and community as clients), nurses and the nursing profession, and methodological issues.

In 1978 Donaldson and Crowley[5] provided the discipline of nursing with a general direction that remains relevant today. They proposed that:

From its perspective, nursing studies the wholeness or health of humans, recognizing that humans are in continuous interaction with their environments. Nursing's perspective evolves from the practical aim of optimizing of human environments for health.

Examples of major conceptualizations are listed on p. 82.

In June 1983 I presented a paper at the Forum on Doctoral Education in Nursing held at New York University. The paper, "Emerging Content in Nursing," was based on a content analysis of 319 dissertations from nursing doctoral programs from 1976 to 1982.[13] Two models were developed for the content analysis, one for the study of clinical nursing and the other for the study of social issues in nursing.

The model for the study of clinical nursing was used to analyze all dissertations in which patients or patient analogs were among the study variables—in most cases, the dependent variable (see box on p. 82). Categories were developed by reading the dissertation abstracts and relating them to the American Nurses' Association (ANA) definition of nursing in *Nursing: A Social Policy Statement:* "Nursing is the diagnosis and treatment of human responses to actual or potential health problems."[2] This definition implies a multivariate model in which all human response systems interact with all actual or potential health problems and

CLASSIFICATION OF NURSING-RELATED DISSERTATIONS BY UNIVERSITY MICROFILMS INTERNATIONAL

1. **Infants***
2. **Children***
3. **Adolescents***
4. **Adults***
5. **Elderly***
6. **Age not specified**

7. **Family**
   Family systems
   Environment
   Health and illness
   Nursing care
   Other professional services

8. **Community**
   Needs and epidemiology
   Access to service and financing
   Occupational health and safety
   Community health programs and services

9. **Nurses and the nursing profession**
   Education
   Licensure and certification
   Nurses
   Nursing practice
   Management of nursing services
   History and image of nursing
   Nursing theory
   Ethical issues
   Legal issues

10. **Methodological issues**
    Psychometrics
    Statistical methods
    Animal models

*Subsystems for categories 1 through 5: person; environment; health/illness; and nursing care/services/intervention.

MAJOR CONCEPTUALIZATIONS IN NURSING

1. Distinctions between human and nonhuman beings
2. Distinctions between living and nonliving
3. Nature of environments and human-environmental interactions from cellular to societal levels
4. Illness versus health and well-being
5. Functioning of the whole human organism versus functioning of the parts
6. Levels of functioning of whole organisms
7. Human characteristics and natural processes, such as consciousness, abstraction; adaptation and healing; growth; change; self-determination, development; aging; dying; reproducing; drive satisfaction; and relating.

From Donaldson SK and Crowley DM: Nurs Outlook 26:119, 1978.

CATEGORIES FOR THE STUDY OF CLINICAL NURSING

A. **Actual or potential health problems**
   1. Developmental life changes
   2. Acute health deviations
   3. Chronic health deviations
   4. Cultural and environmental stressors

B. **Human response systems**
   1. Physical
   2. Emotional
   3. Cognitive
   4. Family
   5. Social
   6. Cultural

C. **Clinical decision making**
   1. Data collection
   2. Diagnosis
   3. Planning
   4. Treatment
   5. Evaluation

From Loomis ME: Nurs Res 34:113, 1985.

with the clinical decision-making process. Despite the obvious inadequacy of the ANA definition in the area of health promotion, one implication of the model is that there is no need for nursing intervention without a human response system interacting with an actual or potential health problem.

The model for the study of social issues in nursing was used to analyze all the dissertations in which nurses, nursing, or social issues were the objects of study (see box on p. 83). The categories were developed by reading the dissertation abstracts and con-

sulting with experts conducting research on social issues. Professional and policy issues (Category D) were defined as questions related to the knowledge base, learning, and science of nursing or to a course of action adopted as expedient. Subcategories included studies in which education, socialization and

---

**CATEGORIES FOR THE STUDY OF SOCIAL
ISSUES IN NURSING**

D. Professional and policy issues
 1. Education
 2. Socialization and role
 3. Ethics
 4. Organization
 5. Economics
 6. History
 7. Politics

E. Unit of analysis
 1. Individual
 2. Group
 3. Organization
 4. Profession
 5. Culture
 6. Nation

F. Social decision making
 1. Documentation of existing conditions
 2. Diagnosis of problem areas
 3. Planning for social and collective action
 4. Policy implementation and planned social in-
    fluence
 5. Evaluation-maintenance-revision

From Loomis ME: Nurs Res 34:113, 1985.

role, ethics, organization, economics, history, or politics were included in the theoretical formulation of the research.

The units of analysis or dependent variables in the study of social issues in nursing were individuals, groups, organizations, professions, cultures, and nations. The social decision-making process used for this analysis was a modification of a more detailed model of the social policy proposed by Rose.[19]

The results of the content analysis were published in *Nursing Research*[13] and elaborated in the second edition of *Current Issues in Nursing*.[14] For the purposes of this chapter I would like to focus on the changes I have made in the original classification system and subcategories, based on my experiences in conducting the original study and on feedback from colleagues.

RECENT MODELS

To begin with, I have attempted to expand the ANA definition of nursing. Hall and Allan[11] have proposed a definition of nursing that acknowledges the two dis-

tinct realms of illness and health: "Nursing is concerned with the phenomena of human responses to illness and health." More recently Schlotfeldt[20] asserted, "Nursing is the appraisal and the enhancement of the health status, health assets, and health potentials of human beings." This definition focuses the discipline of nursing entirely on health.

The model with which I am currently working is based on a series of new assumptions and definitions. The primary definitional change is that nursing is the science of health and healing (see Fig. 11-1). Nursing science includes empirical observation, basic theory, and application theory. Therefore all professional nurses should be engaged in the development of nursing science. Nursing science can be subdivided into (1) the study of clinical nursing therapeutics and (2) the study of social issues in relation to nursing.

Clinical therapeutics is concerned with health-related human responses and nursing interventions as they apply to all client populations in all private and public settings (see Fig. 11-2). Clinical therapeutics can be conceptualized along several interrelated dimensions: (A) human responses and related nursing interventions, (B) client populations, and (C) the health environment. These dimensions correspond with nursing's metaparadigm concepts of health, nursing, person, and environment in a set of relationships that emphasize the multivariate nature of health and nursing interventions, persons across the life span within the family context, and the health environment.

The relationship between human responses and nursing interventions is especially important. Health-promotion interventions must be studied and implemented in light of what is considered to be normal growth and development for selected client populations within a specific health environment. Health-restoring interventions are directed toward the responses of individuals and families to acute health deviations. Health-supporting interventions are dircted toward the responses of individuals and families to chronic health deviations. Of course in the real world of clinical practice holistic nursing care might consist of a combination of preventive, restorative, and supportive interventions as required for a client in an acute episode of a chronic illness who is also engaged in tasks appropriate to a particular stage of growth and development.

Social issues in nursing are concerned with health-related responses that extend beyond the individual

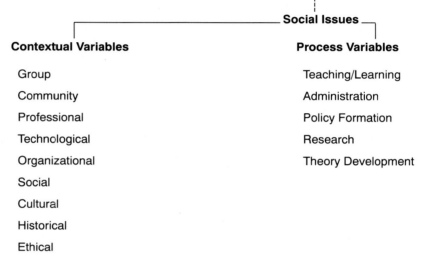

Fig. 11-1 Model for the development of nursing science.

and family (see Fig. 11-3). This model is less developed because clinical therapeutics is my area of expertise. I think it is important, however, to acknowledge and develop our understanding of the various contexts in which nurses practice health and healing and the various processes by which we attempt to influence the health of individuals, families, groups, and societies. We must continue to examine the interfaces among the science of health and healing and theories from the humanities and social sciences to understand and influence health in the larger political, social, and international contexts.

The subcategories of health issues have been left blank to allow for the changing nature of what constitutes a health issue. Genetic engineering, surrogate mothering, euthanasia, and organ transplants are among the most relevant health issues today. Tomor-

row's issues may be entirely different, but will also require consideration in the contexts of groups, professions, technologies, societies, cultures, history, and ethics. The process variables of teaching and learning, administration, policy formation, research, and theory development refer to areas of derived application theory that nurses must learn and apply to the study of health-related social issues.

Both of these categorizations can be used to classify the research in which nurses are engaged. At the 1987 inaugural meeting of the Southern Nursing Research Society I was able to classify the 45 research presentations and posters using either the model for the study of clinical therapeutics or the model for the study of social issues in nursing. For example, a study titled "Post-Surgical Recovery and the Use of Self-Regulatory Strategies" was classified as A-2, B-2, and

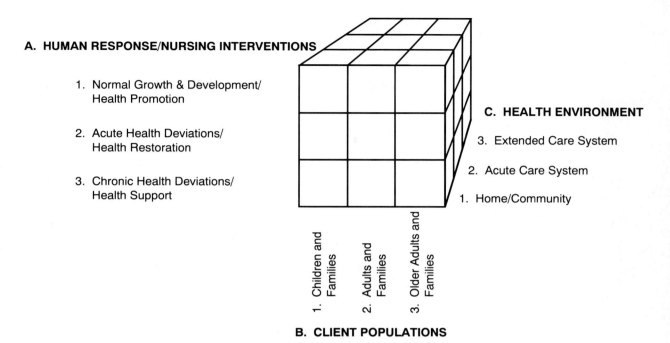

A. HUMAN RESPONSE/NURSING INTERVENTIONS

1. Normal Growth & Development/
   Health Promotion

2. Acute Health Deviations/
   Health Restoration

3. Chronic Health Deviations/
   Health Support

C. HEALTH ENVIRONMENT

3. Extended Care System

2. Acute Care System

1. Home/Community

1. Children and Families
2. Adults and Families
3. Older Adults and Families

B. CLIENT POPULATIONS

Fig. 11-2 Model for the study of clinical therapeutics.

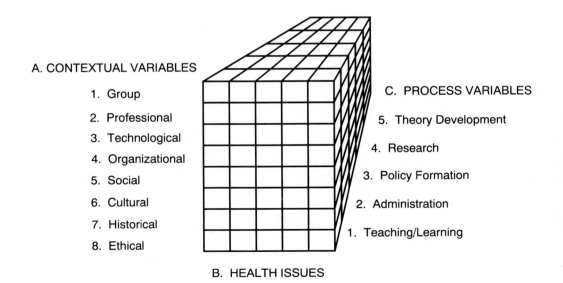

A. CONTEXTUAL VARIABLES

1. Group
2. Professional
3. Technological
4. Organizational
5. Social
6. Cultural
7. Historical
8. Ethical

C. PROCESS VARIABLES

5. Theory Development

4. Research

3. Policy Formation

2. Administration

1. Teaching/Learning

B. HEALTH ISSUES

Fig. 11-3 Model for the study of social issues in nursing.

C-2 on the clinical classification grid. Another study, "The Influence of Esther Lucille Brown on Nursing Education: An Oral History," was classified as D-1, E-4, and F-4 on the social issues classification grid. I found these classification schemes fairly easy to apply and hope that they will prove useful in the future.

In summary, the development of classification systems that can be used to organize nursing knowledge is an important endeavor. There has been debate as to whether a uniform classification system can be developed to categorize the practice of nursing and nursing research or whether two separate classification systems are required. My experience suggests that it is possible to develop a single classification system, and I believe that we should conceive of nursing research and practice as convergent.

Several years ago the faculty of the School of Nursing at the University of Wisconsin at Eau Claire revised their curriculum based on the Loomis-Wood model[15] (the original version of Fig. 11-2). Many Eau Claire faculty and graduate students have conducted their research using this model, and Luther Hospital in Eau Claire is currently organizing their nursing assessment and care planning according to the model. My contact with the nursing community in Eau Claire has been exciting, stimulating, and humbling.

It is my hope that others will experience this excitement and intellectual stimulation and will contribute to development of a uniform classification system for the discipline of nursing.

REFERENCES

1. Abdellah FG: Overview of nursing research, 1955-1968, parts 1, 2, and 3. Nurs Res 19:6-17; 151-162; 239-252, 1970.
2. American Nurses' Association: Nursing: a social policy statement, Kansas City, Mo, 1980, The Association.
3. Barnad KE and Neal MV: Maternal-child nursing research: review of the past and strategies for the future, Nurs Res 26:193, 1977.
4. Brown AF: Research in nursing, Philadelphia, 1958, WB Saunders Co.
5. Donaldson SK and Crowley DM: The discipline of nursing, Nurs Outlook 26:113, 1978.
6. Ellis R: Fallibilities, fragments and frames: contemplation on 25 years of research in medical-surgical nursing, Nurs Res 26:177, 1977.
7. Gortner SR, Bloch D, and Phillips TR: Contributions of nursing research to patient care, J Nurs Adm, p 23, March-April 1976.
8. Gortner SR and Nahm HE: An overview of nursing research in the United States, Nurs Res 26:10, 1977.
9. Gould SJ. The mismeasure of man, New York, WW Norton Co, Inc., p. 21.
10. Gunter LM and Miller JC: Toward a nursing gerontology, Nurs Res 26:208, 1977.
11. Hall BA and Allen JD: Sharpening nursing's focus by focusing on health, Nursing and Health Care 7(6):315, 1986.
12. Highriter ME: The status of community health nursing research, Nurs Res 26:183, 1977.
13. Loomis ME: Emerging content in nursing: an analysis of dissertation abstracts and titles—1976-1982, Nurs Res 34:113, 1985.
14. Loomis ME: Emerging nursing knowledge. In McCloskey JC and Grace MK, editors: Current issues in nursing, ed 2, Boston, 1985, Blackwell Scientific Publications Inc.
15. Loomis ME and Wood DJ. Cure: the potential outcome of nursing care, Image: The Journal of Nursing Scholarship 15(1):4, 1983.
16. Notter LE. Essentials of nursing research, New York, 1974, Springer Publishing Co.
17. O'Connell KA and Duffey M: Research in nursing practice: its present scope. In Chaska NC, editor: The nursing profession: views through the mist, New York, 1978, McGraw-Hill Book Co.
18. Roberts MM. American nursing: history and interpretation, New York, 1954, Macmillan Publishing Co.
19. Rose R: The dynamics of public policy, Beverly Hills, Calif, 1976, Sage Publications.
20. Schlotfeldt RM: Defining nursing: a historic controversy, Nurs Res 36:64, 1987.
21. Sigma Theta Tau International, Directory of nurse researchers, Indianapolis, 1987.
22. Sills GM: Research in the field of psychiatric nursing, Nurs Res 26:201, 1977.
23. Simmons LW and Henderson V: Nursing research: survey and assessment, New York, 1964, Appleton-Century-Crofts.

CHAPTER 12

Classification of nursing research

RUTH M. BARNARD

Classification of the knowledge developed by nurse researchers is essential to efficiently share that knowledge with others and to promote its further development. Until relatively recently no system, other than bibliographic indexes, was available to aid in this classification. Bibliographic indexes using keywords are familiar to many nonlibrarians and can be used by specialists to search for library material. However, these indexes were developed to classify articles rather than to encompass entire research programs. Recent changes to these classification systems make them more attractive for categorizing nursing research. Many scholars would like to see a system unique to nursing. This goal may not be feasible or even desirable. The focus should be on the problem, rather than on the professional credentials of the researcher. Classification of nursing research will help researchers to locate possible collaborators, doctoral students to locate potential mentors, and practitioners to locate research related problem areas.

Several criteria describe a classification system:

- Categories and labels are well defined, allowing high reliability of classification
- Terminology is understandable and used by professionals in the discipline
- The highest levels in the classification are the broader, more global terms, with subcategories subsumed
- There is a means available to add additional categories and subcategories
- Retrieval of meaningful information is possible with reasonable flexibility.

NURSING CLASSIFICATION SYSTEMS

Different systems of nursing research classification have been described over the last few decades. One of the earliest was developed by Henderson and others

---

HENDERSON'S NURSING RESEARCH CLASSIFICATION SYSTEM

A. Historical, philosophical, and cultural (9 subcategories)
B. Occupational orientation and career dynamics (9 subcategories)
C. Specialties in nursing by occupational categories (6 subcategories)
D. Nursing organizations and organizations including nursing (3 subcategories)
E. Administration of nursing services in hospitals, clinics, public health, and other agencies (5 subcategories)
F. Nursing care (6 subcategories)
G. Patients' reactions and adjustments to identifiable variables related to their illnesses (6 subcategories)
H. Interaction patterns among nurse, patient, patient's family, other nurses, physicians, and other members of the health team (5 subcategories)
I. Nursing education (8 subcategories)
J. Conducting research—facilities, personnel, support, and method (12 subcategories)

From Simmons LW and Henderson V: Nursing research: a survey and assessment, New York, 1964, Appleton-Century-Crofts.

---

in the late 1950s to classify research projects as part of the Nursing Studies Index. In their project, funded by the National Institutes of Health (NIH) to survey and assess studies in nursing, identify omissions and gaps, and appraise developing trends and research potential, Simmons and Henderson[8] provided essentially the first classification system for nursing research (see box above).

Many of the nursing studies up to this time were primarily educational, administrative, or occupational; there were few clinical nursing studies. The largest number of subcategories occurred under the "conducting research" category. The subcategories under nursing care were especially interesting, and included *medical* specialties such as "maternal and child care"; "procedures and techniques, considered without reference to a particular ailment"; a subcategory "focused on certain patient states (body constitution), or conditions, and without reference to a particular disease, such as anoxia, fever, and insomnia;" another subcategory called "special aspects of nursing care applicable to most patients" such as "assessing patients' nursing needs" and "helping patients to relieve, control, or tolerate pain;" and a subcategory on "studies in the evaluation of nursing care." Henderson's system is most impressive, but retrieval of information may pose a problem. As with most systems, it is easier to put things in places than to find where you put them. However, it is possible that this classification system may have been adaptable for the Sigma Theta Tau classification had we been aware of it at the time.

In 1973, 1980, and 1984 the American Nurses' Association (ANA) published a *Directory of Nurses with Doctoral Degrees*[1-2a] featuring two indexes, one by major area of doctoral study and the other by current research or academic activities. The earlier editions included some broad categories with subcategories, although there was some overlap. In the 1984 Directory[2a] the Index of Current Research or Academic Activities was changed to eliminate the broad categories and consisted of 179 separate categories, ranging from "Acute care" to "Women's issues." Some categories have many nurses listed, such as "Gerontology," which has 394 nurses. Other categories, such as "Physics" and "Transplants," have only one or two nurses listed. No definitions were provided. The words or phrases identifying the categories are self-evident, although it is not clear how one would choose one category over a similar one. For example, someone looking for persons focusing on family planning would have to consider the nurses listed under "Maternal health," "Women's health," or possibly "Attitudes and beliefs." Someone looking for persons focusing on AIDS patients would probably have to consider the nurses listed under "Infections" or "Immunology." As with any categorization system, it is hard to know when to add new categories and what terminology to use so that usage is up to date.

Ozbolt and others[7] recently developed categories for classifying nursing-related dissertations for University

---

UMI CLASSIFICATION OF NURSING-RELATED DISSERTATIONS

1. Infants*
2. Children
3. Adolescents
4. Adults
5. Elderly
6. Family
7. Community
   a. Needs/epidemiology
   b. Access to service/financing
   c. Occupational health and safety
   d. Community health programs/services
8. Age unspecified and indeterminate
9. Nurses and the nursing profession
   a. Education
   b. Licensure and certification
   c. Nurses
   d. Nursing practice
   e. History and image of nursing
   f. Nursing theory
   g. Ethical issues
   h. Legal issues
10. Methodological issues
    a. Psychometrics
    b. Biophysical measures
    c. Statistical methods
    d. Animal models

From Ozbolt JG *and others*. In Nursing: a catalog of selected doctoral dissertation research, Ann Arbor, Mich, 1986, University Microfilms International.
*Categories 1 through 6 and 8 have the following subcategories: a, person; b, environment; c, health/illness; and d, nursing care/services/intervention.

Microfilms International (see the box above). They used developmental stages as the major categories, with the nursing metaparadigm—"Person, Environment, Health, Illness, and Nursing Care/Services/Intervention"—under each major heading. In addition to the developmental stages, three other major categories were used, each with several subcategories. Dissertations can be classified according to this system because dissertation titles tend to be long and complex. However, retrieval from this system is problematic. Unless one knows what age to search under, it will be difficult to locate either nursing or medical diagnoses. The attempt to use a nursing framework is laudatory; however, the way it is applied under each developmental heading does not facilitate the search for information.

INDEX MEDICUS AND CINAHL SUBJECT HEADINGS

A. Anatomy
B. Organisms
C. Diseases
D. Chemicals and drugs
E. Analytical, diagnostic, and therapeutic techniques and equipment
F. Psychiatry and psychology
G. Biological sciences
H. Physical sciences
I. Anthropology, education, sociology, and social phenomena
J. Technology, industry, agriculture, food
K. Humanities
L. Information science and communication
M. Named groups
N. Health care

From Cumulative Index to Nursing and Allied Health Literature 23(1), Jan-Feb 1988; and Index Medicus 29(1), part 2, January 1988.

BIBLIOGRAPHIC INDEXES

Bibliographic indexes, primarily used for categorizing published articles, also were considered for the Sigma Theta Tau classification. The Sigma Theta Tau classification was to provide a method of classifying an investigator's research program, but these indexes were used mainly to classify journal articles into two or three categories. Each article typically represents only a small part of an investigator's program. Most research programs encompass or fit into many more categories.

Index Medicus,[6] published by the National Library of Medicine (NLM), uses medical subject headings (MeSH) that are maintained and revised by the NLM. The major headings are shown in the box above. Nursing is a subcategory under a few of these headings. Most nursing subcategories have a few subcategories listed under them. Many categories appropriate to categorize nursing research are included under other headings, because the categorizations are not unique to nursing. The current listing is an increase from the 1979 listing (which was considered for the Sigma Theta Tau classification), when only about 25 categories were included under "nursing." The appropriate context for a subheading is not always evident to the classifier, or perhaps even to a nurse in another field. Part of the

problem with classification is that the language and categories are not always part of the existing systems. For example, in *Index Medicus* nursing diagnosis is equated with nursing assessment and is placed under "health services administration, health care."

Obviously, much of the research done by nurse researchers would not be listed under the limited MeSH heading "nurse or nursing." MeSH uses medical terminology for labels and the medical model for structure. New headings are added to the MeSH by the NLM[6] according to their policy:

"Criteria for selection of subject headings are: frequency of term usage in the medical literature; recognition of need for the term by various users of MeSH; recommendation by advisory panels on terminology; and the ability to assign relatively clear and precise definitions to the term.

There are efforts underway to expand these classifications and to incorporate additional nursing terminology. It is interesting to note some of the classifications that are part of the MeSH system. For example, in MeSH "nursing theory" is categorized under "health occupations, biological sciences" (G2). The category "mental/visual/guided imagery" is not yet included in *Index Medicus*. The closest classification appears to be "imagination," which falls under "psychological processes and principles, Mental Processes, Cognition" (F2).

The *Cumulative Index to Nursing and Allied Health Literature (CINAHL)*, started in 1956 as the first index to nursing periodicals, has evolved a thesaurus of more than 3600 index terms.[5] Each term is linked with one or more of the 14 primary headings, the same as the headings used by *Index Medicus*. Approximately 30% of the terms are unique to nursing or the allied health professions. *CINAHL* underwent significant changes in reconstructing its subject heading list in 1983, prior to allowing computer access in 1984. They instituted a numbering system resulting in a tree structure for retrieval very similar to that of *Index Medicus*. They also identify and include many non-MeSH and non-*CINAHL* headings. Changes are made annually to improve the indexing of headings and to add new headings. The changes made to the 1988 subject heading list included very substantive improvements. One welcome addition was to change "models, theoretical" to "nursing models, theoretical" and to list each of the well-known nursing theorists with the name of the theory. However, it is difficult to understand why

Mental states (5 subcategories)
Parent-infant health/parenting (10 subcategories)
Physiological states (18 subcategories)
Women's health (6 subcategories)

Cultural research (6 subcategories)
Environment and health (13 subcategories)
Historical research (11 subcategories)
Methodological research (5 subcategories)
Nursing care
Assessment (5 subcategories)
Interventions (33 subcategories)

Nursing education (11 subcategories)
Nursing philosophy (6 subcategories)
Professional issues (14 subcategories)

Systems research
Multisystem issues (13 subcategories)
Patterns of care (16 subcategories)

From Barnard RM, Kiener ME, and Fawcett J, editors: Directory of nurse researchers, ed 2, Indianapolis, 1987, Sigma Theta Tau.

Persons completing the questionnaire were asked to mark all the categories describing their current research and to be as descriptive as possible. The "other" category was used by many. Sometimes a new category was added, but many times the suggested category duplicated one already in existence. Refinements were made. For example, the original category of "women as caretakers" was modified to "caretakers." It remained under the heading "women's health" and should be moved in future uses.

Self-classification using controlled vocabulary can lead to problems. Definitions were provided only for

classification system, we were unaware of Henderson's work on classification. Although our categories do not cover exactly the same areas, several similarities are evident. Henderson's "interaction" category is covered in the Sigma Theta Tau "clinical topics, health promotion, interpersonal relationships" category and in the "nursing care, interventions" category. One might argue that the Sigma Theta Tau listing does not adequately cover research related to interactions among professionals, such as nurse-physician relationships. Considerable research on professional relationships was conducted in the 1950s and 1960s, as compared to the 1970s and 1980s. There seemed to be no need for that category, judging by the responses of the persons completing the Sigma Theta Tau questionnaire. An area covered less by Henderson is the Sigma Theta Tau category of environment and health. This, too, may reflect the difference in research emphasis over time.

Reference was made previously to retrieval emphasis. Although some advisors did not support the inclusion of disease or syndrome categories, we believed it was important to be able to identify researchers working with patients in selected disease or syndrome categories. Whatever the client's disease, syndrome, or developmental stage, the investigator must understand its impact on the problem being studied in order for their research to be helpful to researchers looking at other problems in the clients. For example, research being conducted on problems associated with Alzheimer's disease might be classified using categories such as "impaired skin integrity," "sleep pattern disturbance," or "coping." A researcher studying other problems associated with Alzheimer's would be unable

CINAHL classified nursing models under "physical science" (H1).

SIGMA THETA TAU CLASSIFICATION

In 1979 the Sigma Theta Tau Research Committee was charged by Sigma Theta Tau President-elect Carol Lindeman with developing a research depository and a directory of nurses with their research activities and interests. The directory and the depository were to serve as a source of information to facilitate communication and promote collaboration among nurse researchers. The responsibility to lead this effort fell to me, as chairperson of the committee. It was evident from the outset that a system of classification would be needed either for a depository or to identify activities and interests. A survey of available classification systems included several of those mentioned above as well as the system used by the Southern Regional Education Board (SREB). The SREB had collected unpublished research abstracts for a few years. Their classification system was seen as insufficiently complex for the large-scale endeavor visualized for Sigma Theta Tau. The SREB work sensitized us to the significant editorial load of handling unpublished abstracts. Their experiences helped us decide to put the depository on the back burner and to develop a classification system to be used with a directory of nurse researchers. We did incorporate into the Directory listing a marker where the researcher indicated an abstract to share on given topics, but chose not to handle the abstract itself at least for the time being.

At that time neither *Index Medicus* nor *CINAHL* provided the kind of categorization for nursing research that we thought desirable or adequate. The development of nursing diagnoses was just under way and not ready for consideration as part of the Sigma

CLASSIFICATION USED IN 1983 (DIRECTORY OF NURSE RESEARCHERS)
Biological (27 subcategories) Clinical (132 subcategories) Environment and health (14 subcategories) History of nursing (15 subcategories) Nursing care delivery (22 subcategories) Nursing education (20 subcategories) Nursing philosophy (8 subcategories) Research methodology (10 subcategories) System research (21 subcategories)

From Barnard RM, editor: Directory of nurse researchers, Indianapolis, 1983, Sigma Theta Tau.

lection of data for the 1983 Sigma Theta Tau *Directory of Nurse Researchers*.[3] Mary Kiener and Jacqueline Fawcett joined me as coeditors of the second edition. Later into the project Marie Sparks was appointed as Director of Library and Information Service for Sigma Theta Tau and was very helpful to us. We modified the 1983 categories by consolidating and renaming them and by adding two new categories, "cultural research" and "professional issues," for the 1987 *Directory of Nurse Researchers*.[4] The classification used in the later edition is shown on page 91.

The emphasis of the classification continued to be on retrieval. Efforts were made to categorize a person's research activities so that retrieval would be possible from several points of view. The general focus was identified as well as additional areas. For example, because it could be helpful to know certain characteristics about the research being conducted or planned, categories were included such as the nursing model used, the ages of subjects, the type of human subjects (clients or patients, students, etc.), the species of an-

to identify these studies as being concerned with Alzheimer's patients, because the listed nursing problems are not necessarily unique to persons with Alzheimer's disease. Another example is research being conducted on problems associated with acquired immunodeficiency syndrome (AIDS). The nursing problems being studied might be classified under the same categories as above—"impaired skin integrity," "sleep pattern disturbance," or "coping." Again, these problems are not unique to persons with AIDS. Before researchers can retrieve nursing research being conducted on problems associated with AIDS, a categorization must be included in the data base.

The example using the AIDS diagnosis points out an additional problem—the addition of new terminology to the field and the changing of existing terminology. The NLM added AIDS to its classification in 1983, but in 1988 changed it to HIV. The changes in knowledge and uses in the field must be incorporated into the classification system. In order to assist the searchers in locating the desired topic, the addition and change in terminology must be carefully recorded and referenced as changes occur.

Our efforts pinpointed three kinds of clinical nursing research: research focused on a particular problem, on a particular assessment or intervention, or on a pattern of care. We categorized these three areas as follows: the particular problem focus was put into "clinical topics," the intervention focus was put into "nursing care," and the focus on pattern of care was put into "systems research." The "clinical topics" classification needs substantive refinement. The 11 secondary headings helped organize this research, but

much more work needs to be done to make categories that are appropriate and will allow efficient information retrieval.

It was difficult to use any nursing framework to organize research headings and categories. Because of the variety of approaches taken by nursing theorists, no single nursing model was adequate. Although there was some desire to use nursing categories, nursing labels are not inclusive of all questions under investigation by nurse researchers. Many medical labels are used by investigators to identify their research and are more meaningful, at least at the present time, in categorizing research programs.

SUMMARY

Developing a classification of nursing research is difficult and tedious. It is important to nursing that some improved system be available to categorize the expanding amount of research, to facilitate retrieval and sharing, and to help identify areas needing research. The categories developed for Sigma Theta Tau are being used by Knowledge Access International of Mountain View, California, to classify research for a project sponsored by the National Center for Nursing Research and to develop a Nursing Research Alert (NRA) to facilitate access to nursing information resources. Sigma Theta Tau is revising the 1987 classification system described above, organizing it under the framework of Person, Health, Environment, and Nursing. I hope these endeavors will contribute to the evolution of a system for classifying nursing knowledge.

REFERENCES

1. American Nurses' Association: Nurses with doctoral degrees, Kansas City, Mo, 1973, The Association.
2. American Nurses' Association, Nurses with doctoral degrees, Kansas City, Mo, 1980, The Association.
2a. American Nurses' Association: Directory of nurses with doctoral degrees, Kansas City, Mo, 1984, The Association.
3. Barnard RM, editor: Directory of nurse researchers, Indianapolis, 1983, Sigma Theta Tau.
4. Barnard RM, Kiener ME, and Fawcett J, editors: Directory of nurse researchers, ed 2. Indianapolis, 1987, Sigma Theta Tau.
5. Cumulative index to nursing and allied health literature 33(1), Jan-Feb 1988.
6. Index medicus 29(1), part 2, January 1988.
7. Ozbolt JG and others: Classification of nursing-related dissertations, in nursing: a catalog of selected doctoral dissertation research, Ann Arbor, Mich, 1986, University Microfilms International.
8. Simmons LW and Henderson V: Nursing research: a survey and assessment, New York, 1964, Appleton-Century-Crofts.

CHAPTER 13

New knowledge from old truths

Problems and promises of historical inquiry in nursing

OLGA MARANJIAN CHURCH

Learning from history is never simply a one-way process. To learn about the present in the light of the past means also to learn about the past in the light of the present. The function of history is to promote a profounder understanding of both past and present through the interrelation between them.

E.H. CARR, *What is History?*

To understand the lessons to be learned from our past, we must first ask for the facts. For the most part, until recently the facts of nursing's history were ignored, neglected, undiscovered, or simply unknown. Although organized nursing in the United States has been in existence for well over a century, the legacy of the nurse in our society during this time has not been adequately examined. Handlin describes history as "the distillation of evidence surviving from the past. Where there is no evidence, there is no history."[10] Without history we would suffer a fate similar to a patient with amnesia; unable to rely on our past to guide us in the present, we could not go forward either. We would be in a state of perpetual confusion.

Fortunately, historical inquiry by nurse scholars such as Lavinia Lloyd Dock (1858-1956) and Mary Adelaide Nutting (1858-1948) was a legitimate pursuit at the turn of the century.[16]

The pioneers' sense of history provided them with a firm foundation for their professional identity and activities. Indeed, this may be the first lesson to learn. That is, historical awareness, a sense of history, can provide a broad framework within which to view nursing as an experience and as a profession. As O'Connell and Russo[17] note:

We look to history for many things: for guidance, for inspiration, for trends that help us understand the present and predict the future, for links that help establish self identity.

The study of our history promises to serve as a vital connection to our collective experiences in the name of nursing. Such connectedness can enhance a sense of continuity in our ongoing development. Exploring the works of our pioneers reveals the relevance of their efforts to our own, and often we come to recognize that the burning issues of today may have been smoldering for decades past. Whether such issues were addressed or allowed to smolder and when and where they came up provide vital data as well. Historical awareness should be viewed as a prerequisite to a professional mentality and identity.

History, broadly defined as the search for truth, relates to our need for knowledge and understanding of the human condition. Eisenstadt[5] refers to historical study as a form of self-consciousness and self identification. "Like every work of scholarship and thought, [the study and writing of history] require that the scholar and thinker come to grips with his society and his age." In other words, historical study promises self-knowledge and becomes the "indispensable first step toward a meaningful inquiry into the present." The implications for nursing were obvious to Ashley[1]:

> Without knowing history, one cannot approach knowing truth . . . Without historical thinking, science can all too easily become a fiction, an illusion, a social lie told with no regard for what is true.

The historical perspective then can provide the knowledge and understanding of our collective past. The awareness of our roots, including past weaknesses, strengths, aspirations, and failures, makes for a mature foundation from which to build our future. The responsible acknowledgment of all that has gone on before in the emergence of our discipline promises an enlightened and credible assertiveness. To hold ourselves accountable to true ownership implies the public commitment required of every professional group, and is fortified by that vital benchmark, autonomy.

Another promising lesson acquired from the actual pursuit of historical inquiry is that historiography, or historical methodology itself, teaches us to develop a healthy skepticism. For just as conclusions and analyses in the experimental or traditional methodologies of research change as more evidence is gathered, so too do historical interpretations. Acknowledged truths of one generation may be discarded by later generations, but this in no way reflects on the truth in its time. Tuchman[20] states that "the story and study of the past, both recent and distant, will not reveal the future, but it flashes beacon lights along the way and it is a useful nostrum against despair." Christy[4] alludes to this when she speaks of the hope that history offers. When discussing the "usable past," Handlin[10] speaks of history's

> capacity for advancing the approach to truth [and maintains that] Truth is absolute. It does not exist because individuals wish it to anymore than the world exists for their convenience. . . . Truth is knowable and will out if earnestly pursued; and science is the procedure or set of procedures for approximating it.

The knowable truth, that is, the available data that can be collected and processed as objectively, accurately, and systematically as is humanly possible, requires some measure of interpretation. Furthermore, the evaluation and synthesis of evidence should result in defensible conclusions. The process includes asking *what* happened (the search for facts) as well as *why*—thus the interpretive task. In addition to the above, historians attempt to satisfy what is commonly referred to as the "so-what factor." This refers to the issues of implications and relevance. Given the complexities inherent in the human condition, historical interpretations are fraught with multiple causation. Tuchman[20] speaks of

> the unknowable variable—namely man [maintaining that] human beings are always and finally the subject of history. History is the record of human behavior, the most fascinating subject of all, but illogical and so crammed with an unlimited number of variables that it is not susceptible of the scientific method nor of systematizing.

Whether one agrees with Tuchman or Handlin about the scientific nature of historical inquiry is not as important as recognizing that the quest for truth is paramount. In addition, "the greater our knowledge of the present, the more relevant can be our inquiries into the past. There is thus a reciprocal relation between historical and current studies."[2] Nevins[15] clearly acknowledges this basic reciprocity when he states that "it is as true to say that current events cast their shadows backward as that coming events cast their shadows before."

The proliferation of developments on all fronts currently impinges on our impulse to "search for implications from the past . . . historical events are explored for their similarities and applications to our current confusion and dilemmas."[11]

Yet the rapidly increasing technological advances in today's society impress us with the need for innovative responses. Some of the patterns of the present may be comprehended through the measured detachment that history provides. Viewing the record of a people or a profession, says Nevins,[15] often clearly reveals that

> immediate results are frequently of slight account compared with the remote results. . . . Those who prefer principle to expediency in the conduct of human affairs are usually right. . . . respect for tradition, the value of continuity in affairs, the importance of dependable habits to a community as to a man, the close connection between principle and rectitude—all this weighs heavily in the balance.

The importance of what we learn from history cannot be overemphasized. A collective sense of history can provide the profession with ideas and options from past encounters with similar issues. Modified, recreated, refined with time and wisdom, our responses can contribute to the evolution of our discipline toward its professional destiny.

We may not find specific answers to nagging questions because history deals best with generalities. Today our resourcefulness is challenged by unprecedented developments in recent history, such as the bomb, the tube, the pill, and the box.[19] We are continually impressed with the awesome power in such developments, but we have yet to measure their impact in any meaningful way.

The bomb, which in the 1940s propelled us into the atomic age, has evolved into the nuclear era of today; the tube began the media blitz of the 1950s, as television increasingly invaded the privacy of our homes and continues to shape our perspective on the world; and in the 1960s revolution was brought about by pills as much as any other development. The Pill transformed the sexual mores of society, and, along with other chemotherapeutic agents, fostered a drug-oriented culture that affects our daily lives. And finally, the box—the computer—has those of us who did not grow up with it struggling to catch up, for we have entered the information age and we are bombarded by too much to fast to assimilate it. With an informed sensitivity to our place in history we may find the strength and the wisdom of humility and patience to proceed along the untraveled path ahead.

We must accept historical truths as they become revealed to us. Ownership of our past includes the acknowledgment that we have not kept up with the vision of those pioneers in nursing at the turn of the century. They saw nursing as more inclusive and involved with educational and preventive aspects of health care.

Stewart, in describing the work of Isabel Hampton at the turn of the century, points to her expectation that nurses possess a broad cultural background. According to Stewart, Hampton urged nurses to have a "familiarity with current events, a knowledge of what is going on in the world of art, literature, and even science."[18]

As for concerns with the preventive aspects of health care, the pioneering work spearheaded by Lillian Wald at the Henry Street Settlement in New York was carried on by nurses throughout the country in the name of public health nursing. For example, when Lystra Gretter[5] became director of the Detroit Visiting Nurse Association, she pointed to the "growing demand for the trained nurse's help in social reform and philanthropy and in scientific protective and preventive work."

Yet in order to keep up with the advances in patient care, nursing has become increasingly narrow and specialized. In the first decade of this century, nursing was not fragmented but inclusive—more inclusive than seems possible to any single practitioner today. The simplicity of the nurse's role was balanced by its numerous responsibilities. The nurse's domain was the family and the community. Home nursing included the health care of all ages, as well as all bodily and mental concerns. The graduate nurses of the early twentieth century could be found in medically unserved and underserved communities, working interdependently with physicians and as advocates for health care consumers.

During the Great Depression the transition of the nursing work force from homes and communities into institutional settings redefined the nurse's role and responsibilities. According to Melosh,[14] the transition to modern nursing in the hospital from its earlier counterpart in the community took less than two decades.

In 1927, nearly three quarters of hospitals with training schools relied exclusively on students for ward nursing services; a decade later, most reported that they had begun to employ some graduate staff nurses. By 1940, nearly half of all nurses were employed in hospitals, and by the end of World War II, a decisive majority of active nurses held hospital jobs.

Although there were certainly advantages to the hospital milieu, it also served to limit opportunities for furthering the development of the nurse's autonomy. This institutionalization of its work force accounts for nursing's narrowing focus and special interests, a result of the influence of the medical model that prevailed in the hospital setting. As long as nursing activity was confined to institutional settings and administered by nonnurses, the nurse's autonomy and development would also be limited.

Consider then the following pragmatic lesson to be learned from history with regard to autonomy and self-determination. Our history is replete with examples of nonnursing experts who were ready and willing to guide and control the development and practice of nurses and nursing. Some were more successful than others. The availability of such "experts" persists today. Yet the promise of shaping its own destiny continues to challenge the profession. Current efforts to establish a national agency for nursing highlight the chronic problems of control and an adequate power base so necessary to self-determination. As Dumas and Felton[7] write:

At various times in the history of professional nursing, we have sought to develop stronger power bases to enable us to determine the direction of our future and to negotiate in our best interest. Success in these endeavors will not be achieved without more solidarity among our ranks. We must pull together to resist forces that threaten to keep us dependent upon conceptions of what others believe to be in our best interest.

The call for solidarity among our ranks has a familiar ring. The nursing pioneers who gathered together at their first meeting at the 1893 World's Fair in Chicago echoed the same sentiment. Edith Draper's words[6] became a ready slogan: "To advance we must unite!—Otherwise factions will arise and stagnation result." And Isabel McIsaac,[13] concerned with what we today might refer to as networking, spoke of the benefits of establishing alumnae associations:

It needs no argument to convince us that "in union lies strength" and "in knowledge, power!" We have for ourselves a most honorable calling, one which compels respect of all mankind. We are just beginning to realize how much higher we may go. . . .

We have fought for firm footing. We can by united effort lift ourselves to honorable permanency. "United we stand, divided we fall!"

Thus there has been a recycling of burning issues dealing with the image, the attitudes, and the power base for nursing. All are interconnected and each relates to the potential advancement or regression of the discipline[7]:

Whatever we do, fulfilling the aspirations of the profession requires internal cohesion, strong collective organization and demonstration that nursing's interest are indeed in the public interest."

Historical inquiry reveals old truths about nursing's past and sheds light on the process of its emergence, helping to determine whether as a profession it has grown up or only grown older. The resurgence of interest in nursing history bodes well for the profession. The old truths to be found will contribute to the ongoing quest for new knowledge. Ultimately the examination and understanding of the historical imperatives in nursing should serve to define its future endeavors.

To be recognized as a viable methodological option for nurse researchers, the historical inquiry of nursing's past must satisfy the so-what factor. Specifically, the relevance of historical research to the practice of nursing must be explicit if the research is to be recognized, supported, and funded. This assumption is based on the current position taken by the National Center for Nursing on prioritizing fundable research.

As a practice-oriented profession nursing may never have the luxury of supporting history for history's sake—but the study of its history for the profession's sake is an imperative increasingly recognized by those who seek a comprehensive approach to understanding nursing's role and function in society.

The challenge for historians is to unequivocally demonstrate the relevance of their efforts to nursing care today and to clearly portray the contributions of the past, both positive and negative, to our present state of affairs. The challenge is not new and must be taken seriously.

For the present, history provides a broad perspective enabling us to be as well informed as possible—to possess the self-knowledge that will enable us to think and act rationally when engaged in decision making with regard to policies that define our discipline.

Looking back, one may be tempted to lay blame elsewhere for obvious shortcomings. Yet in the final analysis, Santayana's advice is worth following: "We must welcome the future remembering that soon it will be the past, and we must respect the past remembering that once it was all that was humanly possible."

REFERENCES

1. Ashley J: Foundations for scholarship: historical research in nursing, Adv Nurs Sci 1:30, 1978.
2. Bellaby P and Oribabor P: The history of the present. In Davies C, editor: Rewriting nursing history, Totowa NJ, 1980, Barnes & Noble.
3. Carr EH: What is history? New York, 1963, Alfred A. Knopf.
4. Christy TE: The hope of history. In Fitzpatrick ML, editor: Historical studies in nursing, New York, 1978, Teachers College Press.
5. Deans AG and Austin AL: The history of the Farrand Training School for Nurses, Detroit, 1936, Alumnae Association of the Farrand School for Nurses.
6. Draper EA: Necessity of an American Nurses' Association. In Nursing of the sick: 1893, New York, 1949, McGraw-Hill Book Co.
7. Dumas RG and Felton G: Should there be a National Institute for Nursing? Nurs Outlook 23:22, 1984.
8. Eisenstadt AS: The craft of American history: selected essays vol 2, New York, 1966, Harper Torchbooks.
9. Hampton I: Training schools for nurses. In Proceeding of the Seventh Annual Conference of Charities and Corrections, Baltimore, 1890.
10. Handlin O: Truth in history, Cambridge, Mass, 1979, Belknap Press of Harvard University Press.
11. Harvey S: Why today's films turn to history, The New York Times, section 2, p 1, Aug 28, 1893.
12. Krug MM: History and the social sciences: new approaches to the teaching of social studies, Waltham, Mass, 1967, Blaisdell Publishing Co.
13. McIsaac I: The benefits of alumnae associations. In Nursing of

the sick: 1893, New York, 1949, McGraw-Hill Book Co.

14. Melosh B: The physician's hand: work culture and conflict in American nursing, Philadelphia, 1982, Temple University Press.

15. Nevins A: The gateway to history, rev ed, Garden City, NY, 1962, Doubleday & Co, Inc.

16. Nutting MA and Dock LL: A history of nursing, 4 vols, New York, 1907-1912, GP Putnam's Sons.

17. O'Connell A and Russo NF, editors: Models of achievement: reflections of eminent women in psychology, New York, 1983, Columbia University Press.

18. Stewarts IM: The education of nurses: historical foundations and modern trends, New York, 1943, Macmillan Publishing Co.

19. Tuchman B: Historical clues to present discontents. In Practicing history: selected essays, New York, 1982, Ballantine.

20. Tuchman B: Practicing history: selected essays, New York, 1982, Ballantine.

CHAPTER 14

A comparison of nursing journals established before and after 1981

KAREN A. O'HEATH
ELIZABETH SWANSON
JOANNE COMI McCLOSKEY

Publishing has become an established means for nurses to convey information, research findings, opinions, and ideas. In addition, publication is expected in all areas of nursing, including administration, education, and clinical settings. Over the past 10 years, many changes have occurred in nursing journals that may affect the way they are perceived by nursing professionals. The purpose of this chapter is twofold: to provide information about multiple aspects of nursing journals and to identify similarities and differences between nursing journals established prior to 1981 and those established between 1981 and 1986.

Many new nursing journals have appeared since McCloskey and Swanson's 1982 survey,[2] thus the distinction in time period established for this paper. The information that follows was taken from the 1986 survey reported by Swanson and McCloskey.[3] As the details of the survey are reported elsewhere, only a brief review is provided here.

Data were collected from October 1985 through February 1986. The sample included nursing and health care journals previously surveyed, as well as others listed in the 1985 Cummulative Index to Nursing and Allied Health Literature. After the first questionnaire and cover letter were mailed, nonresponding editors received a reminder postcard, followed by a second questionnaire, and then a telephone call. Journals were categorized as nursing journals if at least 50% of the audience were nurses. They were grouped into the following content categories: administration, education, general practice, specialty practice, professional development, and research. The specialty practice journals were further categorized by content focus: community, critical care, gerontology, maternal-child,

mental health, nephrology, oncology, operating room, and other specialties.[3]

For this analysis the authors compared the 60 nursing journals established prior to 1981 with the 25 nursing journals established between 1981 and 1986 (Tables 14-1 and 14-2). Content and speciality areas were the same as those used previously.

YEAR ESTABLISHED

The year each journal was established is presented in column 1 of Tables 14-1 and 14-2. The oldest journal is *Midwives Chronicle*, an English journal established in 1887. The oldest U.S. journal is the *American Journal of Nursing*, which was founded in 1900. It is interesting to note that during the 10-year span from 1970 to 1980 36 journals were founded, more than all those established in the previous 82 years. In the first 6 years of the 1980s, 25 journals were founded, 9 of them in 1984 (Table 14-3). This proliferation of journals is indicative of the knowledge explosion in the health sciences.

CIRCULATION

The number of paid subscribers for each journal as of 1985 is listed in column 2 of Tables 14-1 and 14-2. The mean circulations of journals are shown in Table 14-4. The mean circulation for journals established prior to 1981 is 285% larger than those founded in 1981 or later. The circulation ranges within each group are also quite varied. For the journals begun in 1981 or after, the range of circulation is 500 (*Journal of the Association of Pediatric Oncology Nursing*) to 175,000

Text continues on page 106.

Table 14-1 Nursing journals established prior to 1981

Name of journal	1 Year began	2 Circulation	3 Issues per year	4 No. of pages	5 % research	6 Review* procedure
Administration						
Journal of Nursing Administration	1971	14,000	11	12-15	15	3
Nursing Administration Quarterly	1976	3500 [3500]§	4	14-16	25	3
Nursing Management	1970	120,000 [2000]	12	10-15	15	4
Education						
Journal of Continuing Education in Nursing	1969	—	6	10-15	5	3
Journal of Nursing Education	1969	—	9	8-15	25	3
Nurse Educator	1976	4000	6	12-15	15	3
Nursing and Health Care	1980	19,000	10	8-15	10	3
General practice						
American Journal of Nursing	1900	314,000 [6500]	12	10-12	8	3
Australian Nurses' Journal‡	1962	48,198	11	6-8		2
Journal of Practical Nursing	1950	23,000	4	8-12	20	1
The Nurse Practitioner	1975	10,700	12	20	5	3
Nursing '85	1971	511,148 [2672]	12	6-15	0	3
Nursing Times‡	1905	60,000	51	8	0	2
RN	1937	275,000	12	6-12	0	2, 4
Topics in Clinical Nursing	1979	2664	4	20-30		3
Nursing Clinics of North America	1965	7735	4	20	20	4
Nursing‡	1979	15,000	12	7-15	10	1
Specialty practice						
Community						
AAOHN Journal	1951	11,000 [2000]	12	10-15	10	3
Health Visitor‡	1927	15,800	12	10	50	2
Critical care						
Cardiovascular Nursing	1958	AHA mem.	6	15	40	3
Critical Care nurse	1980	26,200 [2000]	6	15-20	5	3
Heart and Lung	1972	60,000	6	12-15	60	3
Journal of Emergency Nursing	1975	18,198	6	6-10	25	3
Gerontology						
Geriatric Nursing	1980	28,000	6	8-10	5	3
Journal of Gerontological Nursing	1974	11,000 +	12	10-12	40	3
Nursing Homes	1950	4500	6	10	10	1
Perspectives	1977	1200	4	5-7	5	1
Maternal-Child						
Birth	1974	—	4-5	10	25	3
Children's Health Care	1971	4500	4	20	40	3
Issues in Comprehensive Pediatric Nursing	1974	1640	6	15-20	5	3
Journal of Obstetric, Gynecologic and Neo- natal Nursing	1972	26,148	6	12-15	35	3
Journal of Nurse-Midwifery	1955	4300	6	15-20	30	2, 4

7 Authors† informed	Time for		Readers' educational background (%)				
	8 Acceptance	9 Publication	10 AD	11 DIP	12 BSN	13 MA	14 PhD
3, 4, 5	6-8 wk	10 mo	20	0	23	45	12
4	2 mo	4 mo		5	10	50	35
2, 4, 5	8 wk	Varies	5	30	40	20	5
3, 4	6 wk	12 mo			20	70	10
3, 4	6 wk	6-12 mo			25	25	50
3, 4	6-8 wk	10-12 mo			10	80	10
2, 4	4-6 mo	2-24 mo	20 BSN or less			60	20
2, 3, 4, 5	2-3 mo	6-12 mo	←40→		60 BSN or higher		
2, 3	2-6 wk	Up to 1 yr					
3, 5	1-2 mo	1 yr	5	2	2	1	
2, 4	6-9 mo	6-12 mo	3	13	31	46	1
2, 4	2-12 wk	4-12 mo	—	—	—	—	—
2, 3, 4	3 mo	6 mo					
2, 4, 5	4-6 wk	6-12 mo	20	40	25	←20→	
2				5	10	80	5
2, 3, 4	Varies	Varies	25	25	25	20	5
3, 4	4-6 wk	3-6 mo	—	—	—	—	—
	1 mo	9-12 mo					
3, 4, 5	4-6 mo	4-6 mo	20	20	20	20	20
2, 3, 4, 5	3-4 mo	6-12 mo	80% BSN or below			15	5
2, 3, 4	6 wk	4-6 mo	21	26	41	10	2
2, 3, 4	2-4 mo	4-6 mo	11	48	29	9	1
2, 4, 5	3-4 mo	1-2 yr	9	29	29	19	1
2, 4	8-10 wk	4 mo +	5				
3	1-2 wk	Unknown	40	10		20	30
3	1 mo	1-12 mo		75	24	0.5	
4, 5	1 wk-6 mo	1-12 mo				60% + PhD	
2, 3, 4	4 mo	6 mo	5	5	60	25	5
4, 5	3-4 mo	1-3 mo	10	20	40	30	
2, 3, 4	4 mo	12-18 mo	13	32	35	18	1
2, 4, 5	2-3 mo	3-6 mo	20	20	25	25	10

Continued.

Table 14-1 Nursing journals established prior to 1981—cont'd

Name of journal	1 Year began	2 Circulation	3 Issues per year	4 No. of pages	5 % research	6 Review* procedure
Maternal-Child—cont'd						
MLN: The American Journal of Maternal/ Child Nursing	1976	38,000 [2500]	6	15	33	3
Midwives Chronical‡	1887	2550	12	10		3
Pediatric Nursing	1975	9750	6	10-12	35	3
Mental health						
Canadian Journal of Psychiatric Nursing‡	1961	5000	4	6-8		4
Issues in Mental Health Nursing	1978	700	4	18-20	60	3
Journal of Psychosocial Nursing and Mental Health Services	1962	13,000	12	4-12	25	3
Nephrology						
Am. Nephrology Nurses' Assoc. Journal	1974	3600	6	10-15	25	3
Oncology						
Cancer Nursing‡	1978		6	10-20	50	3
Oncology Nursing Forum	1974	8100 [1100]	7	12-15	33	3
Operating room						
AANA Journal	1933		6	20	22	3
AORN Journal	1960	33,000	12	15-20	5	3
Point of View Magazine	1963	[52,000]	3	8-12	2	1
Today's OR Nurse	1979	8000	12	8-10	20	3
Other specialties						
American Journal of Infection Control	1973	8075	6	10-20	40	3
Journal of Enterostomal Therapy	1980	2730	6	9-21	15	3
NITA	1977	5400	6	10-20	40	4
Rehabilitation Nursing	1975	5064	6	4-12	15	3
Plastic Surgical Nursing	1980	995	4	12	10	3
Professional development						
Image	1967	64,160	4	10-14	50	3
Imprint	1968	33,000 [2000]	5	5-8	0	1
International Nursing and Review‡	1954	2,100	6	10-12	20	2
Nursing Outlook	1953	19,000	6	12-16	20	3
Nursing Papers/Perspectives in Nursing‡	1969	875	4	15	75-80	3
Research						
Advances in Nursing Science	1978	4200	4	25	25	3
Journal of Advanced Nursing‡	1976	1880	6	20	50	3
Nursing Research	1952	11,700	6	16	85	3
Research in Nursing and Health	1978	1800	4	15	99	3
Western Journal of Nursing Research	1979	1400	4	<20	95	3

*1, Editor makes decision; 2, editor makes decision in collaboration with associate editor(s); 3, decision is based on reviews from established group of experts mediated by editor; 4, other.

†1, No mechanism used; 2, send postcard to indicate receipt of manuscript; 3, indicate expected date of publication in acceptance letter; 4, authors receive proofs or edited manuscript to check; 5, other.

‡Foreign journal.

§Numbers in square brackets indicate nonsubscription circulation.

7 Authors† informed	Time for		Readers' educational background (%)				
	8 Acceptance	9 Publication	10 AD	11 DIP	12 BSN	13 MA	14 PhD
2, 3, 4	6-8 wk	Up to 1 yr			35	35	5
2, 4	Up to 1 mo	Up to 1 yr					
2, 3, 4	3-4 mo	3 mo	15.8	23	43.6	2.5	0.8
3	<1 yr	2 mo	5	90	5		
2, 4, 5	2-6 mo	6-12 mo					
2, 3	3-5 mo	3-5 mo	1	19	32	43	4
2, 3	3 mo	6 mo	20	30	34	7.5	0.33
2, 3, 4	2 mo	6 mo		20	50	20	10
2, 3, 4, 5	6 wk	6-8 mo	13	24	39	21	2
2, 3, 4	2-5 mo	6-18 mo	14	52.5	30	3	0.5
3, 4	6 wk	6 mo		60	40		
2, 5	2 wk	2 yr	10	70	14	5	1
2, 4	4-6 wk	3-4 mo					
2, 4	6-8 wk	4-6 mo	10	46	25	5	2
3, 4	2-3 mo	5-7 mo	25	33	30	8	4
4	5 mo	14 wk +	25	65	10		
2, 3, 4	12-15 wk	2-4 mo	14	19	39	17	11
2, 3, 4	3 mo	6 mo	10	80	8	2	
2, 3, 4	3-6 mo	2-3 mo		35.6	50.3	8.5	11
2, 4	3 mo	1-2 yr	25	25	45		
2, 3	3 mo	1-12 mo	5	20	25	25	25
2, 4	2-3 mo	1-24 mo	2	4	18.5	60.5	15
2, 3, 4	8 wk	6-8 mo	10	10	35	35	10
2, 3, 4	8-12 wk	5 mo			10	40	50
2, 4	4-6 wk	10-12 mo					
2, 4	4-8 wk	9-10 mo					
2, 4	3 mo	6 mo	2	1	12	25	60
2, 4	6 mo	8 mo					

Table 14-2   Nursing journals established 1981 to 1986

Name of journal	1 Year began	2 Circulation	3 Issues per year	4 No. of pages	5 % research	6 Review* procedure
Administration						
Nursing Economics	1983	6100	6	10	30	3, 4
Education						
Journal of Nursing Staff Development	1985	1000	4	12-16	25	3
General practice						
Journal of Christian Nursing	1984	10,348	4	8-10	2	1, 3
Nursing Life	1981	175,000	6	10-15	5	3
Senior Nurse‡	1984	5000 [5000]§	12	8	30	2
Specialty practice						
Community						
Home Healthcare Nurse	1983		6	15	5-10	3
Journal of the Amalgamated School Nurses' Association‡	1983	1000	2	Varies	Minimal	1
Public Health Nursing	1984	829	4	18-20	>50	3
Critical care						
Dimensions of Critical Care Nursing	1982	6000	6	10-15	20	3
Focus on Critical Care	1983	53,894	6	14	5	3
Maternal-child						
Journal of Pediatric Nursing	1986	6	No limit	50	3	
Neonatal network	1982	9000	6	10+	5	3
Mental health						
Psychiatric Nursing Forum	1984	[20,000]		15-20	100	1
Nephrology						
Journal of Nephrology Nursing	1984	1500 [2800]	6	No limit		3
Oncology						
Journal of the Association of Pediatric On- cology Nurses	1984	500	4	10-20	10	3
Operating room						
Canadian Operating Room Nursing Journal	1983	3200 [2800]	6	8-10	3	3
Perioperative Nursing Quarterly	1984	2000	4	12-15	10	3
Ophthalmology						
Journal of Ophthalmic Nursing and Tech- nology	1981	3000	6	10-12	10	3,4
Ophthalmic Nursing Forum	1985	[5100]		10-12	100	1
Other specialties						
Orthopedic Nursing	1982	7296 [1000]	6		10-15	3

7 Authors† informed	Time for		Readers' educational background (%)				
	8 Acceptance	9 Publication	10 AD	11 DIP	12 BSN	13 MA	14 PhD
3, 4	8 wk	12 wk	1.93	9.80	28.9	51.6	7.65
2, 3, 4	8-10 wk	Up to 1 yr					
2	3-4 mo	3-18 mo	24.1	14.2	33	8.9	1
2, 3, 4	2 mo	6-12 mo	40	30	20	5	5
2, 3, 4	4-6 wk	1-6 mo					
5	3-4 mo	6 mo					
3	2 wk	<6 mo					
2, 4	<2 mo	6 mo					
2, 3, 4, 5	6 wk	6-10 mo	5	20	40	30	5
2, 4	3 mo	9-12 mo	20.6	25.4	41.6	8.79	0.16
	9 wk	6 mo					
2, 3, 4	2 mo	6 mo	41	5	43	6	1
3, 4, 5	2-3 mo	4-6 mo					
2, 3, 4	6-8 wk	2-8 wk	28	14	46	12	1
3	2 mo	3-4 mo	20	10	50	10	1
4, 5	3 mo	3 mo			60	35	5
3, 4, 5	6 wk	1-9 mo	30	60	10		
2, 4	6-8 wk	4-5 mo					
	2-3 mo	4-6 mo					
2, 4	12 wk	6-8 mo	17.5	43.2	31.5	7.5	0.3

Continued.

Table 14-2 Nursing journals established 1981 to 1986—cont'd

Name of journal	1 Year began	2 Circulation	3 Issues per year	4 No. of pages	5 % research	6 Review* procedure
Professional development						
Computers in Nursing	1984	5500	6	15-20	40	3
Journal of Professional Nursing	1985		6		33	3
Nursing Success Today	1984	3000	12	4-10	5	1
Scholarly Inquiry for Nursing Practice	1986		3	20		3
Research						
Australian Journal of Advanced Nursing‡	1983	1500	4	8-24		3

*1, Editor makes decision; 2, editor makes decision in collaboration with associate editor(s); 3, decision is based on reviews from established group of experts 4, other.

†1, No mechanism used; 2, send postcard to indicate receipt of manuscript; 3, indicate expected date of publication in acceptance letter; 4, authors receive proofs or edited manuscript to check; 5, other.

(*Nursing Life*). In contrast, the circulation range for journals established prior to 1981 is 700 (*Issues in Mental Health Nursing*) to 511,148 (*American Journal of Nursing*). In addition, approximately 16% of the journals established from 1981 to 1986 have circulations of 1000 or less (*Journal of Nursing Staff Development, Journal of the Amalgamated School Nurses' Association, Public Health Nursing,* and *Journal of Pediatric Oncology Nursing*), whereas only 5% of the journals established prior to 1981 have circulations of 1000 or less (*Plastic Surgical Nursing, Issues in Mental Health Nursing, Nursing Papers/Perspectives in Nursing*). These differences in circulation can be attributed, in part, to the recent establishment of the newer journals and to the fact that they tend to be specialty journals with smaller readerships.

ISSUE FREQUENCY AND MANUSCRIPT LENGTH

The majority of nursing journals in both categories publish 6 times per year or less (column 3 of Tables 14-1 and 14-2). The mode for issue frequency of both categories of journals is 6 times per year (Table 14-4).

The range of annual issue frequency for journals established in 1981 or later is 2 (*Journal of the Amalgamated School Nurses' Association*) to 12 (*Nursing Success Today, Senior Nurse*). The range of annual issue frequency for journals established prior to 1981 is 3 (*Point of View Magazine*) to 51 (*Nursing Times*). Issue

frequency clearly affects the number of manuscripts published annually.

Although preferred manuscript length varies (column 4, Tables 14-1 and 14-2), most editors prefer a typewritten manuscript of between 8 and 20 pages. With an increase in the number of manuscripts submitted for publication, journal editors may be trying to set shorter submissions so that more articles may be published. In addition, as publishing requirements play an increasing role in nursing service, education, and research, editors may be forced to limit manuscript lengths in order to accommodate more submissions. It is also possible that a decrease in the length of manuscripts enables authors to generate more articles from the same piece of research. The differences in issue frequency and manuscript length are minimal between journals established prior to 1981 and those established from 1981 to 1986.

PERCENT OF RESEARCH ARTICLES

The mean percentage of research articles for each category of journals is found in Table 14-4. As can be seen, the means for the two groups are fairly similar. In addition, each group has approximately the same percent of journals in which 50% or more of the articles published are reports of research. Of the journals established prior to 1981, 17.8% publish articles that are research based 50% or more of the time. Similarly, 17.4% of the journals established between 1981 and

7 Authors† informed	Time for		Readers' educational background (%)				
	8 Acceptance	**9** Publication	**10** AD	**11** DIP	**12** BSN	**13** MA	**14** PhD
2, 3, 4	2 mo	6 mo +	10	10	10	40	30
2, 3, 4	2 mo	2-4 wk					
2, 4	1 wk	1 mo					
	90 days	<12 mo					
3, 4	6 wk	3 mo					

‡Foreign journal.
§Numbers in square brackets indicate nonsubscription circulation.

Table 14-3   Year journal established, 1887 to 1986

Year	Frequency	% of total
Prior to 1981		
1887	1	2
1900-1909	2	3
1910-1919	0	
1920-1929	1	2
1930-1939	2	3
1940-1949	0	
1950-1959	8	14
1960-1969	10	17
1970-1980	36	59
TOTAL	60	100
1981 to 1986		
1981	2	8
1982	3	12
1983	6	24
1984	9	36
1985	3	12
1986	2	8
TOTAL	25	100

Table 14-4   Journal characteristics

1981 to 1986	Prior to 1981
Circulation	
Mean: 11,590.6	Mean: 34,041.2
Range: 500-175,000	Range: 700-511,148
Issues per year	
Mean: 5.6	Mean: 7.8
Range: 2-12	Range: 3-51
Mode: 6	Mode: 6
% Research	
Mean: 25.8%	Mean: 27.7%
Time for acceptance	
Mean: 8.3 wk	Mean: 11.1 wk
Range: 1 wk–3-4 mo	Range: 1-2 wk–6-9 mo
Time for publication	
Mean: 20.5 wk	Mean: 32.7 wk
Range: 2-4 wk–3-18 mo	Range: 2 mo-2 yr

1986 publish 50% or more of their articles as reports of research (also see column 5, Tables 14-1 and 14-2). However, these research articles are distributed among varying types of journals. For the group of journals established before 1981, 6 of the 10 with 50% or more of their articles based on research are in the categories of "professional development" and "research" (*Image,*

Nursing Papers/Perspectives in Nursing, Journal of Advanced Nursing, Nursing Research, Research in Nursing and Health, and *Western Journal of Nursing Research*). The remaining 4 journals in which 50% or more of their published articles are research based are found in the specialty practice category (*Health Visitor, Heart and Lung, Issues in Mental Health Nursing,* and *Cancer*

Nursing). In contrast, in the group of journals established between 1981 and 1986, all of those in which 50% or more of the published articles are research based are found in the category of specialty practice (*Public Health Nursing, Journal of Pediatric Nursing, Psychiatric Nursing Forum,* and *Opthalmic Nursing Forum*). It appears that there is an increasing tendency to report research findings in journals other than those designated as research journals. More specifically, an increasing number of published research reports are disseminated through specialty practice journals.

REVIEW PROCEDURE AND AUTHOR INFORMATION

The review procedure for each journal is summarized in column 6 of Tables 14-1 and 14-2. Most acceptance decisions are based on peer reviews (journals usually rely on a group of qualified outside reviewers retained for that purpose) and are mediated by the editor. Editors keep authors informed as to the progress of their manuscripts by a combination of methods (see column 7, Tables 14-1 and 14-2). Both categories of journals provide some form of feedback to authors regarding the progress of their manuscripts through the manuscript review process; this is done primarily by mail.

WAITING PERIOD

The amount of time required for the decision to accept a manuscript for publication is reported in column 8 of Tables 14-1 and 14-2. The average decision time for journals established between 1981 and 1986 is 8.3 weeks, while the time for journals established prior to 1981 is 11.1 weeks. The ranges of acceptance times vary between the groups of journals (Table 14-4). For the journals established between 1981 and 1986, the range is 1 week (*Nursing Success Today*) to 3 or 4 months (*Home Health Care* and *Journal of Christian Nursing*). The range for journals established prior to 1981 is 1 to 2 weeks (*Nursing Homes*) to 6 to 9 months (*The Nurse Practitioner*).

Once the manuscript is accepted for publication, there is a much longer waiting period before actual publication (column 9, Tables 14-1 and 14-2). In addition, the mean publication time is substantially different for each group of journals, with the journals established prior to 1981 taking approximately three months longer for publication (Table 14-4). This dif-

Table 14-5 Reasons for rejection*

Factor	1981 to 1986		Prior to 1981	
	Mean	Rank	Mean	Rank
1. Content inaccurate	4.88	1	4.83	1
2. Content not consistent with purpose	4.78	2	4.45	5
3. Content not important	4.61	3	4.47	3
4. Clinically not applicable	4.30	4	3.38	7
5. Poor research design	4.19	5	4.54	2
6. Content undocumented	4.05	6	4.46	4
7. Poorly written	3.63	7	4.18	6
8. Subject covered recently	3.50	8	3.08	8
9. Content scheduled for future	3.09	9	2.72	9
10. Too technical	2.30	10	2.24	10

*Editor responses: 1, not important; 3, somewhat important; 5, very important.

ference may be partly accounted for by large backlogs of accepted manuscripts, a situation in turn attributable to many nurse authors' greater familiarity with the older journals.

REASONS FOR REJECTION

Factors involved in rejecting a manuscript were rated by editors on a numerical scale. Means were then calculated and rank ordered (Table 14-5). (The most important factors are those with the highest means.) Overall, there was agreement between the two groups as to the most and least important factors contributing to the rejection of a manuscript. One factor that was rated higher by editors of journals established between 1981 and 1986 was manuscript content not consistent with the purpose of the journal. This difference may relate to the more specialized nature of the journals established during this time period and to the fact that prospective authors may not be oriented to the specific focuses of these more recently established journals.

CHARACTERISTICS OF AUDIENCE

The educational background of the journals' readers is presented in columns 10 to 14 of Tables 14-1 and 14-2. The five educational categories were collapsed into two because of the poorer response rate (approximately 48%) for the journals established between 1981 and 1986. The information requested often was not available at the time the editors were surveyed. The two collapsed categories of educational background are (1) associate degree or diploma, and (2) baccalaureate or graduate degree.

For journals established between 1981 and 1986, approximately 35% of the audience are nurses with associate degrees or diplomas, and 65% are baccalaureate nurses and those with higher degrees. *Preoperative Nursing Quarterly* has 90% of its audience composed of associate degree or diploma nurses. On the other hand, 100% of the *Canadian Operating Room Nursing Journal* audience are nurses with baccalaureate or advanced degrees.

Data are comparable for journals established prior to 1981. Diploma or associate degree nurses comprise approximately 40% of the audience for these journals, and nurses with baccalaureate or graduate degrees are approximately 60% of the audience. Three journals have 90% or more of their audiences composed of diploma and associate degree nurses: *NITA* (90%), *Plastic Surgical Nursing* (90%), and *Canadian Journal of Psychiatric Nursing* (95%). Several journals have 90% or more of their audiences composed of nurses with a baccalaureate or higher degree. These journals include *Advances in Nursing Science* (100%), *Nurse Educator* (100%), *Journal of Nursing Education* (100%), *Journal of Continuing Education in Nursing* (100%), *Research in Nursing and Health* (97%), *Nursing Clinics of North America* (95%), *Nursing Administration Quarterly* (95%), and *Nursing Outlook* (94%).

CONCLUSION

The purpose of this chapter has been to provide information about multiple aspects of nursing journals and to identify similarities and differences between nursing journals established prior to 1981 and those established between 1981 and 1986. The information provided is intended to assist nurse authors in selecting a journal that will best match the content of their prospective journal articles. In addition, the information may help authors understand important aspects of the journals of most interest to them, such as reasons for rejection, waiting periods, and audience characteristics.

Differences between these groups of journals center on circulation rates, proportion of research-based articles, waiting time, and reasons for rejection of a manuscript. The circulations of the journals established between 1981 and 1986 are significantly smaller than those journals established prior to 1981, and this can be attributed in part to the fact that the newer journals tend to be specialty journals with smaller readerships. In addition, more reports of research are being published in specialty practice journals established between 1981 and 1986, demonstrating the dissemination of research findings in journals that have a specialized focus and are often practice oriented.

REFERENCES

1. McCloskey JC: Publishing opportunities for nurses: a comparison of 65 journals. Nurs Educ 2:4, 1977.
2. McCloskey JC and Swanson EA: Publishing opportunities for nurses: a comparison of 100 journals, Image 14:50, 1982.
3. Swanson EA and McCloskey JC: Publishing opportunities for nurses: a comparison of publishing policies and practices of 139 journals, Nurs Outlook 34:227, 1986.

CHAPTER 15

The development of nursing service administration as a subdiscipline of nursing and administration in South Africa

PHILDA NOMUSA NZIMANDE

Nursing education in South Africa has made significant strides since the first university chair of nursing science was established in the 1960s. As of January 1986, all professional nursing training previously undertaken by hospital-based nursing schools became affiliated with nursing science departments in universities. In both basic and postbasic nursing education, new perspectives have developed that have had an impact on the discipline.

Nursing has developed numerous subdisciplines; in fact, it is now possible to pursue doctoral study in at least seven nursing subdisciplines in South Africa (see Fig. 15-1).

One of these subdisciplines is nursing service administration, an area drawing on knowledge from both nursing and administration. This chapter addresses issues and education in the developing subdiscipline of nursing service administration.

NURSING THEORY

The accepted definition of nursing in South Africa is a clinical health science practice of persons registered or enrolled under the Nursing Act as nurses or midwives. It is concerned with the diagnosis, treatment, and personalized health care of persons exposed to, suffering, or recovering from physical or mental illness. It encompasses the study of preventive, promotive, curative, and rehabilitative health care for individuals, families, and communities.

Nursing as a science has developed its own body of knowledge derived from practice and research. Nursing practice has a specific philosophical foundation; that is, it embraces a set of values that serve as principal guidelines.

Nursing should be concerned with the individual's physical, emotional, and spiritual well-being. Apart from its instrumental, expressive, and technological functions, nursing also embraces concepts such as compassion, loving care, encouragement, and support.

Nursing is a science grounded in theory. As Thibodeau[7] states, "Every profession has at least, by implication, some pattern to it, that is, it has a prevailing paradigm that should guide its practice, education and research." The nursing paradigm that appears to have universal meaning contains these constant elements: the person or individual; society, in the form of the environment or situation; the health need; and the availability of nursing. As nursing science is a relatively recent discipline, theory development in nursing is in its infancy.

ADMINISTRATION THEORY

Administration theorists and historians agree that administration is involved wherever two or more people take a joint action to achieve an objective. Administration is therefore found in all spheres of human activity.[3,4]

According to Cloete,[3] "Administration thus consists of a wide-ranging set of activities (process) which can be grouped according to their respective function." Administration has many specialized subdisciplines or branches and occurs in a variety of contexts such as health service administration (including hospital administration), social welfare administration, railway

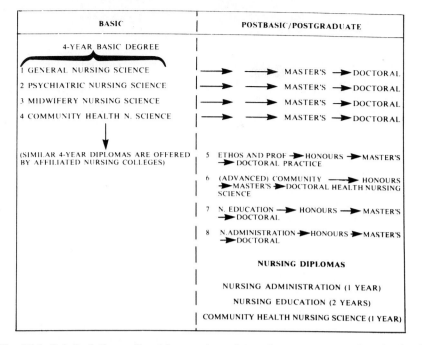

Fig. 15-1 Subdisciplines offered by nursing science departments at university level.

administration, and post office administration, to mention a few. However, all specialized branches of administration must address the same basic issues: policy formulation, organization, financing, personnel, work methods and procedures, and control.

The term *administration* has often been understood in relation to the scientific management movement, which was concerned with the identification of exact scientific principles. This emphasis on exactness and predictability was reflected in the search for scientific principles of administration.

In the private sector the concept of management was identified with the composite of elements contributing to profit maximization. Thus the problems characterizing public institutions were seen as due to the absence of the strategies successfully employed by the private sector. Efficient public administration was thought to require the implementation of principles from the private sector.

Department heads in public institutions, who often come from the ranks of technical specialists, began to call themselves "managers" rather than "public administrators" because of widespread disparagement of the work of the administrator. The perception was that if policy-making could be established as a separate activity, the remaining elements of administration (fi-

nancing, organizing, staffing, work methods, and control) would be susceptible to scientific manipulation. However, this view has not been accepted because exactness and absolute predictability are not the true tests of science. The scientific character of any discipline depends upon a number of other factors, such as methodology. Administration, as a social science, cannot be held to the same standards of exactness and certainty as the physical sciences.

The multitude of definitions of administration can be classified into three main categories: the comprehensive view, the conventional view, and the generic view.

The comprehensive view

In the comprehensive view, administration is perceived as encompassing all group activity aimed at achieving any goal. However, this generalist approach to administration calls for unlimited intellectual ability and practical experience on the part of the administrator, a somewhat unrealistic expectation.

The conventional view

The conventional view of administration occurs in both the private and public sectors. This view is characterized by the dichotomy between specialized and technical work on the one hand and administrative work on the other. On this interpretation the administrator becomes merely a head clerk. Department heads who come from the ranks of specialists, professionals, or technicians are thus more likely to see themselves as "managers" than as administrators. The attempt at an artificial and absolute distinction between administrative and professional personnal often results in serious conflict.

The generic view

In the generic view administration is necessary to maintain job performance in every group effort, and therefore has universal applicability. Thus administration is seen not as the total work of all members of an institution, nor as specifically the work of the "administrative staff," but as an institutional phenomenon directed at the attainment of goals and found in any institutional framework.

Some researchers in South Africa have formulated the following institutional principle:

As individuals rise through any institutional hierarchy their specialized duties (in terms of nature and dimension) decrease in the same rate as their administrative duties increase.[2]

Widespread recognition of this principle has led engineers, geologists, botanists, and other specialists to enroll in courses in public administration. These professionals are heads of departments or institutions and no longer perform their specialized functions on a regular basis. They recognize that their new roles require administrative expertise. Some specialists have actually designed curricula to meet their own particular administrative needs. This is the case in nursing with the subspecialty of nursing administration.

NURSING SERVICE ADMINISTRATION FROM A GENERAL ADMINISTRATIVE PERSPECTIVE

Nursing administration involves the use of generic processes or activities within a nursing situation or health service situation. Arndt and Huckabay[1] define nursing service administration as

the process of setting and achieving objectives by influencing human behavior within a suitable environment. The nursing service administrator, on the other hand, creates the environment that is conducive to the performance of acts by other individuals.

Educators in nursing administration in South Africa share Stevens' view[6] that administration and manage-

ment are not synonymous, but are differentiated on the basis of function. The term *administration* indicates a comprehensive executive role that involves goal establishment, policy formulation, and management. Management in this context is defined as directing the work of others, or facilitating attainment of institutional goals through the use of human and material resources. Thus all administrators manage, but not all managers have administrative power. Some managers are simply responsible for implementing administrative goals and policies that have been determined by others at a higher organizational level.

With respect to nursing administration in South Africa, the prevailing practice is to refer to the nurse who carries on administrative activities as a manager. The nurse at the unit level is referred to as a first-line manager; a supervisor responsible for a group of nursing units is a middle manager; and the nurse who manages all nursing units in the community is a nursing service manager, although she is still occasionally referred to as an administrator.

There is little consistency in the use of the terms *administration* and *management*. Sometimes South African nursing literature states that the two terms are synonymous. If this is so, then a professional nurse in charge of a nursing unit can also be considered an administrator. The discipline of nursing administration should urge greater clarity in the use of these two distinct terms.

NURSING ADMINISTRATION AS A SUBDISCIPLINE OF NURSING

Nursing administration is a collection of activities that enable the practice of nursing. It is carried out, in accordance with predetermined policies, plans, and relevant legislation, when two or more people work together in order to provide the nursing component of health care. Nursing administration is an academic subdiscipline of nursing, and as such its study and research have practical applications for nursing practice.

As previously noted, theory development in nursing is in its infancy. This is particularly true of theory development in nursing service administration in South Africa. There exist a number of individual research projects, but there is as yet no official professional journal dealing with nursing service knowledge, administration theory, and practice in a South African context.

Historically, the position of nursing service administration in South Africa has been based on the European concept of the nurse as a domestic provider and household organizer. Her role was to tend and comfort the sick and to educate others in providing care.

The development of modern hospitals saw a change in the nurse's role that called for educated, skilled people with administrative and leadership abilities. Today the role of the nurse has become very complex due to the demands of the larger health care system. The nurse's role has developed from a mother figure or matron to a nursing service administrator vested with the authority to assume control and to cope with expanding nursing roles. The nursing service administrator, as a leader in the nursing team, must understand the nature of health care needs and problems in a fast-changing society. As services develop, so do the needs of individuals, families, and communities. Nursing service administrators must understand their clientele as well as the environment in which services are provided. Thus the status of health in the society and communities served, the needs and problems of clients, the affordability of services, and the ability to provide services all form important components of nursing administration knowledge.

The view in most developing countries is that hospital-based services cannot meet the vast needs of their populations. The answer has been community-based health services aimed at developing health awareness. Nursing service administration has thus had to focus on policy-making, planning, organizing, coordinating, researching, and evaluating nursing and health care at local, regional, and national levels.

The subdiscipline of nursing service administration is eclectic, borrowing from social, political, and economic sciences. Although this has provided a valuable interdisciplinary base, such an approach also encourages reliance on outdated or irrelevant knowledge. There is therefore an urgent need for nursing service administration to develop the type of theoretical base that reflects its own distinct knowledge and goals.

This raises the distinction between "practice theory" and "theory for practice." The latter is derived from related sciences, while the former has developed from nursing service administrators' own experiences. Practice theory incorporates the following:

Theory development in nursing service administration

Knowledge about the consumer as the beneficiary of service

Knowledge about the providers of care (personnel)

The political system in which nursing service administration is practiced

The legislative process as an enabling factor

Communication skills that enhance service delivery

The ethos of nursing and its relevance to nursing service administration

Systems organization and administration of nursing service

Maintenance of nursing standards

Leadership theory and its practice

Contemporary problems and trends in nursing service administration

Research methodology

Personnel resources and associated problems in nursing service administration

Contributions by nursing service administrators to the education of health professionals

International viewpoints on nursing service administration

Developing and fostering leadership qualities of future administrators is an important component of nursing education. Much of the past effort in preparing nurse leaders, especially those engaged in executive roles in nursing service, was geared toward increasing their knowledge of administration and management. Very little information was provided on the human-relations aspects of leadership, yet this role calls for skill in initiating, developing, and maintaining the caring and productive relationships necessary in any situation involving specific objectives.[5] Effective leaders in executive positions in nursing service are one of the top priorities of nursing education.

FUTURE DIRECTIONS
Research

As in other disciplines, the pursuit of advanced degrees and research skills and experience should be highly encouraged. This development will benefit nursing practice and all levels of administration and supervision. There is a need for supportive knowledge-building facilities, such as an institute for nursing science research. Such institutes already exist for other disciplines, including psychology, law, and medicine.

The need for both theoretical and applied research in nursing service administration cannot be overemphasized. Although there is a wide field available for applied research, three areas in need of investigation may be singled out: personnel or staff research, cost-effectiveness of health care services, and professional relationships.

Personnel or staff research. There is a growing shortage of staff to provide nursing care, compounded by overpopulation and the overcrowding of available health care and nursing resources, particularly in developing regions of South Africa. The objectives of such research should be to develop effective and efficient methods for personnel training, utilization, and development.

Cost-effectiveness of health care services. The cost-effectiveness of health care services and its effects on nursing service administration urgently need attention. Financial resources are an ever-diminishing commodity, and such research could prove valuable in the development of cost-effective measures. There is a need to examine public policy and its implications for nursing philosophy in general and nursing service administration in particular.

Professional relationships. Research is called for into nursing administrators' relationships with other health care professionals and into the extent of their accountability to physicians. The rationale for such research is to address the validity of the arrangement in which a physician is always in charge of a nurse administrator. An issue to be considered here is the specific education and training in administration received by nurse administrators, and the lack of comparable preparation for physicians.

Nursing service administration journal

Nursing in South Africa urgently needs a nursing journal that will facilitate the building of the knowledge bases of nursing administration and other subdisciplines of nursing. Such a journal should focus on issues relevant to nursing and nursing service administration, and should promote the sharing of knowledge.

Collaboration of nurses in education and administration

Nurses in education and service need each other, for the further development of the nursing profession in general and the discipline of nursing service administration in particular. This calls for establishing local, national, and international linkages to benefit from cross-cultural practice and research.

CONCLUSION

Nursing service administration as an academic subdiscipline in South Africa has developed from both nursing science and public administration theories.

Although nursing service administrators in South Africa function in high levels of management hierarchies, there is still much room for building a research- and theory-based nursing administration service. In this way, theory development in the subject will be fascilitated. Personnel shortages, cost effectiveness in health care service, and professional relationships are key issues that face the future nurse administrator in South Africa.

REFERENCES

1. Arndt C and Huckabay LMD: Nursing administration theory for practice with a systems approach, ed 2, St Louis, 1980, The CV Mosby Co.
2. Botes PS, Adlem WLJ, and Uys F: Public administration guide 1 for PBL 100: a guide for PBA 100, Pretoria, 1982, University of South Africa.
3. Cloete JJN: Introduction to nursing administration, Pretoria, South Africa, 1981, Van Schaik.
4. Dunsire A: Administration: the word and the science, Bristol, England, 1973, Western Printing Services.
5. Johnson DW: Reaching out: interpersonal effectiveness and self-actualization, ed 2, Englewood Cliffs, NJ, 1981, Prentice-Hall.
6. Stevens W: Management and leadership in nursing, New York, 1978, McGraw-Hill Book Co.
7. Thibodeau JA: Nursing models: analysis and evaluation, Monterey, 1983, Wadsworth Publishing Co.

PART THREE

CHANGING EDUCATION

Education for Knowledge and Practice

JOANNE COMI McCLOSKEY
HELEN KENNEDY GRACE

Placement of this section on nursing education between those on nursing knowledge and nursing practice is not accidental. Nursing education looks in both directions: nursing educators must provide an atmosphere in which nursing knowledge can be generated and refined and also must prepare competent practitioners. Disagreement within nursing about how best to accomplish these goals has led to the proliferation of different types of nursing programs.

The continuing debate is the question of entry-level preparation for nurses. Even though the American Nurses' Association, the National League for Nursing, and many specialty organizations support the baccalaureate degree as the entry-level requirement, even though most other health professionals educate at the master's or doctoral levels, even though health care is increasingly complex and requires a high level of knowledge by practitioners, nonetheless the requirement for a baccalaureate degree in nursing remains controversial.

In her debate chapter, DeBack presents an overview of the history and issues in the "entry into practice" debate. She points out that although there has been continued opposition to the baccalaureate degree as the minimum educational credential for professional nursing, a shift of focus has occurred. With each new development, however, the opposition has continued to emphasize the possible dire consequences for nurses presently in the profession. One benefit of the continued debate has been the appearance of demonstration sites where nurses practice in differentiated roles. The current nursing shortage may, once again, put nursing leadership's aspirations for a higher level of educational preparation on hold. It is interesting to note that in some countries where decisions are made centrally by governments and are implemented swiftly, this painful change has not occurred. Readers throughout the world may want to debate the merits of planned versus directed change as it relates to the educational preparation of nurses.

The nursing shortage has come about partially because of the declining numbers of students in nursing. The decline is large. According to Naylor, "the total number of new nurses graduating from all types of nursing schools annually is expected to drop from 82,700 in 1985 to 68,700 in 1995." Naylor discusses the reasons for the decline and notes with alarm that the decline in interest in nursing careers is predominately among the most talented women. Naylor outlines the unattractive aspects of nursing: little salary differentials for higher levels of education or experience, requirement for night and weekend work, lack of autonomy in decision making, and a negative public image. She points out that marketing and structural changes (e.g., part-time work and evening courses) have not resulted in increased enrollments in nursing education programs. What is needed, she says, is more financial assistance and a change in the practice and image of nursing. She argues that schools should use this opportunity of decreased numbers to reach out to consumer audiences. Although the going is tough now, Naylor believes optimistically that the potential solutions to the shortage could bring about major and lasting changes in the public image and the practice environment.

Change is also necessary to accommodate the increased number of older adult learners. In their chapter, Rothert, Talarczyk, and Awbrey stress the importance of offering flexible models of nursing education while preserving educational quality. They first discuss the current mandate for innovative flexible scheduling and then give examples of strategies: use of work time for clinical experience, use of preceptors, credit for experience, and use of the computer for decision support. They also recognize and discuss possible consequences of increasing flexibility. For example, as nurses become better prepared, they seek positions and rewards that offer opportunities for continued growth. This is a positive step for the nurses but is a source of stress for the employing agency as large numbers of nurses return to school for more education. The authors emphasize that the key to a successful high-quality, flexible educational program is an enhanced partnership among institutions of higher learning, communities, and the health care industry.

In the next chapter Conway-Welch makes a proposal for minimal preparation for professional nursing at the postbaccalaureate level. A few people in the profession have taken this position for years, but it is only recently, with the impetus of the shortage, that this idea has become popular. First, Conway-Welch lists six events that will provoke dramatic changes in nursing. The future, she says, demands both a paraprofessional nurse, educated at an associate degree level, and a professional nurse, educated at a postbaccalaureate level. According to Conway-Welch, the "bachelor's degree in nursing is history." She reasons that there is too much content to cover in 8 semester hours and also that autonomous practice and financial reimbursement can only be achieved through graduate education. Readers will find this chapter very provocative and at the same time a refreshing and disturbing new twist to the long-debated entry into practice question.

Returning to the more usual progression of education, few professional decisions are more important than choosing a graduate program. Poteet and Hodges discuss nine essential elements to consider when selecting a graduate school. These include faculty qualifications, institutional climate, and availability of teaching and research assistantships. Future directions in graduate education, according to the authors, may include more focused clinical specializations and the preparation of case managers.

More and more nurses are choosing graduate ed-

ucation at the doctoral level. Grace summarizes the development of doctoral education in nursing. With the proliferation of programs in the 1970s and 1980s, the trend has been toward similarity rather than difference. Grace argues that the profession needs doctorally prepared clinicians, clinical teachers, and administrators, as well as researchers. She does not believe that the research doctorate is the best preparation for all people and all roles. She also questions the dilution of quality of some research doctoral programs that have too many students and too little faculty engaged in ongoing research: "Because they try to be all things to all people, they fail in preparing either competent researchers or applied practitioners." She makes the case for three program models: research doctorate, clinical or applied doctorate, and the professional doctorate.

In the last chapter, Affara presents the model for nursing education in Bahrain. Before 1976 nursing in Bahrain confronted many problems: low recruitment, low status, unsatisfactory working conditions, inadequate salaries, and job dissatisfaction. As a result of a move to the College of Health Sciences, nursing education became part of the country's tertiary education system in 1976. The resulting three levels of generalist preparation, organized as a continuum integrated by eight curriculum threads, focuses on community health and primary care. Examples of clinical situations encountered by students are included. Nurses in the United States and other countries will want to compare the differences and similarities in education and the process of change. American nurses will want to note the impact of government change and the importance of community health and primary care in this and other developing countries. Although the details are different, nursing around the world shares many similarities, as this chapter illustrates.

The chapters in Part 3 demonstrate how nursing education is pulled in two directions: toward the education of future scholars and leaders who will continue to advance the knowledge base of the discipline and toward the education of practitioners who need more technical and applied skills. Some interesting solutions to the dilemma of professional education for nurses have been offered in these chapters. The issue that emerges from the dilemma is one of standards versus access. Can nursing have both high standards for accomplishments and easy access into the profession? How many levels of education are necessary to accomplish this, and what should they be? Are standards and access at opposite ends of a continuum? The latest nursing shortage has pushed us again to think more about access to the profession and whether we are doing enough in our educational programs to prepare for practice. The balance for education between scholarship and practice is precarious. A lasting shortage may have serious effects on the development of nursing knowledge and the advancement of the profession.

For several decades now the major issue in nursing has been the one of entry into practice in the educational arena. With the shortage, the major issue now is retention of nurses in the practice arena. The focus of the profession has shifted, and only time will tell what this means for nursing education. The important changes in practice are addressed in Part 4.

CHAPTER 16

Debate

Entry into practice
Will the 1985 proposal ever happen?

VIVIEN De BACK

It may be disconcerting to find out that the changes in educational requirements for nurses that were to have begun in 1985 never happened. What may be even more disturbing, however, is to learn that the 1985 proposal was a reaffirmation of an earlier proposal by the American Nurses' Association (ANA) to the nursing community in 1965.

This chapter will define the issues and present arguments for and against the proposals for educational requirements as they have been set forth by nursing organizations. It will also review the position of the profession on this issue in the 1980s and discuss prospects for the future.

OVERVIEW OF THE ISSUE

In 1965 the ANA, in response to a 1964 request from its House of Delegates, identified two categories of nursing practice and delineated the educational preparation for each category. The minimum educational requirement for beginning professional nursing practice was defined as a baccalaureate degree in nursing (B.S.N.), and the minimum preparation for beginning technical nursing practice would be an associate degree in nursing (A.D.N.). These recommendations were published in a position paper,[1] and they were continuously reaffirmed by the ANA's Delegate Assembly. In 1978 the ANA House of Delegates charged the association with defining competencies for the two categories of nursing practice. In addition, the house approved the recommendation that by 1985 the minimum preparation for entry into professional nursing practice be the baccalaureate in nursing. The ex-

plicit deadline of 1985 for implementing previously accepted resolutions on this subject was the source of a newly coined phrase, "the 1985 proposal," which became a rallying cry for both the supporters and opponents of this change.

On the state level, the New York State Nurses' Association (NYSNA) became the first state association to adopt a resolution to make the B.S.N. the minimum requirement for registered nurse licensure. Although the proposals of ANA and NYSNA were not new ideas but affirmations of recommendations already advanced in the profession, the debate seems to have been fueled by the assignment of a date for implementation—a date within the lifetime of most nurses, of whom 85% held diplomas from educational programs that were expected to close.

ARGUMENTS FOR THE BACCALAUREATE DEGREE

Support for baccalaureate preparation for nurses began with the opening of the first baccalaureate programs, at Teachers College in New York in 1899 and at the University of Minnesota in 1909. Generally, however, nursing education through the 1950s was entrenched in hospital schools. The concept of differences between professional and technical practice would not be addressed seriously until the publication of Montag's work in 1959.[16] The associate degree nursing program described by Montag was developed specifically to prepare nurses for predominantly technical functions. The program expanded in community colleges throughout the country with unparalleled speed.

Montag's "nurse technician" was supposed to (1) assist in the planning of nursing care for patients, (2) give general nursing care with supervision, and (3) assist in the evaluation of the nursing care that had been given.

Before Montag's work, nurse leaders had maintained that nursing education belonged in schools of higher education. Expecting this belief to direct future development, organized nursing envisioned a continued expansion of baccalaureate programs, a quick decline of diploma programs, and a gradual growth of the new associate degree programs. The plan, to assure the public of well-prepared nurses and support personnel, was clear and well articulated in the 1965 position paper. How the plan would be implemented, however, was not at all clear. Although the plans for placing technical and professional nurses into the work setting were not explicit, the work of defining and describing these two categories of nurses continued for twenty years.

The 1978 ANA House of Delegates charged the association with agreeing on a comprehensive statement of competencies for the two categories of nurse.[2] The 1980 House of Delegates received a report and recommendation listing competencies for nurses with baccalaureate degrees and for those with associate degrees.[3] In 1981 the ANA Commission on Nursing Education decided that "further efforts to describe nursing roles from a competency base could best be done in the practice setting."[4] The 1984 House of Delegates adopted the recommendation that the ANA establish the following timetable for implementation of the baccalaureate degree requirement: 5% of the states by 1986, 15% of the states by 1988, 50% of the states by 1992, and 100% of the states by 1995. In 1985, the ANA reaffirmed the educational bases for the two proposed categories of nurse and established titles for each category.

The NYSNA accepted the recommendations in the 1965 ANA position paper. In 1975 a NYSNA Entry into Practice legislative proposal was adopted by the voting body. The Entry into Practice bill was introduced in the New York Assembly and Senate in 1976. In 1981 the NYSNA approved a change in the title of the legislative proposal from "The 1985 Proposal" to "Entry into Practice Proposal" and voted to change the effective date of implementation from January 1985 to January 1986.

During the defining and describing period, the nursing literature was full of articles and research attempting to delineate the roles for technical and professional nurses in the practice arena. In 1966 Johnson stated that the most noticeable difference between technical and professional nurses was the difference in their knowledge.[12] Research related to competencies initially focused on faculty or nursing service perceptions of the performance of A.D.N. or B.S.N. graduates.[6,10] Other studies evaluated graduates' perceptions of their own performance,[19] their educational preparedness,[11] or the extent to which a specific behavior (or behaviors) was demonstrated.[15] Because the clinical settings of most studies had one job description for nurses with different educational backgrounds, studies that looked at what nurses did often found little or no difference in their practice. However, studies that focused on knowledge base and patient outcomes often found differences in the practice of nurses from baccalaureate and associate degree programs.[7,14]

The proliferation of studies regarding professional and technical nursing and the ongoing work of defining competencies and roles kept the subject of two categories of nurse alive and controversial. In spite of the controversy and perhaps because of it, beginning consensus was forming around who the nurse of the future would be. In 1986 the National Commission on Nursing Implementation Project (NCNIP) disseminated a document entitled: "Timeline for Transition into the Future Nursing Education System for Two Categories of Nurse and Characteristics of Professional and Technical Nurses of the Future." The document, approved by the governing board of the project, described the characteristics of the technical and professional nurses of the future and discussed educational transition.[17]

In 1987 the ANA Delegate Assembly accepted the statement of nursing practice developed by the ANA Task Force on Scope of Practice. The statement described the differences between the professional and technical practice of nursing. Those differences were defined by the knowledge base of the nurse, the role of the nurse, and the nature of the client population served.[5]

Using the documents defining competencies and describing future nurses, clinical settings began to develop nurse roles based on education and abilities. Several funded projects increased the momentum of implementation of these standards,[13,20,22] and encouraged the development of differentiated practice sites with differentiated job descriptions for nurses. At these site nurses practiced in professional and technical roles where their practice could be observed and tested. By 1987 more than 20 sites in hospitals, nursing homes, and home care agencies were in operation. For those groups supporting the concept of nursing practice based on education and experience, the move toward demonstration sites was a positive one and seemed to support the belief that the 1985 proposal would become a reality.

ARGUMENTS AGAINST THE BACCALAUREATE DEGREE

The purpose of the 1965 position paper was to end the debate over professional and technical nursing practice in nursing. It was further expected to provide a rationale for the redesign of the nursing education system of multiple levels of nurse. Why the ANA document did not clarify the issue but rather fueled the debate is a matter for much speculation. It is clear that the reasons for the lack of acceptance in 1965 were not the same reasons advanced in the literature in the 1980s.

In 1965 the largest group of practicing nurses who saw themselves as professional nurses had no preparation beyond the original diploma in nursing and felt disenfranchised by the position paper. Coalitions of A.D.N. diploma, and practical nurse groups began to form to block plans for implementation. When the first state, New York, adopted a resolution in 1975 to make the B.S.N. the minimum requirement for registered nurse licensure, the opposition became more entrenched. Nurse licensure is closely associated with nurse identity. This relationship seems to be the result of hiring practices in which nurses have been placed in practice roles based on licensure (minimum level) rather than educational background (optimal level). It should have been expected that threats to a nurse's practice identity (license) would be met with opposition. The New York resolution and subsequent legislation was hotly debated and opposed by the nurses themselves.

In 1981 the ANA Delegate Assembly approved titles for professional and technical nurses: R.N. (registered nurse) for the professional nurse and A.N. (associate nurse) for the technical nurse. Following this action, the national debate became even more heated. Suggesting that an already existing title (R.N.) be awarded in the future only to one of the practicing

groups now using the title served to solidify the opposition and confuse the issues of education and practice with titling and licensure.

Looking back over 30 years, it is clear that an organized approach to planning nursing's future with the cooperation of many nursing groups was not possible in the 1960s. Nursing organizations simply were not ready for a coordinated effort. As a result, the position paper was met with a reactive rather than proactive response, that is, some nurses tried to discredit the paper, and very few took action to implement its suggestions. In later years position papers, recommendations, and study results would become the basis or rationale for organized nursing's **proactive** behavior.

In the 1970s, opposition continued to implementation of plans for professional and technical nurses, but increasing numbers of state nursing organizations, state boards, and specialty organizations were studying competencies and potential differences among categories of nurses. Fourteen organizations supported the baccalaureate degree as the educational requirement for professional nursing practice by 1973.[9] In the 1980s an effort to oppose educational restructuring was organized by the Federation for Accessible Nursing Education and Licensure (FANEL). FANEL is "a single purpose organization dedicated to assuring the continual availability and choice in education leading to nursing licensure.[21]

Although opposition has continued over a 20-year period, a shift of focus has been occurring. In 1965 the concerns about redesigning the nursing educational and delivery systems centered on the loss of professional status and identity for the majority of practicing nurses. Later, opposing groups pointed to a lack of evidence that nurses from different educational programs provide different care.

As the data on differentiation of nursing practice began to develop, a third shift in opposition to the 1985 proposal emerged. The opposition in the 1980s suggests that the "grand plan intends to have B.S.N.'s as technical nurses with master's and eventually doctorate nurses as the professional nurses."[8] In each 10-year cycle, opposition to the restructuring proposal for nursing has continued to focus on dire consequences, such as what could or will happen to nurses who are presently in the profession if future plans were implemented. As the debate continues, many concerns are being resolved. Ongoing discussion does seem to allow opposing groups to consider compromise language and positions.

SUMMARY OF THE ARGUMENTS

Will the 1985 proposal ever become a reality? The evidence seems to suggest that it will but not exactly in the same way it was originally proposed. Change occurs when attitudes change; that is, when a significant number of those who will be affected by the change are convinced that it will occur, behavioral change will follow.

More and more data point to a growing consensus on rationalizing the education system and restructuring the nursing delivery system to include job descriptions based on education and experience. Increasing numbers of diploma schools are translating their educational programs into baccalaureate or associate degree programs.[18] In cooperation with junior or senior colleges, numerous nursing education models have developed as well as some independent *degree-granting institutions*. Practical nurse programs are closing or using their resources to develop associate degree programs in nursing. The organized nursing community has gone on record to support the concept of professional and technical nurses educated in baccalaureate and associate degree programs. Twenty-one nursing organizations were in agreement on this issue in 1988 compared to 14 in 1973. Clinical sites where differentiated practice models are being developed are increasing. The growing body of literature on effective and efficient models of care delivery provides further evidence of "different education equals different role expectation."

The 1985 proposal or "move from four categories to two" includes (1) an educational component, (2) a practice component, (3) a titling component, and (4) a licensing component. The NCNIP timeline and characteristics document mentioned earlier deals with the areas in which there has been growing consensus, that is, the description of educational programs and their continuing transition. In addition, the document describes in broad terms the characteristics of professional and technical nurses of the future. This consensus document, drawn from the literature and the work of nurses themselves, separates the more controversial components of the issue from the academic and practice components.

A second, less controversial component of the 1985 proposal is the development of demonstration sites where nurses practice in differentiated roles. These sites have become the data collecting laboratories, and they provide an opportunity to test ideas before they are fully accepted.

As the education and practice issues are clarified, the titling and licensure issues continue to be discussed. Differences in titling and licensure are not so much at issue as is the kind of title and the type of license. That is, the question is not whether there are differences in the education of associate degree and baccalaureate degree nurses; rather, the debate focuses on the labels and legal parameters to be assigned to the differences. There is also considerable agreement that job descriptions for nurses with different educational backgrounds are needed in the practice arenas. As the important education and practice issues are clarified, titling and licensing issues will be resolved.

THE SHORTAGE

What has been the effect of the nursing shortage (or more accurately, the increased demand for nurses) on the planned redesign of nursing education? The most frequent comment heard in this regard takes the form of the question, How can we encourage change in nursing education during this time of crisis in the labor pool? The answer of course is that nursing is in this crisis because of lack of planning 15 and 10 years ago. The major nursing organizations on the Tri-Council for Nursing (ANA, AACN, AONE, and NLN) have developed short-term plans to address the nursing shortage. Both at the Tri-Council and the NCNIP board table, however, it has been made clear that nursing must continue to plan for the long term to assure the numbers and types of nursing personnel needed for the future.

One organized response to the need to plan for the future is the proposal by the American Medical Association to "solve the nursing shortage" by creating a new level of health care worker called the registered care technologist (RCT). Creating such a new position has been called unnecessary, duplicative, and costly. Nursing groups point out that it may further fragment patient care and seriously threaten quality of care. Although the RCT is a serious threat, it is also a rallying point for nurses and nursing. Nursing has united in its opposition to the RCT and, just as important, nursing's stand has garnered support from many other groups.

Nursing has also used the profession's response to

the proposal to clarify its position on the question of "assistants" to nurses. Registered nurses need assistants that they educate and supervise. Registered nurses need clerical assistants, runners, transporters, and technical support systems. Clarifying the issue of support personnel and services for nurses bolsters the plans for nursing education redesign. Clarifying the various issues—what nurses need in terms of ability, skill, education, and assistants will help set the direction for nursing care delivery systems of the future—systems which nurses design and in which nurses work.

THE FUTURE

The future of health care in the United States is strongly dependent upon a system of high-quality, cost-effective nursing care. The spiraling costs of health care will continue to focus attention on quality, cost, and provider. A redesigned and articulated educational system will provide the types of nurses needed for the community in the emerging health care system. Organized nursing can, in cooperation with other groups, redesign the nursing education and delivery systems. Just as nursing organizations have become aware of the need to work together, individual nurses themselves must learn this same lesson: the lesson of belonging, of involvement, of becoming a part of the process of planning and creating nursing's future.

The redesign of the profession (education and practice arenas) is an opportunity to demonstrate nursing's professionalism, that is, its self-determination. As the plans for that design evolve, we may one day recognize the 1985 proposal as a turning point in our history and the beginning of nursing's new professionalism.

REFERENCES

1. American Nurses' Association: Educational preparation for nurse practitioners and assistants to nurses: a position paper, Kansas City, Mo, 1965, The Association.
2. American Nurses' Association: Summary of proceedings: 1978 convention, Kansas City, Mo, 1979, The Association.
3. American Nurses' Association: Summary of proceedings: 1980 convention, Kansas City, Mo, 1981, The Association.
4. American Nurses' Association: Summary of proceedings: 1982 convention, Kansas City, Mo, 1983, The Association.
5. American Nurses' Association: The scope of nursing practice, Kansas City, Mo, 1987, The Association.
6. Chamings PA and Teevan J: Comparison of expected competencies of baccalaureate and associate degree graduates in nursing, Image 11(1):16, 1979.
7. DeBack V and Mentkowski M: Does the baccalaureate make a difference?: differentiating performance by education and experience, Nursing Education 25(7), 1986.
8. Dolan A: BSN's: nursing elite's technical nurses of tomorrow? Seattle, 1986, FANEL.
9. Hartung D: Organizational positions on titling and entry into practice: a chronology. In Looking beyond the entry issue: implications for education and service, New York, 1986, National League for Nursing.
10. Hayter M: Follow-up study of graduates of the University of Kentucky, College of Nursing, 1964-1969, Nurs Res 20:55, 1971.
11. Hogstel M: Associate degree and baccalaureate graduates: do they function differently? Am J Nurs 77:1598, 1977.
12. Johnson D: Competence in practice: technical and professional, Nurs Outlook 14(9), 1966.
13. Kearns J: WICHE. Improving the preparation and utilization of associate degree and baccalaureate degree nurses, Boulder, Colo, 1985, WICHE.
14. McKenna ME: Differentiating between professional nursing practice and technical nursing practice, Dissertation Abstracts 31:4157-B, 1971.
15. Matthews C and Gaul A: Nursing diagnosis from the perspectives of concept attainment and critical thinking, Advances in Nursing Science 2:17, 1979.
16. Montag ML: Community college education for nursing, New York, 1959, McGraw-Hill.
17. National Commission on Nursing Implementation Project: Timeline for transition into the future nursing education system for two categories of nurse and characteristics of professional and technical nurses of the future and their educational programs, Milwaukee, 1987, NCNIP.
18. National Commission on Nursing Implementation Project: Work Group I, Education. 1987 Invitational Conference Papers, Milwaukee, 1987, NCNIP.
19. Nelson L: Competencies of nursing graduates in technical, communicative and administrative skills, Nurs Res 27(2):121, 1978.
20. Primm P: Associate degree nursing: facilitating competency, Chicago, 1986, MAIN.
21. Wallace T: Facts and fallacies: proposed changes for education, licensure and practice of nurses, Seattle, 1986, FANEL.
22. Waters V: California statewide project for service-education consensus on ADN competencies, Fremont, Calif, 1985, California Organization of Program Directors.

CHAPTER 17

Viewpoints

Recruitment of students into nursing

MARY D. NAYLOR

A severe shortage of qualified nurses exists in the United States that has far-reaching implications for the health of the nation. This situation is compounded by a significant decrease in nursing school enrollments and a dramatic decline in the number of high school and college students interested in nursing. These major changes are occurring at a time when the need for knowledgeable, competent, and caring nurses is more urgent than at any period in the profession's history.

THE SCOPE OF THE PROBLEM

According to a recent American Hospital Association study, the current shortage of staff nurses is a problem in more than 50% of all the hospitals.[6] The average hospital vacancy rate for registered nurses (R.N.s) was 11.4% nationally in 1987. One fourth of all hospitals reported vacancy rates in excess of 15%, indicating a critical need for R.N.s. In long-term care settings, a shortage of R.N.s is interfering with the ability of these institutions to provide quality care. A recent survey of the 9000 nursing homes that are members of the American Health Care Association revealed that 58% of these facilities had R.N. vacancies.[17] One third of these long-term care settings indicated a need for R.N.s just to meet minimum federal standards for staffing. The nursing shortage has its greatest impact on those institutions in which qualified nurses are critically needed to deliver acute and long-term care.

The shortage of nurses that exists today will be severely compounded in coming years as the impact of dramatic declines in nursing school enrollments are felt by the health care system. Since 1983 enrollments in nursing schools have dropped by 20%.[15] All types of basic nursing programs have experienced declining enrollments. Enrollments in baccalaureate programs have dropped by more than 28% in the last 4 years.[4] Between 1983 and 1987 enrollments in associate degree programs declined by 19%.[16] Enrollments in diploma programs have been decreasing for more than 2 decades, and graduates of these programs now account for only 14% of the total number of graduates annually.[15] Programs designed for college graduates have also experienced decreases in enrollments during the past 4 years.[9] The number of new nurses graduating from all types of nursing schools annually is expected to drop from a high of 82,700 in 1985 to 68,700 by 1995.[5]

Changes in the country's demographic profile are partially responsible for declining nursing school enrollments. Since the early 1980s the size of the 18-year-old cohort has been shrinking. The largest part of the demographic decline will occur between 1988 and 1994. Even if the proportion of aspirants to nursing careers had remained stable over the past few years, the number of individuals in the pool of aspiring nurses would have declined because of demographic factors.

The precipitous drop in enrollments since 1983, however, indicates that a much smaller number of high school graduates and college freshman are selecting nursing as a career. The pool of college freshmen interested in nursing peaked in 1976 and has decreased by 50% since then.[8] Between 1983 and 1986 the proportion of aspiring nurses in the college freshman population fell by more than one third from 8.3% to 5.1%. In 1983, 42,000 first-time, full-time, four year college freshmen indicated a desire to prepare for a career in nursing. By 1986 the number of first-time, full-time college freshmen desiring a nursing career had dropped to 19,800.[8]

In addition to the decrease in the number of individuals interested in pursuing a career in nursing, the profession is faced with a significant decline in the quality of the nursing student applicant pool. The College Board recently released data indicating that the SAT scores of high school students interested in nursing careers were well below the national average.[10] Moreover, the report suggested that although the SAT profile of all students was improving somewhat, the performance of prospective nurses was declining. The gap in academic performance between nurses and nonnurses has also widened in recent years. A much larger percentage of high school graduates who express an interest in nursing have earned grade point averages in the C to C+ range.[10] These data suggest that the decline in interest in nursing careers is predominantly among the most academically talented women.

THE CAUSES OF THE PROBLEM

The reasons for the declining interest in nursing are multifaceted. Over the past several years the most significant factors affecting the selection of nursing as a career are changes in the attitudes, values, and career aspirations of women entering college.[7] Attitudinal changes are reflected by much greater support for job equality for women and rejection of the traditional roles of women. Value changes are evident in the widespread endorsement by women of traditionally male materialistic, power, and status goals. As a result of these changes, there have been dramatic shifts in preferences for majors away from traditional female fields, including nursing, and toward business, law, science, and engineering.[7] These shifts have been accompanied by a rising interest in advanced degrees among women. Clearly the women's movement has had a tremendous impact on the career choices of young women. And obviously these women believe that nursing has not responded effectively to the changes in attitudes and values associated with this movement.

The tremendous skepticism of today's youth about the long-term wisdom of a career in nursing is not without merit. High school graduates concerned about their lifelong earning potential seriously question why they should choose nursing. These students know that they could become an engineer in the same 4 years it

takes to become a nurse and with just 6 years of experience have an annual salary 100% higher than that of a nurse.[2]

Individuals selecting careers today look askance at a profession that has a variety of routes to achieve the same position, with little or no recognition or compensation for additional education. Salaries and benefits for nurses are not commensurate with their levels of education, responsibility, experience, or performance.[11] Link reports that the differences in hourly wages for associate degree nurses and baccalaureate degree nurses range from $.61 to $.78 per hour.[12] Using the high end of this range, the difference translates into an annual premium of $1370 per year for a baccalaureate degree as compared with an associate degree. Similarly, advanced education in nursing, years of experience, or scope of responsibility have had little impact on the salaries of nurses. The average starting salary for R.N.s in 1986, for example, was $20,340; the average salary for R.N.s with 10 years of experience that same year was $27,744.[16] The economic return on nursing is poor compared with some other fields.[1]

According to prospective students, a notably unattractive requirement of nursing is that nurses must work nights and weekends.[1] Today's youth question how their chosen career will contribute to the quality of their lives. Other industries that operate on a 24-hour basis offer substantial wage differentials for irregular hours. The differentials offered by most hospitals pale in comparison.

Because of obstacles that are unique to the nursing practice environment (notably hospitals) academically talented students who are interested in careers with recognized status are turning away from nursing. Prominent among these barriers are a lack of autonomy in making decisions regarding patients' care, the absence of a collegial, collaborative relationship between nurses and physicians, and poorly defined opportunities for personal and professional growth.[3]

The skepticism of today's youth about the wisdom of a career in nursing is fueled by nursing's negative public image. Despite the growth and diversification that has occurred in this profession during the past few decades, the public is not able to distinguish the generic "nurse" from nursing assistants or other support personnel. It is as if the professional nurse is invisible. Nursing, as the public knows it, is an anachronism. Clearly the public does not recognize differentiation in nursing roles, such as those assumed by clinical nurse specialists, nurse-practitioners, or nurse researchers. Nursing's public persona fails to communicate what this profession does that makes a difference to our society.

Given these realities, it should not be surprising that young women today, who have many more career options than they have had in the past years, are not choosing nursing. Nor is it surprising that this profession has failed to attract a significant number of men. Many other career options offer comparable or higher economic rewards, have well-defined career ladders, and have effectively communicated the value of their work to the public.

POTENTIAL SOLUTIONS

The changes in the quality and quantity of candidates for a career in nursing are part of larger societal shifts affecting career preferences of women over the past 2 decades. This pattern suggests that the solution to the student recruitment problem in nursing involves long-term strategies, not short-term fixes. The pattern also suggests that the solution does not rest solely with schools of nursing. Although the answers to the student recruitment problem confronting nursing will not come easily, appropriate responses could achieve major and lasting changes in the public's image of nursing as well as in the practice environment where nurses work and are educated. Nursing's ability to capture its share of highly qualified applicants is clearly linked to these changes.

A new public persona

Concern about quality health care in this country is growing. Generational forces suggest that health care will be a major domestic issue for years to come. Baby boomers are now turning 40; their personal needs for health care services will increase substantially in the coming years. Their parents are now entering their seventies. The baby boomers have the potential to live longer than any previous generation and will demand more services for the chronically ill and very old than ever before.

The baby boomers are well educated and have high expectations of health services. This population will want access to the newest and best technology in health care for themselves and their children. At the same time they will expect quality institutional and home care services for their parents. The nursing profession needs to inform the baby boomers that nurses play a pivotal role in addressing their health care priorities. This population must understand that their demands for quality health care services can often most effectively and efficiently be met by qualified nurses.

Nursing needs to actively enlist the support of this new public in addressing the student recruitment problem. Members of the nursing profession must agree on the message for this generation to receive about nursing and devise more effective ways to promulgate the value of nurses' work to society. In addition to the unique contribution nursing makes to health care, this message must communicate the standards of performance the public can expect from nurses. Finally, this message must stress that the public has to pay what it costs to receive quality nursing services. A reasonable share of the health care dollar must be directed to the profession so that nursing can meet the public's expectations.[13]

Aspirants to the profession need to understand the work of nurses—how they spend their days and how their roles and responsibilities expand with advanced education and experience. Aspirants also need to see that they will achieve a reasonable financial return when their work is consistent with the public's and profession's expectations.

Public attention should be focused on those nurses who are designing and offering services that are integral to the solution of major health care problems. The stories of nurses who are making a difference in the care of very low birthweight infants, persons with AIDS, and the frail elderly need to be heard. The findings of nurse researchers who daily are measuring the impact of nursing on the quality and cost of health care must be exploited in all communications concerning the value to society of nurses' work.

Nursing's new public persona needs to be communicated through multimedia public relations campaigns coordinated by national nursing organizations. Nursing organizations, however, are not solely responsible for meeting this communication challenge; every nurse must share this responsibility. The public defines nursing in terms of nurses they know. As the public meets more nurses who are sophisticated, articulate, competent, and caring, expectations will rise. As nurses who are parents, siblings, relatives, and friends of young students talk more about the positive impact of their work, these same youth will be more likely to consider a career in nursing.

Restructuring the practice environment

The profession's ability to recruit its share of bright, talented individuals—men and women—will probably not change dramatically until the work environment of nurses changes. A number of issues are receiving careful consideration as efforts are made to improve nursing's practice environment.

The presence of a differentiated practice system accompanied by a wage structure that recognizes and rewards performance, experience, and education is essential in order to turn the tide of the student recruitment problem in nursing. Aspirants to the profession need be able to identify a career ladder with meaningful growth opportunities as well as multiple career paths for professional development.

A differentiated practice environment would require an examination of the names and terms nurses use to communicate who they are and what they do. As society's needs became more complex, other professions have redefined their work based on areas of specialization and experience. In the legal profession, for example, the public is aware of the unique contributions of constitutional lawyers versus tax lawyers; similarly, the public is aware of the differences between law clerks and senior law partners. The time is ripe to give new names to different kinds of nurses and to move away from the generalist concept of nursing. People who enter the health care system should be able to identify their nurses by name, to recognize the educational preparation and experience level of each nurse by virtue of the nurse's title, and to know what services that nurse is capable of performing.

In addition to initiating models of differentiated practice, a few hospitals are testing other strategies to restructure the role of the hospital nurse and improve the practice environment of nurses. Hospitals have attempted to strengthen nurse-patient relationships through innovative practice models that enable nurses to care for patients throughout their episodes of illness. The case management program at the New England Medical Center in Boston is an exciting example of a model of care that encourages nurses to follow patients through their hospitalization and discharge to home or other health care setting.

Other restructuring initiatives have attempted to foster collegial, professional relationships with physicians. Boston's Beth Israel Hospital has taken the lead in establishing collaborative practice models in which physicians and nurses work as a team. More effective nurse-physician collaboration in hospitals will improve the professional satisfaction of both groups and enhance the status of professional nurses.

Restructuring models have also attempted to remove nurses from the many nonnursing roles they fill and more effectively utilize the clinical expertise of R.N.s. Hartford Hospital in Connecticut has created a multilevel "clinical nursing assistant" program; these assistants provide support to R.N.s by performing some of the nonclinical functions.

Within the limits of available resources, a few hospitals are attempting to address some of the other structural barriers to recruiting qualified individuals into nursing. Valley Community Hospital in Oregon has created a wage differential for undesirable night and weekend shifts. Since 1980, this hospital has provided a modest adjustment in hourly wages for these shifts. In addition, after nurses have worked 1000 hours of night or week-end shifts, they earn an additional $1000. Other hospitals are providing child care to make it possible for some of the 500,000 part-time R.N.s to increase their hours.

Finally, efforts are being made to address more effectively the professional development needs of nurses. Cedars Sinai Medical Center in Los Angeles has implemented in-house clinical training programs, a mobile skills laboratory, and career advancement training.

The mobile skills laboratory was designed to respond to the staff development needs of nurses more effectively and in a manner that recognizes the importance of flexible scheduling. After completing a needs assessment for each nursing specialty, the staff development instructors at the hospital designed videocassettes (10 to 20 minutes in length) to address these needs. The videocassettes and accompanying reference material are wheeled on a cart from unit to unit and nurses avail themselves of these resources as their schedules permit. The staff development instructor is available for follow-up.

The career advancement program at Cedars-Sinai also attempts to address the unique needs of individual nurses. Components of this program include career counseling services, college fairs, and tuition loans for advanced education.

Introducing new structure to nursing care delivery entails a major institutional commitment. The hospitals cited are the many health care settings that are rising to this challenge because they recognize that quality nursing care is the primary reason why patients come to these settings. As the needs of patients become more complex, it is essential to maintain an adequate supply of well-educated, talented, and career-oriented professional nurses. This will only be possible if there is significant change in nursing's practice environment.

Commitment to quality

The current nursing shortage presents a special challenge to schools of nursing. In the face of nursing vacancies that close hospital units and tuition loss that causes retrenchment in educational programs, tremendous pressure is being placed on schools of nursing to increase the number of nurses and the speed at which they graduate. Previously cited data show that increasing numbers in the short term will be achieved only by lowering standards. A "warm body" approach to the student recruitment problem will undermine seriously the profession's ability to recruit academically talented individuals. The challenges facing nurses today and in the future demand bright minds as well as good hearts. Schools of nursing must demonstrate their commitment to quality by recruiting only qualified students and resisting the pressures to lower their standards.

How then can schools of nursing contribute to the solution and still remain viable during this period of enrollment decline? Research findings suggest that investing in costly marketing strategies targeted at both traditional and nontraditional students has not yielded a significant return.[14] Similarly, structural changes in educational programs, such as part-time evening or weekend options, have not resulted in increased enrollment.

Schools of nursing need to join forces to strengthen the financial aid programs available to nursing students. The recent success in the reauthorization of the Nursing Education Act is due, in large measure, to the collaborative efforts of nursing programs. Schools of nursing have the potential to design and seek public and private support for work-study or work grant programs targeted at qualified, financially needy aspirants to nursing. Such programs recognize the nature of the population choosing nursing as a career—often older students with major family responsibilities and limited access to traditional financial aid options.

Schools of nursing should use this opportunity to extend their educational mission to health care settings and consumers. For example, nursing programs could collaborate with hospitals and other health care settings in establishing centers of lifelong learning or professional development for R.N.s. The continued growth of individuals pursuing a career in nursing would be facilitated by such centers. Staff nurses, clinical specialists, and nursing administrators periodically need to renew their skills or develop new skills. In addition, nurses selecting from a variety of career options or attempting to make a move up the career ladder need education, counseling, and support. Schools of nursing are uniquely equipped to promote the professional development of nurses over the span of their careers.

Similarly, schools of nursing have the resources to reach out to consumer audiences and in doing so to strengthen the public's perception of nursing. For example, a school of nursing might identify itself as a resource center for families caring for elderly parents. Faculty and students might offer these families counseling or refer the elderly person and his family to appropriate health or social support systems.

Obviously, during a period of retrenchment, schools of nursing cannot expect universities to support the extension of their educational mission to hospitals and other health care settings or to consumers. Hospitals that are struggling to retain qualified nurses, however, will be very interested in capitalizing on resources in the school that can be used to satisfy the needs of these nurses. In return, hospitals will be more willing to assist schools as they cope with shrinking university support.

Schools of nursing should seek private and public support for programs that will attempt to fill obvious gaps in the delivery of health care. For example, by building a partnership with organizations such as the American Association of Retired Persons (AARP), schools are in a much stronger position to garner private or public support for programs directed at consumers. The benefits that will accrue to schools that reexamine traditional practices and extend their services to a much larger audience will be many. Prominent among these will be the opportunity for students to be exposed to excellent role models earlier in the educational programs, thereby, strengthening their commitment to nursing as a career choice.

Schools of nursing and medicine in academic health centers are in an excellent position to offer educational programs designed to enhance nurse-physician collaboration. Collaborative models of practice will not only have a positive impact on patient care but also contribute immeasurably to the satisfaction and professional status of nurses.

Finally, during this period of retrenchment, schools of nursing should reexamine their programs of study to measure how well their graduates are prepared to lead fulfilling personal and professional lives. Bright students want to develop their minds and become well versed in many areas; they want to pursue a broad-based liberal education and take full advantage of college life. Nursing faculty can respond to this need by collaborating with liberal arts faculty in developing creative programs that link liberal and professional goals or by encouraging their students to complete minors or dual degrees in other fields. Today's students have increasingly global interests; responsive schools will find ways for them to work or study abroad. The tremendous growth in accelerated program options (e.g., direct admission to B.S.N./M.S.N. programs) demonstrates the responsiveness of nursing schools to this discipline's mature student population. Schools of nursing have a pivotal role to play in the resolution of the student recruitment problem. They must take the lead during this crisis by reaffirming the profession's commitment to quality.

SUMMARY

Nursing can play a critical role in addressing the health care challenges of the 1990s and the twenty-first century. To respond to these challenges, nursing requires bright, capable, career-oriented professionals. The quest for solutions to today's student recruitment problem should focus on the public's future needs and expectations. The key elements to this solution should be quality and opportunity. The opportunity exists now to achieve lasting changes in nursing's infrastructure. These changes are essential to enable nursing to capture its share of capable men and women. Capitalizing on this opportunity will lead to the quality of nurses and nursing services that the public needs and the bright future that the profession deserves.

REFERENCES

1. Aiken LH and Mullinix CF: The nurse shortage: myth or reality? N Engl J Med 317(10), 1987.
2. Aiken LH and Mullinix CF: Recurring hospital nursing shortages: explanations and solutions, Am J Nurs 87:1616, 1987.
3. American Academy of Nursing: Magnet hospitals: attraction and retention of professional nurses, Kansas City, Mo, 1983, American Academy of Nursing.
4. American Association of Colleges of Nursing: Report on enrollment and graduations in baccalaureate and graduate programs in nursing, 1983-1988, Washington, DC, 1988, American Association of Colleges of Nursing.
5. American Hospital Association: The nursing shortage: facts, figures and feelings: research report, Kansas City, Mo, 1987, American Hospital Association.
6. American Hospital Association: Report of the hospital nursing personnel survey, Kansas City, Mo, 1987, American Hospital Association.
7. Astin AW, Green KC, and Korn WS: The American freshman: twenty year trends 1966-1985, Los Angeles, 1986, American Council on Education.
8. Cooperative Institutional Research Program: 1987 freshman survey report, Los Angeles, 1987, Higher Education Research Institute.
9. Diers D: When college grads choose nursing, Am J Nurs 87:1631, 1987.
10. Green K: What the freshman tell us, Am J Nurs 87:1610, 1987.
11. Iglehart JK: Problems facing the nursing profession, N Engl J Med 317(10), 1987.
12. Link CR: What does a b.s. degree buy? An economists view, Am J Nurs 87:1621, 1987.
13. Lynaugh J: The yo-yo ride, Am J Nurs 87:1606, 1987.
14. Naylor M and Sherman M: A description of the effects of current initiatives to attract quality undergraduate nursing students, J Prof Nurs, July/Aug 1988.
15. National League for Nursing: Nursing data review, 1987, New York, 1988, National League for Nursing.
16. National League for Nursing: Nursing student census with policy implications, 1987, New York, 1988, National League for Nursing.
17. Statement of the American Health Care Association, addressing the nursing shortage before the Senate Special Committee on Aging, Philadelphia, April 6, 1988.

CHAPTER 18

Flexible models of nursing education

MARILYN L. ROTHERT
GERALDINE J. TALARCZYK
SUSAN M. AWBREY

Flexible models of education can no longer be perceived as optional approaches to be used by a few innovative programs in nursing. The needs of students, nursing faculty, educational institutions, the profession, and the health care industry dictate a flexible approach to nursing education.

Historically, students pursuing degrees in institutions of higher learning were expected to adapt to the systems, traditions, calendar, and location of the institution. Universities are now faced with adapting to the needs of an increasing number of adult learners with varying backgrounds and experiences. A decline in the number of 18- to 24-year-old men and women seeking college educations has already been noted, and by 1992 half of all college students are expected to be over 25.[16] Trends in nursing are consistent with the national norms. In 1981 Houle noted that the education of professionals was being influenced by three major trends: (1) the increasing age of people entering the professions, (2) an increased willingness to change professions, and (3) the older age at which some people experience the initial desire to learn.[18] Like some other professions, nursing is serving a population of adult learners with needs that are somewhat different than the traditional undergraduate student of the recent past. For example, a survey of registered nurses (R.N.s) who wanted to complete their baccalaureate degree indicated commuting distance, work schedule, lack of funds, and anxiety about returning to school were the major barriers they faced in continuing their educations.[30] These adults expect educational experiences that meet both their intellectual needs and their situational needs.

Not only is the student body older, but it is becoming more diverse: new high school graduates, R.N.s returning for a baccalaureate, first-time adult learners, educationally disadvantaged students, ethnic and gender (male) minorities.[22] These diverse populations require more individualized approaches, flexible educational programming, and increased faculty time. The trend toward enrollment of students with lower grade point averages may also require more faculty attention to time-consuming remedial activities. In addition to facing time constraints resulting from the demands of diverse student populations, nursing faculty are currently faced with conflicting institutional demands. With decreasing funds available to many educational institutions, faculty are expected to contribute more aggressively to their fiscal base by teaching students more efficiently, increasing their research dollar support, and producing more scholarly research.[34]

Universities are reassessing priorities, including the balance between liberal education and professional education. Several recent national studies have recommended the reevaluation of undergraduate education in the United States and have emphasized restoring liberal arts as the central focus and decreasing specialization. The importance of a broad educational background has long been recognized in nursing and was the basic premise for the movement toward baccalaureate education. Recently the American Association of Colleges of Nursing (AACN) reaffirmed this value in their report "Essentials of College and University Education for Professional Nursing," in which they emphasize the inclusion of a broad liberal education in nursing undergraduate programs.[3] The historical controversy over the appropriateness of professional education in the university assumed that practice involved the application of theory with a single and direct path to a single solution. More complex cognitive processes including problem definition and clarification have now emerged as major tasks in many professions, and certainly in nursing.[25]

Many factors have their effects on the educational requirements for nurses. The practice of prospective payment, for instance, has led to shorter hospital stays for some patients and for longer stays in acute care settings (which require better qualified nurses) for more seriously ill patients. The diversity and complexity of health care needs encountered in community health settings and expanded needs with constrained resources in all health care settings require nurses with increased educational preparation to meet the current health care challenges. Both the American Nurses' Association (ANA) and the National League for Nursing (NLN) have, through position statements, supported upgrading educational credentials for entry into practice and a national commission has been established to address implementation.[4,13,26] Although the question of appropriate credentials continues to be debated, there is active lobbying in many states to differentiate technical and professional nursing in the nurse practice acts. Nevertheless, nursing education continues to offer multiple routes for entry into practice, including diploma and associate degrees, which means that large numbers of nurses do not have a baccalaureate degree. Thus, there is a continuing need for flexible baccalaureate educational programs to allow nurses in practice to upgrade their educational qualifications.

The health care industry is feeling the impact of a general nursing shortage while trying to expand the number of better prepared nurses in their agencies. Health care agencies are now looking at ways to attract on-site educational programs to allow their staff to pursue their degrees while remaining employed. However, the cost remains high for a university to provide education at an off-campus site. The health care industry does not currently contribute directly to nursing education. Since nursing education moved out of hospitals into institutions of higher education, teaching of students has been the primary responsibility of the educational institution. Without a pool of private practitioners, such as is available in medicine, clinical supervision becomes a fully paid activity of the educational institution. Although the tuition reimbursement provided by health care agencies to their staff has been helpful to nurses in educational programs, it does not alleviate the high cost to universities of clinical education. A fully collaborative model between industry and education has yet to be developed.

When discussing flexible models of education and the needs mandating them, there are three basic areas of concern: conservation and allocation of time, location, and resources. Issues related to time include student time off from work, travel time to educational site, integration of classes into personal and family schedules, and service hours of clinical sites. Issues of location may refer to proximity of educational site from home and work for students and from the main campus for faculty. Resource issues include availability of agency support for staff who are in school; student finances; availability of community clinical sites; qualified community faculty and preceptors; and university resources related to finances, faculty, educational policies, and systems to support innovative, flexible modes of education. This chapter will discuss how these concerns are currently being addressed through flexible models for curriculum, educational delivery, and support services in nursing education and also will identify controversies surrounding the implementation of these models.

DESIGNS FOR FLEXIBLE LEARNING

Flexible systems will not be successful unless they are based on sound educational principles that examine the entire educational system including curriculum and delivery methods as well as the necessary support services.

Curriculum and delivery innovations
Clinical approaches

Clinical courses are an essential component of nursing education, but they represent a financial burden for the educational institution and a considerable time commitment for both faculty and students. Institutions would like to cut the costs associated with faculty time, and students would like to master the content of their courses in shorter periods of time, scheduled in ways that permit them to meet their multiple responsibilities. Strategies must be considered to meet these needs without sacrificing educational quality. One approach is the use of the work site and work time for required clinical experience. Health care agencies may support the concept of work time serving as an educational experience or the use of the work site for educational practice. These strategies have historically been viewed with caution by nursing educators, whose primary concern is with the quality of the educational experience, and the trade-offs continue to be reassessed.[17,29]

Another approach is the development of a cooperative association between education and service through which resources are shared. Nurses employed by a health care agency who meet established criteria are able to share clinical education responsibilities for students through the role of preceptor. Numerous reports of the success of this and similar models have been published. The model is typically used for master's level students and for special leadership assignments for undergraduate students.[1,15,19,20] The preceptor model has the potential to free faculty time, provide more flexible scheduling for students, and broaden the types of clinical experiences available to students.

Credit for experience

As the diversity of students applying to nursing programs increases, the question of credit for prior learning is raised more often. The 1987 statement by the National League for Nursing supports credit for prior learning *within the policies of the educational institution*. Possibilities usually include transfer of credit, standardized tests (for example CLEP, ACT-PEP, NLN tests), teacher-made tests, and simulated or actual clinical performance evaluations.[21] However, as older students with varying life experiences, previous education, and work experiences apply for degree programs, nursing educators may need to redefine the kinds of prior learning that document attainment of educational objectives. These objectives may be met through experiences in the workplace, workshops, and in-service programs. The Council for Adult and Experiential Learning has developed guidelines that can be used to implement this option, and those who have implemented it in nursing are beginning to report their experiences in the literature.[9]

Delivery innovations
Technology

Effective instruction demands a systematic method of designing, implementing, and evaluating the total process of learning and teaching based on research and specific objectives. Such effective learning systems require the selection of a combination of human and nonhuman resources to bring about optimal delivery.[28] As Scupham[33] points out in his report on the Open University of the United Kingdom, "The unique character of the teaching obviously resides not in the use of any or all of these teaching media, but in the degree of integration achieved and in the organic relationship between the planning of course content and the planning of teaching methods for each course." Building an effective learning system requires consideration of the learner characteristics as well as the instructional setting. As student demographics in higher education change, the methods of delivery must be reassessed and modified to meet student needs. Nursing educators can use innovative educational technologies to deliver experiences that require students to become actively involved problem solvers rather than passive receivers of information.

Technology has undergone dramatic changes. In 1900 the Mercedes-Benz Company did a study from which they concluded that worldwide demand for automobiles would not exceed 1 million because of the limitation of available chauffeurs.[7] The evolution of the automobile is much like that of the computer. The computer went from a complex, costly mainframe machine operated by specially trained experts to a democratized microcomputer costing a few thousand dollars with software that eliminated the need for expert operation.

The microcomptuer and videodisk technology have allowed the combination of video and print media with levels of interaction and feedback that are almost instantaneous. A 1986 survey of NLN-accredited baccalaureate nursing programs showed that traditional media such as videotapes and slides with tapes are still commonly used in nursing education, but new innovations such as videodisk are emerging.[5] Computers today can be used not only for simple drill and practice but also for simulations that allow the student to experiment with situations too hazardous and costly to duplicate in real life. Students can also use computers to manipulate data and test hypotheses through the use of artificial intelligence. For example, the COMMES project at Creighton University used artificial intelligence to create an expert system that acts as a decision support tool to guide patient care planning and to instruct nursing students.[11]

In addition to its use for direct or supplementary instruction on campus, technology can help bridge the locational gap for students at remote sites. Through computer and satellite networks students and faculty can be brought together. Michigan State University has experimented with CONFER, a computer conferencing system that allows faculty members on campus to advise students at a remote site through electronic mail.[27] Such two-way communication can help off-campus students overcome feelings of isolation.

The use of distance education to create a cost-effective, quality learning environment outside of the parent institution is an innovative approach that allows both individualized and mass instruction. Locational barriers can be effectively addressed through systems such as the telecommunications model use by Indiana University's School of Nursing to reach 1800 students on seven campuses.[6] Savings in both faculty and student commuting time are substantial.

The use of technology in nursing education can increase flexibility for students and enrich the learning experience while maintaining quality. Numerous research studies on the use of technology in instruction indicate that experimental learning technologies compare favorably with traditional classroom teaching when student achievement is examined.[31] Students show evidence of substantial time savings in learning over a wide range of content and types of learning via individualized modes such as computer assisted instruction CAI. Studies have also shown that students with lower aptitude show greater cognitive achievement with the use of technology.[10]

In a 1986 study for the Corporation for Public Broadcasting, Raymond Lewis conducted discussions with 173 faculty from eight colleges and universities who had used audio, video, and computer technologies for on-campus instruction. The faculty identified ways in which the technologies had enhanced effectiveness: by eliminating repetitive tasks and shortening course management, by speeding up student learning, by motivating the students (e.g., through video's ability to involve the student emotionally more than other approaches), and by expanding the learning environment.[14]

Flexible scheduling

Nearly 70% of practicing nurses in the United States have not achieved the baccalaureate level of education. Time constraints and inflexible work schedules create substantial barriers for nurses seeking to complete a baccalaureate degree. A recent U.S. Department of Health and Human Services survey of registered nurses indicated that more than 75% of licensed nurses are employed in nursing, and approximately 67% of these are working full-time. Almost 70% of the licensed nurses are married.[8] Innovative methods of curriculum packaging can assist in overcoming the barriers of time and location caused by employment and personal commitments, but these adjustments must be done in a way that preserves the educational quality of the program. For example, arrangements such as the California State University Statewide Nursing Program that divide undergraduate and graduate courses into one- and two-unit modules can help provide opportunities to nurses with difficult schedules.[23] Programs using evening and weekend classes have also provided options for registered nurses as well as for beginning professional students, many of whom are also employed full-time.

Supportive services
Financial aid

The rising cost of a college education has made financial support more important than ever for adult learners. Creative approaches are necessary for nurses seeking financial aid because their employment status makes them ineligible for most packages. Family and personal financial obligations require RN students (as well as those in other disciplines) to maintain employment and still seek additional financial assistance to cover educational expenses.

Agencies may be willing to allow concentrated time away from work for professional development that could be used for degree completion using a concept similar to sabbaticals given to educators.[12] Such leaves would diminish financial strain, relieve stress from role conflict, and shorten the educational program. Financial aid can also be made available through loans or tuition reimbursement. Such arrangements are beneficial to employers because they foster recruitment and retention of well-educated nurses. Communities can also assist students through scholarship programs such as the one developed as part of the Michigan State University Battle Creek Project for RNs completing their baccalaureate degrees. In this project a community nursing leader has taken the initiative to obtain the funds from local industry. The scholarship program is coordinated and administered locally, and in the first two classes 13 students received financial assistance.[30]

Other support services

Because older students bring diverse backgrounds of work and educational experiences, flexible educational programs require a strong support mechanism for advising and career development. The educational system is structured to handle traditional students. The bridge between the student and the university must be made through advising. Nontraditional students also need to be assisted in overcoming personal and situational barriers through socialization into the student role. This requires targeted strategies such as extended orientation efforts and bridge courses or activities designed for students as they begin their educational experience and as they complete an educational program.

ISSUES RELATED TO INTRODUCTION OF FLEXIBLE MODELS INTO HIGHER EDUCATION

Although we have identified the current mandate for innovative flexible models of nursing education and examples of strategies designed to meet this demand, implementation of such programs creates both challenges and opportunities for the institutions involved. Unless addressed, the challenges can become barriers to developing and implementing innovative educational strategies.

Universities

Most universities are built on tradition. The framework and systems of the established institution are not designed to give priority to and support flexible models of education. Lynton and Elman[24] cited the importance of reexamining the structure of the university because of the significant changes that have occurred over the past 40 years. This includes the shift from a traditional college-age population to an older population with previous work experience. Success in addressing these issues depends on the extent to which certain policies, procedures, values, and norms can be changed within the university itself. For example, the concept of offering credit for prior learning is important for adult learners with rich and varied backgrounds, yet it is difficult for institutions to assess the comparability of life experiences to classroom experiences. Tracking the educational progress of adult learners who have earned credits from multiple institutions, advising students who drop out and return to a program several times, and finding the number of enrolled students changing daily due to personal exigencies are some of the considerations that arise when implementing nontraditional programs.

As the university is asked to reassess priorities in a time of fiscal constraint, it is important to acknowledge that universities cannot be all things to all people. Diluting the university mission to a level that jeopardizes quality of instruction serves no one. What is called for is the provision of a quality university education in a mode and manner that serves a population not previously targeted.

Developers of flexible educational models have struggled with the issue of quality, because only quality educational programs can meet the needs of students. Flexible educational programs must be built on a sound research base and must be evaluated periodically. Faculty have a major responsibility for curriculum planning and commitment to quality education. Development of innovative programs requires a faculty commitment to development to gain the knowledge and skills, imagination, resources, creativity, scholarly effort, and time. There must be incentives for talented faculty to participate in the creation of such programs, and a means by which such activities can be credited toward promotion and tenure in the academic system. Although in the long run innovative models such as use of technology can ease faculty time pressures, in the initial period faculty find it difficult to schedule the time to develop such cost-effective teaching materials. The Lewis study[23] found that many of the barriers to the use of technology by faculty were institutional: lack of funds for software and equipment, institutional policies, lack of faculty time and rewards for production, and confusion over copyright and royalty policies. New approaches such as the peer review of software being developed by EDUCOM, a computer consortium of more than 500 colleges and universities, are being sought by institutions.[32] However, much work remains, and the problems are not yet resolved.

Community agencies and the health care industry

A key to successful implementation of innovative models of education is enhanced partnership among communities, the health care industry, and institutions of higher learning. The dilemmas in health care delivery, including the nursing shortage and cost containment strategies, must be addressed from multiple perspectives. To be successful, the community, profession, and educational institution must share a common goal and intent to support the individual pursuing professional education. Historically, nursing has not developed such a partnership, but mutual needs and limited resources require a reassessment of strategies. This partnership must include collaborative planning and development of strategies to address financial support for educational programs and for students; sharing of clinical resources; scheduling and flexible packaging of programs to accommodate employment; and providing a quality, accessible, feasible educational program. Agencies face both administrative dilemmas, such as scheduling of staff and support for staff members experiencing role conflicts as workers and students, and fiscal dilemmas as staff request tuition reimbursement and educational leaves.

A word must be said about the challenges facing community health care agencies as nurses succeed in gaining their baccalaureate or graduate degrees. The educational process is more than the process of acquiring credentials; it is a process of growth. As nurses change their professional perspective, skills, and knowledge, these changes are brought to the agencies in which they are employed and are reflected in the autonomy of nursing practice. Although positive, such changes must also be recognized as sources of stress and as factors that must be addressed. Better prepared nurses will seek positions that reward them and offer them opportunities for career advancement. Many nurses who have experienced higher education will also seek graduate degrees. These changes represent challenges to agencies that have already felt the stress of staff completing their undergraduate educations.

The needs of the profession, health care industry, and educational institutions require flexible models of nursing education. All three areas must work together to address the issues related to successful implementation of innovative educational strategies.

REFERENCES

1. Adams DE: Agency staff facilitate student learning, Nurs Outlook 28(6):382, 1980.
2. Aiken L: Nurses for the future: breaking the shortage cycles. In Am J Nurs supplement: nurses for the future, December 1987.
3. American Association of Colleges of Nursing: Essentials of college and university education for professional nursing, final report, Washington, DC, 1986, The Association.
4. American Nurses' Association: American nurses' association first position on education for nursing, Am J Nurs 65(12):106, 1965.
5. Awbrey S: Technology and distance education in nursing. Technology in nursing education conference, Detroit, June 1987.
6. Billings DM: Teaching at a distance using telecommunications technology. Technology in nursing education conference, Detroit, June 1987.
7. Brand S: The media lab: inventing the future at MIT, New York, 1987, Viking.
8. Brimmer P, editor: Facts about nursing, Kansas City, Mo, 1985, American Nurses' Association.
9. Bunkers S and Geyer C: The nursing portfolio of prior learning: access and credibility for the RN, J Nurs Educ 27(6):280, 1988.
10. Chang BL: Computer-aided instruction in nursing education. In Werley HH, Fitzpatrick JJ, and Taunton RL, editors: Annual review of nursing research, vol 4, New York, 1986, Springer Publishing Co.
11. Cuddingan J: COMMES—an artificial intelligence-based expert system. Technology in nursing education conference, Detroit, June 1987.
12. Curran CR: Sabbaticals: not for teachers only, Nurs Outlook 33(2):92, 1987.
13. DeBack V: The national commission on nursing implementation project: report to the participants of nurses in agreement conference, J Prof Nurs 3(4):226, 1987.
14. Dirr P: Using technology to serve distance learners. Technology in nursing education conference, Detroit, June 1987.
15. Dobbs KK: The senior preceptorship as a method for anticipatory socialization of baccalaureate nursing students, J Nurs Educ 27(4):167, 1988.
16. Farrell J: Recruitment planning in light of changing student profiles. In Patterns in nursing: strategic planning for nursing education, New York, 1987, National League for Nursing.
17. Fields SK: Nurses earn their B.S. degrees—on the job, Nurs Outlook 24(3):169, 1976.
18. Houle CO: Continuing learning in the professions, San Francisco, 1981, Jossey-Bass, Inc, Publishers.
19. Joel L: The Rutgers experience: one perspective on service-education collaboration, Nurs Outlook 33(5):220, 1985.
20. Keen MF and Dear MR: Mastery of role transition: clinical teaching strategies, J Nurs Educ 22(5):183, 1983.
21. Lenburg CB: Nontraditional nursing education. In Werley HH, Fitzpatrick JJ, and Taunton RL, editors: Annual review of nursing research, vol 4, New York, 1986, Springer Publishing Co.
22. Lenhart RC: Faculty burnout and some reasons why, Nurs Outlook 28(7):424, 1980.
23. Lewis R. Research notes, no. 11, Corporation for Public Broadcasting, Office of Planning and Policy Development, Washington, DC, 1987.
24. Lewis JM and Cobin JT: Mediated learning: a new pathway to the BSN. In McCloskey JC and Grace HK, editors: Current issues in nursing, ed 2, Boston, 1985, Blackwell Scientific Publications, Inc.
25. Lynton EA and Elman SE: New priorities for the university, San Francisco, 1987, Jossey-Bass, Inc, Publishers.
26. National League for Nursing: Position statement on nursing roles—scope and preparation, Pub No 11-1893, 1982.
27. Parnes R and Bernstein MA: The beginner's guide to confer II, Ann Arbor, Mich, 1986, Advertel Communication Systems, Inc.
28. Percival F and Ellington H: A handbook of educational technology, London, 1984, Kogan Page.
29. Planchock N: RN education: working and learning in the community hospital. In Pathways to practice: reports of seven demonstration projects on RN education, Atlanta, 1982, Southern Regional Education Board.
30. Rothert ML and others: Joining forces to meet the needs of the RN learner, Nursing and Health Care 9(5):261, 1988.

31. Schramm W: Big media, little media, Beverly Hills, Calif, 1977, Sage.

32. Sculley J: The relationship between business and higher education: a perspective on the 21st century, EDUCOM Conference, Los Angeles, October 1987.

33. Scupham J: The open university. In Mackenzie NI and others, editors: Open learning, Paris, 1975, The Unesco Press.

34. Slaughter S: From serving students to serving the economy: changing expectations of faculty role performance, Higher Education 14:41, 1985.

CHAPTER 19

Emerging models of postbaccalaureate nursing education

COLLEEN CONWAY-WELCH

NATIONAL INITIATIVES FOR CHANGE

The year 1988 will be remembered as a benchmark year for nursing. Several recent publications, projects, and proposals will provoke dramatic changes in nursing, for better or for worse. Those events are (1) the publication and review of the work of the first two years of the Kellogg-funded National Commission on Nursing Implementation Project (NCNIP) and the production of three documents entitled "An Introduction to Timeline for Transition into the Future Nursing Education System for Two Categories of Nurse,"[11] "Characteristics of Professional and Technical Nurses of the Future and Their Educational Programs,"[10] and "A View of the Immediate Future"[9]; (2) the interim report of Secretary Bowen's Department of Health and Human Services Commission on Nursing; (3) the recommendations about nursing of the *Presidential Commission on the HIV Epidemic*[12] (1988); (4) the acceptance by the Advertising Council of a project to market nursing and its image on a sophisticated national level; (5) the proposal of the American Medical Association for a new type of low-paid, low-skill bedside worker known as a registered care technician (1988); and (6) the publication of the *Sixth Report to the President and Congress on the Status of Health Personnel in the United States*[14] (1988).

The Sixth Report's section on nursing ends with these prophetic words:

A national initiative is needed to address the problem of declining nursing school enrollments. Continuing enrollment declines noted in nursing and in other health care professions raise concerns about the ability to replenish and augment the supply of nurses, thus causing an aging nurse population and shortages as we progress into the 21st century.

Continuing national initiatives are required to ensure the appropriate preparation of nurses. Current health care needs, as well as the changes in the population of the country and the changing locus of the settings in which health care is delivered, requires that there be an adequate number of nurses prepared to provide and manage care in a variety of settings, and to serve as expert clinicians, teachers, administrators, researchers and consultants.[14]

This need for national initiatives for change occurs in the midst of a nursing shortage that is not just the usual cyclical shortage but the result of many new disturbing elements that are negatively influencing nurse recruitment and retention. These include reduced interest among prospective applicants in nursing as a career, confusion about the career opportunities for nurses, concern about salary compression, and dissatisfaction with the workplace.

THE APPROPRIATE LEVEL FOR THE FIRST PROFESSIONAL DEGREE

Few other professions have used the word *profession* so loosely. The fact that five educational routes are available to become a registered nurse (the associate degree, the diploma, the B.S.N., the entry-level master's, and the entry-level doctorate) has made marketing the career opportunities in nursing virtually incomprehensible and therefore almost impossible.

Every profession has its professional and paraprofessional support levels. Physicians have physician assistants, attorneys have paralegals, and dentists have dental assistants. Even with a baccalaureate degree in nursing, however, the nurse remains the least educated member of the health care team. Is it any wonder that frustration, role conflict, stress, and burnout are common?

With the rapid increase in scientific, psychosocial, and biomedical knowledge, nursing education moved into academic settings. Historically, nurses with baccalaureate degrees were required to assume leadership positions because the vast majority of nurses had diplomas. Nurses prepared at the BSN level were generalists. Since 5, and then 4, academic years were utilized to prepare a nurse to function as a generalist in a variety of settings, preparation for leadership and specialization eventually became an outcome of master's level nursing curricula.

However, the demands placed on the nurse of today and tomorrow call on more than the generalist skills acquired in baccalaureate programs. In the future, what will be needed is a paraprofessional nurse, educated at the associate degree level, and also nurses with postbaccalaureate graduate degrees in nursing— the master's of science in nursing (M.S.N.) and the nursing doctorate (N.D.). Regulatory mechanisms need to be reconsidered so that the associate nurse retains the registered nurse (R.N.) title, and the nurse with an advanced degree gets a title that reflects a more specialized position. A comparison of the merits of the A.D. degree with other contrasting degrees is beyond the scope of this article. It is enough to say that the M.S.N. programs of tomorrow will also need to provide foundation, generalist courses for the nonnurse entering the program, along with the M.S.N. specialty content.

Education and engineering are similar to nursing in that they are also having to define where professional level education for the discipline should occur. Jacobsen,[6] discussing the Holmes's report, "called for sweeping changes in what prospective teachers study in college, including an end to undergraduate majors in education and a new emphasis on the 'core disciplines.'" It rejected the typical bachelor's degree program of teacher education and stated that "the undergraduate major must be abolished in our universities." It concluded with the idea that "greater coherence and dedication to the historic tenets of liberal education is . . . essential to the improvement of teacher education." The report recommended that the title *professional teacher* would be the first full professional certificate. It would be granted only to teachers who had completed a master's degree in teaching. Recent articles about engineering have also documented

a concern about the validity of educating the professional at the baccalaureate level.

Samuel Jay Keyser,[7] Associate Provost for Educational Policy and Programs at Massachusetts Institute of Technology, states that "among the engineers, there is a realization that the social and political implications of the technology are as important as the technology itself." Schools of engineering are recognizing that it is not clear how schools can fit both types of courses (engineering and the humanities) into a 4-year program that many agree is already far too brief. Paul Gray,[3] President of Massachusetts Institute of Technology, states: "We should recognize that in four years, we cannot educate an engineering student to the level of a beginning professional. The School's curriculum changes may be a step toward acknowledging that professional training now requires graduate studies."

Eric Walker,[15] Dean Emeritus of Engineering at Pennsylvania State University, states that:

The time has come to admit that four years of undergraduate study cannot produce a fully competent engineer, any more than it can produce a fully competent physician. The undergraduate engineering curriculum should include the basics of engineering, plus the courses required for a liberal-arts education. That preparation should then be followed by specialized studies leading to a graduate degree in engineering. Such a program would strengthen engineer's claim to professional status.

Like engineering, nursing is recognizing that the old models of education and lack of differentiated practice descriptions as they relate to education are not working, and efforts are finally being made by nursing educators and nursing administrators to address these issues. An even more controversial idea is that of the professional doctorate—the N.D. Hecht[4] proposes that:

(1) all who enter the profession of nursing will need a non-nursing baccalaureate degree prior to entry into professional study.

(2) the professional degree will be the professional doctorate, analogous to the M.D. degree. I shall not propose to name the degree here, although the N.D. is used already. The curriculum would probably be three years, although my purpose here is not to outline a course of study.

(3) there will be another level, that of the associate nurse, prepared at the community college level. There would be many more of these nurses than there are now, working under the direction of professional nurses. Similarly, there would be fewer professional nurses than most envision, perhaps five associate nurses to each professional.

STIMULI FOR CHANGE
Diminishing interest in the B.S.N. degree

The bachelor's degree in nursing is history. The need to build a professional nursing education on a strong liberal arts and science base is becoming more and more obvious. A quick review of the "Essentials" document, produced by the American Association of Colleges of Nursing,[2] makes educators tremble about the need to include all that content in 8 semesters. Nor can nurses be prepared for the future described in the NCNIP Futures document (see Appendix A) in 8 semesters. Part of the stimulus for the growth in postbaccalaureate programs is from nurses with associate degrees. Many of them, realizing the constraints their education has imposed on their practice capabilities and recognizing that their education has prepared them to care for patients only with common health problems in medical-surgical units, are returning to school to acquire advanced knowledge about nursing. Given the opportunity, many of them have no intention of stopping at a B.S.N. degree and in fact see it as only a marker on a way to a master's degree. They have provided the impetus for a number of programs to identify ways to make advanced education in nursing on the master's level more easily accessible and to identify ways in which both nurses and non-nurses can begin their professional studies with a strong liberal arts and science base.

Changing demographics of the minority populations in the United States

By the year 2005, one in three Americans will be of African, Asian, or Hispanic descent.[5] Yet many women and men in these minority groups who have an interest in health care are being counseled into types of nursing that require the least amount of education and pay the lowest salaries, for example, as licensed practical nurses and as nurses with only associate degrees. Assuming current trends, as the patient population becomes more ethnically diverse, the number of care givers who have ethnic backgrounds similar to their patients will decrease, and those working will not have the sophisticated skills necessary to care for people in an increasingly complex health care system.

Many minorities who want a college education are not considering nursing as a viable career option. With effort and scholarship support, they see themselves obtaining a baccalaureate degree in liberal arts and sciences and then getting an advanced degree in a more lucrative and autonomous field such as law, medicine, business, dentistry, or engineering. To many of minorities nursing is seen as a low-paid, thankless, dead-end occupation.

Changing work environment

The nurse of the future must be able to think, work, organize, communicate, and learn. Therefore, people needed in nursing must possess a well-developed aptitude for conceptual and critical thinking rather than just factual knowledge. These qualities will be essential for success in the next century.[13]

The twenty-first century will be a time when vast amounts of available information will require constant shifting and categorization. The health care system will be very dependent on innovation. Care givers will have to be able to create new technologies, new ideas, and new services, and to be very comfortable with discarding the old.

Employers now are finding innovative ways to maximize the workforce, for example, using increased robotics and cross-training employees. Health care institutions are recognizing the inevitability of this development as well. We will see the end of departments as we know them and more cross-training of employees.

The ability to think and conceptualize rather than simply memorize and recall facts will be recognized by the health care industry as a desirable skill for employees. Computers, not nurses, will be charged with brute memorization of facts. Nurses must learn to use technology as a tool. The computer saves time, which means that nurses will have more time to express their ideas and realize their full potential.

In the future it will not be uncommon for people to change careers four or five times. Nurses will continue to be lost to nursing unless there are a number of different career paths available to them within nursing and educational opportunities as well. Many schools of nursing have already established postmaster's option programs, which allow nurses who hold master's degrees in nursing in one specialty to cross-train and prepare for certification in another nursing specialty. The most successful nurses will be those who enjoy taking risks, who can deal with many ideas simultaneously, and who bring a broad perspective to solving problems.

Sculley[13] talks about the age of "know how," which will be dependent on the thinking and conceptualizing talents of people, not on the years of experience they have had doing the same thing. So much information is available today that we need discerning individuals to figure out what is important, what is useful, and how it can be understood. We need nurses with strong communication skills and a broad view of the world.

Sculley[13] also predicts that more emphasis will be put on collaborative work. Much of what students do in school is individualized; students need to be encouraged to work in groups while developing concepts. Team learning, team building, and team discovery help strengthen conceptual skills when comparing, contrasting, and analyzing. Nursing students who are educated with a foundation in the liberal arts and sciences can challenge the ideas of the past, discover the wisdom of others, explore knowledge, and stretch their minds.

Sculley[13] emphasizes that college is the last place in which to be pragmatic. This is a time when people should be most inquisitive and exposed to ideas, and career training should be a low priority. In the 21st century, a well-rounded education is going to be far more practical and desirable than we can imagine today.[13]

Changing student body

In addition to attracting more minorities into nursing, nursing programs must be presented as a challenging opportunity to men, to older students, to part-time students, and to college graduates (both non-nurses and nurses) who seek the level of autonomous practice and financial reimbursement that can be achieved with a master's degree or a nursing doctorate.

Nonnurses entering directly into master's study are a new source of students for nursing. Nursing education must find pathways into the profession at the master's level for people who do not have a baccalaureate degree in nursing.

These nontraditional programs are becoming more and more plentiful. They are categorized as either combined programs or accelerated programs.[8] Combined programs are those that bypass the B.S.N. and combine generalist and advanced nursing content in a course of study that culminates in an M.S.N. or N.D. These programs can be found at Vanderbilt University, Case Western Reserve University, University of Tennessee-Knoxville, Yale University, and Massachusetts General Institute. Vanderbilt University School of Nursing offers a bridge to a specialty master's degree. Nurses and nonnurses who have accumulated the equivalent of 6 semesters of liberal arts and sciences (and preferably a college degree) can enter the

"bridge," where the generalist undergraduate nursing content is taught. On completion of the bridge, they do not receive a B.S.N. but move directly to the specialty master's and graduate with a master's degree. A nonnurse can complete this program in 6 semesters or 2 calendar years; a nurse can complete it in less time by getting "credit by exam" for some of the nursing courses. Case Western Reserve University School of Nursing offers a different kind of program, based on a college degree, which awards an N.D., or nursing doctorate (analogous to the M.D.) after 3 academic years. Yale, University of Tennessee-Knoxville, and Massachusetts General Institute offer programs of study in basic nursing and a nursing specialty of choice leading to an M.S.N.

Accelerated programs allow a student with previous college credits and/or a degree to accelerate to the B.S.N. These programs are offered at Barry University in Miami Shores, Florida; Columbia University in New York City; Creighton University in Omaha; Fairleigh Dickinson University in Rutherford, New Jersey; Pace University in Pleasantville, New York; St. Louis University; University of Pennsylvania; University of Colorado in Denver; University of California, San Francisco; and Georgetown University in Washington, D.C. This list of schools with combined and accelerated programs is not meant to be exclusive, because many schools are considering offering these options.

Even a cursory review of the "Futures" document of the NCNIP[11] will convince the casual reader that we need to do things differently to prepare students to practice nursing in the next century. Those future nurses are now in elementary school. Phasing out the B.S.N. degree, restructuring the associate degree to a true 4-semester educational offering, and emphasizing direct entry to the profession at the postbaccalaureate level are ideas that need to be moved to the center of our stage.

REFERENCES

1. American Medical Association basic program to prepare bedside personnel, Report of the Board of Trustees CC(I-87), Chicago, 1987.
2. Essentials of college and university education for professional nursing: final report, Washington, DC, 1986, American Association of Colleges of Nursing.
3. Gray P: MIT's study of its undergraduate program: preparing students for the new milleneum, Chronicle of Higher Education, Dec 3, 1986, p. 42.
4. Hecht A: The post-baccalaureate doctorate model. Paper presented at the fall semi-annual meeting of the American Asso-

ciation of Colleges of Nursing, Washington, DC, Oct 25, 1988.

5. Hodgkinson H: All one system, Washington, DC, 1985, The Institute for Educational Leadership, Inc.

6. Jacobsen R: Universities asked to help reform teacher education, Chronicle of Higher Education, April 9, 1986, p. 21.

7. Kingston J: Future engineers getting more humanities requirements, The New York Times, p 26, July 19, 1987.

8. Krauss J: Generic master's degree in nursing. Paper presented at the fall semi-annual meeting of the American Association of Colleges of Nursing, Washington, DC, Oct 25, 1988.

9. National Commission on Nursing Implementation Project: Invitational conference. A view of the immediate future, 1986.

10. National Commission on Nursing Implementation Project: Invitational conference. Characteristics of professional and technical nurses of the future and their educational programs, 1986.

11. National Commission on Nursing Implementation Project: Invitational conference. Timeline for transition into the future nursing educational system for two categories of nurse, 1986.

12. Report of the presidential commission on the human immunodeficiency virus epidemic, Rep No 0-214-701:QL 3, Washington, DC, 1988, US Government Printing Office.

13. Sculley J: Perspective on the future: what business needs from higher education, Change 20(1):1, 1988.

14. Sixth report to the President and Congress on the status of health personnel in the United States, No. HRP0907200, Washington, DC, 1988, US Department of Health and Human Services.

15. Walker E: Our engineering schools must share the blame for declining productivity, Chronicle of Higher Education, Dec 2, 1987, p. A52.

16. Watson J: The professional doctorate as an entry level into practice. In National League for Nursing: Perspectives in nursing 1987-89, Pub No 41-2199, New York, 1988.

APPENDIX: NATIONAL COMMISSION ON NURSING IMPLEMENTATION PROJECT: A VIEW OF THE IMMEDIATE FUTURE

To plan well, it is necessary to have an understanding of the present and a view of the forces that will shape the immediate future.

The Governing Board of the National Commission on Nursing Implementation Project agreed to accept the challenge of proposing a view of the next five to fifteen years. That view would be used as the basis for the work of the project.

The board recognized the difficulty of predicting the future in an age of expanding knowledge and a time of turbulence in what was once the relatively stable system of health care. The board also recognized that one of its strengths was the fact that it included persons representing a number of disciplines, who brought a variety of perspectives and long-standing commitment to health care. After studying current trends and a variety of future projections, board members participated in a consensus exercise to create a composite view of the future.

While board members consider their view to be the thoughtful effort of responsible people, they recognize its fluidity. This view is expected to change as the future becomes the present, as new trends emerge and as better projections become available.

Major forces

The Governing Board identified the following major forces that they believe will be most important in shaping nursing's role in the health care environment of the next several years.

- Shifting payment systems
- Increased proportion of the aged population
- Increased competition among health care providers
- Increased complexity of client needs and severity of client conditions
- Government intervention in cost containment

Future predictions

The Governing Board also examined the interaction of these major forces to predict those that would most impact the profession of nursing.

These immediate future predictions are not unique. Many futurists and forward-thinking organizations are predicting the same. However, the Governing Board predictions are different in that they were selected as being the most influential for the immediate future of nursing. The predictions were viewed from three perspectives: the health care delivery system, consumers, and nurses/nursing.

The health care delivery system

The business orientation will continue in the health care industry. The profit motive will drive the changing system, resulting in structural changes as well as delivery changes. Shifting payment systems as well as government intervention to contain costs will fuel this movement.

The business orientation in health care will require more precise justification for costs and substantive data on results of interventions. It appears that the fundamental measure of the economic performance of the health care delivery system will be productivity. In such a situation, the monitoring of quality of care becomes increasingly important. These developments highlight the need for data on the cost/benefit outcomes of nursing care.

The shifting payment system and the explosion of technology will cause client populations to shift away from acute care hospitals. This shift will produce new combinations of in-patient and out-patient services. Another outcome may be increased development of multi-tiered systems of care and the continuing problem of uncompensated care. To lower the costs of long-term care, services for management of chronic illness will be in demand. The need for home care services will increase dramatically.

Consumers

The profile of the consumer of health care will continue to change during the next fifteen years. The proportion of elderly consumers will increase significantly. The numbers of elderly persons and others for whom uncompensated care must be provided will escalate. The need for nurses prepared to meet the physiological, psychological and sociological needs of the elderly will continue to rise. An expected change in the proportions of ethnic populations suggests a greater need for health care professionals with second language skills and an understanding of ethnic diversity.

Although some observers predict that self-care and wellness services will increase, it is not clear whether consumers will take advantage of these services. Further, it is expected that some people will not be able to exercise self-care or will not choose to do so. They will remain dependent on the health care system for illness care. Futures literature suggests that growing numbers of consumers will become involved in developing a more responsive health care system. Whether this will happen in the immediate future is not yet clear.

In situations where clients, families and health care providers are making decisions about use of procedures or equipment to support extension of life, a key consideration will be the quality of life that will follow the procedure. Ethical issues will be part of such decisions.

Nurses and nursing

The government role in health care is expected to continue. This suggests that nurses must be adept at influencing public policy. The future role of major nursing organizations will clearly require constant involvement in the public arena for the purpose of affecting policy. This will be true whether the arena is the nurse's workplace, the community, the state legislature or Congress.

The changing settings for the delivery of health care will demand that a larger number of nurses be prepared to give service outside of acute care organizations. At the same time, traditional settings will require a greater proportion of nurses with advanced preparation to manage the increasingly complex needs of clients. Because the health care system as we know it is changing, it is expected that the environments in which nurses work will be dramatically different. As nursing services begin to respond to this change in the system, there will be a growing need for retraining and cross training nurses.

The evolving need for more highly educated nurses who can function in future environments that are different from what presently exists is the direct result of a number of socioeconomic-political forces. Primary among these forces are shifting payment systems, the explosion of technology, increased competition among health care providers and increased interest in self-help and wellness.

Because of the future needs of the community, nurses will need educational preparation that is *different* from the education of nurses today. It is expected that there will be a shortage of baccalaureate prepared nurses and an oversupply of associate-degree prepared nurses. This suggests the need to embrace a dramatic change in the system that educates nurses. The change must be implemented in such a way that the supply of appropriately prepared nurses does not dwindle during the transition period. In addition, it is critical that the planned change include the shifting of monies from one educational system into another.

The future nurse's practice will be based on greater use of scientific and research data. This projection is directly related to forces such as the technology explosion and further supports the need for educational remapping.

Because of changes in the way health care will be delivered, it is expected that nurses will provide a greater diversity of health care services in a greater variety of settings. Nursing services may be arranged through contractual arrangements, private practice, professional collaboration, consultation and other entrepreneurial endeavors. These types of systems will respond to the business orientation of health care services.

Summary

A view of the immediate future is a necessary "first step" if action strategies for that future are to be formulated. The future as defined here, is considered a fluid one with expectations for change as time goes on. However, the vision set forth by these forces and expectations will provide the framework for action to guide nursing and other health care efforts toward planning nursing's contribution to the health care system for the year 2000.

BIBLIOGRAPHY

Abramowitz K: The future of health care delivery in America, New York, 1985, Sanford C. Berstein & Co.

American Nurses' Association: Long range, strategic and business planning for the American Nurses' Association, Kansas City, Mo, 1986, The Association.

Detmer S: The future of health care delivery systems and settings. Paper presented at the conference on nursing in the 21st century sponsored by AACN and AONE, Aspen, Colo, July 1985.

Franz J: Challenge for nursing: hiking productivity without lowering quality of care, Modern Healthcare 14(12):60, 1984.

Goldbeck W: A new force for change in U.S. health policy, Bell Atlantic Quarterly 2(4), 1985.

Health Insurance Association of America: The health care system in the mid 1990's. Study conducted by Arthur D. Little, Inc, Washington, DC, 1985.

Health Insurance Association of America Technical Advisory Committee: Report on uncompensated care to the HIAA federal programs committee, Washington, DC, 1985.

Health Network of America: Forecast '86. Developed by Center for Health Management Research, Lutheran Hospital Society of Southern California, Los Angeles, Calif, 1985.

Milio N: Telematics in the future of health care delivery: implications for nursing. Paper presented at a conference on nursing in the 21st century sponsored by AACN and AONE, Aspen, Colo, July 1985.

Nathanson M and Bazzoli F: Bedside terminals will save work, cut staff, Modern Healthcare 15(9):44, 1985.

Schlotfeldt R: A brave, new nursing world: exercising options for the future, Prof Nurs 1:244, 1985.

Studin I, Coile C, and Strum D: Future of hospital-based nursing explored, Hospital Forum 27(4):65, 1984.

Styles M: The future marketplace, regulation of health care providers, and education of nurses. Paper presented at a conference for nursing in the 21st century sponsored by AACN and AONE, Aspen, Colo, July 1985.

Toffler A: The Third Wave, New York, 1980, Bantam.

CHAPTER 20

How to choose a graduate program

GAYE W. POTEET
LINDA C. HODGES

One of the most critical decisions a nurse will make is whether to attend graduate school. The second most important decision is where to attend graduate school. No matter whether one is considering entering a master's or a doctoral program, a commitment to graduate education at either level represents a considerable investment of time, energy, and financial resources. In most instances it also involves personal sacrifices on the part of the individual and that individual's significant others. The choice one makes about graduate education determines in large part the course of career development over a lifetime. At the same time one considers personal factors, one also needs to consider marketplace forces that will affect current and future employment opportunities and educational preparation.

Downs pointed out in 1978 that graduate education is preparation for scholarship and that demonstration of scholarship occurs through a consistent pattern of productivity. Therefore, the choice of a program in which to acquire the knowledge and skill during the preparation phase is crucial.[5]

HISTORY

The first master's degree in nursing was awarded in 1916 by the Department of Nursing Education at Teachers College, Columbia University, in New York.[2] Early programs were designed to prepare administrators and teachers to serve as directors of nursing services and nursing education programs.

Frances Richter coined the term *clinical nurse specialist* in the early 1940s to refer to a nurse with advanced knowledge and expertise in a specialized area of clinical practice.[6] Preparation for this role had as its primary focus the improvement of patient care.

Since that time more than 128 schools of nursing have developed accredited programs leading to a master's degree in various specialties.[7] These programs range from broad areas such as community health nursing to narrow fields such as adult oncology. For example, the University of Alabama offers opportunities for major areas of concentration in clinical specialization, nursing service administration, and nursing education and also offers 14 subspecialty areas.[8]

The first program to award a doctoral degree in nursing was also Teachers College in New York. This program was designed to prepare nursing educators and was based upon the Ed.D. model. The second doctoral program in nursing was at New York University in the nursing science program. Its Ph.D. was modeled on the Ph.D. from N.Y.U.'s College of Education. In 1960 the first doctoral program with a practice discipline focus was developed at Boston University. Graduates of these programs were awarded the D.N.Sc.[9] Nurses choosing to attend doctoral programs in nursing in 1960 had only four choices. By 1988 the number had grown to 45.[11]

Graduate nursing education has grown rapidly during the last 3 decades. This growth occurred at both the master's and doctoral levels. In addition, the opportunities for specialization multiplied, and a variety of degrees were chosen to be awarded for completion of the various programs. In 1988, 22,259 students were pursuing graduate nursing degrees, 20,182 the master's degree and the remaining 2077 the doctoral degree.[11]

TYPES OF DEGREES

The proliferation of graduate degrees has created less confusion at the master's level than at the doctoral.

Whether the master's degree is a Master of Science in Nursing (M.S.N.), Master in Science (M.S.), Master in Nursing (M.N.), or Master of Arts (M.A.) is a practical matter. At this level it is commonly understood and accepted that the end result is preparation for practice, whether it be administration, education, or advanced clinical practice.

Degrees at the doctoral level are usually classified within two categories, academic and professional. Academic degrees are generally designed to prepare the individual for knowledge development. The professional degree is awarded following a program designed to prepare practitioners. In some instances the choice of the degree for a nursing doctorate rests more on the choices open to nursing faculty on individual campuses than on the actual differences in the curriculum plan for the various programs leading to a nursing doctorate.

The preparation of researchers in any discipline takes place at the doctoral level, and the Doctor of Philosophy degree is recognized as the "mark of highest achievement in preparation for active scholarship and research" by the Council of Graduate Schools in the United States.

The doctoral program is designed to prepare a student for a lifetime of intellectual inquiry that manifests itself in creative scholarship and research, often leading to careers in social, governmental, business, and industrial organizations as well as the more traditional careers in university and college teaching.[4]

CONTINUING YOUR EDUCATION: WHY GRADUATE SCHOOL?

Professional practice implies a commitment to life-long learning. With the rapid growth of knowledge, continuation in a career demands continued updating and development of new skills and knowledge. This can be done either through formal degree-granting institutions or through informal continuing education. The choice is not whether one continues to learn but rather by what method one chooses to learn.

For those committed to a career, advantages of acquiring advanced degrees through formal education programs are many. Nursing has developed a professional model of practice that, in many instances, requires a master's degree in nursing for attainment of positions such as head nurse or for advancement via a career ladder. Holding the formal credential provides access to advanced positions, increased salary, key positions on institutional committees, and increased status in the organization.

Most often the people who advance in professional organizations are those who hold advanced degrees. Enrollment in a formal advanced degree program puts one in touch with other potential leaders in nursing— classmates who can form a close personal and professional network and who in later years are in a position to assist in career development. Additionally, formal degree-granting programs bring the student in contact with mature professionals who are committed to the advancement of bright and eager graduate students. Most likely, it is in the master's program that the student acquires the skill for formal presentation and scholarly writing so necessary for overall career success.[10]

Perhaps the best reason for returning to graduate school is that of personal fulfillment and professional commitment. When motivated to acquire an advanced degree only to qualify for a job, the goal becomes paramount, often to the exclusion of enjoying the journey. The student with limited motivation often fails to become immersed in a field of study, its literature, and the scholarly inquiry process. For these persons, the goals of graduate education become a series of checkoffs—products produced and designated hurdles jumped—rather than the acquisition of knowledge for professional enhancement and personal fulfillment. The learning that occurs from being a participant in the academic community is lost.

Many educators in practice disciplines support the position that a period of time as an active practitioner is needed in order to internalize the theories and skills learned so that practice and clinical decision making become automatic.[1] In the past, nurses seeking degrees have tended to complete doctoral programs at a later age than females completing doctorates in other fields.

Potential candidates often arrive at the decision to commit to graduate study when they feel capable of handling the challenges of their present position and begin to experience a sense of stagnation. Potential applicants verbalize this sense of frustration and boredom with statements such as:

> "I have learned all I can in this job."
> "The mold is beginning to grow."
> "Is this all there is?"

Formal educational programs offer the opportunity and challenge for personal and professional develop-

ASSESSING ESSENTIAL ELEMENTS IN GRADUATE NURSING EDUCATION
1. Accreditation status (NLN, regional, speciality) 2. National standing 3. Admission requirements 4. Faculty qualifications 5. Institutional climate 6. Resources 7. Clinical facilities 8. Assistantships 9. Program requirements

ment necessary for those committed to career advancement.

CHOOSING A PROGRAM

Many variables need to be considered when choosing a program of graduate study. The most critical factor is to have formulated a career idea of "what it is that you want to be when you grow up." One cannot prepare for all areas of study or nursing roles in a single program. The danger in choosing too broad a field of study is being unemployable because of a lack of expertise in a particular area. This mistake is more commonly made at the master's level.

Once a definable career goal is in mind, the next step is identifying graduate programs that offer the chosen area of study. Desirable programs should also seem feasible given individual considerations such as finances, family and personal responsibilities, commuting distance, and the need to work. One's previous academic record and general academic ability should also be considered.

When shopping for the ideal graduate program, 9 factors should be considered. Individual needs and interests will modify and refine this list, but every potential student should consider each of the items listed in the box above.

One of the first elements to be determined when selecting a quality graduate program is the program's accreditation status. Brochures and catalogs should list National League for Nursing Accreditation and regional accreditation status. Speciality accreditation, such as that granted by the American College of Nurse Midwifery for graduate nurse midwifery programs, is

a prerequisite for writing for certification on graduation.

Another dimension to be considered is the national standing of the school and the university. Those schools that are prominent nationally generally have attained that status through the presence of outstanding facilities, faculty qualifications and scholarship, outstanding students, and a cadre of alumni with nationally recognized achievements. Information about the national standing of schools of nursing can be found in the Gorman Report, although some individuals have questioned its authenticity. Recent nursing research studies have also addressed the relative status of schools of nursing.[3,12]

Admission standards tell you not only whether you are likely to be accepted or rejected, but also what kind of classmates you are likely to have. Potential applicants should pay particular attention to requirements for a minimum grade point average and the minimum scores on the graduate record examination.

Underlying the belief system of graduate education, especially at the doctoral level, is the premise that the student has the opportunity to be guided by an active scholar. Thus nonproductive faculty whose only qualification are doctoral degrees and completed dissertations do not meet the qualifications for teaching at the graduate level. A graduate faculty composed primarily of junior faculty members is not likely to meet the needs of doctoral students.

Senior faculty with recognized records of scholarly productivity are essential if doctoral students are to realize their full potential. The caliber of the faculty can be determined by first inspecting their credentials as listed in the catalog. Many schools of nursing also publish lists of faculty research interests and expertise. Additionally, the more recent NLN self-study report provides detailed information about faculty experience and scholarly accomplishments. If the NLN accreditation is several years old, this source may be out of date. In that case, an author search would provide a check on faculty productivity.

The student who has previously identified an area of study should determine whether faculty with similar interests and expertise are available to direct student research. This is particularly important at the doctoral level.

To assess the climate that prevails in an individual institution, the best source of information is other students or alumni. Key questions should include:

1. Are relationships characterized by supervisor/ subordinate roles or by patterns of mentoring?
2. Are opportunities available for students to work with faculty on research projects?
3. How accessible are faculty for advising?
4. To what extent are faculty involved in classroom teaching, as opposed to research assistants and guest lecturers?
5. Can students challenge existing opinions without fear of retribution?

Adequacy of institutional resources is best demonstrated by the presence of statistical consultants, computer services, facilities to support presentation (instructional aides development), and the availability of student study space and lounges. A simple walk through the library to assess the nursing and related holdings is advisable.

An environment rich in clinical facilities provides the learning laboratory for master's programs whose purpose is the education of the advanced practitioner. At the doctoral level, access to patient populations for clinical research can be essential to the development of a dissertation and the identification of a career-long focus for research. Although contractual arrangements offer many successful affiliations, the university hospital and associated clinical services generally provide opportunities and advantages not always found in patient-care oriented institutions. For example, a primary mission of the university hospital is the conduct of research. Faculty and students in associated health professional schools are involved in research and can facilitate, and often times collaborate on, nursing student and faculty projects.

When assistantships are available, it is advisable to explore the responsibilities and opportunities the position provides prior to making a commitment. Generally, assistantships are available in two areas—teaching and research. Graduate teaching assistantships usually require a designated number of hours of classroom or clinical teaching, primarily in undergraduate programs. Research assistant responsibilities vary according to both institutional policy and the needs and preferences of individual faculty to whom the assignment is made. Traditionally, these positions are considered opportunities for the development of abilities outside of classroom work. Unfortunately, in some instances, faculty take advantage of teaching and research assistants, and students find that instead of acquiring additional skills, they are doing boring, tedious

jobs that the faculty want to avoid. If teaching or research assistantship is necessary to support one's education or desire for personal growth, it is advisable to assess the nature of these positions before agreeing to serve.

The last element to be considered when selecting a graduate program are the program requirements. At the master's level the number of hours required, whether a thesis option exists, and requirements for comprehensives are key factors often considered. Potential candidates are wise to check into time requirements and curriculum organization along with the flexibility of practicum requirements before enrolling. Of paramount importance is the average length of time it takes a full-time student and a part-time student to complete the program requirements. For example, some programs are advertised as a year in length for full-time study, but in fact few are able to complete it in one year.

At the doctoral level, special attention should be given to determining the number of hours required for the degree and whether hours earned at the master's level can be counted toward the total. The qualifying process should also be explained to determine the nature of comprehensives within the graduate school. Other requirements to check into include demonstrated competencies in computers, statistics, and foreign languages. As with the master's level, the prospective student is advised to investigate the average length of time to complete the program requirements.

PERSONAL CONSIDERATIONS

Depending upon preferences, other factors to be considered include the availability of social and cultural events and student organizations. These opportunities are of differing importance to more mature students, but graduate education does provide the opportunity to demonstrate leadership and build on undergraduate achievements. Graduate student organizations and involvement on university committees provide additional experience in leadership roles that are important for career development.

Other factors that many students must consider when choosing a graduate program is how they will manage family and employment responsibilities, the scheduling of classes, and commuting. Increasingly, students returning for master's degrees and doctorates require flexible programs that allow part-time study and evening or back-to-back classes. For students who must work as well, ease in scheduling is essential.

FUTURE DIRECTIONS IN GRADUATE NURSING EDUCATION

New opportunities for different specializations at the master's level and innovative dual degrees, such as the M.B.A. Ph.D., are now available. Numerous programs across the country are developing R.N. to master's programs to facilitate graduate studies for bright returning nurses educated earlier in diploma and associate degree programs. As market demands for specialization change, innovative programs, such as the University of Maryland's master's degree in nursing informatics that features a multidisciplinary approach, have been developed. Upgrading of credentials required by ANA and specialty organizations such as the American College of Nurse Midwifery and the American Association of Nurse Anesthetists are moving preparation for these roles into the mainstream of graduate nursing education.

Other specializations at the graduate level can be anticipated as graduate education in nursing moves away from the medical model to a nursing model. In the future, concentrations may be developed in areas such as pain and incontinence management. For example, incontinence is the single most important factor that prompts institutionalization of an elderly person. Incontinence and the restoration to normal functioning is nursing's domain. As the population ages, this area of specialization will likely become increasingly important.

The role of case manager has emerged with the advent of prospective payment and the move by third-party payers to insure cost effectiveness. Nurses are more prepared to handle the comprehensive nature of this role than social workers or physicians. The ranks of staff nurses are being depleted by insurance companies and industries to manage patients' holdings disability claims and those with chronic health care problems. Graduate nursing education has not responded to the need to prepare nurses for this advanced role. Within the next few years, case management will take its place with clinical specialization, administration, and education.

Doctoral education in nursing can also be expected to change. More and more often advertisements appearing in the *Chronicle of Higher Education* call for candidates holding the Ph.D. in nursing. It seems likely this preference will continue. Additionally, the increasing complexity in the health care environment will require innovation in programming to meet the need for nurse executives to manage multifocused health care corporations. One such program is the University of Pennsylvania/Wharton School of Business Ph.D./M.B.A. program.

It is anticipated that as the patient population becomes more acutely ill and the technology becomes more and more advanced, there will be a need for the preparation of a clinician researcher who will be capable of dealing with clinical problems in the highly complex health care setting. Because of the emerging preference for the Ph.D., it is anticipated that this preparation will also award the Ph.D.

SUMMARY

Choosing a graduate program has emerged as the most important career decision a nurse can make. Graduate studies represent huge investments of time, energy, and money. The wise professional should assess carefully the human resources and the intellectual climate of the school before making a commitment. A program of studies is greater than the curriculum outlined in the catalog. It also includes the learning that occurs in the relationship between student and teacher and activities occurring in the study environment. Quality and standards of excellence vary among graduate programs. The wise professional will gather data and base a decision on the best fit between professional and personal needs.

REFERENCES

1. Benner P: From novice to expert: excellence and power in clinical nursing practice, Menlo Park, Calif, 1984, Addison-Wesley Publishing Co.
2. Brown JM: History of master's education in nursing in the United States, 1945-1969, New York, 1979, Teachers College, Columbia University.
3. Chamings PA: Ranking the nursing schools, Nurs Outlook 32(5):238, 1984.
4. Council of Graduate Schools of United States: The doctor of philosophy degree. No ED 153 546, Washington, DC, 1977. Council of Graduate Schools.
5. Downs FS: Doctoral education in nursing: future directions, Nurs Outlook 26(1):56, 1978.
6. Edlund BJ and Hodges LC: Preparing and using the clinical nurse specialist: a shared responsibility, Nursing Clinics of North America 18(3):499, 1983.
7. Guide to programs in nursing in four-year colleges and universities: baccalaureate and graduate programs in the United States and Canada, New York, 1987, Macmillan Publishing Co.

8. National League for Nursing: Master's education in nursing: route to opportunities in contemporary nursing 1986-1989, New York, 1986.

9. Parietti E: Development of doctoral education for nurses: a historical survey, New York, 1979, Teachers College, Columbia University.

10. Poteet GW, Edlund BJ, and Hodges LC: Consider this . . . support scholarship in the health care system, JONA 17(9):4, 1987.

11. Report on enrollment and graduations in baccalaureate and graduate programs in nursing 1983-1988.

12. Wandelt MA, Duffy ME, and Pollock SE: Profile of a top-ranked school of nursing. Pub No 41-1990, New York, 1985, National League for Nursing.

CHAPTER 21

Issues in doctoral education in nursing

HELEN K. GRACE

During the last decade there has been a dramatic increase in the number of doctoral programs in nursing and an accompanying increase in the number of doctorally prepared nurses. Given this increase, are the types of doctoral programs available to nurses sufficiently diverse to address the needs of a practice-based profession? This chapter first provides a brief summary of the development of doctoral education within nursing. With this as a framework, the question of "doctoral preparation for what?" is posed. Arguing that nurses with doctoral preparation are needed in a variety of leadership roles within the profession, the case for a variety of program models for doctoral education is made.

DEVELOPMENT OF DOCTORAL EDUCATION IN NURSING

Although a few nurses earned doctoral degrees (mainly in education) early in the twentieth century, modern doctoral education in the United States is now some 25 years old. The number of doctoral programs in nursing has grown dramatically in the 1970s and 1980s, with approximately 40 programs now in place. Given this stage of development, it is appropriate that this be a time for taking stock and setting future directions.

To understand current patterns of doctoral education it is useful to review the progression of nurses into doctoral study both in and out of nursing. Nurses earned their first doctoral degrees primarily in schools of education, an environment receptive to a practice discipline. The focus of doctoral study was on methods of teaching rather than on the substantive content of the field of nursing. These programs focused on such things as teaching and learning theories, curriculum construction, instructional methodology, and evaluation. Research as part of the educational doctorate was

focused on educational issues and not on building a knowledge base for the field of nursing.

Following World War II, with impetus from the GI bill, many nurses entered institutions of higher education for academic preparation in nursing. A number subsequently entered graduate study in a variety of fields. This trend was accelerated by the Nurse Scientist program, which provided scholarships for nurses to study in a variety of fields. With support from this source a number of nurses studied in the natural and behavioral sciences, joining those who had earlier completed doctoral study in the educational fields. These nurse-scientists were trained in the research traditions of the behavioral and natural sciences. On completing their doctoral studies they became faculty members within schools of nursing. This corps of faculty became the designers of doctoral programs in nursing and the researchers and faculty for these programs. As doctoral programs began to evolve, one of the difficulties encountered was reaching agreement on their substantive content. The nursing leadership, the deans and directors of programs, was primarily prepared at the doctoral level in the field of education. The newly graduated nurse-scientists came into schools of nursing with built-in traditions and biases from their different scientific disciplines. For example, those coming from the natural sciences had been trained in a research-mentorship process where research is learned through doing. Those trained in behavioral science fields were familiar with mastering a body of theoretical knowledge, learning research methodology and statistics, and then conducting their own independent research under guidance from a faculty researcher. Faculty coming from diverse orientations toward doctoral study brought these perspectives to the dialog about the content and structure of doctoral education in nursing.

At the same time as the nurse-scientist approach

was being fueled by federal funding, support for specialization in psychiatric nursing at the graduate level was accelerating preparation of nurses in this clinical specialty area. Based on the national concern for mental health as a priority, graduate programs were developing in schools of nursing throughout the United States. As a natural part of this development, a clinical specialty doctoral program in psychiatric nursing developed at Boston University. Although this program is no longer operational, it is important to note that in the late 1960s and early 1970s there were three distinct program models for doctoral education in nursing: (1) the older functional specialty model for preparation in nursing education and administration, (2) the research model emerging out of the nurse-scientist perspective, and (3) the clinical specialty professional doctorate.

As doctoral programs in nursing proliferated in the 1970s and early 1980s, there was a trend toward increasing similarities in their structure and content. A theory strand, a research component, and an integrative science piece were common across programs. Most doctoral programs built on clinical specialization achieved at the master's level. In contrast to other scientific disciplines where the progression is from the most general knowledge base at the baccalaureate level to increasing specialization throughout graduate study, the pattern in nursing was to be prepared as a generalist at the basic level, to become highly specialized in a clinical specialty area at the master's level, and then to move once more to a general perspective at the beginning stages of doctoral study before research specialization. As a result of this pattern doctoral programs, as with all nursing education, became loaded with course requirements in the attempt to build a common knowledge base for the profession as a whole. Integrating the diverse perspectives from the natural and behavioral sciences into the format of doctoral programs in nursing resulted in a large number of broadly based overview courses as prerequisites for pursuing research at the doctoral level. The intent was for nurse-scientists to integrate these diverse perspectives into a common understanding of nursing.

A second characteristic of doctoral programs in nursing was that all were cast in the mold of the research doctorate, although some may have granted the Doctorate of Science in Nursing (D.Sc.N.) degree. The earlier patterns of a clinical doctorate and specialization in the functional areas of administration and education became less visible as the new programs developed in the research mold. Although the overall pattern was that of the research doctorate, faculty members were involved to varying degrees in conducting their own research. A model of research supervision was carried over from master's programs in nursing. In this model, the small number of faculty with research preparation supervised large numbers of students conducting research on a wide range of topics. Frequently the heavy load of thesis advising absorbed most of the faculty members' time, and they themselves did very little research. This research-advising model conflicted with what many of the nurse-scientists had experienced in their own doctoral study, where they had worked in direct collaborative relationships with their faculty mentors.

CURRENT STATUS

What is the net result of these trends? The numbers of doctoral programs have increased dramatically over the past ten years. These programs enroll large numbers of students who are instructed by small numbers of faculty with varying degrees of research productivity. The graduates of these doctoral programs in nursing are becoming faculty of schools of nursing throughout the country. Many of these newly graduated doctorally prepared nurses, knowledgeable of the requirements for promotion and tenure and critical of their mentors, are setting their own research as a top priority, with clinical teaching, administration, and public service as much lower priorities. These doctorally prepared nurses are entering faculty positions at a time of declining undergraduate enrollments and a resurgence of concern within the university for the quality of undergraduate teaching. Second, schools of nursing throughout the country are expressing growing concern about the separation between education and practice. As a result of these factors, increased concern is being voiced over the growing separation of research from other aspects of the faculty role such as teaching, practice, and service. Another concern is for the quality of leadership, both in nursing practice and in nursing education.

DOCTORAL PREPARATION FOR WHAT?

Some would argue that a strong research doctorate in nursing is appropriate preparation as a base for all advanced nursing roles: educator, administrator, clinical practitioner, and researcher. Others take the position that preparation in research is not necessarily appropriate for some leadership roles in nursing and that the diversified nature of a practice discipline requires diversity of advanced preparation.

Drawing from experiences in other practice disciplines such as psychology and education, research indicates that there are characteristic personality differences between those students who do well in a research track and those who are expert practitioners. Clinicians demonstrate integrative and holistic thinking patterns, while researchers tend to be reductionist in their thought processes. Although both patterns of thinking are highly valued in the field, it is accepted that different individuals are more appropriately placed in one track over another. Rarely does an individual attempt to master both basic research and practice. It is acknowledged that the field of psychology needs both experimental and clinical psychologists and that the experimental psychologist needs a beginning understanding of principles of treatment, and vice versa. However, in nursing we tend to adopt the position that one person should be able to be all things, and thus the doctorally prepared nurse should be both a skilled basic researcher and also an able practitioner.

Given the state of development of doctoral education and the diversity of leadership needs in the field of nursing, this may be an appropriate time to examine the question of whether or not there should be diverse options available to nurses wishing to pursue doctoral study. Before considering what these options might be it is important to delineate the varying roles that doctorally prepared nursing faculty now fill in this country.

In addition to nurse researchers, nursing needs administrators both in education and in practice, faculty in clinical nursing as well as in supportive areas, expert clinicians, and even some nurse public policy experts and politicians. Is a generalized nurse doctorate appropriate for all? Although I would argue that all need a grounding in nursing theory, an understanding of nursing practice, and a base for understanding and conducting research, particularly of an applied nature, they also need substantive knowledge in fields supportive of their particular career interests. For example, preparation for administrative roles requires an understanding of organizational theory, the dynamics of small groups, and principles of management. Research conducted as part of such a degree program logically would focus on an administrative problem and would most likely be applied research. An important component of such a program would be an internship with a nursing administrator in service or in education.

In a previous article I have argued for a dual-track approach to the preparation of nursing faculty. Because faculty roles differ according to the level of nursing education, the college or university in which the program is lodged, and the relationship of the educational program to the practice setting, the preparation of someone teaching fundamentals of nursing to undergraduate students needs to be substantively different than for a faculty member teaching research to doctoral students. Both need a general knowledge of nursing, but the clinical faculty member needs to be an expert practitioner, teacher, and applied researcher. On the other hand, the doctoral-level faculty member must be engaged in on-going research and have a depth of knowledge about a particular area of research emphasis.

In addition to the preparation of nurse researchers, administrators, and teachers, the field requires expert practitioners, clinical researchers, public policy experts, ethicists, historians, and humanists. Are all to be prepared at the advanced level in doctoral programs cast in the mold of the research doctorate?

PROPOSED MODELS FOR DOCTORAL EDUCATION

In addressing the diverse needs of the field, three models of doctoral education are needed: (1) the research doctorate, (2) the clinical or applied research doctorate, and (3) the professional doctorate.

The research doctorate

Currently our doctoral programs are a hodgepodge, trying to be all things to all people. While some grant the Ph.D. degree and others the D.N.Sc., the basic structure of all programs is amazingly similar. In the initial stages of doctoral-program development, with faculty resources limited, doctoral programs emphasized independent research to varying degrees. Many became highly structured in course content, limiting the extent of research involvement to the final year of study and leaving the design of research largely up to the student. The rigor of research programs varied widely and was largely dependent on the faculty resources at a particular institution. The end result is a wide range in the quality of the research preparation of individuals completing doctoral study.

Given this state of affairs, it is important that the quality of the research doctorate be given attention. The emphasis within such programs needs to be on developing the thought patterns and discipline of nurse researchers whose primary focus is on building a knowledge base for nursing. To prepare competent researchers, research doctoral programs need to be constructed as total programs that build from the generalist level of basic nursing education to the degree of specialization necessary to add to the discipline's knowledge base. A quality research doctorate should be structured as a total graduate program and need not build on a base of clinical practice specialization, as is currently the design. The research skills of those few who are building a research and teaching career in nursing need to be carefully honed and developed if the knowledge base underpinning practice is to be systematically constructed. Research preparation cannot be tacked on as an afterthought following six years or more of clinical education.

The focus of the research doctorate should be on research and should be built around research-producing faculty who mentor students in their particular areas. Research doctoral programs should carefully limit the number of students admitted to study to ensure that all students will have the opportunity to become competent beginning researchers and to continue on into productive research and teaching careers. The areas of faculty research expertise should be the bases on which the research doctoral program recruits and selects students. In choosing a particular program a student should be confident that the faculty's expertise and ongoing research projects will allow them to develop their own particular research skills and interests.

The clinical or applied doctorate

In contrast to the research doctorate, the clinical or applied doctoral program should build on a clinical specialization base with the primary goal of preparing advanced practitioners and applied researchers. Such programs would prepare not only clinicians but also specialists in the functional areas of administration and teaching, as well as clinical researchers, clinical teachers, public policy analysts and nurse politicians. Within these programs there would be substantive content tracks that provide opportunities for nurses opting for specific career goals to develop the knowledge base that is as necessary to these applied fields as research is to the nurse researcher. Research within these programs would be applied to specific phenom-

ena, such as evaluation research. An example of the type of research conducted might be to test out a model of nursing intervention to address problems of infant mortality in a high-risk population. Research would address the context in which the intervention is undertaken, the process of initiating the intervention and getting mothers engaged in prenatal care, and also the outcome of the intervention. The cost-benefit ratio of a nursing intervention would be an important component of such studies.

A part of doctoral study in a clinical or applied research doctorate program would be an internship with a senior role model in a particular specialty area. Those embarking on an educational or administrative career track, for example, would intern with a dean or department head.

In considering the potential roles of doctorally prepared nurses and the needs of a practice discipline such as nursing, perhaps 10 times as many nurses need preparation in a clinical or applied model as need training in the research model. With both types of preparation mixed in our current models, it is likely that the preparation is inadequate for both tracks.

What of the argument that the research degree is more prestigious than the applied degree and thus is valued more in the marketplace? In this discussion, I have deliberately avoided titling the degrees, because the Ph.D. is traditionally perceived as more prestigious than the D.N.Sc. I would question the validity of the marketplace argument in the first place. Who establishes the marketplace for nursing? Is not the marketplace to be determined by the need for nurses with diverse preparation rather than on the particular label the individual bears? Is the prestige associated with a particular label more important than what the individual is prepared to do? A number of fields have clearly differentiated research and applied doctoral tracks. In some instances both tracks are awarded the same degree; in others, the degree itself differs. The degree offered is not as important as what it is a particular pathway is designed to accomplish. If nursing is clear about the focus of differing career pathways and what particular educational programs are designed to prepare, the marketplace of employment can also be designed to appropriately recognize, utilize, and remunerate those who enter such career pathways.

The professional doctorate

Although some would not include the professional doctorate in this discussion, if we are looking to the future it needs to be given consideration. The professional doctorate is currently offered by several programs throughout the country as a post-baccalaureate, first professional degree in nursing. Some may argue that this is the appropriate model for preparation of the professional nurse, and that in practice such a professional would work with nurses prepared as technicians to deliver high-quality nursing care. Having achieved a professional doctorate the nurse wishing to build a research career or an advanced clinical or applied research career would enter the appropriate post-basic program, much as a medical doctor might enter a Ph.D. or D.P.H. program for advanced preparation.

Building on the general educational background of the baccalaureate program, a professional doctorate program would provide in-depth education in the clinical practice knowledge and skills essential to professional practice in the complex world of health service delivery.

SUMMARY

In this chapter I have traced some of the evolutionary threads that have contributed to current patterns in doctoral education in nursing. Although current programs may differ in the title of the degree offered, all are structured as research doctoral programs. Because they try to be all things to all people, they fail in preparing either competent researchers or applied practitioners. Cluttered with too much general content and lacking sufficient content specific to a student's particular career track, these programs fail to provide an adequate foundation for future career pathways. As a result, preparation is limited for academic and administrative leadership roles, clinical teachers, practitioners, and researchers.

Nursing has a vital contribution to make to the health of the American people. To make it we need to ensure that our researchers are providing a substantive knowledge base for the field, that our leaders in academic and practice fields have a solid knowledge base of nursing coupled with administrative preparation and applied research skills, and that our clinical teachers and practitioners are skilled in their clinical specialties and in applied research in their fields. Finally, we need expert practitioners who deliver and manage truly comprehensive, quality health care services for people in all stages of the health-illness continuum.

CHAPTER 22

Models of nursing education for developing countries

The Bahrain model

FADWA A. AFFARA

INTRODUCTION

Health services in countries in the Arabian Gulf region have undergone a rapid expansion during the past two decades. The state of Bahrain, an archipelago of 30 islands in the gulf with a population of approximately 400,000, has been no exception. Soon after its full independence in 1971, Bahrain undertook a vigorous program to provide free and easily accessible health care for all its citizens. It created a system in which most health care was delivered through a network of health centers. These centers were supported by a modern 600-bed general hospital, a central maternity hospital with five outreach units, a small geriatric hospital, and psychiatric facilities that included hospital, outpatient, and community services.

Concomitant with the evolution of health care was an ever-growing demand for more and better-prepared nurses. That the nursing work force consisted largely of expatriate nurses was accepted as a necessary but temporary stage while the country trained Bahraini nurses. By 1976, however, despite nearly 18 years of providing nursing education, Bahrain was far from being self-sufficient in nursing personnel. Indeed, Ministry of Health figures as recently as 1984 indicated that Bahraini nationals held only 15.5% of the posts in the ministry requiring a minimum qualification of registered nurse.[5] In contrast, nearly all the practical nurse posts were filled by Bahrainis.

Why has it proved difficult to attract nationals in sufficient numbers to the higher grades of nursing? Kamal[9] found a chronic and deep-seated shortage of nurses in most countries in the World Health Organization Eastern Mediterranean Region. Recruitment was hindered by the perception of nursing as a low-status and even morally unsuitable occupation for women. Unsatisfactory working conditions, low pay, and very limited career opportunities added to its lack of attraction. These were compounded by poor teaching in the region's nursing schools, low-level programs, and inappropriate curricula, usually imported from countries with very different health profiles and socioeconomic and cultural patterns.

Two studies investigating recruitment to nursing in Bahrain confirmed Kamal's conclusions.[3,8] Contributing to the unwillingness to consider a career in nursing were family disapproval, shift work and inadequate salary, the physically hard and boring nature of the work, the apparently low entry requirements, and a perception that the final educational achievement was poor. Therefore, it was hardly surprising to find nursing placed consistently last when students selected among the various nursing and allied health programs offered by the College of Health Sciences.[1,8] On graduation the picture was hardly comforting. Al-Hamar found that, of the 14% of college graduates who quit their jobs over a 3-year period, 68% were nurses.[2] Although this phenomenon was hardly unique to Bahrain, its magnitude was alarming because the base from which these nurses were lost was small. In an earlier survey of trained nurses that focused on sources of career dissatisfaction, Bahraini nurses indicated that, although salaries and working conditions were far from ideal, the slow pace of promotion, the lack of a clearly defined career structure, and the scarcity of postbasic and continuing education programs were significant reasons for dissatisfaction.[11] All these factors were directly related to the nature of and opportunities for education for nurses in Bahrain.

The importance of becoming self-sufficient in health care workers was recognized in 1968 when Bahrain began to prepare its first long-range health plan.[6] At that time the only kind of formal education for health care personnel was in nursing. A small hospital school offered a 4-year program in general nursing. Most of its recruits had an intermediate school certificate (9 years). By 1971 the school was able to reorganize and offer an 18-month practical nurse program to intermediate school certificate holders and a 3-year preparation in general nursing to those with full secondary schooling. Therefore, when the Ministry of Health established the College of Health Sciences in 1976, it took a major step toward achieving self-sufficiency in the number of health care personnel.

The college was made responsible for educating all nursing and allied-health personnel in Bahrain. Its strength lay in its newness and consequent freedom from the constraints of tradition. This gave it the leeway to experiment in its educational programs. Moreover, being part of the Ministry of Health placed educators in the college in a favorable position to work closely with service counterparts in developing appropriate programs that would reflect the country's health priorities. Also, as noted by its first dean, the college was not overshadowed by or competing for resources with medical education. Unlike many other countries, Bahrain had made a deliberate choice to build the base of the health care personnel pyramid first, postponing physician education until that infrastructure had been strengthened.[10]

SHAPING THE FUTURE OF NURSING EDUCATION

In the face of rapid social change, a number of challenges faced nursing education. First, it had to fulfill its primary goal of producing enough nurses who were acceptable to and capable of working in the country's health care system. It had to be grounded in the health care needs and the social forces operating in Bahrain. Second, nursing education had to be responsive to the changes occurring in the country's educational system. This sector was growing rapidly, and the number of Bahrainis completing secondary school was rising yearly. The fast-expanding tertiary education system and widening range of job opportunities were matched by increased education and career expectations in secondary school graduates. Therefore, nursing had to introduce sufficient flexibility into its training to take advantage of a future that promised better-educated recruits with high educational and career aspirations. Third, if professional nursing were to become established in Bahraini society, nationals would have to be trained to be its leaders and thinkers, for they would know best how to develop nursing practice that was sensitive to and fitted the health needs of their society.

Two major approaches were selected as the basis for the future direction of nursing education in Bahrain. These were:

1. Moving nursing out of its educational ghetto into mainstream higher education.
2. Developing a comprehensive, open-ended system of education that permitted academic and professional mobility.

Moving to a college setting

In moving to the College of Health Sciences, nursing education became part of the country's tertiary education system. The move also placed it in an environment that facilitated changes in the structure and content of the educational programs. The college founders, concerned that its graduates be equipped with relevant competencies, adopted the systematic approach to curriculum development as the cornerstone of their educational planning.[10] Curricula were developed around the acquisition of a whole range of competencies that graduates were expected to demonstrate at defined levels of proficiency and that would allow them to confront the demands of future jobs. Innovation and experimentation in curriculum design and teaching and learning methods, especially learner-oriented approaches, were emphasized. Student nurses moved from the apprenticeship system of learning to one that conferred full student status. This change freed nursing education from the constraints of balancing learning with service needs and permitted nurse educators to make radical changes in the organization and content of clinical learning.

Developing a system of nursing education

In 1981 the Board of Education of the College of Health Sciences accepted a model for a comprehensive system of nursing education. The proposal reflected the fact that the country required generalist nurses with the capacity and the authority to practice in the

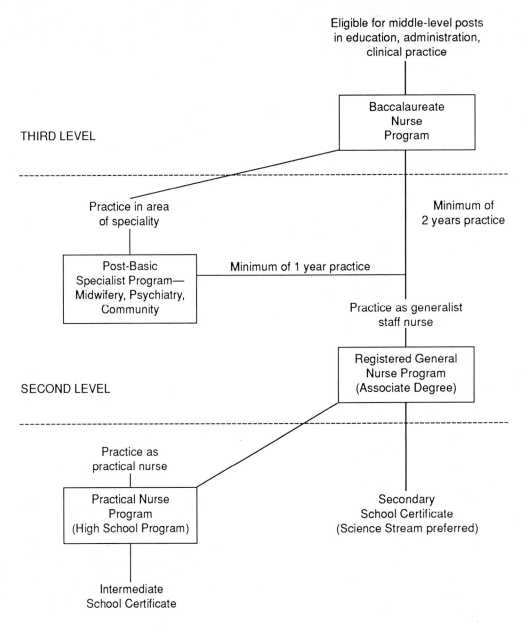

Fig. 22-1 Nursing education model for Bahrain.

primary, secondary, and tertiary settings available in Bahrain. As shown in Figure 22-1, it proposed that these generalists be prepared at three levels through a series of programs that would articulate with one another. Specialist preparation could be developed according to Bahrain's requirements and resource capabilities, but it would be built on the base of competency and authority for generalist practice. Comprehensive preparation in midwifery and psychiatric and community-health nursing were identified as priorities in specialist education.

The three levels of generalist preparation formed a continuum, which was implemented in the following manner:

1. *The Practical Nurse Program (High School Nursing Program)*. Nurses graduating at this level would work with an existing nursing team and under the supervision of a higher-level nurse. The practical nurse would be able to care for persons with uncomplicated health problems and to meet simple illness-prevention and health-promotion needs. The program, also known as the High School Nursing Program, was run in collaboration with the Ministry of Education. Different forms of this type of nurse training existed in several countries in the region and were a result of the diversification of secondary school education after the intermediate cycle. Although the Ministry of Education was responsible for the general education courses, all nursing, life, and social science inputs were under the control of the College of Health Sciences. If successful in all parts of the 3-year program, graduates would earn a secondary school certificate and a practical nurse qualification. At this point they had the option of entering the work force or seeking admission to the next level program.

2. *The Registered General Nurse Program (Associate Degree Nursing Program)*. This program, awarding an associate degree, prepared nurses to work in primary, secondary, and tertiary settings and to deal with more complex health problems and needs than those handled by practical nurses. Graduates would enter the health service at the staff nurse position, the category needed most in Bahrain, and, after experience and relevant postbasic education, could become ward or health-center charge nurses. Because this is an entirely college-based education, entrants were required to hold a secondary school certificate and to pass the college entrance examination. Students with no previous nursing qualifications required just over 3 years to complete their studies; graduates of the High School Program could finish in 2 years.

3. *The Baccalaureate Nurse Program (Post-Associate Degree Baccalaureate Program)*. Whereas the Associate Degree Program focused on training staff nurses, the baccalaureate degree program attempted to prepare a much smaller group of nurses for leadership roles in all sectors of nursing education and service. Its graduates could

function in situations that were less structured and more ambiguous than those handled by the associate degree holders. The 2-year program was open to nurses with an associate degree in nursing (or its equivalent) and with at least 2 years of recent clinical experience.

THE CURRICULUM

The restructuring of nursing education and the opportunity to initiate new programs opened the way for integrating concepts and approaches that would enlarge and enrich the nurses' role in health care provision. To develop programs that were cohesive both in content and process, it became imperative to identify an underlying framework for curriculum design that would provide guidelines for decision making in subsequent educational planning. Figure 22-2 shows the eight integrative curriculum threads that form this framework. They are the backbone of the curricula, providing continuity and coherence among the different program levels. At the same time, they permit incremental program development by expanding the depth and breadth of the knowledge base, broadening skill acquisition, and developing the level of problem solving, judgmental, and decision-making capabilities. Using this model, Bahraini nurses can advance professionally through a series of articulated programs that build on preceding educational achievements and practice experiences.

The most imortant consequence of approaching educational planning in this manner was the opportunity it provided for reflection on the nature and goals of nursing practice. It became evident that institutional health care played a transient and limited role in the health concerns and experiences of most Bahrainis. The traditional medical model based on body systems and diseases dealt little with the key issues in Bahrain. These issues included improving and maintaining the health of the population; enabling individuals to live socially and economically productive lives; promoting self-reliance and independence in maintaining the improving health; and encouraging active community participation in developing health services that were acceptable, just, and in harmony with cultural and social orientations. As a result, the emphasis of the programs shifted from their almost exclusive concern for the hospitalized individual to a broader, community-oriented focus. More specifically, faculty at-

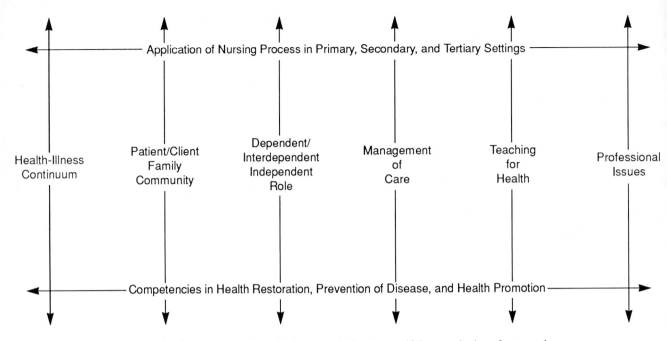

Fig. 22-2 Horizontal and verticular threads forming unifying curriculum framework.

tempted to introduce concepts of primary health care into the programs. These concepts, first elaborated by the World Health Organization at the Alma-Ata Conference in 1978, had been accepted by Bahrain as a fundamental element in the formulation of health policy and strategies for attaining health goals.[16] Therefore, it was crucial that nursing education begin to reflect the fundamental principles and elements of primary health care. Although this redirection of the focus of education occurred before the publication of the World Health Organization's guide for orienting basic nursing education to primary health care and community health, it did incorporate many of its recommendations, particularly at the postbasic and baccalauretate program levels.[14]

The effect of these changes was best illustrated by describing a few of the situations encountered by students during their clinical experiences.

• Assigned to a community setting, a student became interested in working with an extended family that kept appearing at the health center with numerous, often ill-defined, health problems. Having discussed her concern with the community health nurse, she was given permission to observe the family in their home. After several visits she identified overcrowding as a major source of stress in the family. Although the family was not limited financially, it was cultur-

ally unacceptable for the married son to establish a separate home. The student persuaded the father, the head of the household, to build an extension to accommodate his son, the son's wife, and their three children, who had been living in half of a curtained-off room. Building was started within a month, and subsequent visits revealed a marked reduction in tensions and health complaints.

• Convinced that she would not succeed in improving the health of a largely illiterate family unless she made their desperate housing conditions and poverty her first priority, a student investigated all sources of governmental, private, and religious aid available in the community. Having identified the most likely sources of aid, she formulated a plan of action with her teacher and the health care team, wrote letters, and made direct contacts with the agencies. She followed through until the family was rehoused and provided with an income sufficient to meet basic living needs. She learned that resources were available but that the skills of an intermediate such as herself were required to bring them within the reach of illiterate and socially deprived individuals and groups.

• A student practical nurse recognized that dental hygiene was a major problem in his community. He arranged to do some of his clinical experience in the local nursing school and decided to concentrate on this topic. He developed a plan of dental health education for the teachers to use and wrote a song to put over the message. The health education program and the song became a permanent part of the school's teaching curriculum.

- The dramatic recovery of a hospitalized, psychiatric patient occurred when a senior male student, who was also a village leader, intervened on his behalf and settled a land dispute with the municipality.

These few examples demonstrate that students employed strategies scarcely addressed in the previous curriculum. Their approaches recognized that contemporary nursing practice does not confine itself to the resources of the health sector. In their interventions, students learned to reach out and mobilize skills and resources in the nonhealth sectors, the community, and the individual or family.

FACING THE CHALLENGES

A systematic and valid approach to competency identification was clearly fundamental to developing relevant nursing programs. McGaghie and others have identified three major sources for competency elements: an analysis of activities, critical elements of behavior, and the health care needs of the community.[13] However, the use of the majority of the techniques described was beyond the means available to Bahraini nursing at the time the curriculum was being revised.

A partial solution to the problem was found by adapting, with help from external consultants, the Professional Performance Situation Model developed by the Center of Educational Development at the University of Illinois.[13] This model for defining competencies recognized that professional practice must take account of three variables: the client, the problem, and the setting. The interaction of these variables creates the situation that the health practitioner must confront.

To apply this model to Bahrain, a group was formed of teachers and service nurses who were directly involved in clinical practice and who possessed expertise and experience in the settings in which graduates were expected to practice. From real-life situations they developed a series of scenarios describing problems that new generalist nurses should be able to handle. Competencies were derived from these scenarios and organized under the headings of assessment, planning,

implementation, evaluation, and professional conduct. In adapting this model, a useful and efficient tool was created for identifying core competencies for generalist practice in Bahrain. Over time it was validated, modified, and expanded, but this approach to competency identification did lay a foundation for future work.

Surveying the community's knowledge, attitudes, and practices and its expectations of the primary health care system and the community nurse in particular was an example of continuing efforts to identify core competencies.[7] The study generated a group of important competencies for the community health nursing program. It also contributed to the adjustment of the generalist-program competencies so that they better met the real and felt needs of the community.

Among the lessons learned was the importance of including the service sector from the beginning. The process of consultation and working on a common task provided an opportunity to achieve a consensus on the competency profile of the new graduate. This cooperation greatly facilitated future initiatives to reinforce the service role in clinical education and gave an impetus to nursing service reforms that would support practice by graduates with these competencies.

Because care standards in clinical learning sites were critical elements in determining the quality of graduates, teachers were very interested in contributing to the upgrading of nursing services. In extending their responsibilities beyond the student, teachers acted as resource persons supporting efforts to improve nursing practice. They provided professional and educational expertise at the practice sites or in the committees and other structures set up to introduce and monitor changes in the organization and delivery of nursing care.

Equally important in narrowing the gap between education and service was the realization that the context for practice must be defined clearly for education to prepare nurses for it because practice always takes place in the real world. Contextual descriptions were particularly useful in defining limits of practice, identifying the nature of the relationships with recipients of nursing care, and delineating roles and responsibilities with respect to other persons working in the setting.

The move toward competency-based primary health-care-oriented programs called into question many of the educational methods previously considered to be adequate. Two World Health Organization documents examining the education of nurse teachers and managers underlined the importance of this reconsideration.[12,15] The first, a survey of programs in 43 countries, and the second, an expert committee report, exposed severe deficiencies in teacher education programs. Their curricula were little adapted to provide future teachers with the skills to meet the educational challenges of primary health care or to employ the methodologies that would support such a redirection in nursing education. The committee recommended that teachers be better prepared in primary health care practice and the newer educational methodologies, especially learner-oriented approaches, and that they have the confidence to experiment with innovations that "take the classroom to the community."[15]

Teachers in Bahrain, as elsewhere, needed help in making the transition from the traditional book-bound classroom role to one that embraced clinical practice in partnership with the student. Although teachers learned to use participatory, experiential methods and a different approach to evaluation, students, accustomed to teacher dominated, didactic approaches, had to be persuaded that these unfamiliar techniques were worthwhile and encouraged to become active participants in the learning process.

From the ouset, the college authorities realized that good teaching techniques were not enough to guarantee success for their venture. They also had to understand the educational issues, especially as these affected the health profession in Bahrain, and maintain an openness to the options available for solving educational problems. With this purpose in mind, they established the Educational Development Unit to support faculty in institutional, curriculum, and role development. Its primary function was

to assist faculty in addressing and resolving the educational concerns arising from the day to day functioning of educational programs, in assuring their relevance to the needs of the health services, and in maintaining the standard of excellence in the students' performance of the job for which he or she is being trained.[4]

In transferring to the college, nurses had at last achieved access to resources for systematic and appropriate faculty development. Apart from upgrading the skills of faculty already in post, all new Bahraini teachers were assigned for a year to the Educational Development Unit. There they undertook a diploma program in health profession education. Thus new entrants to teaching were introduced to a philosophy and principles of education that were consistent with those underlying the nursing programs at the college. They acquired a thorough theoretical and practical grounding in the educational methodologies they would be expected to follow and were able to learn these skills in the classrooms, laboratories, and clinical sites used by the nursing programs. Also, through Bahraini government and World Health Organization funding, a scholarship program for advanced professional and adacemic study abroad has steadily increased opportunities for development of nursing capabilities. Bahrain can look forward to a future in which national nurses take a leading role in developing the profession and the health services of the country.

CONCLUSION

Bahrain was fortunate to have the resources and political will to take radical action to remedy its shortage of national nurses. Although self-sufficiency in nursing personnel lies some years ahead, indications are that considerable progress has been made toward that goal.

Recruitment has improved significantly. In the space of 4 years, admission to candidates for the associate degree rose from about 40 to just over 100. Three new postbasic programs were introduced and were functioning to their full capacity. As important was the rise in the quality of the associate degree candidates; more had a science background, and the average score of the final school examination rose. Senior nurse managers, initially sceptical that the college-based education would deliver the type of practitioner required by the services, expressed satisfaction with new graduates. By 1986, after evaluating nursing needs, they requested a cutback in practical nurse training. This released much-needed clinical learning places and allowed an expansion in the associate degree program. The prospect of an associate degree entry into practice level may arrive sooner than expected.

Finally, concrete progress has been made towards creating a worthwhile career ladder. Career structure had been determined by a system of job classification that, for nurses, set little more than length of service as the criterion for advancement. Consequently, nurses lacked a strong professional career structure and were severely disadvantaged when it came to setting wage rates. Now that values were changing, academic and professional qualifications were more highly rewarded than longevity of service. The advent

Undergoing a major transition

JOANNE COMI McCLOSKEY
HELEN KENNEDY GRACE

With the dramatic changes occurring in the health care arena, nursing practice is being buffeted from all sides. Pressures to reduce the costs of care result in patients being kept out of acute care hospitals to a later stage in illness. Patients who are hospitalized are more acutely ill and their treatment involves a high level of technological care that requires counterbalancing by "high touch" on the part of nursing staff. With patients discharged into the community at an earlier point in their illness, families are increasingly providing care for family members in home settings. Fragmentation of services and funding sources creates new demands for coordination if individuals and their families are to receive adequate and accessible health care services. As a consequence, nursing practice is undergoing a major transition. The challenge to nursing in the face of these changes is to bring coherence to a chaotic and fragmented system of care. This requires a greater degree of independence and leadership than has been customary in the recent past of nursing practice. This section provides an interesting overview of the dilemmas of nursing practice as viewed from various perspectives.

Opening the section, Lynaugh addresses the question, Is there anything new about this nursing shortage? Historically, there have been a number of nurse shortage situations. The short-term solutions to the nurse shortages of the past have contributed to the long-range pervasiveness of the problem. Creation of a low-cost labor pool has been the traditional solution of the past. Assumptions about health care have inhibited the creation of a rational educational system to prepare nurses to address social priorities. For example, the use of student nurses to provide a free labor pool for hospitals, the immunity of hospitals from attack as exploitative institutions due to their benevolent community service role, and nursing subsidization of

a voluntary sector hospital system are cited as historical examples of ways of maintaining low pay for nurses, the chief underlying cause of nurse shortages. This is a reflection of a broader tendency to underpay or not pay women for their labor. From this premise Lynaugh argues that a change in values related to women's roles in society makes today's a different situation. Society is recognizing the need for nurses, need begets value, and value creates an atmosphere where gender-based economic gaps can be bridged. Whether this occurs rests largely with nursing and nursing's capacity to articulate its message in arguing for patient-centered care and defining and preparing responsible nurses.

Changes in practice are perhaps most evident in hospitals. Noting the effects of changed reimbursement systems on the composition of the patient population in hospitals, Joel succinctly describes nursing in today's hospitals. Enumerating the differences made by skillful nursing in the clinical management of acutely ill patients, particularly the elderly, Joel notes that "hospitals were blind to the inherent value of nursing as they first began to consider approaches to cost-effectiveness." The change in payment systems has increased the importance of nurses in moving patients in and out of hospitals quickly. Joel reports that "three patients each hospitalized for ten days generate more revenue than one patient hospitalized for thirty days." The ability to move patients through the system quickly is largely contingent on the capabilities of nurses to provide expert clinical care. Given the nursing shortages experienced throughout the United States, Joel recommends greater use of assistants in providing nonnursing services, but advocates that these assistants be under nurses' control. She cautions against the use of clinical support systems because of the complex nature of clinical problems of patients.

PART FOUR

CHANGING PRACTICE

of increased access to postbasic and higher education enabled nurses to make a strong case for the revision of their classification scheme, and they successfully negotiated the incorporation of academic and professional qualifications for each step in their job classification grading. In effect, the foundation has been laid for more equitable treatment with respect to renumeration rates and the allocation of resources for more advanced nursing education.

REFERENCES

1. Affara FA: Increasing recruitment to the associate degree nursing program, Bahrain, 1986, College of Health Sciences.
2. Al-Hamar FY: Role of the College of Health Sciences in health manpower development in Bahrain, master's thesis, Champaign-Urbana, 1981, University of Illinois.
3. Al-Omran HA: The experimental use of television in a developing country: widening the social recrutiment into the nursing profession in Bahrain, doctoral thesis, London, 1981, London School of Economics and Political Science.
4. Chawhan AUR: The unit of Educational Development: roles and functions in the College of Health Sciences. In American University of Beirut: Human resources for primary health care in the Middle East, Beirut, 1980, American University of Beirut.
5. Eid A: Nursing manpower in Bahrain. Paper presented at the conference Perspectives in nursing towards the year 2000, Bahrain, November 1984.
6. Fakhro AM: A general description of the health care system in Bahrain. In American University of Beirut: Human resources for primary health care in the Middle East, Beirut, 1980, American University of Beirut.
7. Ghebrehiwet T and Hassan E: Knowledge, attitudes, practice and expectations of primary health care utilizers in Bahrain, Bahrain, 1985, College of Health Sciences.
8. Horsley-Mahmoud K: Career choices in allied health: a survey of College of Health Sciences students, Bahrain, 1980, College of Health Sciences.
9. Kamal I: Nursing manpower development in the Eastern Mediterranean Region. Paper presented at the conference Perspectives in nursing towards the year 2000, Bahrain, November 1984.
10. Kronful NM: Transfer of educational concepts for health manpower development: the Bahrain experiment. In American University of Beirut: Human resources for primary health care in the Middle East, Beirut, 1980, American University of Beirut.
11. Kronful NM and Al-Khalifah H: Career dissatisfaction amongst Bahraini nurses, Bahrain, 1980, College of Health Sciences.
12. Maillart V and Maglacas AM: Report on a survey of post-basic training programmes for nurse teachers (educators) and administrators (managers), Doc HMD/NUR/83.1, Geneva, 1983, World Health Organization.
13. McGaghie WC and others: Competency-based curriculum development in medical education: an introduction, Public Health Papers 68, Geneva, 1978, World Health Organization.
14. World Health Organization: A guide to curriculum review for basic nursing education: orientation to primary health care and community nursing, Geneva, 1985.
15. World Health Organization: Education and training of nurse teachers and managers with special regard to primary health care, Tech Rep Ser 708, Geneva, 1984.
16. World Health Organization: Primary health care: report of the international conference on primary health care, Alma-Ata, USSR, September 6-12, 1978, Geneva, 1978.

Finally, she warns against history repeating itself. In the past, responses to other nursing shortage situations have resulted in an inflation of entrance salaries for nurses, a decrease in expectations regarding qualifications, and an overall compression of the salary scale. This pattern creates an influx into nursing because of the heightened economic incentives for new entrants, but serves as a disincentive over time for those most qualified to provide the expert care that the modern hospital requires.

As the boundaries between hospital and community are increasingly blurred by the rapid transfer of patients back and forth, major problems of discontinuity of care emerge. Baigis-Smith and McKeehan argue that this discontinuity arises from several sources, including highly specialized professional training that focuses on the disease rather than on the diseased person, and the organization of care primarily around hospital acute care settings. Most proposed solutions are directed toward changes in the orientation of health care professionals and in the organization of care, epitomized by the case manager, who acts as an adjunct to the family in obtaining needed care from a fragmented system. Baigis-Smith and McKeehan argue for "tapping the doctor within" each patient and increasing the abilities of individuals and their families to make informed decisions and to manage their own care.

Turning to the community, Salmon and Vanderbush point to the critical leadership role of nurses in community health. With the community as the client for public health nursing, nurses are challenged to provide leadership in creating needed changes at the community level. Leadership interventions are needed in the following domains: (1) social, for example, in shifting the focus away from the treatment of disease to health promotion and disease prevention, in cost-containment efforts shifting financing for health care from the federal government to states and municipalities and in light of demographic shifts, such as the aging society; (2) medical, technological, and organizational, assuring that adequate care is provided by a system progresively driven by financing concerns; (3) environmental, in light of needs for an adequate knowledge base and for interdisciplinary collaborative approaches to addressing environmental concerns; and (4) human and biological challenges, such as those posed by AIDS and the potential of genetic engineering. Community health nurses need to play leadership roles in addressing these issues, requiring vision, con-

viction, the courage to act, and the willingness to work with others.

Traditionally nurses have practiced in organizational settings in which they are salaried employees rather than direct providers of services to individuals. Noting that there have been a number of nurse entrepreneurs over time, Aydelotte describes the current era of independent practice as a relatively new phenomenon. The movement into independent practice is impeded by a number of factors. Some are internal barriers growing out of a long tradition of dependence, such as discomfort with the role of decision maker, a lack of business sophistication, the inability to clearly articulate services to be provided and to place a reasonable monetary value on these services. Other barriers are external, such as the inability to secure sufficient venture capital to begin a private practice, and the lack of direct reimbursement from third-party payers. To overcome these barriers, Aydelotte says that data need to be presented to support results in economy, improved quality, and reduced costs of care.

Picking up on the theme of case management as a way of coordinating care, Zander argues that the control of case management is a matter of considerable concern in this era of cost control. Zander asserts that clinicians are needed as case managers and describes a managed care system implemented at New England Medical Center Hospitals in Boston in which nurses have greater independence and accountability.

The next three chapters shift to a focus on particular specialty areas within nursing: nurse-midwifery, pediatric nursing, and long-term care nursing. Ernst notes that although nurse-midwives have demonstrated the ability to deliver low-cost, high-quality health services, nurse midwifery has never really taken hold in the United States, as reflected by problems in maternity care. The momentum of the natural childbirth movement has created a void in maternity services that poses a particular challenge for nurse-midwifery. Producing adequate numbers of appropriately prepared nurse-midwives is one problem. A second problem is that of constraint of practice and the malpractice insurance crisis. Birth centers are seen as an essential component of low-cost, high-quality maternity care. As birth centers develop they provide opportunities for expanded practice and also serve as training sites for future nurse midwives. Noting that it took half a century to move maternity care into hospitals, Ernst projects that the third-party reimbursement system will be the force that moves maternity care out of hospitals and into birthing centers.

One of the consequences of our high-technology approach to medical care is the ability to maintain life for infants who otherwise would have died during the neonatal period. Eck and Ryan note the ironic juxta-position of high infant mortality and morbidity resulting from a lack of prenatal care and an increasing number of handicapped children resulting from the technological ability to sustain the lives of severely damaged infants. This high-technology system creates particular challenges for pediatric nursing. The high costs of maintaining life on extensive life support systems contribute to ethical dilemmas of pediatric nurses. In an effort to reduce costs, high-technology care is being transferred from hospital to home settings. This creates a demand for pediatric home care that cannot yet be satisfied. Eck and Ryan propose that individual case management is needed, with nurses working directly with families to identify realistic outcomes. Palliative units such as hospices need to be created as an alternative or a supplement to home care, and greater attention should be paid to the ethical decisions that are essential if resources are to be adequately distributed to address the health care needs of all children.

Turning to the other end of the age continuum, Strumpf argues for greater attention to the health care needs of the elderly. After presenting demographic data regarding the aging U.S. population, Strumpf outlines the problems of long-term care. Temporary and inadequate funding, funding from multiple sources, and the focus on funding for illness care rather than a spectrum of services all contribute to fragmentation. Strumpf proposes a case management model that focuses on functional independence rather than cures. Nursing has a vital role to play in improving care for the elderly. Important reforms include making gerontological nursing a viable and desirable career choice, increasing the emphasis on long-term care in the educational process, and conducting research on the contributions of nursing to an improved quality of life for the elderly.

Concluding this section, Souza provides a valuable perspective on nursing practice in developing countries. She traces the history of nursing education in Latin America, noting the emergence of formally structured nursing education as a post World War II phenomenon. As elsewhere, nurses with formal preparation became concentrated in hospitals and in administration. In recent years, given the limited resources in Latin America available for health care, there has been a conscious effort to focus on primary health care. The large numbers of workers with little formal nursing preparation place a great burden on those few with formal training.

CHAPTER 23

Debate

Is there anything new about this nursing shortage?

JOAN E. LYNAUGH

Can there be anything new about a problem as chronic as a nursing shortage? I argue that there can be, although the underlying historical dynamics are so constant and pervasive as to almost obscure the signs of change or newness in our contemporary situation. The evolution of nursing in American culture helps to unmask hidden elements in this serious and nagging social problem.[1] I'll begin with a story.

A colleague was attending a meeting called for the purpose of recommending solutions to the growing number of vacant nursing positions in a large urban hospital. Comments and suggestions flew. Finally one young physician spoke up in some exasperation. "I don't see what the problem is," he said. "There is plenty of unemployment in Pennsylvania. Let's just send up to the coal country for some of those girls. They will be glad to get the work." His proposal, a ready solution to not just one but two tough problems, has been made and acted on in the distant and not-so-distant past. We have frequently sent away for more nurses, to the farms, to the factories, to the Philippines, or to anywhere we believe we can find people willing to staff our episodically nurse-starved hospitals. It is not really surprising that in 1988 the American Medical Association believed it had found a solution to the nursing shortage in its "registered care technologist" proposal; there is plenty of precedent for that idea.[2]

These impatient calls for quick, cheap fixes, coupled with the "cannon fodder" assumption about candidates for nursing inherent in such "girls from the coal country" suggestions, reflect something of the social priorities, assumptions, and values underlying the American nursing experience.

SOCIAL PRIORITIES IN HEALTH CARE

In the 100 years or so since nursing became a recognized discipline in the United States, at least three social priorities have directed its development: the transfer of the work of caring for the sick from the domestic or home arena to the professional or institutional arena; the implementation of a host of diagnostic and therapeutic activities directed at curing specific diseases or injuries; and the protection of the public from the "dangerous" sick.

The very existence of American nursing is grounded in the nineteenth-century decision to transfer part of the work of caring for the sick from the home and family to the hospital and trained attendant. As the country grew and became more affluent in the years after the Civil War, Americans turned their attention to health and illness in their communities. Between 1880 and 1920 more than 7000 hospitals were established. Some were temporary; a significant proportion, however, became essential community institutions supported and used by all segments of the population.

Two essential elements of these new social institutions were the nurse superintendent and the training school for nurses. It was important to the middle class that the care givers in these new institutions be as reliable, respectable, and clean (in all senses) as the mothers or sisters who formerly had been charged with nursing responsibility.

Hospitals also had to be as safe as home, especially if they involved the care of children and women, as they came to do at the turn of the century. Thus the invention of American nursing was tightly linked to the success of the modern hospital. The concept of the intelligent, respectable woman heading an institution under the guidance and control of a socially responsible hospital board (usually all male) fit very well with American domestic ideals of the late nineteenth century. The hospital school, where nurses could be fitted for a life of needed service while at the same time reducing the cost of the hospital through their free labor, blossomed in the pragmatic reform climate of the time.

Over the first few decades of development, nurse superintendents and their pupils assumed responsibility for the care of those suffering from infectious disease, the chronically ill, injured industrial workers, the alcoholic and the insane, the aged, and later on, the sick or injured child and the laboring mother. Initially these patients were poor or without family resources. As the century drew to a close, however, hospitals became more and more popular as agencies of first resort for the sick and injured of all classes.

A revolution was also occurring in beliefs about disease and its treatment or prevention. By the 1880s the concept of disease as specific in origin and amenable to specific treatment began to spread. The power of germ theory in explaining the origin of infectious diseases such as cholera, diphtheria, and later, tuberculosis, captured the imagination of the public by 1900.

Linkages between physicians and science attained greater public notice when microbiology and chemistry began to offer physicians real tools to understand, prevent, diagnose, and eventually treat frightening infectious diseases. Even more visible was the surgeon's new freedom to repair the body, using anesthesia to prevent pain and relying on antisepsis or asepsis to prevent infection.

The medical revolution swept into the hospitals where domesticity had so briefly reigned. Good medical practice, once home and office based, began to require regular access to hospital beds. The physician's work was transformed from the holistic nineteenth-century encounter between an advisor and a patient to a twentieth-century search for a specific disease and the selection of treatment. As historian Charles Rosenberg puts it, the physician was "hospitalized"; in the process, the nurse and the hospital were conscripted into the service of this revolution.[3]

Both the work and the mission of the nurse shifted. The hospital had proved safe and attractive as a substitute for home during illness. The nurse created order out of the chaos of sickness, provided food, cleanliness, and nurturance, and relieved families of some of the burden of illness. Now was added the task of managing the temple of science that promised successful treatment and cure of illness rather than relief of suffering and a peaceful death.

Nurses became the implements of twentieth-century medical care. They created an antiseptic and, where necessary, aseptic environment; regularized prescribed treatments; enforced medical rules; oversaw laboratory testing; and dispensed drugs. Meanwhile nurses continued to feed, clothe, and nurture patients. By 1920, however, control of the patient's hospital experience was in the hands of the physician.

Hospital boards, nurses, and physicians wholeheartedly accepted biomedical strategies as the framework for their work. Conversion of the hospital to the tasks of searching for disease and trying out treatments left little place for the chronically ill, the marginally dysfunctional, or the aged. Both nurses and physicians arranged their priorities to give maximum attention to the compelling task of conquering disease.

For the nurse, however, the prize was small and the price high. As implementors rather than conceivers of the new medical strategies, nurses were thought to require only training instead of expensive college educations. Once that training was completed, the nurse was sent into private duty nursing, usually in the patient's home. As nurses left the training hospital their places were taken by new pupils. Perversely, the growing popularity of hospitals steadily undermined the private duty practice of the graduate nurse, as patients who would have paid for home care went instead to their local hospitals.[4]

Some nurses, however, were attracted to the third social health priority: health teaching for children and their mothers and protecting the public from the dangerous sick. Nineteenth-century city slums were breeding places for disease. Religious impulse inspired some citizens to try to alleviate the difficulties of city life. Although benevolent organizations had existed from colonial days, nurses entered the scene in the 1880s when they were recruited by the founders of what came to be called visiting nurse societies.

Visiting nurse movement

The visiting nurse movement grew slowly at first, but then spread rapidly across the country from Buffalo, Philadelphia, New York, and Boston. The central idea was to bring to the poor or isolated person instruction, cleanliness, comfort, and sometimes material aid. Visiting nurses were remote from physician influence. Their early alliances were with the middle-class women who founded and financed the visiting nurse societies. By the turn of the century their focus was on teaching the laws of health, preventing the spread of infection, supervising child care, assisting the chronically ill, and aiding sick workers and their families.

Their approach sought Americanization for the immigrant, urged work and self-reliance, and discouraged dependency. The introduction of school nursing by Lillian Wald in New York City, for example, was fueled by evidence that school nurses could reduce truancy and absence among immigrant children. Thus visiting nurses were agents for the social mores of their times.

Although rural visiting nursing developed later, it was the problems of urbanization that created public and philanthropic support for the visiting nurse movement. Fear of the poor, particularly the immigrant poor, and of infectious disease, particularly infant diarrhea and tuberculosis, caused the public to look with favor on these progressive women who risked their lives on city streets to bring health care to the downtrodden.

Education for this role was gained on the job, since most nurses were trained in the hospital system. Few special programs were available to prepare public health nurses before the late 1920s. Nevertheless, visiting nurses, school nurses, industrial nurses, and tuberculosis nurses became something of an elite corps among the rapidly burgeoning profession.

The visiting nurse movement overlapped with the urban reform movement of the Progressive Era and relied on the same faith in experts, government involvement in social problems, and education. Leaders in visiting nursing joined some of the nurse superintendents in large hospitals to agitate for better educational opportunities for nurses.

Although American society developed many institutions to enable the transfer of care of the sick away from home, although it embraced the achievements of biomedical strategies for identifying and treating disease, and although it admired and respected the work of the visiting nurses who protected the public from the dangerous sick, American assumptions about health care still inhibited the creation of a rational educational system to prepare nurses to address these social priorities. This was true despite the fact that other "female" occupations such as teaching and social work, which developed at the same time as nursing, found educational niches in the American college system.

SOCIAL ASSUMPTIONS THAT AFFECT NURSING PRACTICE

Four somewhat overlapping assumptions about care of the sick have contributed to the American failure to come to grips with the realities, intellectual and fiscal, of educating nurses.

Free labor pool

Our hospital system was founded in an essentially private voluntary sector not originally vulnerable to collective political influence. During the first 30 years of hospital development, laissez-faire community government was the norm. Hospitals were completely free to fix the rules of competition and the conditions of labor. There was no central planning of any kind at local or state levels and certainly not at the national level.

Nurses, with their complete reliance on hospitals, became in a sense the victims, educationally, of their own success. The founders of hospital training schools created a formula perfectly suited to the underfinanced, marginal institution operating in an almost totally unregulated environment. What industry would willingly give up a free labor pool?

Religious and benevolent missions

Added to the absence of any outside political influence was the fact that the health care institutions of the late nineteenth century were dominated by religious, benevolent, or professional groups. Standards in community hospitals at first were based on their religious or benevolent missions, and nurses' training schools were intended to serve the hospital mission. No mention was made of the hospital's obligation to its students. After the turn of the century, when serious efforts to improve education for nurses began to surface, no one really attacked the conflict between the hospital's interests and the interests of its students. It is surely fair to speculate that the hospital's immunity from attack as an exploitative institution was due in part to its benevolent community service role.

By 1910 leaders in nursing education in the hospitals began to rate schools according to hospital size, the number of years of training per nurse, and affiliations with national nursing organizations. These informal standards, promulgated in national nursing meetings, succeeded earlier ad hoc religious or benevolent criteria but still failed to criticize the hospital training system. Thus nursing seemed to be subsidizing the voluntary sector hospital system and apparently was willing to do it.

Generating hospital revenue

There was a good economic reason for clinging to the hospital system for educating nurses. These schools generated their own revenues through student labor, often creating income for the hospital by charging patients for special care by students. Later, in the 1930s and 1940s, the schools' costs were passed along to patients through direct billing, or to insurance companies through negotiated rates.

For the first 75 years of organized nursing the hospital school system made it possible for healthy Americans to completely ignore the economic implications of educating a large supply of nurses. This odd, interesting method of using an educational system to provide the labor for a quasi-public service delivered by private institutions endured for years without serious challenge. It meant that hospitals were staffed by a constantly rotating pool of workers called students.

Surplus of nurses

Another persistent element in the American attitude toward nursing is a preference for abundance, if not oversupply. Whenever it appears that an abundant supply of nurses is not waiting in the wings, calls are made for speeding up the production of trained nurses, adding minimally trained assistants to staff hospitals, sending overseas for nurses, sending to the equivalent of "the coal country" for unemployed women, or recalling unemployed nurses to the wards.

Despite the fact that the number of nurses per capita has risen steadily since 1890 and has, in fact, doubled since 1950, there is an almost traditional cyclical lament about the nursing shortage. Before and during World War I, for example, when the number of nurses

peaked for the first time, there were recurrent worries about shortage. "Waning Nurse Supply in America," proclaimed one headline in a 1907 issue of the *National Hospital Record*. In 1921 Adelaide Nutting, a renowned nurse leader, worried about the "scarcity of applicants" in the *Proceedings* of the 26th meeting of the National League of Nursing Education. Five years later, with the supply of nurses still increasing rapidly, the *Transactions* of the American Hospital Association decried the "paucity of nurses as one of the chronic ills of a hospital."

But by 1928 the professional literature was filled with stories of the nurse surplus, and nurses began to swell the ranks of the unemployed. In the 1920s and 1930s there was a shortage of students to meet increased demands for hospital care and a surplus of graduate nurses turned out by the training schools into a glutted private-duty market. When in the late 1930s graduate nurses finally began to be employed in hospitals, some of the surplus problem was alleviated.

Shortages were again reported during and after World War II, followed by surpluses of nurses in the early 1960s. But students still provided much of the nursing care in hospitals, so from the hospitals' point of view it was undesirable to cut back on their numbers. Until the 1960s, Americans assumed that nursing should be a low-cost service. Even after World War II, when federal money began to be used to support the creation of a university-based educational system, funds also went to hospital-based schools, guaranteeing low salaries and a surplus of nurses.

But part of the story is still missing. After all, people choose to work in health care for a number of reasons. To some degree Americans support health care for altruistic reasons. Values, both explicit and implicit, enter into social decision making. Often indirectly expressed, values are always difficult to deal with—but how else to explain the paradox presented by a society that frets over nursing shortages for 80 years but still supports an idiosyncratic system for nurse preparation? Even now, neither nursing education nor nursing practice is adequately financed and fairly remunerated.

One conclusion that can be drawn from American health priorities and assumptions about nursing is that the present nursing shortage is no different from any other experienced since nursing was invented. However, it may well be that the values influencing nursing are changing and, therefore, that this shortage will not be like all the others.

VALUES THAT INFLUENCE NURSING

Nursing entered the culture on a newfound American enthusiasm for freedom from the onerous tasks of caring for the sick, an enthusiasm fueled by sufficient affluence to make that freedom possible. Nursing was identified with economic growth, cleaning up the cities, reform by the so-called earnest classes, and self-improvement. Nurse reformers could envision a new wage-earning role for women of educated intelligence. When, during this era of reform, the idea grew of education as a means to upward mobility, nursing did not fully participate. The strategy of upward mobility through education operated only in a limited way for nurses because most were women and their gender alone restricted opportunities for advancement.

As we are seeing today, one cost of denying nurses access to upward mobility through education is skepticism among the young as to the long-term wisdom of the nursing career choice. On the other hand, nursing is now enriched by the presence of thousands of nurses prepared at the highest levels of the American educational system. Creation of a critical mass of well-prepared, influential people in the profession who can conceive and execute effective solutions to personnel supply problems will help to resolve the present shortage. This important change in nurse education grew out of a mid-twentieth-century shift in American thinking about education for women. The process of extending full educational opportunities to women and minorities, although slow, has proceeded far enough to alter nursing's role from supplicant for assistance to negotiator at all levels of policy-making.

Nursing has been very much caught up in the ebb and flow of American faith in science and technology. The highly technological, aggressive interventionism so long characteristic of American medical practice still absorbs much of nursing's energy, as it has since physicians moved into hospitals.

With varying degrees of success nursing has clung to its own nurturing, supportive, holistic attitude toward its clients. But, to this day, the siren song of cure sounds sweeter to Americans than the gentler refrain of comfort and care. It is the vacant positions in the acute care hospitals that raise the cry of nursing shortage, not the 40:1 patient-to-nurse ratio in the nation's nursing homes. Nursing's own values are persistently undervalued in our high-tech society. But as criticism mounts of twentieth-century reductionist concepts of biomedicine, nurses and laypeople find they share many health care values. Disappointment with biomedical approaches to chronic illness coupled with the AIDS crisis has created an environment in which it is easier for nurses to reassert the centrality of the care-giving role. As Americans grapple with the idea that many illnesses stem from lifestyle and diet, and as aging affects a larger proportion of the population, the value Americans place on nursing is likely to escalate.

When other values are accounted for, though, we must return to the issue of gender in American life. Feminist and nurse Lavinia Dock put it simply enough in 1920. "The status of nursing . . . depends on the status of women."[5] Throughout its history nursing, both as a discipline and as a profession, has been defined by its "female" character. But ironically, that femaleness would not matter if nursing itself were not so important. The vital role of nursing in relation to American health care priorities has led, in my view, to our reluctance to come to grips with the worth of its work. As long as nurses were willing to subsidize through their low wages the development of institutions, high-technology care, and care of the poor these priorities could expand at a relatively low cost.

The techniques employed to avoid paying nurses for the care we want are a testimony to American ingenuity. We have used students instead of trained nurses to care for patients. We have created turnover by refusing to employ married nurses. We have labeled women's wages "supplemental." We have allowed hospitals to fix wages in communities. We have excluded nurses from direct insurance-based reimbursement. And, most recently, we have argued that we cannot afford to entertain the concept of comparable worth. Throughout the history of nursing, Americans have not wanted to pay women what it costs.

Now we will see if American values actually have changed. As this shortage is played out we will discover whether the public once again will settle for nonsolutions. Its decision this time will be based on a different level of information, expressed in forums where nursing's own voice was rarely heard in the past. In 1987 and 1988 articles such as that by Aiken and Mullinix in the *New England Journal of Medicine*, Colman McCarthy's columns in the *Washington Post* and the *Philadelphia Inquirer*, Suzanne Gordon's pieces in the *Boston Globe Magazine*, front-page coverage in the *New York Times*, and debates on public television and in other forums kept the issue before us.[6] I argue that society recognizes its growing need for the services that nurses provide, that needs beget values, and that values create an atmosphere in which the gender-based economic gap can be bridged.

NURSING IN THE 1990s

The end of the first 100 years of American nursing is an appropriate time to take note of nursing's resilience. Although economically undervalued, nursing continues to grow and diversify. Nursing is fundamentally gratifying and engrossing. It is work that generates positive personal regard from others. Although the science and technology used by nurses change with new knowledge, the encounter between nurse and patient is always intimate and significant to both parties. It is work full of complications and emotional strain.

Often intellectually demanding, nursing requires making important decisions with incomplete data. When nurses make mistakes the consequences are serious. Nursing can be disgusting and tedious. It also can be frightening to deal with human beings under stress, out of control, in pain, or near death.

Both because of and despite all this, nursing attracts and holds very competent people. This will no doubt continue to be true, but currently the issue is one of an appropriate match between society's demands for health care and available nursing services.

The demands will be great, judging from past experience. Increased longevity among Americans will create a rising demand for care givers for the chronically ill and the elderly. Previous experience with devastating infectious disease warns us that AIDS will seriously challenge nursing's resources.

The American public will continue to demand access to new technology in health care; management of that technology is and will continue to be nursing's domain. Although there is now much interest in home care, it is likely that the institutional solution will continue to be favored for major acute care as well as for the growing number of the dependent chronically ill.

When nursing was new it promised safe hospitals, health reform, healthy babies, and relief for families. Today Americans are unclear about what it is that nurses do; nursing applicants really don't know how nurses spend their days either. The personal care, emotional support, education, and comfort practices of nursing have been hard to explain. Nursing's domestic origins tend to obscure its social contribution both for nurses themselves and for the public.

Part of the problem is the limitations of the scientific metaphors shared by nursing and its public. Traditionally, nursing studies delivery systems, techniques, and practitioners. Nurses hesitated to study ordinary responses to illness, the effect of knowledge on recovery, or other questions that did not seem to fit the scientific method. It is only in recent years that nurses have begun to feel confident enough to question, analyze, and argue the basically moral, humane functions that are at the heart of nursing.[7]

It is not so much that nursing does not need and use both basic and social sciences; rather, the sciences are not enough. To convey the promise or mission of nursing clearly, nursing needs to exploit all the explanatory devices of scholarship. After all, most pressing health care problems that we face, such as care of the aged and of AIDS patients, carry significant technological and moral choices.

Nurses have a responsibility to do for their patients those things that patients cannot do for themselves. One thing many patients cannot do for themselves is manage the health care system to their own advantage. Should the infant in Newark with AIDS remain in intensive care until its death, or should it be sent home to be sung to by its grandmother? Nurses make these choices but few are aware of it. To fully articulate the mission of nursing requires that nurses strive for person-centered health care and a place for nursing in policy formation. To the extent that nursing acts on its own broad mission, it will attract bright and active people to its ranks. Should we fail to accomplish that mission, we will dwindle as most irrelevant groups do.

Another means of ensuring that nursing remains a strong discipline is to make a share of the health care dollar directly available to the practitioner. Aspiring nurses should be assured of good working conditions that make appropriate use of their skills and training and that allow self-realization, both professional and economic. Nurses need work systems that support nursing values and that offer a fair financial return.

One promising strategy is the "nursing firm" or "nursing corporation" in which nursing services are contracted to hospitals, home care agencies, businesses, and schools. These firms have one objective: to provide nursing care to patients. There is no obligation to the institution beyond patient care. Thus the practitioner is employed in a system with a nursing goal and patient-care priorities. Now that direct payment to nurses through third-party payers is becoming a reality, nursing may be emancipated from its entanglement in hospital budgets.

The history of nursing is a history of conflicted loyalties. Nurses constantly juggle two sets of demands—those of patients and those of the hospital. At one time, of course, most nurses worked directly for individual patients. Private duty nurses were most likely driven out of business by nursing surpluses and hospital competition. I am not arguing for a return to the private duty system, but rather for a return to a more accountable nursing care system where the money spent on nursing care goes directly to the nurse or her firm.

Defining and preparing the responsible professional nurse is the third essential task for nursing. No general professional mission can succeed unless it is reflected in the actions of the practitioners of the discipline. And no nursing firm can meet its obligations unless its members adhere to a standard of performance shared by the group and acceptable to the public. As the public encounters more nurses who recognize and respond effectively to care needs using the best of current information and skills, expectations of nurses will increase.

The inescapable analogy is the improved public service offered by physicians as their training and skill repertoires were expanded after 1900. Admittedly the care, comfort, and education services provided by a skilled nurse are more subtle and abstract to the consumer than a well-performed appendectomy. Enthusiastic public acceptance of nurse-practitioners, nurse-midwives and psychiatric nurse clinicians, however, shows the positive impact of the right service delivered well.

What remains to be clarified is the standard of performance for the professional nurse. Ensuring a reliable standard of performance requires the careful selection of nursing candidates credible measures of skill attainment, and careful clinical training. All of these will be difficult to achieve and to maintain in the face of pressures to increase nursing's numbers.

One of the lessons of the history of nursing is that quick fixes for shortage situations aggravate the long-range problem by undermining the standard of performance expected by the public. Nurses and our supporters will have to be very clear about standards for professional practice if we hope to attract the best applicants in the 1990s.

There is something new about this nursing shortage, even though the causes leading to it are depressingly familiar. That something new is the environment in which the shortage is being perceived. A full and detailed dialog between the participants is vitally important to restate the social contract between nursing and society. There is no issue more important and no task more necessary to our collective welfare.

NOTES

1. This essay is based on a discussion paper prepared for Nurses for the future: an Invitational conference, sponsored by the University of Pennsylvania School of Nursing and the Pew Memorial Trust, Philadelphia, June 28-30, 1987.
2. American Medical Association Board of Trustees: Implementation of report CC (I-87), January 29, 1988.
3. Rosenberg C: The care of strangers, New York, 1987, Basic Books, Inc, p 175.
4. Reverby S: Something besides waiting: the politics of private duty nursing reform in the depression. In Lagemann E, editor: Nursing history: new perspectives, new possibilities, New York, 1983, Teachers' College Press.
5. Dock L and Isabel Stewart I: A short history of nursing, New York, 1920, GP Putnam's Sons, p 338.
6. A sampling of these includes Aiken LH and Mullinix CF: Special report: the nursing shortage—myth or reality? N Engl J Med 317:641, Sept 3, 1987; McCarthy C: The AMA's bad pill for nurses, The Philadelphia Inquirer, p B6, July 13, 1988, Suzanne Gordon S: The crisis in caring, Boston Globe Magazine, p 22, July 10, 1988; Holcomb B: Nurses fight back, Ms, p 72, June 1988, New York Times, p 1, July 31, 1988.
7. A particularly cogent example of this work is Benner P and Wrubel J: The primacy of caring: stress and coping in health and illness, Menlo Park, Calif, 1988, Addison-Wesley Publishing Co.

CHAPTER 24

Viewpoints

Changes in the hospital as a place of practice

LUCILLE A. JOEL

Burgeoning technology, advances in medical science, shifts in demography, and the economics of health care have dramatically changed hospitals and hospital nursing practice. This chapter establishes a historical perspective to allow a better understanding of nursing practice in contemporary hospitals. Given an idea of what exists and why it has come to be, the reader will be able to distinguish current trends and what nurses can expect under a variety of circumstances.

THE ORIGINS OF CHANGE

The conquest of infectious disease and advances in the treatment of traumatic injury and acute illness have created a world where chronic conditions are common. Medical science and technology, coupled with reimbursable services to the elderly through Medicare, have caused a dramatic shift in demographics. Medicare has created a healthier old age. By the year 2030, 20% of Americans will be over the age of 65 and many will be over 75 years old. In 1900, 4% of the elderly were 85 years or older; by 2050 that figure will be 25%.[6]

Where health care coverage is provided through the workplace, reimbursement has begun to favor treatment in community settings; however, public-entitlement programs such as Medicare continue to be biased toward traditional hospital- and physician-based models of service. Given these factors it is no surprise that 40% of hospital admissions are Medicare recipients and 60% of hospital days are Medicare days.[5] The elderly predominate among hospital patients, and unstable or acute exacerbations of chronic illness are the most frequent clinical situations. Ready access to state-of-the-art technology and an extremely litigious environment create circumstances in which aggressive therapy has become more the rule than the exception.

The changes attributable to medical science, an aging population, and expanded access to services pale next to the manner in which hospitals have been reshaped by economics in the last decade. By end of the 1970s the federal government began to feel uneasy about the magnitude of its financial obligation to Medicare and Medicaid recipients. By 1980 cost-effectiveness in health care reimbursed through public-entitlement programs was mandated by the government. Hospitals, the most costly element in the delivery system, were targeted for cost containment. In a sequence of events from 1980 through 1983 hospital rates and fees for in-patient ancillary services paid by the Medicare program were negotiated downward, and related expenses such as capital improvements, interest payments, and the cost of care to the indigent were disallowed. In October 1983 the Medicare prospective pricing system (PPS) was instituted for hospitals. This system awarded a fixed-dollar amount for an episode of illness based on a cluster of variables found to be highly predictive of hospital resource use (diagnosis, complications, surgery, age). The taxonomy of diagnosis-related groups (DRGs) provided the reimbursement categories for PPS. To ensure fiscal solvency hospitals were obliged to influence the prescriptive practices of physicians. Reducing the length of stay and the use of ancillary services became critical. The use of proprietary as opposed to generic drugs and defensive diagnostic testing for protection in a litigious milieu both create serious financial liability for hospitals. From another perspective, physicians construe the need to be judicious in their ordering practices as an administrative intrusion into clinical management. The reaction has been for physicians to favor treatment of patients in the community and to choose hospitalization only as a last resort.

PPS has been described as the ultimate in both regulation and deregulation. Cost-benefit decisions were decentralized to the facility level, and the hospital was able to predict the dollar amount of Medicare revenue based on its historic case mix. Further, by striking reimbursement rates according to the average cost of treatment in a category, PPS intended hospitals to assume some risk for patients who consume resources in excess of the usual. The industry's response has been less humanistic, often denying admission to patients who appear to be a financial liability. Such cases often become the charge of public sector facilities.

The efficiencies imposed by Medicare and, in most instances, state Medicaid programs, shifted some of the costs of doing business to patients who paid out-of-pocket or were reimbursed by private sector insurers, predominantly through the workplace. In order to safeguard their premium payments, insurance intermediaries and employers began to limit reimbursable treatment options and to monitor clinical management practices. Community care was favored over hospitalization except in the most serious instances. The effect of these complementary private and public sector trends has been unprecedented severity and aggressive treatment both to speed discharge and as a therapeutic response to acutely ill patients. Clinical intensity is also affected by the need to maintain high patient volume and maximum occupancy rates. In today's reimbursement environment, three patients each hospitalized for ten days generate more revenue than one patient hospitalized for thirty days. Each new admission requires assessment, development of a plan of care, and subsequent implementation and integration of a therapeutic regimen. The increased demands on nursing are obvious.

NURSING IN TODAY'S HOSPITALS

In the midst of a hospital environment where the physician continues to be the gatekeeper and reimbursement focuses on medical management, nursing has become the singular most essential service. There are few if any medical conditions that cannot be treated in the community. An increasing number of surgical procedures are appropriate to free standing surgical centers or day-of-admission programs. Patients come to hospitals for nursing. They come because of the need for monitoring and surveillance on a continuous basis. They come because of self-care deficits and compromised functional statuses. They come for teaching, counseling, coordination of services, development of community support systems, and preparation of the family to cope with an individual's changed health status. Consumers have begun to distinguish the roles that hospitals and physicians play in promoting the return to health. Consumers are more judicious in selecting their hospitals as well as their physicians. This choice is often based, either consciously or unconsciously, on the perceived quality of nursing.

Competent nursing is also critical to the financial integrity of hospitals. Skillful clinical management of the acutely ill elderly can minimize functional deficits and avoid costly disposition problems. Advancing the patient's diet on a meal-to-meal basis, furthering self-care as motivation appears, seizing the opportunity to teach and counsel at the moment of receptiveness, all contribute to reducing the length of stay and shortened lengths of stay contribute to the financial well-being of the hospital. Documenting complications at the first detectable clinical signs and immediately instituting a corrective regimen may increase short-term costs but may also avert the need for a protracted hospital stay. Skillful clinical observation can reduce the need for testing. Careful coordination of hospital services can speed diagnosis, treatment, and stabilization of the medical regimen. Cash flow concerns and maximizing reimbursement demand thorough documentation executed with a cost-conscious eye. Chart completion and the establishment of a principal diagnosis are critical for reimbursement. Nurses' notes often provide information overlooked by physicians. Given the potential clinical and financial benefits of sophisticated nursing, regionalization and organization of clinical services based on nursing specialties is more prudent than consolidation reflecting the medical model.

Hospitals were blind to the inherent value of nursing as they first began to consider approaches to cost-effectiveness. Early in the days of cost containment nursing departments, as labor-intensive centers, were targeted for downsizing. The hospital budget was often balanced off the back of nursing, most notably by reducing the numbers of registered nurses. Those nurse executives who had the foresight to document increased resource consumption by patients were the most successful in maintaining their staffs. As hospital patients became more acutely ill, the wisdom of decreasing the number of registered nurses became suspect. Instead, hospitals began to cut back on the support services available to nursing and to thin the ranks of other provider professionals in such areas as pharmacy, physical therapy, and respiratory therapy in favor of increasing the number of nurses on staff. Nurses were recognized as extremely versatile workers, ready and able to assume the duties of a wide variety of other skilled and unskilled workers. Nursing practice in hospitals began to be characterized by all-registered nurse (RN) staffs. In truth, there was a lack of appreciation for what nurses could contribute as nurses. There are two issues hidden here: the use of nurses to perform nonnursing activities, and nurses performing clinical duties below their skill levels. The latter situation, at least, has been well documented.

Management studies have found that up to 40% of a nurse's time may be invested in nonnursing functions.[4] Research in New Jersey in the late 1970s indicated that 23% to 48% of the nurse's time is invested in work inappropriate to the role.[7] Great variation exists in the creation of support systems for nurses that allocate more professional nursing time to the bedside. The "unit assistant" created at Rush-St. Luke's-Presbyterian Medical Center in Chicago is one example. The unit assistant takes on a variety of nonnursing tasks rather than operating exclusively as a messenger, a transporter, or a clerical worker. This approach is based on the fact that because the needs of each hospital unit are different, it is unwise to create specific categories of supportive workers or to detail their tasks. The essential role that nurses play in coordinating and integrating the hospital routine makes it prudent to place support workers under the control of nursing. Ideally the money for these positions should come from the nursing budget and the support worker should be assigned consistently to one registered nurse. This arrangement creates the best environment for shaping the support role and allows the nursing philosophy of care and work ethic to be clearly communicated and modeled by the responsible superior. Similar nonclinical, nursing-designed, unit-based models have been reported at Providence Medical Center in Seattle and at Miami's Children's Hospital.[1] In a recent survey of hospitals conducted by the American Nurses' Association (ANA) and the Association of Nurse Executives (AONE), 84% of the respondents reported creating support personnel to perform non-

nursing duties.[2] The result is an increase in the amount of time nurses can devote to patient care.

The question remains, is there is a role in hospitals for personnel who can assist nurses with direct care? The condition of the hospital patient is the critical element in this debate. Clinical circumstances have limited the hospital job market for licensed practical nurses and others who in the past have assisted the registered nurse with direct care. This is not to deny the need for assistant clinical workers in long-term and home care. Decisions on the need for clinical support personnel and their level of training are best made by nurses at the facility level, based on the complexity of patient needs.

The reader is cautioned about the danger of moving too quickly to embrace clinical support systems for nursing before adequately assessing the nonnursing duties that have become part of the nurse's role. It is also necessary to lobby for hospital policies that allow nurses to control the introduction of support personnel and that establish the nurses' authority over their work. In recent years nurses have accepted new categories of clinical workers in specialty areas with little protest, viewing each incident as an isolated occurrence. Specific examples can be cited in dialysis, critical care, emergency services, anesthesia, and the operating room. This trend gained little attention until the American Medical Association proposed a new class of caregiver, the registered care technologist (RCT), as its response to the nursing shortage.

Both personnel utilization patterns and compensation have been positively influenced by the current nursing shortage. The market for nursing responds to supply and demand. Nurses' salaries have increased significantly in some geographic areas. Hospital nurses, as the most visible group, have profited the most. Starting salaries have often been increased at the expense of economic growth within existing nursing positions. The AONE suggests a 100% range between beginning and maximum salaries. Establishing unrealistic entry salaries creates future problems in the attempt to solves present ones. Salary compression creates a serious obstacle to nurse recruitment and retention.

The tendency to pay more for personnel during a shortage has always been the first step in a vicious cycle. Nursing salaries have always been increased in times of shortage. The high cost of nursing then prompts a more cost-efficient use of nurses and the introduction of support systems to take over non-nursing duties and those less-skilled activities commonly delegated to nurses. A nursing surplus gradually develops and salary gains are slowed, at which point it becomes feasible to hire nurses rather than less-skilled workers. This returns us full circle to a demand-driven shortage.

Benefits have also been reshaped by the nursing shortage to address personal and professional needs. Over 93% of the respondents in a recent ANA/AONE survey of 1065 hospitals offer flexible work schedules for nurses seeking degree education. More than 81% of these hospitals provide financial assistance to licensed practical nurses (LPNs) and licensed visiting nurses (LVNs) enrolled in RN-educational programs, and almost 81% subsidize baccalaureate and graduate courses for registered nurses. Nurses who take on less-desirable work schedules are rewarded financially by 63% of the hospitals. Clinical excellence and productivity are identified as the bases for promotion by 52.4% of the respondents. On a more negative note, there is a positive correlation between more flexible, creative, and professional employee policies and the degree of nursing shortage experienced by the hospital. Where there is little or no shortage there is little openness to change.[2] This is unfortunate and demonstrates the need for progressive hospitals to publicize their incentives and practice programs to attract nurses. Market competition may be the most effective tactic to restructure hospital nursing.

OUR PREFERRED FUTURE

I have already offered examples of how hospital nursing is being restructured to promote professionalism. The nursing shortage has been the catalyst. Moving beyond salary and benefits, it will be the practice programs and role relationships in hospitals that provide status and prestige. Hospital nursing can only flourish in an environment of status and prestige. The elements critical to a preferred future have been thoroughly described by organized nursing.[3,8,9]

A preferred future must include the ability to distinguish nurses according to education, seniority, experience, supervisory and peer evaluations, and certification, as well as any other appropriate variables. Either job descriptions, clinical ladders, or both may be the vehicles to formalize these distinctions. It is critical that role expectations change as a nurse's role

changes within any system of differentiation and that salary and benefits are tailored to recognize these levels of personal growth and accomplishment. Ideally there is a hierarchy of clinical competencies that complements the variations in patient complexity seen in the hospital. A staff hierarchy also accommodates variable demands in the areas of research and innovation, mentoring, and institutional involvement.

Dissatisfactions with hospital nursing are closely associated with the growing fragmentation of practice and the consequent loss of control over plans of patient care. The intimacy and holism that lie at the core of nursing have been seriously compromised by attempts to accommodate more profoundly ill patients, technology, specialization, and rapid discharge. Hospitals that successfully retain their nurses organize service delivery to reinstitute continuity, comprehensiveness, and control of the clinical nursing regimen. The principles are the same whether we talk about primary nursing, case management, district nursing, or a variety of other models. The role of the nurse as patient advocate, systems coordinator, and integrator of the total hospital experience is surfacing as logical and cost effective.

The decentralization of clinical authority and the establishment of systems of reward based on competence demand that nurses be accountable to and for one another. A practice council becomes the forum in which interdisciplinary clinical management can be discussed. Practice councils allow the resolution of problems between groups of provider professionals; this resolution is achieved without administrative intrusion but with administration serving in an advisory capacity and offering a broader perspective on operations. A nursing staff organization provides the self-governing structure to develop and institute a program of peer review.

The reporting relationships and responsibilities that have been described can only flourish in an environment where the chief nursing executive has the status of other major department heads. This individual must be secure enough in status and ability to recognize that one cannot be an expert in all areas. One must have the self-assurance to allow people to fail, to delegate authority as well as responsibility, and to give people some latitude in approaching their responsibilities.

There is no single best structural and functional design for hospital nursing services. Modeling must be done at the facility level within a system of participatory management. Individuals invest highly in systems that they help to develop and will have to live by. A tertiary provider institution with high levels of clinical intensity and well-developed specialization will require a different organization and mix of resources than a community hospital with a simpler patient population.

In effect, the test of any system is to look at outcomes. Are patients discharged in fewer days? Is recidivism lower? Are iatrogenic occurrences less frequent? What about drug errors and accidents? Is staff turnover less? Is research a part of everyday life? Is the facility a desirable place for students? Do faculty from affiliated schools participate readily in staff development activities? This is not an exhaustive list, but it does begin to identify critical indicators against which to measure our preferred future. Moving beyond guild issues, hospital nursing will flourish only to the extent that it makes a difference to sick patients and to the institutional health of the hospital.

REFERENCES

1. American Hospital Association: Restructuring the work load: methods and models to address the nursing shortage, Chicago, 1989, The Association.
2. American Nurses' Association: Nursing practice update, Kansas City, Mo, December 1988, The Association.
3. American Nurses' Association: Magnet hospitals: attraction and retention of professional nurses, Kansas City, Mo, 1983, American Academy of Nursing.
4. Ernst and Whinney: Personal communication to the American Nurses' Association, June 1988.
5. Joel L: Geriatric imperative: the acutely ill elderly, Journal of the Medical Society of New Jersey 81(8):655, 1984.
6. Koop EE: The strengths and needs of the elderly. In Issues and Strategies in Geriatric Education, McLean, Va, 1985, The Circle, Inc.
7. New Jersey Department of Health: A prospective reimbursement system based on patient case mix for New Jersey hospitals, 1976-1983, 2nd annual rep, vol 1, Trenton, December 1978, State of New Jersey Department of Health.
8. Nursing Summit statement on short-term strategies to address the nursing shortage, Washington, DC, May 1988.
9. Secretary's Commission on Nursing: Interim report, Washington, DC: July 1988, US Department of Health and Human Services.

CHAPTER 25

Continuity of care across hospital-community boundaries

JUDITH BAIGIS-SMITH
KATHLEEN M. McKEEHAN

Each person carries his own doctor inside him. They come to us knowing this truth. We are at our best when we give the doctor who resides within each patient a chance to go to work.

ALBERT SCHWEITZER

Continuity between hospital and community in the delivery of health care services is one of the most important patient care issues confronting the present generation of nurses. Discontinuity in the care process is closely linked to a number of related concerns: prospective payment mechanisms, institutional interest in saving money, strict malpractice regulations against discharge without adequate follow-up, and the therapeutic effect that early hospital discharge has for many patients. This chapter focuses primarily on discontinuity in the care process itself. We state our views on the causes of discontinuity of care and emphasize the active role patients need to take during discharge planning based on a unique approach to decision making. This approach should smooth the often fearful transition between hospital care, home care, or other types of community-based care. Since patients would be participating in goal setting, it may also facilitate their recuperation.[18]

THE CAUSES OF DISCONTINUITY OF CARE

Discontinuity of care is a break or gap in any phase of the health care process that can limit a patient in reaching a healthy level of functioning.

Discontinuity of care is most frequently identified as a reflection of deficits in the preparation of practitioners and of related problems in the organization of health care services.

Specialization, by practitioner and by site, is one main cause of the discontinuity of patient care across hospital-community boundaries. The growth of science in the nineteenth century and the development of scientific health care were major events in narrowing the scope of practice in medicine and nursing.[35] The growth of the hospital as a center for research and practice contributed to this process.[31] The medical and nursing literature in the United States had begun to address continuity of care issues arising from the ascendancy of specialists and hospitals as their practice bases in the early decades of the twentieth century.[10,11,20,34] Paul Starr[36] points to three economic factors that increased the rate of specialty practice among physicians in the first decades of this century: (1) the rise of specialty board-certifying examinations with no limit on the number of physicians who could sit for them, (2) incentives for hospital-associated specialty training programs, and (3) reimbursement of specialists through government subsidies and health insurance. Nursing, for its part, modeled nursing school curricula on those of the medical schools. Nursing students are taught to have an intensive concern with various diseases, their treatment, and the nursing care specific to those diseases. The result is an emphasis on specialty nursing practice in both hospitals and other practice sites.

The effects of discontinuity of care

The negative side of specialty practice in both nursing and medicine has gradually emerged. Nurses and physicians, by concentrating their attention on particular parts of the body such as the heart or the lungs, are seen as lacking interest in the whole person. They have increasingly concentrated on the person's disease rather than on the diseased person. Thus the result is a narrowing of the scope of contemporary nursing and medicine. This narrowing of scope is reflected in case reports of patients who have been discharged from hospitals without reasonable follow-up plans made for self-care, health education, or adequate supervision even when those services are available in the community.[20,42] These reports have come to be viewed as classic examples of patients who have "fallen through the cracks" because the nurses and physicians responsible for their care do not have the big picture, that is, a view of the patient within the context of family and community. To help rectify such problems, the elements of successful discharge planning programs have been identified.[8,22,24,28,37] There are growing research activities in continuity of care examining hospital discharge planning models,[14,17,27,32] the impact of discharge planning on length of hospital stay,[7,9,21] and the impact of hospital discharge planning on patient outcomes.[15,33,38] (There are also significant problems in ensuring continuity across levels of care for the poor, those without adequate health insurance, and those who live in communities with limited services for the ill and infirm. Although such situations are not directly related to the negative side of specialty practice, our suggested solution may be of use to some people in those circumstances.)

FROM DISCONTINUITY TO CONTINUITY OF CARE

There are several ways of dealing with the problems created by discontinuity in the care process. The first is through the introduction of a category of professional that counters the trend toward specialization. Medicine has done this with the introduction of the family practice physician. This physician is trained to administer to all age groups and to coordinate the medical care for families. Similarly, nursing has introduced the family nurse clinician, whose job is to coordinate primary care for all family members and to treat minor acute conditions and monitor chronic stable conditions in those families. Since these professionals are still in short supply, another solution is to reinstitutionalize a generalist perspective in graduate education that would further move nursing education away from its specialty focus.

The second way to deal with discontinuity of care is through the introduction of discharge planning consultants—generally nurses or social workers based in hospitals—who work with the different health care disciplines involved in patient care to facilitate the transition of that care from one setting or level of care to another.

The third and, from our perspective, most important way is through the involvement of the patient. Although the responsibility for *implementing* the patient's continuing care falls to health professionals, enhancing the patient's decision-making abilities for *selecting* care improves continuity of care across settings.

Decision making in continuity of care

An untapped resource for improving the discharge planning process lies in our patients, that is, in their capacities to make quality decisions. We can assist them in their decision making during discharge planning through appropriate counseling.

Decision making is the most deliberate and voluntary aspect of social conduct.[16] Despite the attention to theoretical models of decision making during the past several decades, health professionals have only recently begun to view patient counseling for decision making as an important approach to the discharge planning process. There are many theoretical models of decision making.[1,5,6,19,23] Of these, the conflict model of decision making by Janis and Mann[15] is viewed as the most important for influencing decision making in the discharge planning process,[14,25] and it has been a useful framework for research in discharge planning.[13,25] This model describes "when, how, and why psychological stress generated by decisional conflict imposes limitations on human rationality,"[19] and specifies antecedent conditions related to the variables of hope, risk, and time that lead to a particular level of stress, evoking patterns that result in either defective or quality decision making.

Decision making is defined as "that thinking which results in the choice among alternative courses of action."[40] Unfortunately, the choices during discharge planning are often limited by the availability of both community resources and options. One effective way to extend options is to give patients the name and phone number of either a continuity of care consultant or a primary nurse, for use in case the chosen course of action does not work out. Often, this approach helps patients to relax and to commit themselves to the alternatives or options chosen because they have that contingency plan. Many continuity of care consultants have found this approach to be successful, with very few problems occurring and little need for the patient to call.

Research results thus far indicate that health care providers need to become more skilled in the techniques of helping their patients tap into what Albert Schweitzer called "the doctor within." Reaching the doctor within—that is, one's personal explicit and implicit knowledge—is the key to quality decision making. This idea is explored in several Eastern systems of philosophy and psychology,[4,30,39] but one that offers a very practical approach for using personal knowledge in decision making is yoga.

Yoga perspectives on decision making

In the Yoga tradition, quality decision making requires the ability to calm the mind and body. This can provide insights into ways to achieve personal physical and psychological health. An important technique for calming the mind and body and gaining these insights is through appropriate breathing. Yoga texts on physical and psychological health emphasize that breath is the essence of life.[29] Calming one's breathing has a calming effect on the mind. In other words, calm breathing enhances the ability of individuals to focus their energy to make responsible decisions. It can also have a relaxing effect.

According to a review of the scientific literature, breathing may be a significant variable in most, perhaps in all, relaxation techniques.[2] The reason breathing is essential to relaxation is that it has a special relationship to the autonomic nervous system. Breath control is directly related to a hypothalamic response that can balance the parasympathetic and sympathetic nervous systems.[26] When patients' energies are already depleted through illness the process of decision making is stressful. Stress often clouds one's perceptions and interferes with the ability to make responsible decisions. Thus any technique that reduces stress when important decisions have to be made contributes to beneficial outcomes.

Characteristics of optimal breathing patterns emphasized in yoga texts include a breath pattern which is nasal, diaphragmatic, regular with no pauses or jerks, slow, deep, quiet, within one's comfortable capacity.[12,30] Appropriate use of the breath is defined here as the conscious observance of these patterns. Most of the patterns are self-explanatory; however, the pattern of diaphragmatic breathing warrants further discussion.

Diaphragmatic breathing

In diaphragmatic breathing patients lie on their backs with a pillow under their heads. One hand is placed on the upper part of the abdomen with the little finger near the navel and the thumb under the breastbone. The other hand is placed on the chest. As the patient inhales, the hand on the upper abdomen should rise; during exhalation, it falls. The hand on the chest remains relatively motionless, signifying the absence of chest movement during respiration. To develop skill in diaphragmatic breathing, it should be practiced twice a day. After the basic technique is learned, the hands do not need to be placed on the torso.

If the breath is consciously guided into a diaphragmatic pattern of breathing, and if the other patterns of breathing previously mentioned are used, a state of alert relaxation can readily emerge. This state of relaxation can sharpen the capacity for critical thinking and the ability to accurately weigh the pros and cons of alternatives when making decisions. It can lead to what several schools of Eastern psychology call the "witness stance," that is, the ability to stand back and objectively observe the entire situation surrounding decisions. Achieving a state of relaxation and the witness stance can also help in conserving already limited energy.

Stress management in discharge planning

Research findings indicate that when individuals make decisions involving their own vital interests they enter into potential decisional conflict that can affect the quality of their decision making behaviors.[19] For this reason and because of the stress of illness itself, stress management training should be an integral part of all discharge planning with patients and families. Relaxation techniques are an integral part of all stress management programs and proper breathing is a foundation for relaxation. Complete relaxation is achieved when one mentally focuses on relaxing the muscle groups of the body in a gradual and systematic way.

This is often best achieved lying on one's back in a supine position with the legs 14–16 inches apart and the arms 6–8 inches from the body, with palms facing up. However, it may also be done in a sitting position with the head, neck, and trunk straight. Refer to Samskrti and Veda[31] for an in-depth description of systematic (complete) relaxation. This formal relaxation technique can be done one to two times per day for 10 minutes, but the goal in breathing is to develop the habit of constant diaphragmatic breathing.

Although the techniques of diaphragmatic breathing and relaxation are relatively easy to learn and teach, there are a few points to keep in mind:

1. To teach the techniques properly and to recognize the levels of subtlety reached, the nurse needs to gain proficiency in these techniques.
2. Breathing should be natural and relaxed, with a rhythm and duration comfortable for the individual. There is no need for perceptible muscular effort and there should be no sense of strain.
3. Because diaphragmatic breathing is a general foundation for relaxation, consistent use of this breathing pattern should reduce the stresses that aggravate the signs and symptoms of disease. Thus medication levels (for example, antihypertensive drug levels) may have to be reduced. Patients need to be monitored for this benefit.
4. When learning these techniques, a few people may experience a sense of tension associated with the process of breathing itself. Changing to a relaxation technique, such as the systematic (complete) relaxation technique, should help.[29] Then the technique of diaphragmatic breathing can be reintroduced.
5. Rarely, an individual may become anxious from the relaxation process itself. If this should happen, shorten the time and depth of relaxation. The depth can be shortened by, for example, opening the eyes or sitting in a chair.

CONCLUSION

The American Nurses' Association's Social Policy Statement specifies that "[patient] deficiencies in decision making and the ability to make personal choices are a focus for nursing interventions."[3] Nurses are in a good position to assist patients in making decisions for continuing health care. The essence of the nurse's counseling is helping patients to maximize their strengths so they can make responsible decisions. A necessary condition for accomplishing this is a quiet or calm mind, which can be achieved through appropriate use of the breath.

The following questions are raised to stimulate directions for further research:

Is calming the patient's mind preferable to stimulating it (e.g., by reading the patient the Patient's Bill of Rights)?

How do we know when the patient is using a "calm mind" to make decisions as opposed to merely being passive or resigned? How can the clinician recognize the witness stance?

Why and how does a calm mind lead to responsible decision making? What is the relationship between informed decision making and the yoga approach?

How does one distinguish between decision making due, for example, to the patient feeling more involved in his or her care and that due to calming the mind?

What is the patient's role in decision making? What are the boundaries of the patient's decision making and who sets them?

Health professionals have tried to acknowledge the patient's autonomy and the need for the patient's informed consent as a condition of practice. When patients are in the hospital, however, they often feel passive, incompetent, and unable to make decisions. Nevertheless, they are often more competent than they realize. For example, imagine a patient who has been discharged from the hospital to his home and needs a caretaker. From the professional's view, the patient's spouse would not be the ideal caretaker. The son or daughter are more competent and responsible. But the patient may prefer the spouse for continuity of care reasons: that is, he shares his life with this person; this is the person who has always taken care of him. If the patient is involved in health care decisions, these decisions may reflect a concern for continuity of care rather than a concern solely for competence. We can also see why patients feel that they cannot make these kinds of decisions. They often think they are meddling in nursing or medical care. So responsible decision making is an instructive matter for both patients and health professionals. Realizing that responsible decision making by patients is fundamental to discharge planning is the initial step in really achieving continuity of care across hospital-community boundaries.

ACKNOWLEDGMENT

We thank John Clarke, M.D., Chairman of the Himalayan International Institute in Honesdale, Pa., for his comments on yoga perspectives and diaphragmatic breathing.

REFERENCES

1. Abramson LY, Seligman ME and Teasdale JD: Learned helplessness in humans: critique and reformulation, J Abnorm Psychol 87(1):49, 1978.
2. Arpita, S. The role of breathing in current clinical interventions. Research Bull 1982: 4(1):22, 1982.
3. American Nurses' Association. Nursing: a social policy statement. Pub. Code NP63-35m. Kansas City, MO: The Association, 1980, p. 10.
4. Arya U. Yoga-sutras of Patanjali. Honesdale, PA: Himalayan International Institute, 1986.
5. Atkinson JW and Birch D: The dynamics of action, New York, 1970, John Wiley & Sons, Inc.
6. Blau PM: Exchange and power in social life, New York, 1964, John Wiley & Sons, Inc.
7. Boone CR, Coulton CJ, and Keller SM: The impact of early and comprehensive social work services on length of stay, Soc Work Health Care 7(1):1, 1981.
8. Bristow O, Stickney C, and Thompson S: Discharge planning for continuity of care, Pub No 21-1604, New York, 1976, National League for Nursing.
9. Cable EPC and Mayers SP: Discharge planning effect on length of hospital stay, Arch Phys Med Rehabil 64:57, 1983.
10. Cannon IM: Social work in hospitals, New York, 1913, Russell Sage Foundation.
11. Carn I and Mole EW: Continuity of nursing care, Am J Nurs 49(6):388, 1949.
12. Clarke, J. Characteristics of the resting breath pattern. Research Bulletin Fall 1979; 7-9.
13. Coulton C *and others:* Discharge planning as a decision-making process, Health Soc Work 7:253, 1982.
14. Coulton C and McKeehan KM: A systems approach to program development for continuity of care in hospitals. In McClelland E, Kelly K, and Buckwalter KC, editors: Continuity of care: advancing the concept of discharge planning, Orlando, Fl, 1985, Grune & Stratton, Inc.
15. Donabedian A and Rosenfeld LS: Follow-up study of chronically ill patients discharged from hospital. J Chronic Dis 17:847, 1964.
16. Etzioni A: Mixed-scanning: a "third" approach to decision-making, Public Administration Review 27:385, 1967.
17. Feather J and Nichols LO: Hospital discharge planning for continuity of care: the national perspective. In Hartigan EG and Brown DJ, editors: Discharge planning for continuity of care, rev ed, New York, 1985, National League for Nursing.
18. Hefferin E: Health goal setting: patient-nurse collaboration at veterans administration facilities. Milit Med, p: 812, Dec 1979.
19. Janis IL and Mann L: Decision making: a psychological analysis of conflict, choice, and commitment, New York, 1977, Free Press.
20. Jensen F, Weiskotten HG, and Thomas MA: Medical care of the discharged hospital patient, New York, 1944, Commonwealth Fund.
21. Marchette L and Holloman F: Length of stay: significant variables, Journal of Nursing Administation 16(3):12, 1986.
22. McClelland E, Kelly K, and Buckwalter KC, editors: Continuity of care: advancing the concept of discharge planning, Orlando, Fla, 1985, Grune & Stratton, Inc.
23. McGuire WJ: The current status of cognitive consistency theories. In Feldman S, editor: Cognitive consistency: motivational antecedents and behavioral consequences, New York, 1966, Academic Press, Inc.
24. McKeehan KM, editor: Continuing care: a multidisciplinary approach to discharge planning, St Louis, 1981, The CV Mosby Co.
25. McKeehan KM: Decision making by clients planning for continuing health care, doctoral dissertation, Cleveland, 1985, Case Western Reserve University.
26. Nuernberger, P. Freedom from stress: a holistic approach. Honesdale, PA: Himalayan International Institute, 1981.
27. O'Hare PAP: Examining the discharge planning process: an evaluation of two models in an acute care community hospital, doctoral dissertation, Baltimore, 1984, The Johns Hopkins University School of Hygiene and Public Health.
28. Previte VJ: Continuing care in a primary nursing setting: role of a clinical specialist, Int Nurs Rev 26(2):53, 1979.
29. Rama S, Ballentine R, Hymes A. Science of breath: a practical guide. Honesdale, PA: Himalayan International Institute, 1981.
30. Rama S, Ballentine R, Ajaya S. Yoga and psychotherapy: the evolution of consciousness. Honesdale, PA: Himalayan International Institute, 1976.
31. Samskrti and Veda (1985). *Hatha yoga manual I.* 2nd ed. Honesdale, PA: Himalayan International Institute.
32. Schuman JE, Ostfeld AM, and Willard HN: Discharge planning in an acute hospital, Arch Phys Med Rehabil 57:343, 1976.
33. Schuman JE and Willard HN: Role of the acute hospital team in planning discharge of the chronically ill, Geriatrics, p 63, February 1976.
34. A field nurse for old Bellevue, Charities and the Commons 17:125, 1906-1907. Quoted In: O'Hare PA and Terry MA, editors: Discharge planning. Rockville, MD: Aspen, 1988.
35. Smith JA: The idea of health: implications for the health professional, New York, 1983, Teachers College Press of Columbia University.
36. Starr P: The social transformation of American medicine, New York, 1982, Basic Books, Inc.
37. Steffl B and Eide I: Discharge planning handbook, New Jersey, 1978, Clarles B. Slack.
38. Steinwachs DM *and others:* Impact of hospital discharge planning on patient outcomes, Baltimore, The Johns Hopkins University School of Hygiene and Public Health, book in preparation, 1989.
39. Tigunait R. Seven systems of Indian philosophy. Honesdale, PA: Himalayan International Institute, 1983.

40. Taylor, D.W. (1965). Decision making and problem solving. In J. March (Ed.). *Handbook of organization*. Chicago: Rand-McNally.

41. Vogel M: The transformation of the American hospital, 1850-1920. In Reverby S and Rosner D, editors: Health care in America: essays in social history, Philadelphia, 1979, Temple University Press.

42. Wensley E: Nursing service without walls, New York, 1963, National League for Nursing.

CHAPTER 26

Leadership and change in public and community health nursing today

The essential intervention

MARLA E. SALMON
PATIENCE VANDERBUSH

The focus of this chapter is on leadership as an essential intervention for change in the practice of public and community health nursing. Leadership has come to mean many things in our society and has numerous definitions. For the purposes of this chapter, leadership is defined as the ability to envision and communicate a changed future and to foster a dynamic that mobilizes and catalyzes the efforts of many toward that end. In this definition the dynamic between leader and follower is "leadership"; it is not simply what the leader does.

Leadership has been a theme in the literature and professionalization of nursing; it is viewed as the hallmark of professional nurses. For nurse administrators and supervisors, leadership is an integral component of the managerial and administrative strategies used to optimize clinical practice. For the overall profession, leadership is seen as a means of advancing the professionalization of nursing. Leadership, however, has not been viewed as a key intervention strategy for the direct practice of nursing. Nursing care plans or other documentation of the nursing process generally do not include leadership as an intervention. With one critical exception, the clinical practice of individual nurses can proceed on a day-to-day basis without any consideration or utilization of leadership as an intervention strategy. The exception is the practice of public and community health nursing.

Public and community health nursing practice differs from all other nursing practices in a number of significant ways. The departure point for practice, particularly for public health nurses, is public mandate and responsibility for the health of the public. This mandate translates into a focus on the prevention of premature death and disability and the preservation of health. The client is the public or community; advocacy is for the public and community good. This form of advocacy and focus of practice demand that interventions involve both the formal and informal structures of society and communities. In other words, the policies, organizations, institutions, and other components of the community infrastructure are the foci for action; the community is the client. The tangible, reassuring, here-and-now character of other types of clinical nursing practice is not a constant dimension of public and community health nursing. While the practice for the entry-level practitioner of public health and community health nursing may involve predominantly hands-on nursing care, the raison d'être is the well-being of the community and public. Advanced practice, which may appear indirect relative to other forms of nursing, is quite direct in the domain of moving the health status of communities and populations.[18] To accomplish this, nurses must effectively use leadership as an applied clinical strategy.

THE CLIENT'S CURRENT CONDITION

The nature of leadership as an essential strategy for public and community health nurses is best emphasized by examining the condition of the client. Currently there are some key factors or determinants of health in communities and American society in general that seriously affect the health of their members. These determinants constitute the domain of public health and community health nursing practice and require that interventions address them directly, rather than focusing only on the person whose health is affected. The determinants are classified in four general categories:[18] (1) social, (2) medical/technological/organizational, (3) environmental, and (4) human or biological. The common theme in all these determinants is that the ability of individuals to affect them on behalf of communities and society is greatly enhanced by the leadership in public policy and social institutions. For public and community health nurses to play a role in these arenas, leadership must also be their key intervention.

SOCIAL DETERMINANTS OF HEALTH

One significant social trend affecting the health of people today has been the emergence of concern for health promotion and disease prevention. In 1979 the federal government published *Healthy People: The Surgeon General's Report on Health Promotion and Disease Prevention*.[4] It was the first report of its type and clearly outlined a national agenda for health promotion and disease prevention. This report and subsequent related documents reflect two major social phenomena: Americans' realization that lifestyle is a major determinant of health, and the escalating costs of health care, particularly to businesses through health benefits packages.[16]

Although the trend toward health promotion and disease prevention is clearly in keeping with the goal of public health nursing and has given community health nurses new opportunities to expand the scope of their practice, it does pose challenges to the public health nursing leadership. Ostwald and Williams,[12] for instance, have written that community health nurses are in an excellent position to capitalize on national trends toward wellness promotion and cost containment by contracting with local companies to provide health-promotion programs for their employees. However, they also warn that community health nurses must understand the rationale for development of these programs and that the organizational structure of the workplace may compromise individual autonomy and the goal of optimal health. Cost containment and wellness promotion can be, but are not always, complementary; to be so requires significant influence through leadership at policy levels within and outside the organizations in which such initiatives are formulated.

Cost containment has itself become a major social determinant of health. In recent years U.S. health care costs have risen faster than the inflation rate. Now at 12% of the gross national product, they are expected to reach 15% by the end of the century.[19] The biggest factors in these rising costs have been the costs of advanced technology and hospital care.[16] The ramifications of increasing costs are many. Society will have to consider difficult trade-offs.[19] A challenge for the public health nursing leadership is to become actively involved in that debate, to ensure that the good of the public is paramount in these considerations.

One response to problems of cost containment has been the federal fiscal policy of the Reagan administration, including the Omnibus Budget Reconciliation Act of 1981 (OBRA) and the Tax Equity and Fiscal Responsibility Act of 1982 (TEFRA). According to Milio,[11] this legislation has been the single most important policy action affecting Americans' health in the early 1980s. Linked to the growing federal deficit, the stated aims of this legislation were to bring federal spending under control, to transfer responsibility to the states in the form of block grants, and to reduce regulation to allow the marketplace to efficiently allocate resources and thus reduce health care cost inflation.[11]

As a result of these federal initiatives, cuts were made in many programs. States have commonly responded to these cuts (in concert with recession) by cutting or ending services, the eligibility of certain groups, or provider payments. Over two thirds of the states are now attempting long-term reforms, such as providing home or community-based care in place of institutional care. These actions reflect leadership at all levels of government; they are examples of opportunities for public and community health nursing involvement that have far-reaching health consequences.

At first glance the consequences of these cost-containment strategies may appear to enhance public and community health nursing practice. An immediate outcome of these actions has been greater reliance on publicly funded health agencies, with an accompanying push toward preventive and alternative health services strategies. Milio contends that these changes may be a cloud with a "silver-yet-gray lining."[11] It is increasingly obvious that restricted state and local budgets are not sufficient to support the rapid development of the alternative preventive and health-promotion strategies that are needed. In addition, those people with existing health problems are often only minimally affected by preventive strategies that could have only worked prior to the onset of the problem. The confusion that has resulted from this shift of financing from the federal government to local and state authorities, with an accompanying shift in the ostensible focus of services from curative to preventive, is also a confusion about who is responsible for providing these services. Those who are lost in this confusion are generally people who have the greatest need for services and the fewest resources to purchase them.

Other social factors affecting the health of communities include some major demographic changes, such as the increase in the older population. With extension of the lifespan and the movement of the baby boomers into middle age, there is a rapidly increasing demand for services relating to chronic and other diseases associated with aging. Another important factor is the increase in minority and ethnic populations in the United States and the need for traditionally white, middle-class institutions to become responsive to the needs of these people. In addition, while resources to support services are becoming increasingly scarce, unemployment, teenage pregnancy and suicide, violence, and drug and alcohol abuse are on the rise in this country. The "shrinking" of the globe and the crucial interrelations with the world community, particularly with respect to peace, also are critically important health considerations. All these and many other social factors determine the condition of the client and what public and community health nurses do. To have any significant impact on these determinants, nurses must be able to master the leadership of society and its institutions.

MEDICAL-TECHNICAL-ORGANIZATIONAL DETERMINANTS OF HEALTH

The nature of medical technology and services and how they are organized and financed reflect the values, resources, and nature of society in general. Too often, however, these factors are not considered to be key determinants affecting the health of communities and their members. Recent rapid and large-order changes in the medical-technical-organizational domain have had major effects on who receives services, who provides services, what types of services are available, and who is responsible for ensuring the quality of such services. The common theme of recent innovations in health services financing and delivery systems has echoed the overall social and political climate: reduce and contain costs! Diagnosis-related groups (DRGs), health-maintenance organizations (HMOs), and emergency care centers[10] are all reflections of the finance-driven nature of the health services systems. An accompanying theme has been the "corporatization" and

"commodification" of health services, where health and illness are variables in the equations of the marketplace and are targets for the generation of profit.

These new health care delivery systems provide nurses with practice opportunities in both ambulatory and home settings and thus contribute to the demand for more nurses. But they also challenge public and community health nurses to look at the systems from a broader perspective than their immediate effect on the nursing profession. In the face of a finance-driven delivery system, it is essential to assess more than the savings. The equation must be one of cost-effectiveness (rather than cost efficiency) and must include careful appraisal of the quality of service, the response of providers to these varying economic incentives, and the overall performance (both financial and qualitative) of different types of organizations relative to their social and health-related responsibilities.[19] It is essential that public and community health nurses play leadership roles in these evaluative and regulatory functions; they are key factors in shaping the health of communities. Nurses must, at the very least, be able to do so relative to their own practices.

One area in which these regulatory roles for public and community health nurses are of acute importance is home health services, particularly home care. Prospective payment under Medicare, DRGs, and the expanding elderly population have contributed to a tremendous growth in home care. Although home care has been a traditional domain of community health nursing, both the increasing complexity and extent of home services have provided greater opportunities for nurses in the community. Yet in many states there is little if any regulation of home care, and many experts are concerned that quality may seriously deteriorate as services expand.[6]

One reason the quality of home care is increasingly threatened is the growing need for nurses to have the knowledge and skill to manage seriously ill clients, particularly those requiring high-technology interventions and equipment.[16] Not only have the numbers of patients requiring home care increased, but the majority of them are older, sicker, and require more complex care.[13] Community health nurses are experiencing changes in their clinical, counseling, and coordinating roles,[13] reflecting more sophisticated technical interventions. Clients and their families also require more counseling and teaching, because they are sharing the burden of the complex direct care being provided in their own home. As case managers in the home setting, community health nurses need outstanding organizational and interpersonal leadership skills to effectively patch together a productive collage of services from the myriad of unrelated community resources. This is particularly challenging in cases where financial resources are minimal.

One particularly difficult aspect of this concentration of the need for nursing services in home care is the extent to which this diverts resources from preventive programming, particularly in official public health nursing agencies. The competition for scarce resources between caring for the sick and preventing morbidity and mortality in healthy populations challenges public health nurses to provide leadership in developing creative and collaborative approaches to generating and allocating resources within and outside their own agencies.

Federal reimbursement systems, while contributing to the growth of home care services, also present a challenge to quality assurance programs.[13] Medicare doesn't pay for most long-term home care—only for skilled assistance, as from a physician or nurse.[6] According to Rogatz, to meet the increased level of need among patients discharged from hospitals, governmental third-party payers must broaden eligibility standards, benefits ranges, and reimbursement levels. Current home delivery models have led to problems of access and fragmentation.[7] The responsibility for seeing that clients are not dropped from care and that they receive maximum reimbursement is being assumed by many staff nurses in home health agencies.[13]

Public and community health nursing leaders must work to ensure that the federal government and others supply sufficient resources to meet the growing demands on health care. One way to do this is to define the elements of a home visit in such a way that it can be priced appropriately for various buyers.[2] Nurses should participate in developing patient classification systems; in describing and measuring clinical care, counseling, coordination, and other activities; and in collecting data on the cost-benefit ratio of prevention to make a compelling argument for resources for preventive practice.[13]

Another challenge to public and community health nursing leaders is in their capacities as advocates for the good of society. The changes in our health care delivery system are already threatening to pit corporate interests against those of the public and society at large. Third-party payers and profit incentives are exerting increasing influence on the for-profit health sector. This pressure has resulted in moves to provide services only to paying clients, dumping high-risk, costly, nonpaying clients into the already straining public sector, and skimming off those clients with resources who could help offset the cost of others. This phenomenon, while contributing to the health of the corporation, is creating a two-tiered care system that is devastating to the overall health of the public. Vertical integration is a part of this corporatization of health care.[17] Providers are organizing in groups of increasing size, corporations are managing or providing their own health care, and major for-profit entities are taking an increasing share of the health care business or industry.[5] One advantage to nursing may be that because nursing services are more cost-effective than physician services, many cost-conscious health care organizations could be persuaded that nurses get the job done more efficiently.[5] However, this again places nurses in the ethical dilemmas posed by conflicts between the needs of clients and the requirements of the corporation.[19] These dilemmas can only be resolved through creative and responsible leadership at policy levels within and outside these organizations. Unless nurses are involved in such leadership, the advocacy and social concern required for enlightened decision making may well be lacking.

Another determinant in the medical-technical-organization domain of health is what has been called the "mechanization" of health care. This is defined as the growing orientation of U.S. health care toward technology—the drugs, devices, and medical care and the organizations and supportive systems within which such care is provided. In the current atmosphere of cost containment, there is a greater need to assess whether technology has sufficient advantages to justify its costs, and to explore its social and ethical implications for our health care system.[5] Public and community health nurses, increasingly asked to use new technologies in nonhospital settings, must understand and also be able to evaluate the new technologies, including the broader values, principles, and roles of this technology, if they are to be involved in the decision-making process.[5] They must also be included in forums where the costs and benefits of the technology of "care and cure" are weighed against those of preventive strategies. These discussions, which occur at all policy levels, are critical intervention points that have far-reaching effects on health. The effective practice of public and community health nursing in this context again demands leadership as one of its intervention strategies.

Leadership is also required to ensure that nurses are educationally prepared to practice effectively within this rapidly changing health services system. In their recent study of public health nursing education and practice, Jones and colleagues emphasize the gap between what nurses are educated to do and what their actual practice entails.[8] The Institute of Medicine's 1988 "Study on the Future of Public Health"[3] also emphasizes that current public health workers are generally not prepared in public health. Lack of preparation in public health, including the skills required for leadership intervention, has serious implications for this rapidly emerging finance-driven high-tech health services system.

ENVIRONMENTAL DETERMINANTS OF HEALTH

In terms of impact, the environment may be the single most important determinant of health in the very near future. It is also the determinant about which nurses perhaps know the least. The nursing literature on environmental health and the role of public and community health nurses vis-à-vis the environment is alarmingly sparse. Environmental problems of concern to community health nurses include the disposal of hazardous waste, including toxic industrial waste and radioactive-contaminated materials; acid rain; urban lead poisoning; inadequate solid waste disposal; noise pollution; air pollution; and water pollution.[16] Global concerns include the depletion of the ozone layer, with its accompanying weather changes and warming of the oceans. And most critical of all is the threat of thermonuclear war.

Part of the leadership required of public and community health nurses is the task of educating themselves and others about what environmental health issues are and how to intervene effectively. Clearly, all of the environmental issues relate to the state of environmental policy and regulation. Nurses must learn to insert themselves into the debates surrounding these policies and regulations, at the same time becoming involved in the specifics of environmental exposures in their own clientele. Macinick and Macinick[9] suggest some action guidelines for nurses to begin to help solve the problems of our environment, including the fol-

lowing: being willing to admit to the idea of asymptomatic, subclinical toxicity and the multiple-effects disease model; being aware that environmental toxicology is a politically charged issue involving the world of high finance and corporate egos; being able to accept disbelief and even anger toward not only the message but the messenger; and being aware that almost no research on the synergistic effects of low-level toxins has been done, leading to downplaying of their importance. They suggest that the nurse's most helpful coping mechanism is knowledge, which will also enable the nurse to begin educating the community about the effects of low levels of pollution.

One of the key leadership strategies relating to the environment is that of interdisciplinary, collaborative action. While this is also a key intervention strategy with other health determinants, it is most critical in dealing with environmental issues because of the specialized knowledge required to address and monitor action in this area. Although nurses generally do not possess sophistication in this area, they can provide the generalist leadership and health knowledge necessary to catalyze health-committed action relating to the environment.

HUMAN AND BIOLOGICAL DETERMINANTS OF HEALTH

The human and biological health determinant, probably the most familiar and comfortable to nurses, is one in which significant public health issues have emerged in this last decade. We have observed the appearance of devastating and exotic infectious diseases such as AIDS, toxic shock syndrome, herpes, and Legionnaires' disease. More than any other disease, AIDS,[1] coupled with the reemergence of new strains and epidemics of diseases formerly thought to be under control such as syphilis, gonorrhea, mumps, measles, diphtheria, and flu, has radically altered the course of public health in this nation. The global eradication of smallpox in the 1970s signaled a new era in public health in which there was great optimism that the age of infectious disease was coming to an end. This hope has been erased; public health practitioners are faced with challenges greater than ever in infectious diseases, as well as the challenges of chronic disease associated with growing numbers of the elderly. The increasingly grave and diverse disease picture in public and community health has not been accompanied by an increase in resources or systems to address these problems. Again, the development of effective strategies must involve the leadership of public and community health nurses to be appropriately responsive.

Public health practitioners are also confronted with the promises and threats to society inherent in the reality of genetic engineering. The ethical, moral, legal, social, and economic questions surrounding developments in this area fall squarely in the domain of public health. Society will confront these issues in all arenas: individual, family, community, state, and national. How these issues are resolved depends greatly on who provides the leadership. The inclusion of public and community health nurses in these debates is essential to an outcome sensitive to and respectful of the public good and the public health.

A final concern is the challenge of enabling people to optimize their own health. Although the lifestyle movement certainly provides answers for the middle and upper classes, which have options associated with their financial resources, it does not address the needs of those people who are less fortunate. Questions of how to ensure that all people are equipped with the advantages of a healthy fetal and early childhood experience, adequate nutrition, immunizations, exercise, and the skills of self-development, are not easily answered through most of the current lifestyle programs. Children are still bearing children, destroying themselves and others through drug abuse, suicide, and other forms of violence. These questions clearly cannot be addressed solely at the one-to-one level. They require the leadership of those who are close to the problems, committed to the good of the community, and skilled in understanding the relationship between the health of the individual and the broader society.

THE NEXT STEPS

Although the condition of the client—our communities and society—is clearly grave, it is not without hope or an agenda for action. One of the intriguing and perplexing aspects of the problems that we face today is that we already know many of the answers. Never before have we known as much about health as we do now; what we don't know is how to put this knowledge into action. Again, this requires leadership.

In the July 4, 1988, issue of Newsweek[14] a special report portrayed a number of "unsung heroes." The common theme in these stories was the unwillingness of each of these "heroes" to accept the status quo; each took action and effected change. Each person, while not trained to accomplish what they undertook, had a vision of a better situation and pursued this vision with personal commitment and courage. Of all of the attributes of leadership, these are perhaps the most important. Another noteworthy theme in this report was that for each of these individuals, people were the primary means for achieving change. These leaders relied on themselves and others as the means for effecting change; they did not wait for technical or economic answers.

The message here for public and community health nurses is that leadership is necessary and attainable. The lessons from the unsung heroes—vision, conviction, and the courage to act—are an excellent departure point. Another worthwhile lesson was their willingness to work with others. Finally, the reason that these heroes are "unsung" is that they did things in their own backyards and communities; their actions were local, beginning at home.

The next steps for public and community health nursing are to focus on nursing's leadership interventions. Understanding the condition of the client and the factors creating this condition is only the beginning. The future health of the client, our communities and society, relies greatly on the development of leadership as the key strategy for public and community health nursing. The challenge is perhaps best stated by an aphorism from the 1960s: If you aren't part of the solution, you are part of the problem. If public and community health nurses aren't part of the leadership required to enhance the health of society, then we are, in fact, contributing to its decline.

REFERENCES

1. Fineberg HV: The social dimensions of AIDS, Scientific American, p 128, Oct 1988.
2. Griffith EI: The changing face of home health care, Public Health Nurs 4(1):1, 1987 (editorial).
3. The future of public health. Report of the Institute of Medicine Committee for the study of public health, Washington, National Academy Press, 1981.
4. Healthy people: the surgeon general's report on health promotion and disease prevention, Washington, DC, 1979, US Department of Health, Education, and Welfare.
5. Herdman RC: Health care technology and the changing health care system, NLN Publication 41:15, 1985.
6. Hey RP: The challenges of caring for a relative at home, Christian Science Monitor, p 3, May 26, 1988.
7. Humphrey CJ: The practice of home care nursing, Public Health Nurs 4(2):79, 1987.
8. Jones DC, Davis JA, and Davis MD: Public health nursing:

education and practice, Springfield, Va, 1987, National Technical Information Service.

9. Macinick CG and Macinick JW: Toxic new world: what nurses can do to cope with a polluted environment, Int Nurs Rev 34(2):40, 1987.

10. McCreight LM: The curriculum of the future: adapting to changing demands in community health, NLN Publications 41:144, 1985.

11. Milio N: Chains of impact from reaganonomics on primary care policies, Public Health Nurs 1(2):65, 1984.

12. Ostwald SK and Williams HY: Community health nursing in workplace health programs: rationale and ethics, Journal of Community Health Nursing 4(3):121, 1987.

13. Phillips EK and Cloonan PA: DRG ripple effects on community health nursing, Public Health Nurs 4(2):84, 1987.

14. Special report: a holiday for heroes, Newsweek, p 34, July 4, 1988.

15. Rogatz P: Perspective on home care, Public Health Nurs 4(1):7, 1987.

16. Spradley BW, editor: Readings in community health nursing, Boston, 1986, Little, Brown and Co, Inc.

17. Starr P: The social transformation of American medicine, New York, 1982, Basic Books, Inc.

18. White MS: Construct for public health nursing, Nurs Outlook 30(9):527, 1982.

19. Winkenwerder W and Ball JR: Transformation of American health care: the role of the medical profession, New England Journal of Medicine 318(5):317, 1988.

CHAPTER 27

Entrepreneurs

Issues and barriers to independent practice

MYRTLE K. AYDELOTTE

The number of nurses operating as entrepreneurs is unknown, but one study has identified 1298 nurses engaged in independent practice in the United States.[2] The concept of entrepreneurship is not new, the term having been introduced by Cantrillon, who considered an entrepreneur an uninsurable risk.[3]

Since 1970 the growth of entrepreneurship in the United States has been phenomenal. the "entrepreneurial explosion" has been identified by Naisbitt in his book *Megatrends*.[4] Women have played a large role in the movement, their participation in self-employed businesses growing at a faster rate than that for men. Among these women are nurses who have set up independent practices.

HISTORY OF ENTREPRENEURSHIP IN NURSING

The concept of entrepreneurship is difficult to describe because no single definition appears in the literature. Such factors include risk, the nature and purpose of the undertaking and the growth to be expected, the presence of new ideas, the combination of ideas, the life of the business, the reason for starting the business, and whether the business is old or new have all been mentioned. There is general agreement in the literature that risk is a major component of the concept.

In the nursing literature the definition of *entrepreneur* is intertwined with the terms *independent nursing practice* and *private practice*. These terms are used interchangeably. Although the current era of independent nursing practice is usually dated from 1971, when Lucille Kinlein established her practice, nurses were engaged in this type of practice from a much earlier date. Independent nursing practice is characterized by (a) the beginning of a new business or venture (b) the

synthesis of new ideas or combinations of ideas for the market (c) the anticipation of profit and growth (d) the involvement of risk and (e) the ultimate responsibility for decisions residing with the legal owner of the business.

Although not all these features are apparent in the practices of some of the early pioneers, they are still considered entrepreneurs. Among them are such persons as Lillian Wald, Mary Breckenridge, Margaret Sanger, and the many unknown early midwives and private duty nurses who operated independently until changes in technology, science, and health care delivery led to care in the hospital instead of in the home.

The revival of interest in independent nursing practice introduced by Kinlein was accelerated by changes in nursing education. The development of programs preparing nurse-practitioners and clinical nursing specialists and the emphasis on liberal arts and autonomous decision making in undergraduate programs served to change the perception of nurses themselves from dependent and subservient workers to autonomous decision makers capable of self-direction.

Changes in nursing education, and an increasing number of publications describing how individual nurses established their practices and offering advice to others, have contributed to the growth of nurse entrepreneurs. Associated with the trend, however, are serious problems and issues faced by nurses engaging in private practice. The issues have been identified by various authors as relating to ethical and legal questions, the appropriateness of nurses engaging in private practice, and the control and regulation of the practice. Other issues relate to funding sources and the lack of direct third-party reimbursement. The fact that many of the issues remain unresolved contributes to the barriers confronting nurses who wish to engage in private practice as entrepreneurs.

The barriers to the establishment of independent practice go beyond unresolved issues. The lack of adequate preparation to conduct business, the inability to take risks, and the failure to recognize and seize opportunities are barriers which exist within nurses themselves.

ISSUES CONFRONTING THE ESTABLISHMENT OF PRACTICE

The issues are subjects of debate and discussion among nurses, the public, and other disciplines. Each issue enters on a set of questions that to date remain unanswered. First are problems of the acceptance of private practice nurses by other nurses, other professionals, and the public. Is it appropriate for nurses to engage in this type of practice and run their own businesses? If a nurse engages in such practice, what are the regulatory and control mechanisms that should be in place? What is a reasonable remuneration for such services? Is making a profit acceptable? How does the nurse relate to other sectors of the health care delivery system?

The problems of appropriateness and acceptability thus include several complex issues arising out of an understanding of nursing practice and its legal scope, the ethics of practice, the relationship of nursing to other disciplines, the relationship of nurses to other health professionals, the capitalist system, and the role of women.

Unfortunately, many members of the public, other professionals, and nurses themselves do not understand or accept what nurses by law are allowed to do. These individuals continue to view nursing practice as dependent on physician orders and direction and, as a result, question the right of nurses to establish themselves in independent practice. The role of the physician as gatekeeper for health and medical services is widely accepted in our society and is one of the barriers to change in the health care system. Physicians themselves believe that they are authorities on all matters of health and access to services, including nursing services.

Some nurses are uncomfortable in the role of decision makers accountable for their own actions. These nurses are not risk takers and are more comfortable in a role that they believe protects them from liability, although in fact it may not. They may question the effrontery of nurses who wish to run their own business and may view the nurse in independent practice as in competition with physicians, not recognizing that nursing and medicine differ in essential content and purpose.

In the process of socializing nursing students and novice nurses, faculty, mentors, and peers unwittingly may create conflict for these individuals entering the profession. In the socialization process the student is indoctrinated with an ideology leading to a professional identity that emphasizes altruism, caring, advocacy, and service. The professional identity requires giving of the self, in that the professional expends psychological and physical energy in performing the service. Since nursing historically grew out of monastic orders and under the influence of Florence Nightingale, who viewed nursing as a calling, relatively little emphasis has been placed on the right of the individual nurse to establish a monetary value for her or his services and to expect monetary payment in return for the expenditure of time, energy, and skill in providing those services. In most nursing education programs, students are not taught to view nursing services as generating income for the institution. Nor are they introduced to the concept that it is appropriate for the nurse in independent practice to generate income for a self-owned business. The employed nurse views the institution as owing the nurse a salary, not recognizing that, in reality, it is sharing earnings that the nurse has helped to generate.

This lack of understanding about the right to expect remuneration based on one's contribution to the income of an institution through the expenditure of energy, coupled with the inculcation of a socially accepted identity of giving, may lead to distorted perceptions of the appropriateness of a nurse in independent practice establishing fees and collecting money from clients.

Most nurses are employed in hospitals, and thus few are familiar with the business aspects of profits and losses, income, expenses, and financial investments. Because of this lack of business sophistication, many do not relate the venture of the nurse entrepreneur to the free enterprise system or embrace that effort.

Although more women are engaging in entrepreneurship than ever before, the phenomenon is relatively recent. Little research has been conducted on women entrepreneurs, but studies have shown that they differ from men in that they tend to be older, educated in the liberal arts instead of business or other majors, engaged in a service occupation, average fewer hours in the business, and earn less. The acceptance of women as entrepreneurs is likely to depend on the type of business they are engaged in and the assests they have available to raise venture capital. There continue to be few women as heads of major corporations or in executive positions in large businesses. Whether it is appropriate for a female nurse to operate her own business remains questionable in the minds of many individuals.

This questioning is subtle. It is reflected in the reluctance of physicians and nurses to support other nurses by referring clients to them or by granting hospital privileges to nurses in independent practice, and in the hesitancy of banks and lending institutions to loan money for beginning a venture. The image of nurses as lacking legal authorization for nursing practice, as dependent on physicians, as possessing no right to engage in free enterprise, and as lacking business acumen, presents problems and barriers to those who wish to engage in independent practice.

Ethical and legal issues are intertwined with those above. Is it ethical to engage in private practice that provides a service to patients and clients and to set charges that cover more than cost? How does one conduct oneself ethically? If one sets a limit on the services provided because of specialization and time, what is the obligation to provide continuity of services? What constitutes a benefit package? Can it be limited?

These questions may arise in large part because of the nurse's education. Although nursing education has embraced specialization and the treatment of selected population groups such as the poor, the elderly, and children, it has not adequately addressed the ethical obligations of the practitioner to the clientele served. Nurses are taught to provide holistic care and are uncomfortable if they must curtail their services because of religious beliefs or limitations on their own knowledge, time, and energy. The American Nurses' Association's *Guidelines for Implementing the Code for Nurses*[2] are useful, but the nurse in independent practice is confronted with dilemmas concerning the extension, referral, or termination of services to clients. Further, she or he has no access to a process involving peers who may assist in making those decisions.

The issue of regulating and controlling the nurses who engage in private practice has not been fully articulated. A license to practice is the current minimum legal requirement. Some states have issued regulations governing the reimbursement and practice of nurse-practitioners, nurse-anesthetists, and midwives, but no universal credentialing mechanism has been established beyond state licensure to assure the public that the private nurse practitioner is knowledgeable and competent. Slightly over half the nurses in one recent study were certified by a national organization.[2] The problem is compounded because the public is not well informed about nursing credentials. The regulation of independent practice is managed by state incorporation laws, and some practices are regulated by state boards of health or state boards of nursing, but there is no universal standard for control. Because the license to practice sets only minimal standards for safe practice, there are questions as to whether evidence is needed that the individual practitioner is competent beyond that level and whether a special license should be granted. If the answer is yes, on what credentials should the license be based? What kind of review process is indicated to ensure that the practice meets standards, and what are those standards? What kind of quality assurance system is needed for nurses in independent practice, and how will it be monitored and by whom? Quality assurance systems can be introduced for nurses receiving payment through governmental programs and contracts with insurers, but how can systems be put in place for those nurses serving clients who pay directly?

These issues of appropriateness and acceptability, ethical and legal questions relating to practice, the regulation and control of services, and the need for quality assurance have not been addressed fully in the literature. The barriers to practice have been more frequently mentioned by various authors. The major emphasis has been placed on the lack of financial reimbursement directly to the nurse, especially from governmental agencies and private insurers.

BARRIERS TO PRACTICE

The barriers confronted by the nurse entrepreneur are of two kinds: those arising from personal limitations and those imposed externally by institutions and the community.

Barriers due to personal limitations

Establishing a private practice requires a set of personal abilities and characteristics that are not always dependent upon one's experience and educational background. One analysis[2] of financially successful nurse entrepreneurs indicates that recognizing and seizing opportunities are of primary importance. This implies that the nurse has the abilities to envision what nurses can provide a population and to tolerate risk and ambiguity as the vision is acted on. Coupled with this is the ability to clearly and convincingly communicate to others what nurses do, the effects of their actions, and how nursing differs from medicine. The ability to take the long view and to forecast results is essential. Unfortunately, many nurses are oriented to immediate action and are unable to tolerate uncertainty, risk, and possible failure. Nursing educational programs do not always tolerate innovation or the maverick student but instead emphasize conformity, conservatism, and certainty. A major barrier to the establishment of an entrepreneurial venture, then, resides within the individual's own psychological makeup.

The second personal limitation serving as a barrier is one that can be partly eliminated through self-education. To become an entrepreneur requires knowledge and skill in the business arena, as well as political acumen. Business skill involves the abilities to conduct a marketing analysis, design a benefit package or service to fit the analysis, establish reasonable fees, negotiate contracts, write a business plan, raise venture capital, make use of available resources, and secure support and acceptance of the venture. Political acumen is also necessary to convince others of the soundness of the proposal and to build coalitions for support. Unfortunately, few students have the experience of working with an entrepreneur and the majority have limited business and political skills.

Barriers due to external conditions

The barriers most frequently mentioned in the literature are related to the lack of third-party reimbursement directly payable to the nurse or the nursing service. Several difficulties contribute to the complexity of the issue. First, the policy underlying direct reimbursement is unclear, and whether nurses seek full competition with all other health professionals in providing service has not been fully articulated. Compounding the problem of reimbursement is the lack of uniformity regarding the definition of reimbursable services and the lack of documentation of actual costs of nursing services provided to the noninstitutionalized customer.

The current economic environment and the pressures by private and governmental payers to keep costs down serve as barriers to change that may encourage the entrepreneurial movement. Although the payment of nursing services has been on the agendas of phy-

sicians and nurses for several years, the debate has extended to individual public members and private payers. However, current reimbursement systems will probably not change until data are presented that support results in economy, improvements in quality or at least continuation of the same quality of services, and the reduction of overall costs. The responsibility for obtaining direct third-party payment rests with the profession and with nurses engaging in independent practice.

The lack of legislation providing for third-party payment, although perceived as a barrier to establishing a practice, need not be one. Nurses can explore the financial mechanisms of grants, contracts, and private payment. Several sources of funding are encouraged. Obtaining grants requires proposal-writing abilities, and pursuing contracts demands negotiating abilities and assertive marketing.

A second barrier is the problem of securing money for the capital venture and for operations until the business is well established. The ability to raise money is in part a business skill. It also depends on the attitudes toward women and nurses held by bankers and lending institutions. Building coalitions and support groups can assist in overcoming the hesitancy of lenders. The Small Business Administration, women's support groups and networks, and the resources of a university or college can be drawn on to plan a strategy for obtaining financial assistance. Some entrepreneurs maintain part-time work until the business becomes more secure.

There is no lack of counsel or advice for new businesses. The problem is knowing what help is needed and how to approach those individuals who will be useful. A perceived barrier is the lack of knowledge about a community, its power structure, and the means of access to powerful individuals. This barrier can be met by nurses becoming active in community affairs and laying a network prior to the actual negotiations that involve money, advice, and other necessary resources.

SUMMARY

The issues and barriers confronting the nurse who wishes to become an entrepreneur are exceedingly complex. Several of the issues orginate in the perceptions that individuls have of nurses and nursing practice, while others stem from the task of assuring the public that the services provided are legitimate and of high quality. The barriers can be located in the psychological makeup of the nurse and her or his educational preparation and experience. The financial barriers, although annoying and potentially obstructive and defeating, are not insurmountable. Several financial mechanisms and sources can be employed, but this requires energy and perseverance. As the entrepreneurial movement continues and more nurses become involved, the barriers and issues will be addressed and gradually overcome.

REFERENCES

1. American Nurses' Association: Guidelines for implementing the code for nurses, Kansas City, Mo, 1980, The Association.
2. Aydelotte MK, Hardy MA, and Hope KL: Nurses in private practice: characteristics, organizational arrangements, and reimbursement policy, Kansas City, Mo, 1988, American Nurses' Foundation.
3. Martin S: Exploring the concept of enterprise, Nursing Economics. 12:406, 1984.
4. Naisbitt J: Megatrends: ten new directions transforming our lives, New York, 1982, Warner Books.

CHAPTER 28

Case management

A golden opportunity for whom?

KAREN ZANDER

Case management, generically a "system of health assessment, planning, service procurement/delivery/ coordination, and monitoring through which multiple service needs of clients are met,"[1] is on the bidder's block. Because of the potential financial consequences of putting case management into operation, it seems to many to be a golden opportunity in the otherwise gloomy health care game. Competition is running high for control of the industry, and case management seems to offer much promise. This chapter argues that nursing must seize the opportunities offered by case management, though the competition is keen and the profession is besieged by other priorities.

BACKGROUND

Historically, case management has been used in social service agencies, public health nursing, insurance companies, and rehabilitation settings. With the use of prospective reimbursement in the form of diagnostic related groups (DRGs), case management has entered the acute care environment. It has proven an effective means to target specific patient populations (often the catastrophically ill or aged) for concentrated attention by physicians, nurses, and key support departments. Case management entails an intense focus and frequently a restructuring of the way clinical work is organized and processed. In turn, there is usually a need for better clinical and financial information systems, clarity of standards, improved integration of operations, incentive programs for those creating positive results, and other profound changes. In addition to the decreased fragmentation of care and improved effectiveness of that care, case management augments an institution's ability to enter into managed care contracts and augments its quality image to the community.

THE INSURERS OR THE PROVIDERS?

The war for control is being waged by the providers of health care and the insurers of those needing care, with the government setting the rules. It could be characterized as a complex and sometimes hostile interrelationship in which the providers woo patients, physicians, and insurers, and the insurers and the government set the limits. The providers have considerable leverage and prestige. The 1960s and 1970s were characterized by a concern about the impact of technology on the human business of caring. The 1980s are marked solely by a concern for the high costs of an industry seemingly out of control, yet one that followed the "more is better" mandate of the two previous decades and produced remarkable innovations. Currently prospective payment methods first instituted by the government for Medicare patients are forcing an evaluation of resource utilization and quality. No doubt historians will equate the change-agent power of penicillin in the first half of the century with the power of diagnosis-related groups (DRGs) in the second half.

To make an analogy, the providers are in the driver's seat of the health care business as long as the gasoline from the insurers and government keeps flowing. The administrative arm of the providers is acutely aware of the potential problems of a gasoline shortage and does whatever it takes to keep driving. Although government and insurance money drives the system, the providers drive the business. Providers hold enormous control even though they will never have total control. Ironically, in the final analysis, the passenger (client) drives the money as both insurance purchaser and voter.

Unfortunately, the complexity of the interrelationships displayed in Figure 28-1 makes it difficult to locate accountability for either financial or clinical per-

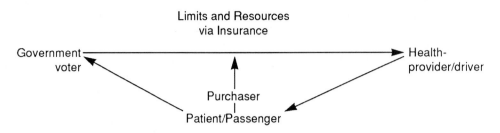

Fig. 28-1 Interrelationships between consumer, provider, and government/insurer.

formance. Services are fragmented for the consumer, and insurers and providers blame each other for lack of services and funds. Indeed, although everyone supposedly wants cost-effective health care, those who set the limits do not understand the business, and those who know the business—the providers—are still determining how best to restructure. The client, of course, wants the same standard of care without giving up anything.

As a result, the health care environment is full of ambiguities. McCaskey[5] characterizes ambiguous, changing situations as those in which there is an unclear and shifting notion of the "problem"; the amount and reliability of information is insufficient; there are multiple interpretations and political clashes; contradictions and paradoxes abound while time, money, and attention are lacking; and roles are vague, and traditional hierarchies are in flux. Because of the ambiguities, professional nursing is in a position to assert its inherent strengths and rightful position in the management of care.

HEALTH CARE ADMINISTRATORS OR CLINICIANS?

The rules have changed in health care, and the providers' responses to the rules vary within a range of predictability. In other words, when an institution is threatened with financial survival, it will probably apply increased control to its expenses and take fewer risks. This is an understandable approach and could go unchallenged except for two main issues: (1) There is a tendency to review costs and make key decisions in a vacuum from the actual clinical implications; and (2) A nursing department is traditionally vulnerable to cost cuts because it is the largest department and is viewed as a cost center.

Health care administrators in acute-care settings usually do not have backgrounds as clinicians and therefore lack the instincts and technical training of physicians, nurses, and other direct care givers. Being one step removed from the process of actual care delivery, they do not have to deal with the family who is angry at the suggestion that grandpa, who has had a stroke, go to a nursing home before he is allowed into rehabilitation, or the new parents who cannot understand why their premature baby must be transferred from a medical center to a community hospital before coming home because of their HMO plan.

Because they allocate approximately 80% of a hospital's resources,[8] nurses and physicians are in the best position to anticipate, interpret, and reorganize the health care they directly provide. They are perfectly capable of making necessary changes if they believe that quality will not be sacrificed for cost. They also need administration's support for potentially high-impact ideas, such as opening certain services on weekends or providing some traditionally inpatient procedures on an outpatient basis.

Are physicians case managers? Yes, to a point. They have the invaluable perspective on a case type throughout the institution rather than on only one unit (as do nurses). They write orders that have major cost and quality implications, and they care about their patients. They care about their relationship with the institution and the community. Although physicians are not happy with increased regulation, they are willing to investigate strategies for dealing with current regulation and preventing more.

Nurses, too, need to be involved in hospital administration. Although individual nurses traditionally are not as conscious about costs of care as they are about quality, nurses are becoming increasingly aware of changes in their work environment related to the effects of prospective reimbursement. Because nursing is "the glue"[4] that pulls and holds a hospital together, nurses know firsthand when the delivery system is working well and when it is stressed or dysfunctional.

Nursing is sometimes overlooked by administration as a potentially powerful ally in case management.

Physician practice is usually reviewed first, because the pivotal function of professional nursing has not been clearly articulated or promoted in a manner that administration understands and responds:

Contrary to popular opinion, the nursing function is task-centered but also outcome-driven. Patient problems addressed by nursing are "dynamic, *nonserial*, multi-functional, and time-critical."[7] Unfortunately, the often literal, task-oriented interpretation of systems such as nursing acuity has done nothing to enhance nursing's professional image internally. As a result, many nonnurses do not understand that when length of stay is shortened, the intensity of the nursing process increases.[3] If nursing weren't inherently outcome-driven, there would be no increase in intensity. DRGs mean that the same outcomes must happen in less time. Because of the lack of acknowledgement of the outcome-driven nature of nursing, it is more vulnerable to the simplistic view that the "glue" can either be diluted or replaced with a cheaper substitute.

Logically, physicians and nurses together hold the knowledge necessary for administrators to make the most prudent decisions regarding cost-effective yet quality services. Because nurses and physicians have great stakes in the restructuring of care delivery systems, they need to be actively involved with administrators from the beginning. Whatever an institution's decisions at the administrative level, the clinicians will be expected to follow through in practice. If the clinicians do not mobilize for case management, administrators will be desperate enough to form a new group of nonclinician players to oversee care delivery.

NURSES OR PHYSICIANS?

Because case management entails the coordination and sequencing of care, all clinicians need to be involved.

Case management may involve many professional disciplines, including nursing, social work, mental health, and medicine. In fact, depending upon program policies and client needs, it is often preferable to have an interdisciplinary team participate in the planning and delivery of care. However, even if a team approach is used, one member of the team is usually designated as the case manager for a specific client. The manager then collaborates in the delivery of care with other professionals as well as family members, the client, and others providing services.[1]

Nurses are in a unique position to provide case management in collaboration with physicians and the in-stitution because they have intimate access of patients and families over extended time periods.

In addition, there are nurses in almost every care delivery area, from intensive care units through home health care, and they have all had formal training in every segment of health care. Nurses continually apply knowledge from the biologic and psychosocial sciences, as well as communication, collaboration, and advocacy skills. They are instrumental in achieving practical and desired outcomes of care. An astute nursing action can produce multiple outcomes and prevent costly complications.

In summary, nurses are the generalists; they are the detail people, and they excel in managing care. They are at the juncture of cost and quality, and they know the human implication of trade-offs such as early discharge, patient education in groups, or the use of new technology. Most important are two underlying elements: (1) Nurses use the formal nursing process, which is directly analogous to the process of case management; and (2) Nurses are committed to the welfare of the institution and, with support, are willing to assume more authority in the smooth, integrated management of patient care.

The resolution to the issue of whether physicians or nurses provide case management is that both professions need to agree on process and outcome standards, as well as to design monitoring and documentation tools. If case management is structured as a collaborative practice from the beginning, nursing can reasonably commit to a lead role.

WHOSE DEFINITION?

The ideal case management would be provided by an expert clinician with advanced educational preparation who traveled with a patient throughout the episode of care, giving direct care 24 hours a day! Obviously this ideal situation is unrealistic on all counts.

To make case management in acute care a reality in our lifetime, New England Medical Center Hospitals in Boston has defined and established new practice patterns. Beginning in January 1985, the Department of Nursing determined that patient care across an episode of illness is a production process with a product, that is, a definable, measurable patient outcome. The outcomes are the clinical resolutions of the patient problems (i.e., nursing diagnoses) most often seen in relation to a DRG or its subset (i.e., Abdominal

Aortic Aneurysm Repair as part of DRG 110, Major Vascular Surgery). Both outcome and process standards within DRG-allotted lengths of stay were agreed on by nurses and attending physicians and were written in documents called case management plans. An abbreviated version of them, called a critical pathway, can be seen in Figure 28-2. After much experimentation, managed care became the foundation for case management.

Managed care is unit-based care that is organized to achieve specific patient outcomes within fiscally responsible timeframes (length of stay) while utilizing resources that are

	Patient				Case Type	Myocardial Infarction	
	MD						
	Case Manager				DRG	122	
	Date Critical Path	**MYOCARDIAL INFARCTION**			Expected LOS	7 Days	
	Reviewed by MD	**CRITICAL PATHWAY**					
	Date						
	Day 1	Day 2	Day 3	Day 4	Day 5	Day 6	Day 7
ICU				6S			
Consults		Cardiac Rehab. Dietician				Copy of Low Chol. No Added Salt Diet	
Tests	EKG	EKG	EKG Receive MBs R/I or R/O MI Holter if nec. on Day 5		Holter ETT Cath. if nec.		
		ETT if nec. for Day 6 Echo, Muga, if nec.					
Activity	BRP w/ Commode		OOB Chair		Amb in Rm/Hall w/Asst	Up Ad ⟶ Lib Stairs	
Treatments	O₂ ⟶ > D/C O₂					D/C Monitor p negative Holter	
	Cardiac Monitor						
	I & O qd ⟶ >					D/C I & O qd wt, unless CHF	
	IV ⟶ Heparin Lock ⟶ >					D/C Heparin Lock	
Diet	No Added Salt, Low Chol. Diet ⟶ >						
Discharge Planning			VNA		Check w/ Attending RE:D/C Date	Discharge Orders	Discharge before 12 Noon
Teaching	Angina, MI, PN., Med, Teaching Plan in Chart	Begin MI Teaching Plan	3 discharge classes Formal Med tx				Amb Classes Re:Risk Factors Diet & smoking

Admission Date _____   Discharge Date _____   Discharge Time _____
Days in ICU _____   Stress test date _____
Days in Routine bed _____   Thalium _____   Cardiac cath. date _____
Routine _____
Holter date _____

Copyright: New England Medical Center Hospitals 1987, Department of Nursing

DATE	VARIATION	CAUSE	ACTION TAKEN

(Reverse side of Critical Pathway form shown above)

Fig. 28-2 Critical pathway: myocardial infarction.

appropriate in amount and sequence to the specific case type and to the individual patient. Outcomes are the patient's discharge condition, stated in measurable terms, that result from the activities of nurses, physicians and other health care providers. The term "unit" refers to the geographic area in which the patient receives care. The focus of managed care is on redesigning tools and systems, the outcomes and processes of care are identified on a daily basis; hourly in areas such as the Emergency Room or the Operating Room; by visit in ambulatory settings. This facilitates identifying those patients who are deviating from the expected early enough to take corrective action.

Because managed care does not change the fundamental role of the nurse, it can be used in any nursing care delivery system. It is therefore, appropriate to incorporate the precepts of managed care into delivery systems as diverse as functional nursing and primary nursing.[2]

Building on the base of managed care, case management is defined as a model and technology for producing financial and clinical outcomes for an episode of care within allotted and appropriate time frames, brought about by a formally prepared collaborative practice of specific staff nurses and specific attending physician(s) for patients in specific case types. The case manager is a primary nurse who works with the patient, family, and health care team to coordinate care in the hospital and after discharge. The case manager is a member of a collaborative practice that includes the physician and selected inpatient and outpatient nurses.

WHO IS ACCOUNTABLE?

In nursing case management in acute care, the individual staff nurse is accountable to the point of eventually being audited for outcomes. The staff nurses and attending physician succeed because of the coordination and relationships within the collaborative practice and the institution. In the future the collaborative practice could receive a bonus for the financial savings to the institution resulting from good management. For the past 20 years nursing has been ambivalent about expecting accountability for outcomes at the staff nurse level. Primary nursing was the profession's best opportunity to practice the interpersonal skills and unit structures underlying the notion of accountability, but only a relative minority of institutions permanently implemented the model so aptly defined by Mundinger as "individual accountability, shared care."[6]

There are many reasons, including the equation of primary nursing with total patient care or other unwieldy care-delivery modes and the lack of administrative support of managers and manager expectations and support of staff.

To nurses, managers, and administrators who never tried or succeeded with primary nursing, case management will seem like a quantum leap. Managed care is an interim step to help departments that are either plateauing with primary nursing or firmly entrenched in shift-based delivery systems make the transition to case management.

Using clinical specialists as case managers may be an interim step if there is already solid primary nursing in place and if a plan to develop the staff nurse as case manager has been outlined organizationally. Otherwise, clinical specialists will succeed with case management, but the authority base of a staff nurse in the institution will never really be altered. If anything, it may be diminished due to the addition of another level.

SUMMARY

Case management is in the process of development and presents opportunities for the nursing profession to address the issues of allocation of resources, effectiveness of care, cost containment, and accountability. Further, as a vital component of the health care system, case management can encompass the conceptual framework of individual practitioners and facilitate personal practice model development. Case management differs from traditional delivery systems that often influence the practitioner to adopt the agency's designated framework for nursing. Case management has the potential to increase the nurse's level of satisfaction and sense of autonomy as a health care provider.[1]

Case management in the formal sense is new to acute care and cannot occur without institutional sanction because the implications of building systems from the caregiver level upward can be enormous. It is not perfect, but if nursing waits for other groups to perfect it, the other groups not only will own it, but also will control the domain of practice that is nursing.

REFERENCES

1. American Nurses' Association: Case management: a challenge for nurses (draft), Kansas City, Mo, 1988, The Association.
2. Bower K: Managed care: controlling costs, guaranteeing outcomes, Definition 3(3):1, 1988.
3. Gross K: Length of stay: impact of the nursing process. Con-

ference on developing cost and quality standards for nursing, American Hospital Assn, Fall 1986.

4. Grossman J: The nursing challenge, Massachusetts Medicine, p. 1. Sept/Oct 1987.

5. McCaskey M: The executive challenge: managing change and ambiguity, Marshfield, Mass, 1982, Putnam Publishing Co.

6. Mundinger M: Autonomy in nursing, Rockville, Md, 1980, Aspen Systems Corp.

7. Rosenberg V: Technology to protect the nursing identity. Unpublished proposal, Center for Nursing Case Management, Boston, 1987.

8. Zander K: Revising the production process when more is not the solution, Health Care Supervisor 3:47, 1985.

9. Zander K: Nursing case management: resolving the DRG paradox, Nurs Clin North Am 23(3):503, 1988.

CHAPTER 29

Nurse-midwifery

A nursing challenge

EUNICE K.M. ERNST

Organized midwifery in the United States began at the Frontier Nursing Service in a remote rural region of the Appalachian Mountains in southeastern Kentucky in 1925. After careful study of nursing in the United States and midwifery in Europe, Mary Breckenridge determined that rural families would be served best by combining the talents of the public health nurse and the midwife. In 1931 the Maternity Center Association in New York City came to much the same conclusion after investigating options for education for midwifery. It opened the first school of nurse-midwifery in 1931 in affiliation with its urban nurse-midwifery clinic and home birth service for poor and immigrant women. The outstanding records of these two pioneering services are well documented and well known.* Similar demonstrations of the effectiveness of midwifery care, of nurse-midwives and physicians working together in a common commitment to improve care for childbearing families, have been replicated in a variety of settings in the United States over the past 60 years. In large medical centers, small community hospitals, and freestanding birth centers in rural and urban areas and in public service and private practice, nurse-midwives have provided safe, high-quality, cost-effective care and have increased access to primary care in a wide variety of settings not adequately served by the present medical care system.[7,11,15,16]

Yet nurse-midwifery has never really taken hold. Perhaps if it had, the problems of maternity care in the United States would be less severe. The infant mortality rate is shamefully high. One out of four women are being delivered by cesarean section (half of which operations may be unnecessary). Obstetrical malpractice claims are terrorizing providers of mater-

nity care and causing physicians to drop obstetrics from their medical practice. The availability of prenatal care and access to it are chronic problems. The wealthiest nation in the world has insufficient funds to guarantee even the simplest care to all women who are bringing forth and nurturing a new generation.

Nurse-midwives working together with physicians can help to solve these problems. National and state health policymakers have begun to recognize the potential of nurse-midwifery care and have recommended expansion of nurse-midwifery services.[5] Former U.S. Surgeon General, Julius Richmond, in a symposium on nurse-midwifery in 1986, exhorted nurse-midwives to stand firm in the face of barriers to their profession and to recognize their invaluable contributions to improving the health status of women and infants, especially minority women. He said, "To a large degree it lies in your power to realign the national and local debate to include issues of social justice, equity and compassion. Perhaps more than any other health profession, midwifery has been able to inject human values into the provision of health care." This is a broad challenge to nurse-midwifery and nursing. Decisions on how to meet this challenge raise issues about nurse-midwifery and freestanding birth centers and their role in the evolving system for health care delivery.

BACKGROUND

Demands for change began as early as the 1940s and came first from consumers seeking "natural childbirth." At the same time, the postwar demand for greater access to medical care spawned publicly funded expansion of medical education and construction of hospitals. Third-party reimbursement, which paid only for physician and hospital services, became avail-

---

*References 2, 6, 9, 17, 19

able to almost everyone and supported the development of what President Dwight D. Eisenhower called the medical-industrial complex.

In 1959 Maternity Center Association, in keeping with the shift to university-based nursing education, moved its School of Nurse-midwifery into Downstate Medical Center of the State University of New York at Kings County Hospital and closed its home birth service. In the 1960s and 1970s 24 educational programs in universities opened across the country. Nurse-midwives were sought by hospitals and public clinics to supplement physician care to women with low incomes.

At about the same time, the natural childbirth movement gained momentum. Informed and insured women began to ask for alternatives to a physician-hospital system of care. In 1971 Booth Maternity Center in Philadelphia, a medically overserved area, successfully demonstrated the readiness of middle-class America for family-centered nurse-midwife care.[4] Availability of nurse-midwife care to insured women raised new issues of direct third-party insurance payment and changes in hospital medical staff bylaws to grant practice privileges to nurse-midwives.[3] The relationship of nurse-midwives to physicians and hospitals was changing. Private nurse-midwifery practices and partnerships with physicians were established.[18] Freestanding birth centers, developed primarily by nurse-midwives and sometimes owned and operated by nurse-midwives and nurses, became licensed health care facilities and also became eligible for third-party reimbursement. In spite of these advances, the profession remained unable to produce enough nurse-midwives to meet the growing need for their services, which perhaps accounted for the resurgence of lay midwifery and home births.

WHO WILL MEET THE CHALLENGE?

It has taken 60 years to bring nurse-midwifery near the mainstream of health care in the United States. Those who have worked to demonstrate the contribution that nurse-midwifery could make to the health and welfare of childbearing families know that it has been an uphill climb all the way.

Constraints to education

The most effective constraint on the expansion of nurse-midwifery has been limitations imposed upon educational programs. When nurse-midwifery edu-

cation moved into the university teaching centers, the clinical teaching sites came under the control of medicine. Student nurse-midwives, who have made a career commitment to serve childbearing women, stand at the end of a long line for clinical teaching experience. Medical students and interns, who may never again care for a woman in childbirth, are given priority. This single factor more than any other has restricted the number of nurses admitted to nurse-midwifery education programs and therefore the number of nurse-midwives in practice. The one other significant constraining factor was the temporary loss of the profession's liability insurance coverage, which caused a temporary but serious reduction in enrollment. Prospective students had to reconsider the expense of preparing themselves for a clinical specialty that they might not be able to practice.

Obstetrical nurses continually express a desire to become nurse-midwives. The most common barriers are personal and financial: family responsibilities and limited financial resources for graduate education. Most would have to relocate to enter a nurse-midwifery program, placing undue hardship on their families. The salary of a nurse-midwife would probably not compensate for the lost income and expenditures required.

Constraints to practice

Constraints to the practice of nurse-midwifery have included the myths about the safety of midwifery care, the reluctance of hospital medical staffs to grant practice privileges, denial of third-party reimbursement for services, denial of obstetrical specialist consultation and referral agreements, denial of prescription-writing priviledges and rulings by state nursing boards that nurses may take orders only from physicians.[14]

The most serious current constraint to practice is the malpractice insurance crisis that affects all providers of maternity care services. Although the American College of Nurse-Midwives was able to obtain an affordable insurance program for its members, obstetricians working with nurse-midwives or serving as consultants to freestanding birth centers have been penalized by surcharges or threats of discontinuation of their insurance coverage. The comprehensive care that childbearing families seek cannot be provided by nurse-midwives without nursing support and medical consultation and referral services. Presently, insurers for professional liability seems to support the fragmentation of maternity care services that contribute to liability problems rather than the development of the interdependent practices needed to provide comprehensive services on a continuum. Nurse-midwifery has grown in spite of these constraints largely because of consumer demand but also because of federal funding for education, the negotiation of a joint practice statement with the American College of Obstetricians and Gynecologists, state and federal legislative mandates for reimbursement, interim liability coverage during the insurance crisis by the American Nurses' Association, and support from individual physicians and health care facilities.

Nursing prerequisite challenged

Over the past 2 decades, also in response to women seeking alternatives to physician-hospital services, there has been a resurgence of the lay midwife, the empirically trained midwife. Like the maligned "granny midwife" of old, she is a mother who became a self-taught midwife by responding to calls from women giving birth at home. Unlike the granny midwife, today's lay midwife is usually middle class, well educated, and articulate; she is also now questioning the need for the prerequisite of nursing for midwifery education.

There has not been a serious study of nurse-midwifery versus direct-entry midwifery education in the United States. Whether nonnurse midwife services produce the same quality, cost-effective care that organized nurse-midwife services have reported for more than half a century is not known. It is also not known what conflicts would arise between obstetrical nurses and nonnurse midwives seeking practice opportunities in a hospital setting. It is unclear whether physicians would view these nonnurse midwives as competitors, as they do nurse-midwives, or as more manageable, cost-effective physician's extenders. Nor is it known whether public funds would be available to support direct-entry education.

Nurse-midwives themselves have avoided taking a stand on whether it is essential to be a nurse to become a midwife. Most say that it is not but that it certainly helps. Nurse-midwifery educators have expressed concern about starting a student with no previous preparation in the health sciences.

Organized efforts already exist to separate midwifery from nursing, a separation that proponents of direct-entry midwifery education say is essential. They argue that nursing today is not relevant to education for midwifery, and the emphasis on pathology and medical technology is negative preparation for the practice of midwifery. They further argue that the current alleged shortage of midwives supports consideration of direct-entry programs rather than drawing from the already shallow reserves of nursing.

Empirically trained midwives have been able to practice legitimately in a number of states. There is one recognized educational program for direct entry to midwifery education. Loosely structured apprentice programs are offered by groups in several states, including Texas, California, and Colorado. The emergence of this new midwife is a clear sign that there are gaps in the present system of care that nurse-midwives and physicians are either unable or unwilling to fill.

Other countries exploring more efficient and effective models for delivery of maternity care are also looking at midwifery education and practice. The Ministry of Health in the province of Ontario, Canada, reacting to consumer pressure for midwifery care and intense lobbying by articulate women's groups and lay midwives, conducted an exhaustive study of midwifery education in Europe and the United States.[10] After reviewing the findings, a decision was made to open a four-year, university-based, direct-entry midwifery education program that would include essential elements of nursing. Also in response to consumer demand, the Ministry of Health has established four hospital-based birthing centers. Reports from England reveal a resurgence of advocacy for the direct-entry midwifery education abandoned several decades ago.

All of these events notwithstanding, most of the hard evidence on midwifery care available in the United States has been generated by nurse-midwives. This evidence has caused policymakers to look at nurse-midwifery as a viable adjunct to improving our system of health care to childbearing families. This 60-year record of nurse-midwives educated in an organized program of study should not be used to make a case for midwives trained in an unstandardized, unevaluated apprenticeship system. Midwives trained in the apprentice system need to apply the same rigorous standards in evaluating their education and services. Then the two approaches can be appraised objectively.

There is a vacuum in the system for providing maternity care that must be filled. If nurses do not move to fill the vacuum, it will be filled by others. How important is midwifery to the profession of nursing? How important is nursing to the profession of midwifery? Will nurse-midwifery expand or will a new midwife evolve?

These questions are unsettling at a time when American nurse-midwives appear to be on the verge of overcoming major barriers to expanding practice opportunities and educational programs. It is clearly the time for nursing to look carefully at the leadership nurse-midwifery has provided for nursing during the past 6 decades. It is also time for obstetrical nurses to examine their role in meeting the challenges posed by women, parents, government, business, and industry for changes in maternity services.

Prudence almost dictates that nurses and nurse-midwives come together in a concentrated effort to build on the foundation for growth that has been carefully laid down over the past 60 years. Direct entry to midwifery education is certainly an option to be explored, but it should not impede the development of nurse-midwifery and the nursing contribution it can make at this critical time.

WHERE WILL IT HAPPEN?
The birth center

Maternity Center Association (MCA) is a 70-year-old voluntary health agency with a commitment to innovative care that is sensitive to the needs of childbearing families. In 1975, perceiving the ferment brewing in the delivery of maternity care, MCA opened the Childbearing Center, a freestanding birth center with a program of care directed at healthy women and families seeking more control, more responsibility, and more participation in their childbirth experience.

Program

The clinical aspects of the program pivot on careful and continuous screening for problems that may require confinement in the acute-care setting, an emphasis on self-care and self-help education in pregnancy, constant attendance during labour and birth, early discharge, and close home follow-up and support. The social and emotional aspects of the program focus on encouraging and preparing the woman's family or friends to participate in pregnancy and birth and to support her throughout the childbearing year.

Safety

After more than a decade of careful evaluation, the freestanding birth center has emerged as a safe, cost-effective place for birth. The data for centers participating in the four annual surveys conducted by the National Association of Childbearing Centers (NACC)

from 1983 to 1986 represent 39,529 mothers admitted to the birth center in labor. There was no maternal mortality. Neonatal deaths occurring in the center were .278 per 1000 live births. Neonatal deaths occurring in the hospital after transfer from the birth center were 1.467 per 1000 live births for a total neonatal mortality of 1.745 per 1000 live births. Most of the neonatal deaths were due to anomalies incompatible with life. Other published studies of birth center care support the data from the national surveys.[10,12,13]

Cost

Maternity is currently the most frequent reason for admission to hospitals and is costing business, industry, and taxpayers more than $15 billion annually. It is estimated that approximately 75% of American women do not need acute care during childbirth. Birth centers participating in the NACC annual survey have consistently reported charges for total care that are up to 50% less than regular hospital stays for normal births and 30% less than short hospital stays. It has been estimated that birth centers could save billions of dollars in the delivery of maternity care.[8]

Potential

Birth centers, like nurse-midwifery, present a compelling argument for major changes in the delivery of care to childbearing families. Birth center programs fit the current focus of third-party payers for a greater emphasis on prevention of disease and education for healthier lifestyles. The birth center removes the major constraint to education of nurse-midwives by providing clinical teaching sites dedicated to the practice of midwifery. It is a place where students will not have to stand at the end of a line for their clinical learning.

The freestanding birth center can greatly improve access to maternity care where it is presently lacking or inadequate. Small community hospitals would do well to convert their obstetrical units to autonomous (freestanding) birth centers. The difference between meeting the national standards for freestanding birth centers and the standards for maintaining an acute-care obstetric-newborn service could represent significant savings in construction and operation and provide a higher level of satisfaction for families served.

The freestanding birth center has been identified as a major catalyst in bringing about changes in hospital maternity care and in opening up hospital privileges for nurse-midwives. In almost every community in which a freestanding birth center has appeared, hospitals have established birthing suites or adopted a short-stay option. In some communities, competition from freestanding birth centers has persuaded hospital medical staffs to open practice privileges to nurse-midwives.

The nursing challenge

The most important consideration for nursing is that the freestanding birth center provides an unprecedented opportunity for nurses and nurse-midwives to take more responsibility and control toward improving care for all women and childbearing families. It can be nursing's contribution to solving the problems of providing maternity care.

HOW WILL IT HAPPEN?

The expanded opportunities for practice are creating an increased demand for nurse-midwives. It is becoming clear that professionals trained exclusively in medical centers are uncomfortable practicing in the birth center setting. If nurse-midwives are to be the primary care providers for childbearing families, and if the birth center is the place best suited to caring for healthy families in childbirth, a new approach to the education and training of practitioners is required.

In 1984 a consortium composed of Maternity Center Association, the Frontier Nursing Service School of Midwifery, Case Western Reserve University, and the National Association of Childbearing Centers (NACC) designed a pilot community-based education program that would allow students to study at their own pace, take a large portion of their credits in a home-study program, and receive most of their clinical training in a freestanding birth center or hospital-based nurse-midwifery practice in or near their home community. The curriculum is based on the mastery learning modular curriculum established by other educational programs. Graduates are eligible to take the national certifying exam of the American College of Nurse-Midwives. Within 6 weeks of the first announcement of the pilot program, over 500 nurses requested information or applications.

WHEN WILL THESE CHANGES OCCUR?

It took more than half a century to move all births into the acute-care setting of the hospital. It was accomplished largely by a third-party system that paid only for hospital and physician services. It is reasonable to expect that the driving force to take normal births out of the acute-care setting will also be a third-party payment system that is struggling to contain costs in a health care system that some feel is out of control. How long it will take depends on how well we are able to evaluate and report to the public the advantages of a shift of this magnitude. NACC will be contributing to this effort in a report of a multicenter prospective study of 20,000 women seeking birth-center care. It will be submitted for publication in the spring of 1989.

As we begin to compare the benefits, hazards, and costs of hospital care versus ambulatory care we can expect to see contraction and centralization of expensive acute-care services and expansion and decentralization of preventive ambulatory services. Both nurse-midwifery and birth centers are in line for this expansion and decentralization. The current issues for nursing presented here pose three questions. Will we take responsibility for expanding nurse-midwifery? Will we take responsibility for developing ambulatory maternity care? Will we take responsibility for containing costs and maintaining quality? If we do not take responsibility, we cannot expect to have control. The ball is in our court.

REFERENCES

1. Bennetts AB and Lubic RW: The freestanding birth centre, Lancet, February 13, 1982.
2. Browne H and Issacs G: The Frontier Nursing Service, Am J Obstet Gyn 124:14, 1976.
3. Ernst EKM: The evolving practice of nurse-midwifery, Health Law Project Library Bulletin 4(a):289, 1979.
4. Ernst EKM and Forde M: Maternity care: an attempt at an alternative, Nurs Clin North Am 10:2, 1975.
5. General Accounting Office: Better management and more resources needed to strengthen federal efforts to improve pregnancy outcome, Washington, DC, 1979, General Accounting Office.
6. Laird M: Report on the Maternity Center Associates, New York, 1931-1951, Am J Obstet Gyn 69:178, 1955.
7. Levy B, Wilkinson F, and Marine W: Reducing neonatal mortality rate with nurse-midwives, Am J Obstet Gyn 109:50, 1969.
8. Lubic RW: Birthing centers: delivering more for less, Am J Nurs, July, 1983.
9. Metropolitan Life Insurance Company, Report on the FNS of Hyden, Kentucky, May 9, 1932.
10. Ministry of Health: Report of the Task Force on the implementation Midwifery in Ontario, Toronto, 1987, the Ministry.
11. Montgomery T: A case for nurse-midwives, Am J Obstet Gyn 105:3, 1969.
12. Murdough Sr A: Experiences of a new migrant health clinic, Women and Health 1(6):25, 1976.
13. Research issues in the assessment of birth settings, Washington, DC, 1982, Institute of Medicine, National Academy Press.

14. Rooks J and Haas JE: Nurse-midwifery in America, Washington, DC, 1986, American College of Nurse-Midwives Foundation.

15. Slone C, et al: Effectiveness of certified nurse-midwives, Am J Obstet Gyn 124:177, 1976.

16. Sharp E: A decade of nurse-midwifery practice in a tertiary university affiliated hospital, Journal of Nurse-Midwifery 29(6):353, 1984.

17. Stewart D: The five standards for safe childbearing, Marble Hill, Mo, 1981, NAPS Publications.

18. Stewart R and Clark L: Nurse-midwifery practice in a hospital birthing center: 2050 births, Journal of Nurse-Midwifery 27(3):21, 1982.

19. Summary of first 10,000 confinement records of the Frontier Nursing Service, Quarterly Bulletin of Frontier Nursing Service 33:45, 1958.

CHAPTER 30

The era of counterbalancing technology in pediatric nursing

SHARON A. ECK
NANCY HANLEY RYAN

John Naisbitt, in his classic book *Megatrends*, identifies the transformation within the United States from an industrial to an information society.[19] The explosion of information has forced extraordinary technologies into our daily lives. Similarly, new technologies have revolutionized pediatric health care. Children who would have died only a decade ago survive today. These health care technologies have permeated not only the acute-care hospital, but also the homes and lives of the American family. Naisbitt describes the way in which we have responded to technology and states, "What happens is that whenever new technology is introduced into society, there must be a counterbalancing human response—that is, high touch—or the technology is rejected."[19] We want to describe the transformation in both the technology and the care of children in the hospital and home settings. The time has arrived, however, for pediatric nursing to go beyond reactively responding to the technology and to begin to actively counterbalance this technology with a human response in practice.

PEDIATRIC TRENDS AND CHARACTERISTICS

The pediatric patients of the 1980s are much sicker than in previous decades. Children are discharged from the hospital much earlier and in much worse shape than ever before, and generally parent(s) must be taught specialized care to perform at home. These trends are similar to existing trends throughout the hospital setting.

There are some characteristics that make the pediatric patient unique. First, the dependent nature of pediatric patients means that another individual must take part or all of the responsibility for providing physical care and for making decisions. Second, because of this dependent nature, ethical decision making is more complicated and challenging, especially because of the potential life span of the child. In most cases decisions must be made keeping in mind that the children have "their whole lives ahead," as opposed to adults who have a lesser life expectancy. Clinical and anatomic features that are unique to children also create some difficulties in ethical decision making. Erlen and Holzman identify controversial issues surrounding the use of organs from anencephalic infants for transplantation.[8] The issues arise from the fact that, "While the anencephalic infant has no cerebral cortex, there is brain stem activity that can maintain the vital functions of the body from several hours to several days."[8] Can organs be taken from a child who still has brain stem activity? Is brain stem activity enough to be considered human? Fletcher, an ethicist, feels that individuals lose their uniquely human characteristics when they lose the thinking functions of the brain. In that case the anencephalic infant would not be considered a unique human being.[10] Further complicating this issue is the controversy over pediatric brain death criteria. In a 1988 *Pediatrics* editorial, Freeman and Ferry state, "The reason given for the caveat is that there is a widely held belief that young children may be more resistant to anoxia and more likely to recover from coma than adults."[11] Thus decisions about termination of high technology interventions become extremely difficult.

The third major characteristic of pediatric patients is that the normal physiology of the child changes dramatically from neonate to adolescent. The neonate starts life with immature organ systems that change very quickly and often with little warning to more adultlike body functions. The diseases and conditions that affect children are often quite different from those that affect adults. Similarly, the same entity may be exhibited quite differently from the child to the adult. Finally, illness in children interrupts the normal growth and development of the child. This results in the need for additional specialized resources to help the child attain normal developmental milestones.

TECHNOLOGY IN PEDIATRICS

Technology has revolutionized survival of the infant and child with major medical problems. These advances in care have become so commonplace that our society has forgotten just how dramatic these changes actually are. For example, the number of neonates weighing less than 1500 g that survive for at least 1 month doubled between 1960 and 1980.[28,29] Children with malabsorption, short-gut syndrome, and other gastrointestinal problems now survive for years due to recent advances in the delivery of parenteral nutrition. The survival of neonates, infants, and children with congenital heart disease has been dramatically improved due to advances in pediatric cardiac surgery. Development of multilumen intravenous catheters has provided a mechanism for the simultaneous delivery of multiple medications into the tiny veins of infants and children. Pharmacological development of drugs that can be used in the treatment of the smallest of human beings has greatly increased their survival rates. The use of high-pressure, high-frequency ventilation has improved survival of children with acute and chronic respiratory problems. Advances in chemotherapy have greatly improved the life expectancy of childhood cancer victims. Development of pediatric trauma centers and improvements in pediatric transport teams have improved survival rates for pediatric multiple-trauma victims. It is likely that technological advances will continue to increase the survival chances of children with severe medical problems. New challenges will include advancements in fetal surgery, multiorgan transplantation, and care of AIDS victims. For example, the number of American children with AIDS is expected to rise from 584 children in 1987 to 10,000 to 20,000 in 1991.[27]

An example of a new and sophisticated technology in pediatrics is extracorporeal membrane oxygenation (ECMO). This is a mechanism for systemic life support for full-term infants with acute respiratory failure. The pioneers in ECMO have determined very specific guidelines for case selection based on the children most likely to benefit from this intensive technology. Currently the survival rate with ECMO is 75% to 83%.[23]

Without ECMO, 80% to 90% of these children would die.

HIGH TECHNOLOGY

Now the focus must turn to the problems and issues that have arisen from the successes of sophisticated technology. Some children remain hospitalized for months to years because of a dependence on equipment available only in hospitals. These hospitalizations can exhaust a family's financial resources. In times of severe shortages of intensive-care and step-down-care beds, these chronically ill children take up precious bed space that could be used for acutely ill children who may require only short-term interventions. Further compounding the problem are the severe shortages of nurses and other health care professionals to provide direct care.

One of the major solutions to these long-term, high-technology hospitalizations has been to move high-technology care into the home. Handy describes three motivations for moving toward high-technology home care: (1) wanting to decrease health care costs, (2) having the ability to provide the technologies at home, and (3) fulfilling the consumer demand for home care.[13] Specifically in pediatrics, a fourth incentive for home care is in decreasing the adverse effects of the hospital environment. For example, recent studies in neonatal intensive care units (NICUs) suggest that bright lights and noise levels may have a permanent ill effect on the infant's sight, hearing, and motor ability.[3,12]

It is estimated that 10 million children in the United States have chronic illnesses, and approximately 2% to 5% (200,000 to 500,000) of these children are in need of home care services.[7] Although the population needing home care has grown fairly large, the development of pediatric home care is relatively new to the home health care industry.[4] The 1984 Ad Hoc Task Force on pediatric home care defined the goal of a home care program as the provision of comprehensive, cost-effective health care in an environment that maximizes individual capabilities and minimizes the effects of the disabilities.[1] [The primary decision-making force in high-technology pediatric home care is the family's desire and ability to care for the child in the home.] Much nursing literature describes the critical family assessment and teaching strategies for high-technology pediatric home care.[2,15-17,21,25,30]

The sophisticated technology has led to a small but

growing number of children who are technology dependent. The Senate Labor and Human Resources Committee and the House Energy and Commerce Committee recently commissioned an Office of Technology Assessment (OTA) Task Force to examine the problems of these children in the United States. In the 1988 published report of the OTA, the technology-dependent child is defined as one who requires both a medical device and ongoing nursing care.[22] It is estimated that approximately 100,000 children are dependent on high-technology care in the home.

COST OF HIGH TECHNOLOGY

What are the costs of this high technology for society and for the individual family? Is it more cost-effective to provide care in the hospital, the home, or an alternative setting? In the United States, approximately 10% to 15% of all children have some level of chronic illness.[6] These children use significantly more of our health care services than other children. The most recent surveys available indicate that 4% of all (noninstitutionalized) children under the age of 17 have some activity limitations.[20] This small percentage of children was responsible for 19% of all hospital discharges for children, 30% of all hospital days, and 9% of all physician visits.[14]

Accurate figures for the actual costs of health care for these children are difficult to determine. Newacheck and McManus state, "Total charges for the health services . . . averaged $760 per child limited in activity compared with $263 for other children during 1980."[20] Thus in 1980 the costs of health care for children limited in activity were 2 1/2 times the cost of other children. It is reasonable to assume, based on current consumer price indexes for medical care, that this trend will continue to increase the variance in cost between these two groups of children.

Newacheck and McManus also describe the out-of-pocket expenses incurred by these families. These expenses include insurance deductibles, travel expenses, home renovations, increases in utility bills, medications, and any other uninsured care costs. The authors point out that "On average, out-of-pocket expenses for children limited in their activities were about twice as high as those for other children."[20] Among the children who are limited in their activity, there are wide variations in the distribution of out-of-pocket expenses.

The skewed distribution of out-of-pocket expenses—10% of disabled children accounting for 63% of total direct patient payments—indicates that financial burdens were unevenly shared by families of chronically ill children. Children without any insurance faced the greatest financial risks, but those with intermittent or part-year insurance also faced substantial financial risk.[20]

One may also assume that there was wide variation in types and amounts of services required by individual children in this small group, which may contribute to the uneven distribution of costs.

In 1980 the total national cost for physician visits and hospitalization for children with activity limitations was about $1.6 billion. Approximately two thirds of these costs were for hospitalization.[24] Low-birth-weight infants, which are accounting for an increasing percentage of children with activity limitations, had an annual NICU cost of between $16,000 and $250,000 per neonate in the early 1980s.[26] Low-birth-weight infants are twice as likely, and very-low-birth weight infants are 4.5 times as likely, to be rehospitalized, as normal infants.[18] Thus it is clear that high-risk children are consuming the overwhelming majority of child health care dollars.

Technologies in the home vary in complexity and cost. There are conflicting reports on the reimbursement for home care; however, reimbursement for home care in the early 1980s remained significantly less than that for hospital care. Recently, there have been changes in these practices and movements toward higher reimbursement for home care, including reimbursement for catastrophic illness.

Much of the literature in home care speaks to the significant financial incentives of home care versus hospital care. Many of these reports, however, have not been substantiated with actual data. Further complicating these comparisons are the variety of methodologies for calculating costs of care. For example, a study may or may not state whether direct nursing care costs are included in the estimates, and these costs may affect significantly the total actual costs. Many families assume a portion of the total responsibility in the provision of home nursing care. Although care provided by the family decreases the amount spent on the child's health care, it is certainly a major burden on the family and must be considered in describing the costs. For example, Feinberg describes the severe stresses of pediatric home care on the family, which have created an array of new psychosocial concerns for the health profession.[9]

Three examples of high-technology pediatric care are apnea monitoring, phototherapy, and ventilator support. Norris and Hutchins describe the 1986 costs of individual infant apnea monitoring and estimate a 1-year cost to be approximately $4175.[21] This is an example of a common home care technology. The infants require hospitalization only for stabilization, diagnostic testing, and teaching. Phototherapy is a technology that remains controversial and uncommon. Heiser reported, in a small study, that phototherapy can be managed effectively at home at a cost savings of $300 per day compared to hospitalized management.[5] The highest technology care in the home is provided to ventilator-dependent children. The OTA compares the home vent start-up costs of $1200 with average monthly costs of $10,000 to the estimated $25,000 per month cost for such care in a hospital setting.[22] Although difficult to compare, most data suggest that with appropriate family support and resources, pediatric home care is significantly more cost-effective than hospital care.

OUTCOMES OF HIGH TECHNOLOGY

The cost of this high-technology health care is often justified by the outcomes. The family members of critically and chronically ill children generally cite the child's mere survival as being the single most important outcome of the technology. The days and months of anguish and uncertainty are worth it if the child survives. In general, the loving relationships within these families, and the fact of maintaining some level of family interaction at all, is an outcome that is impossible to measure.

Perrin estimates that there are 1 million severely impaired children living in the United States.[24] A small percentage of children with severe limitations are using the majority of monies spent on health care. The question for society is whether this is an appropriate distribution of health care dollars.

Despite the successes of high technology and the tremendous improvement in survival rates of infants and children with serious medical problems, there is still much concern about mortality rates of normal-birth-weight infants. Wise and others report a rise in infant mortality in the Boston area in the early 1980s.[31] They relate the statistically significant rise in the mortality rate of normal-birth-weight infants to a stabilization in mortality rates of low-birth-weight infants and to a lack of prenatal care. So while vast amounts of dollars and resources are being spent on a small number of severely disabled children, children are still being born to women who do not receive the prenatal care necessary to prevent childhood disability or death. This problem emphasizes the greater need for primary care, which may lessen some of the need for high-technology tertiary care.

Other questions related to the outcomes of high technology are difficult to describe and to evaluate. These questions are specifically related to the individual and the family yet have significant implications for society. What is the quality of life of the surviving child? Who determines what that quality is? When, if ever, does the quality not justify the cost in suffering, dollars, and resources? What is the quality of life of, and long-term effects on, the parents and siblings? How does the predicted quality of life affect the decision making about using high technology on children, and who makes those decisions?

IMPLICATIONS FOR PEDIATRIC NURSING

Society and the American family face the problems arising out of the successes of applied technology. The individual consumer or the parent demands all that technology has to offer. These consumer demands are exceeding the supply of resources. Most people do not wish to pay more for health care, however, and in fact are demanding reductions in health care expenditures. Now is the time to counterbalance this high technology with a greater human response. Consumers of health care in concert with pediatric physicians and nurses, insurers, legislators, and ethicists must begin to struggle with the reality that being able to save a child's life cannot be the single determinant of whether or not to do so. People must determine how to redistribute resources to maximize the capabilities of the children with the greatest potential to be productive members of society. Pediatric nursing must organize toward effectively influencing the way in which children's health care is managed, distributed, and provided. Ideas for nursing's active human responses to counterbalance technology are presented below.

Participating in application of technology to children

Individual case management of critically and chronically ill children is probably the single most important area in which to consider the consequences of high technology intervention on the quality of the child's life. It is also the single most difficult area for health team members. Nurses, as direct-care providers, must take a much more assertive role in the case-by-case decisions regarding the applications of technology. Through relationships with the family and colleagueship with physicians, nursing is in a unique position to influence directly the application of the human side to the technology. Nursing can help the family and other health team members to examine critically the options for care as they relate to potential outcomes. What is the anticipated length and quality of life compared to the resources and technology required to produce the outcomes? For instance, will the child be a productive member of society or one of the 1 million severely disabled children who use the overwhelming majority of child health care dollars and resources? Will the child ever walk, talk, go to school, or get dressed independently?

Nurses must also take a direct role in the realistic identification of those children who will die or whose functions will be severely limited. Thus nurses must learn to recognize and help the family and physician identify the appropriate time to change from high technology intervention to palliative or hospice care. More generally, nurses should work toward further expansion of hospice care for children.

Nursing should become actively involved in the creation of units or other settings that provide alternative types of care, such as palliative or hospice care. They should focus on comfort and care that will allow a dignified death, perhaps through the withholding of traditional interventions that prolong life.

Nursing must develop greater expertise in the area of health care ethics to provide the family and other health team members with the insights necessary to make the difficult clinical decisions. Nursing must also keep abreast of current technology to maintain an up-to-date understanding of the consequences of applying technology to cure certain pathologies. In this way nurses will be an invaluable resource to the family and other health team members when difficult decisions must be made.

Model development in application of high technology to children

Current and future technologies must be examined to determine which patients would benefit most from them. The mere ability to provide the technology should not mean it will be used when there is little evidence that the patient's quality of life will be high.

Nursing must take an active role in prospective and retrospective research related to appropriate case identification. Through research findings and direct-care expertise, nursing must collaborate to develop models for appropriate application of high technology to children. The ECMO model of case identification is a unique example of this type of sophisticated application of high technology. This type of case selection model will be necessary in other areas as technology continues to develop. We must ask, "Who is most likely to benefit from this technology?" rather than, "Who might benefit in some way from this technology?" Through model development, nursing will be applying the human touch to the technology.

Maximizing the abilities of chronically ill children

Nurses must take an active role in the identification of resources needed by chronically ill children to reach their optimal level of functioning. Perrin describes a comprehensive program to provide the resources necessary to increase the productivity of chronically ill children.[24] Nursing needs to further identify and develop interventions to maximize directly the individual child's capabilities, for example, to care for themselves, attend school, and develop relationships. Continued expansion and research in the area of pediatric home care should suggest possible intervention. For example, the innovation by Brooten and colleagues in the early discharge of very-low-birth-weight infants with nurse specialist follow-up is a remarkable accomplishment, with a potential $334 million annual national savings.[5]

Influencing American social policy in the financial distribution of children's health care resources

Pediatric nursing must develop a strategy to influence health care policy at both the state and federal levels. We must examine critically the cost-effectiveness of both the settings and providers of care for chronically ill children. To do this effectively, standardized cost analysis and comparisons must be established. In a united voice we must describe new approaches to providing comprehensive care to children. Emphasis should be placed on resource appropriation to increase the abilities of the 9 million children who have great potential. Perhaps with continued expansion of home care, the dollar savings can be redistributed for comprehensive program development. Much emphasis needs to be placed on expanding reimbursement patterns to support new and creative approaches to health care. Greater access to prenatal care continues to be a central issue and one that directly affects the lives of children. Nurses who care for children are in one of the best positions to be their advocates and to articulate clearly to legislators and insurers not only the needs of this population, but also the ways in which these needs can be met most effectively.

The technologic explosion that Naisbitt predicted has created the demand for the human response in the care of children. Nurses and physicians along with families must develop knowledge and wisdom to deal with our new wealth of technology. Pediatric nursing is positioned well to provide leadership in establishing the directions for the future of children's health care. Naisbitt summarized our challenge well, "Technology and our human potential are the two great challenges and adventures facing humankind today. The great lesson we must learn from the principle of high technology/high touch is a modern version of the Greek ideal—balance."[19]

REFERENCES

1. Ad Hoc Task Force on Home Care of Chronically Ill Infants: Guidelines for home care of infants, children, and adolescents with chronic disease, Pediatrics 74:434, 1984.
2. Andrews MM and Nielson DW: Technology dependent children in the home, Pediatric Nursing 14(2):111, 1988.
3. Bess FH, Peek BF, and Chapman JJ: Further observations on noise levels in infant incubators, Pediatrics 63:100, 1979.
4. Brault GL: 1980's reorientation to home health care, J Pediatr Health Care 1(1):8, 1987.
5. Brooten D and others: A randomized clinical trial of early hospital discharge and home follow-up of very-low-birth-weight infants, N Engl J Med 315(15):933, 1986.
6. Butler J and others: Health care expenditures for children with chronic disabilities. In Hobbs N and Perrin J, editors: Issues in childhood chronic illness, San Francisco, 1985, Jossey-Bass, Inc, Publishers.
7. Cabin B: Cost effectiveness of pediatric home care, Caring 4:48, 1985.
8. Erlen JA and Holzman IR: Anencephalic infants: should they be organ donors? Pediatric Nursing 14(1):60, 1988.
9. Feinberg EA: Family stress in pediatric home care, Caring 4(5):38, 1985.
10. Fletcher J: Humanhood: essays in biomedical ethics, Buffalo, 1979, Prometheus Books.
11. Freeman J and Ferry P: New brain death criteria in children: further confusion, Pediatrics 81(2):301, 1988.
12. Glass P and others: Effect of bright light in the hospital nursery on the incidence of retinopathy of prematurity, N Engl J Med 313:401, 1985.
13. Handy CM: Home care of patients with technically complex nursing needs, Nurs Clin North Am 23(2):315, 1988.
14. Health characteristics of persons with chronic activity limitation, US Department of Health and Human Services Pub No 82-1565, Hyattsville, Md, 1981, National Center for Health Statistics.
15. Heiser CA: Home phototherapy, Pediatric Nursing 13(6):425, 1987.
16. Jackson DF: Nursing care plan: home management of children with BPD, Pediatric Nursing 12(5):342, 1986.
17. McCarthy MF: A home discharge program for ventilator assisted children, Pediatric Nursing 12(5):331, 1986.
18. McCormick ML, Shapiro S, and Starfield BH: Rehospitalization in the first year of life for high-risk survivors, Pediatrics 66:991, 1980.
19. Naisbitt J: Megatrends, New York, 1982, Warner Books.
20. Newacheck PW and McManus MA: Financing health care for disabled children, Pediatrics 81(3):385, 1988.
21. Norris-Berkemeyer S and Hutchins KH: Home apnea monitoring, Pediatric Nursing 12(4):259, 1986.
22. Office of Technology Assessment Task Force: Technology-dependent children: hospital vs. home care, New York, 1988, JB Lippincott Co.
23. Ortiz R, Cilley R and Bartlett R: Extracorporeal membrane oxygenation in pediatric respiratory failure, Pediatr Clin North Am 34(1):39, 1987.
24. Perrin JM: Chronically ill children in America, Caring 4(5):16, 1985.
25. Schreiner MS, Donor ME, and Kettrick RG: Pediatric home mechanical ventilation, Pediatr Clin North Am 34(1):47, 1987.
26. Shankaran S and others: Medical care costs of high-risk infants after neonatal intensive care: a controlled study, Pediatrics 81(3):372, 1988.
27. Smith K: Legislative update, Pediatric Nursing 14(1):54, 1988.
28. US Department of Health and Human Services, Public Health Service: A study of infant mortality from linked records by birth weight, period of gestation and other variables, Pub No (PH5) 79-1055, Hyattsville, Md, 1972, National Center for Health Statistics.
29. US Department of Health and Human Services, Public Health Service: Advance report of final natality statistics, 1984, Monthly vital statistics report 35(4, Suppl):37, 1986.
30. Wildblood RH and Strezo PL: The how-to's of home IV therapy, Pediatric Nursing 13(1):42, 1987.
31. Wise P and others: Infant mortality increase despite high access to tertiary care: an evolving relationship among infant mortality, health care, and socioeconomic change, Pediatrics 81(4):542, 1988.

CHAPTER 31

Long-term care

Fulfilling promises to the old among us

NEVILLE E. STRUMPF
KAREN KAUFFMAN KNIBBE

In rewriting this chapter for the third edition of *Current Issues in Nursing*, we have considered what is as accurate today as 5 years ago and also what has changed. The earliest chapter contained several statements that are still compelling and relevant as we prepare for the next decade:

1. Nursing remains a potentially powerful force in the planning and humane execution of care for older people.
2. Reform of, and alternatives to, the existing system of long-term care are urgently needed.
3. The presence of a growing number of older persons likely to need some care is an opportunity for nursing to demonstrate its political and social maturity as a profession.

Any discussion of the challenges of long-term care must now, however, also consider the impact of a widening national concern for the costs of care, perceived limitations in material and human resources, changing priorities about the use and distribution of technology and sophisticated interventions in health care, a growing proportion of older people who are quite vulnerable because of their frailty and have reduced financial means, and a shortage of health care workers, especially professional nurses, to care for the aged. The character of a society and its professions is mirrored in the response to those in need. The Social Policy Statement formulated by the American Nurses' Association states that nursing is "owned by society" and "must be perceived as serving the interests of the larger whole of which it is a part."[1] Fulfilling that promise, as it pertains to the old among us, is the central challenge in long-term care.

In Lynaugh's discussion in this volume of the nursing shortage, she identifies the consequences of a wholehearted acceptance of biomedical strategies as the framework for the health professions: "Little place for the chronically ill, the marginally dysfunctional, or the aged."[34] She adds that the "siren song of cure sounds sweeter to Americans than the gentler refrain of comfort and care," and she reports a "40 to 1 patient-to-nurse ratio in the nation's nursing homes" to prove it. Thus one of the most pressing health care problems remains care of the very old, which has attached to it the burden of technological and moral choices likely to shape the availability and the quality of health services well into the twenty-first century.

For purposes of this discussion, long-term care refers to a range of health and support services that are carried out over an extended period of time, in a variety of community or institutional settings, for individuals lacking some or all ability to care for themselves. This chapter provides background essential to understanding long-term care: changing demographics, a fragmented system of health care, needed reforms, and the role that must be taken, as Lynaugh has argued elsewhere, if nursing is "to take hold of aging the way medicine took hold of disease."[33]

DEMOGRAPHY AND OLD AGE
Statistical data

According to statistics compiled by the U.S. Senate Special Committee on Aging,[56] the source of all demographic data included here, the pattern of age structure in the United States has changed dramatically in recent decades. Approximately 29.2 million persons are 65 years old or older. In 1986 one in five persons was at least 55 years old, and one in eight was at least 65, with a median age of 31.8. By 2040 about 20% of the population will be 65 or older. Other startling figures are the projections for the old-old: by the year

2000, half of the aging population will be 75 or older.

These shifts are the result of increased life expectancy along with recent declines in the birth rate. On average, females can expect to live longer than males (78.2 years versus 71.2 years), with white females having the longest life expectancy (78.7), followed by black females (73.7), white males (71.8), and black males (65.3). Overall, older women now outnumber older men three to two, and the disparity is even greater at age 85-plus, when there are only 40 men for every 100 women.

Despite some general improvements in the economic status of older people, analyses for 1986 show that 12.4% of persons 65 and older still have incomes below the poverty level, with the poorest of those being 85 years and older. Close to half of the aging population hovers at a financial level allowing for few expenses beyond the minimum required for food, shelter, and some health care. Nearly three out of four aging poor are women. Regardless of sex, nonwhite older individuals have substantially lower incomes than their white counterparts. In 1986, 90% of all older people received some income from Social Security, and 14% relied on it entirely, making it by far the single source on which the largest proportion of older people must depend.

Seven out of 10 persons over the age of 65 describe their health as "good" or "excellent" compared with others their age. Not until age 85 and older does about half the population report limitations in activities because of chronic illness. More than 90% of the noninstitutionalized population over 65 are able to manage their daily needs. Nevertheless, the majority report at least one chronic health problem, and multiple conditions are commonplace. In addition, mental health problems are significantly more frequent in later life and can influence considerably the course of physical illness. Alzheimer's disease and other organic mental disorders affect more than 6% of older adults, and cognitive impairment, whether from Alzheimer's or other causes, is one of the principal reasons for institutionalization. Suicide is a more frequent cause of death among older adults than among any other age group; however, the majority eventually die from heart disease, cancer, or stroke, with heart disease the major cause of death.

The number of people in nursing homes is expected to rise with the increase in the population of very old. Although about 5% of aging persons are in nursing homes at any given time, the rate of institutionalization still has doubled since the implementation of Medicare and Medicaid programs in 1966. Current projections indicate that the nursing home population will increase to 2 million persons by the year 2000 and will probably double again by 2040. Nursing home residents are characteristically very old, female, white, and without a spouse, family, or others able to provide informal support for health and maintenance.

More older persons now live in the suburbs than in cities, and almost half of the older population lives in eight states: California, New York, Florida, Pennsylvania, Texas, Illinois, Ohio, and Michigan. The United States is distinguished among the nations of the world in the size and growth of its older population; in numbers it is exceeded only by China and India.[55] Forty years from now, it will be home to one of the oldest populations in the world. What remains unknown about this large group of future older Americans is the nature of their unique health problems and the results of changing environmental and social conditions and risk factors over time.

Implications of statistical data

Shifts in age structure are beginning to have profound consequences and will definitely affect planning for future health care. The significant increase of persons older than 75 means a greater incidence of functional disability or debilitating illness and increased use of both acute- and long-term care services. Most people over 75 are women, who, in addition to facing problems created by ageism and sexism, are also seriously constrained by unusually high poverty levels. Minkler and Stone[40] report that the poverty rate among older women is 19%, the highest for any group in the United States.

The chance of developing one or more chronic conditions or disabilities increases with age. About 23% (6 million) of the noninstitutionalized older population have functional limitations in one or more of several areas, including personal care and home management.[14] Of this number, approximately 850,000 older people residing in communities live with varying limitations, a figure that exceeds the 600,000 severely limited people currently in nursing homes.[31] The ability of older people to get help with activities is an important factor in determining whether they can continue to reside in the community or they have to move to a long-term care setting. One estimate of the cost of noninstitutional care is $4.2 billion annually.[12] Of this figure $1 billion was paid as out-of-pocket expenses by the care recipients themselves. A prolonged high level of personal expenses results in an economic burden posing another significant risk factor for institutionalization.

Published estimates by the Department of Health and Human Services for recent total expenditures for all long-term care services list an annual figure of $32.3 billion.[23] Nursing home expenditures are increasing at an average annual rate of 10% and are expected to reach $55 billion per year in 1990.[24] With annual nursing home costs of $22,000 or more per person per year, with little coverage under public programs, and with no significant private insurance coverage available, chronic illness can emotionally and financially destroy thousands of American families each year.[44] Many people are destitute within 13 weeks of entering a nursing home.[25] Initially, nursing home payments are private, direct, out-of-pocket expenditures; not until individuals "spend down" their resources are they eligible for Medicaid, the state-administered health program for the poor. Medicaid is increasingly assuming responsibility for long-term care of the elderly and is now the major third-party payer for long-term care.[54]

The latest figures from the National Center for Health Statistics (1986) report 26,380 nursing and related-care homes with 1,770,206 beds and 1,609,419 patients.[50] These numbers represent 4.3% of the population aged 65 and older in nursing homes and .4% in residential facilities. Since 1974 the numbers of nursing homes and beds have increased by 22% and 38%, respectively, with general operating capacity of the homes at 92%; 75% of the homes are proprietary, 20% are not for profit, and 5% are operated by federal, state, or local governments.[52] By the year 2000, 3 million nursing home beds may be needed, a 103% increase from 1980.[43] With financial constraints facing many state governments, however, pressure to hold down the number of nursing home beds to reduce Medicaid expenditures will probably be considerable.

Nearly 30% of all expenditures for medical care are for persons aged 65 and older. As Kovar[30] points out, (1) the proportion of money spent to care for older people is large relative to their proportion in the population, and (2) a large proportion of money spent on the care of older people is from public funds. This focuses considerable attention on the aging population in any discussion of the cost of care. At the same time, aging members of society must not be made into scapegoats for consuming what appears to be a disproportionate share of available resources. Although the average amount spent on health care for those 65 and older is greater than that spent for people under 65, expenditures vary with health status, and the majority of older people have modest expenditures during most years. For those older persons who do experience hospitalization, poor health, or institutionalization, however, the expenditures are significant, whether paid for with personal or public funds. Thus, for obvious reasons, the need is tremendous to promote the maintenance of functional ability and independence for as long as possible and also to provide community-based and institutional supports that are high quality, economically feasible, and equally accessible. The current system of long-term care falls far short of these ideals.

THE SYSTEM OF LONG-TERM CARE
Current problems

T. Franklin Williams, director of the National Institute on Aging, argues that a comprehensive care system for older people must offer a full range of integrated services, including "primary care, preventive and maintenance care, acute hospital care, extended care, home support services, and long-term care services, tailor made for each individual."[57] In general, we have failed to appreciate the fact that the chronic impairments of older people are often more complex than the problems experienced by other age groups. The current approaches to care by both providers and the health system itself have not been entirely responsive or sensitive to this important point. The persistent efforts of many health providers, agencies, family members, and advocacy groups are often required to find the necessary services or to coordinate them for one individual. The present system, or more accurately nonsystem, satisfies no one.

The central problem facing long-term care in the United States is its makeshift and inadequate financing. Existing mechanisms for eligibility and reimbursement for health care continue to emphasize an institutional model of care with its related biomedical and technological "solutions." Dealing with acute illness is favored over more comprehensive approaches to care, with the result that short-term hospitalization or nursing home placement are virtually the only choices available to older people and their families. In their excellent examination of care for the disabled elderly, Rivlin and Wiener summarize the major problems in long-term care: (1) The burden falls heavily on persons unlucky enough to need extensive care and on their families; (2) Public costs are rising rapidly, primarily in Medicaid, leaving poor families with children and the frail elderly to compete with one another for limited funding; (3) A two-class system of long-term care, especially in the case of nursing homes, is perpetuated by dependence on individual out-of-pocket spending or Medicaid as the chief means of reimbursement; (4) Access to care is often limited, with patients capable of paying privately preferred over those who must rely on public funds; and (5) Reimbursement for home care services is limited, and financing those home care services that are available is extremely fragmented.[45]

The current system of long-term care is characterized by multiple public funding sources (Social Security, Supplemental Social Security, Medicaid, Medicare, Title XX, and the Older Americans Act) and multiple agencies (hospital, nursing home, home health agency, adult day health care, homemaker service, meals on wheels), each with its own eligibility and service provision requirements.[5] The "unresolved catastrophe," to use Brody's apt phrase, is the need, despite this maze of funding sources and agencies, to achieve continuity of care for the multiproblem client. Brody[8] describes continuity of care as moving through three stages: (1) acute care, usually representing a hospital stay; (2) short-term long-term care, which is the brief time period, often less than 90 days, following a hospital stay that allows for transition to community living; and (3) long-term long-term care, which may be intermittent, of varying intensity and locations, but continuous.

Several highlights of the current system of financing health services for older people are essential to understanding the gaps in providing such continuity of care. Medicare, a federal entitlement program for all persons aged 65 and older, covers mainly acute care, even after passage of the Catastrophic Insurance Bill in 1988.[4] A growing portion of the costs for Medicare are borne by older individuals themselves through increased monthly premiums and a surtax on federal taxes. For the most part, the law does not address the problems of paying for extended or nursing home care.

Since 1983 Medicare has paid for hospital care with essentially a fixed rate per discharge, depending on the diagnosis-related group (DRG) in which the patient is classified. Prospective payment, intended to curb soaring medical costs, may forever change the structure and function of the long-term care system, because reduction in length of hospital stay has dramatically increased the practice of discharging patients "quicker and sicker." As a consequence of the early discharge of many older patients, nursing homes have been forced to accept a heavier-care case mix to accommodate those needing posthospital extended care.[48] The reliance by hospitals on nursing home care following early discharge may, however inadvertently, be contributing to unnecessary or even permanent institutional placement. Hospitals also continue to have few incentives for establishing specialized geriatric evaluation units, although these have been shown to **increase functional status** and decrease institutionalization.

Unlike Medicare, Medicaid is a means-tested welfare program for the poor, financed by individual states and the federal government. It now accounts for about 40% of all nursing home reimbursement, usually at a fixed per-patient-day rate that varies greatly among the states[25] but averages less than $40 and $50 per-patient-day for intermediate and skilled nursing services, respectively.[78,27]

As an alternative to the customary method of Medicaid reimbursement, experimentation with the case-mixed payment systems in nursing homes, based on functional capacity, medical condition, and/or service intensity of patients, is under way in several states. Among the more promising of these methodologies is resource utilization groups (RUGs). Funded by the Health Care Financing Administration, RUGs classifies patients with similar needs, rather than similar diagnoses, into one of 16 resource groups and allows payment levels to be established for each group. It could simplify the regulatory process by eliminating arbitrary definitions of levels of care; eliminating financial penalties for admitting sicker patients; and providing incentives for rehabilitation, discharge, and better patient outcomes.[18] Many questions remain unresolved about case-mixed payment systems, including equitable payment schedules and the needs of selected categories of patients, particularly the demented.[27] In a powerful ethnographic description of the nursing home, Diamond[15] criticizes all such reimbursement schemes as further obliteration of the individuality of the patient, who is conceptualized and acted on purely in terms of activities of daily living and the cost of each activity.

What should be obvious from the above description of two of the primary sources of reimbursement for health services for older people is the lack of organization among the five essential components of a long-term care system: (1) the client, (2) informal support services, (3) formal direct services, (4) linkages, and (5) the financing mechanism itself.[32] To insufficient reimbursement mechanisms for the health care of older people can be coupled some additional reasons for sub-optimal conditions in the existing set of long-term services: poor public and provider attitudes toward aging persons, inadequate education about the clinical problems of older people, perceived lack of stature and attractiveness of careers in gerontology and geriatrics, and a low level of expectations from both patients and society regarding the therapeutic potential of older adults.[51]

Although the provision of adequate health care for older people must be considered from the standpoint of a continuum of service ranging across settings from home to hospital to long-stay institution, the nursing home continues to dominate and symbolize the problems and dilemmas of long-term care. The influence of Medicare and Medicaid programs serves to reinforce the ambivalent position of nursing homes as second-class hospitals performing both medical and social functions.[28] The populations in nursing homes remain heterogeneous in their needs and include those who require care for terminal illness (among them a growing number of AIDS patients), short-term convalescence, intensive rehabilitation, skilled nursing, mental illness, developmental disability, or shelter and home-making services. We still have to identify what the role of nursing homes ought to be: housing and support for frail older people with nowhere else to go, sophisticated rehabilitative services after hospitalization, protection for the cognitively and functionally impaired, or places to die. The financial reality in most nursing homes is that a large proportion of the residents use up their entire personal savings in less than a year. Completely impoverished, with Medicaid payments to the home the resident's sole means of support, discharge is impossible even if health improves. Thus little incentive exists for nursing homes to emphasize rehabilitation or discharge; at the same time, Medicaid reimbursement for the continued care of these residents is pitiably low. This lack of funds in turn affects the quality of care and the ability to attract and to pay professional staff, two more serious problems in many American nursing homes. At a moment when prospective payment systems have increased the number of nursing home residents who are severely ill, the fiscal and human resources to care for these elders is at its lowest ebb in 20 years.

Directions for reform

According to Rivlin and Wiener,[45] the objectives of any reform of long-term care are to (1) reduce the uncertainty and anxiety that now surround paying for long-term care, (2) enable older people to remain at home as long as possible, and (3) improve the quality of care and the flexibility and efficiency of the delivery system. Both private- and public-sector strategies are needed to achieve these objectives, but given a capacity to spend 10% or more of its gross national product on health care, it is certainly possible for the United States to do so. The greatest challenge is discovery of a way to integrate and coordinate long-term care services in a cost-effective and compassionate manner. The creation of a comprehensive system of long-term care is frequently linked to case management, defined by Arnold[5] as a "process of assessment and service provision that is conducted within a system of service organization." Who will get to be case managers remains to be seen, although the best candidates are nurses and social workers.

A case management model would have as its framework a focus on functional independence rather than cure, an interdisciplinary team approach, equal access to a range of services, support for families, and maintenance at home for as long as reasonably possible. Critical to the success of a case management model will be the ability of managers, through their respective agencies, to have some control over resources and access to care. Several successful models exist for such case management approaches, for example, the On Lok Community Care Organization for Dependent Adults in San Francisco, California, the Veterans Administration's system of long-term care for elderly veterans, and the social health maintenance organizations in several states,[5] along with the channeling experiments.[7]

The pressure to control costs will be impossible to ignore in any attempt to design better methods of delivering long-term care. This is already apparent in discussion or development of private and public long-term care insurance, continuing care retirement communities and life care at home,[54] block grants, expanded home care,[21] liberalized approaches to Medicaid, hospital-based skilled nursing facilities,[29] and public senior citizen housing.[49] Although few would question the goal of comprehensive and coordinated community-based service delivery systems, Estes and Wood,[17] nevertheless, identify a growing national trend toward decentralization "away from a primary concern for community and access to care, in the name of containment and cost effffectiveness." It will thus challenge us politically, socially, and morally to devise a system that allows for access to care and quality of life in a fiscally responsible and ethical manner.

As changes in the delivery of long-term care are considered, the allocation of resources to older people is likely to be debated further. Two arguments for the rationing of health care by age have recently been put forward by Daniels[13] and Callahan.[9] If their proposals are basically untenable, we must still accept the fact that a form of rationing does exist in the United States, namely, access to care based on the ability to pay. Churchill[10] lucidly argues that we must struggle to overcome our misguided commitments to very expensive, high-technology interventions and consider the universality of our collective vulnerability to disease, disability, and death. "A realization that we are in the same circle biologically and geographically should clarify our need for policy that puts us all in the same circle in health care as well." We cannot deny that difficult decisions about the allocation of societal resources in general and health care dollars in particular will have to be made,[11] but we must also beware the pitfalls of benefit and cost analysis in geriatric care.[6] As Strumpf[53] has written elsewhere, the intersection of the competing forces of ethical care and cost containment presents nursing with unique challenges and an opportunity to help reshape long-term care.

THE ROLE OF NURSING IN LONG-TERM CARE

Demographics, reimbursement structures, need for a more comprehensive approach to the care of older people, and a growing concern for a reformed, morally just, and efficient system of long-term care form both background and context for the role of the nurse in gerontology.

The framework for gerontological nursing practice is delineated in a statement on standards and scope prepared by the American Nurses' Association.[3] The standards call for quality care at a level beyond that required by minimal regulatory criteria and serve as a model for basic and advanced professional practice in the areas of organization of services, generation and testing of theory as a basis for clinical decisions, data collection, health assessment, planning and continuity of care, intervention, evaluation, interdisciplinary collaboration, research, ethics, and professional development. Emphasis is placed on maximizing functional ability in activities of daily living; promoting, maintaining, and restoring health, including mental health; preventing and minimizing the disabilities of acute and chronic illness; and maintaining life in dignity and comfort until death.

Given the existing state of long-term care, nursing can make its most significant contributions by:

1. Increasing the pool of baccalaureate, master's, and doctorally prepared nurses in gerontology
2. Participating actively in the delivery of health services specifically aimed at the enhancement of accessibility, management, and continuity of long-term care for older people
3. Improving care in nursing homes
4. Conducting research documenting impact by the nurse on quality care for older people

The selection of a career in gerontological nursing has been hampered by negative societal images about aging and beliefs that care of older people is unglamorous, unrewarding, less intellectual and sophisticated than other specialties, and ultimately hopeless in the face of chronicity, decline, and death. Gradually, a more enlightened public and profession is recognizing the diversity and capacity of persons in their later years, as well as their unique needs for a range of health care services spanning community, hospital, and nursing home. Interest in and commitment to the older population also profoundly affects the type of care and resources available to older people. The National League for Nursing continues to reiterate its belief that the incorporation of gerontological content into undergraduate and graduate nursing programs can make a difference.[42] Indeed, the efforts of a pool of faculty at the University of Pennsylvania with expertise in gerontology and affiliations with a wide variety of agencies providing services for older people in every conceivable setting have demonstrated that such integration is possible and, furthermore, that students can be recruited with the understanding that they are preparing for a future characterized by creative and meaningful practice.

Throughout most of the United States, however, the nursing shortage remains critical in long-term care settings, particularly in nursing homes. Only 7% of all registered nurses are employed in nursing homes.[52] Less than 1000 certified gerontological nurse-practitioners are spread across the country,[41] and only about 3% of nurses in nursing homes have master's degrees.[52] Major barriers to be overcome are the limited supply of nurses capable of entry-level (baccalaureate degree) and advanced (master's degree) practice in gerontology, salary inequities favoring employment in acute- over long-term care settings, and failure in most instances to obtain direct reimbursement for nursing care.

A number of trends indicate a significant role for nursing in regard to accessibility, management, and continuity, including an increase in the variety and availability of experimental and established community-care options as an alternative to institutional care; shifts in accountability and decision making among health care providers responsible for long-term care; and realignment of the customary functions of hospitals, nursing homes, and home care agencies in regard to long-term care.[37] As these adjustments and realignments take place, nurses will need to respond quickly to the care requirements of older people in many settings and at all levels of health. Expert assessment, timely intervention, and continuity of the client-nurse relationship will be essential; willingness to have a major role in coordination, creation of policy, and advocacy will also be important.

Because of changes that will inevitably occur in long-term care as the number of older people requiring services increases, nursing will need to negotiate its role with other providers. Shifts in accountability and decision making need to occur as medicine and nursing work out a "cooperative agenda" that will keep both professions technically expert and humane.[35] Nurses have the authority to act in matters within their sphere of competence, and this includes assessment and management of a wide range of problems typically experienced by older people.

As already noted, reform of nursing home care will remain a special challenge. Efforts by nursing and consumer advocacy groups, as well as the study by the Institute of Medicine on improving the quality of nursing homes,[26] helped pave the way for the Nursing Home Quality Care Amendments of 1987.[16] Their intent is improved care for nursing home residents, including better resident assessment; more intensive training for nursing assistants; increased staffing by licensed nurses; strengthened provisions for residents' rights; a stronger ombudsman program; stricter anti-

discrimination policies, especially for Medicaid beneficiaries; greater availability of records and survey reports; and stiffer penalties for failure to comply with regulations. It is critical that professional nurses be part of survey teams evaluating adherence to these new federal regulations.

The presence of nurses in nursing homes is still impeded by the underfinancing of long-term care; those nurses present in nursing homes or familiar with their problems will need to be vocal about the outcomes, in human terms, of such underfinancing. Largely as a result of prospective payment systems, the typical nursing home resident is far sicker than in the past, and staff in many nursing homes often function like their counterparts in acute-care settings.[20] Professional nurses need to hold administrative positions in nursing homes to develop or use effectively quality monitoring tools documenting the need for increased staffing.[46] The American Nurses' Association recommends that nursing home staffing be based on levels that ensure the safe and effective delivery of care and that the expertise of clinical nurse specialists or nurse-practitioners be available.[2]

The experience of the teaching nursing home and the use of gerontological nurse-practitioners in some nursing homes has been an experiment in change demonstrating the benefits that can be achieved by increasing the presence of professional staff in long-term care.[38] Among those benefits are improved assessment and management of ongoing chronic problems, for example, incontinence, confusion, falls, and pressure sores; reduction in use of medications and restraints; reduction in transfers to the hospital; an increase in the number of discharges back to the community; greater support for ancillary staff caring for a frail population of residents; the initiation of special programs and units, for example, day care and hospice; and enhancement of staff morale with less turnover. It seems likely, as Rossman[47] has observed, that "all the great problems of chronic illness—long-term care, convalescent care, and finally, terminal care—will come to a head in the nursing home."

This brings us, finally, to the need for research documenting the contribution of nursing care to the health and well-being of older people. Rivlin and Wiener[45] suggest that the most desirable solution (or partial solution) to the problems of long-term care would be breakthoughs in reducing disability. Many alterable health-related problems associated with aging (nutrition, smoking, stress control, misuse of alcohol and drugs, accident prevention, exercise and fitness) lend themselves to the health promotion–disease prevention framework that characterizes professional nursing practice. Minkler and Pasick[39] note, however, that lack of follow-up and evaluation impedes the generation of valid and reliable data about health promotion in general and for older people in particular. Limited resources and narrow research focuses often lead to development and testing of interventions on an isolated and singular basis. Minkler and Pasick conclude that if research in health promotion continues to focus on individual behavior changes, public policy will reflect this emphasis, and the major preventable health problems, especially for the older population, will continue unabated.

As Harrington[22] points out, public policymakers and officials face difficult choices when attempting to raise nursing care standards, given growing federal deficits and ever-expanding expenditures for health care. The choices are all the more difficult because they are often made without data demonstrating the improvements in quality of care that result from expert nursing. Thus it is of the utmost importance that nurse researchers continue to devote themselves to those clinical problems affecting the functional status of older people that are amenable to nursing intervention: problems in cognition, mobility, nutrition, elimination, drug taking, sensory impairments, skin care, loss, and response to institutionalization. This is by no means an exhaustive list but an outline that is of keen interest to both the National Center for Nursing Research and the National Institute on Aging of the National Institute of Health at the federal level and to numerous private foundations dedicated to improving health care for older people.

CONCLUSION

An ideal community ensures the personal liberties of older people, protects their individuality, and enhances the integrity of the aging experience.[19] The nurse who chooses long-term care will be expected, above all, to contribute to the preservation of these values. At the same time, this nurse will also be living in a nation with a growing percentage of older people, a fragmented system of health care, and a finite supply of human and material resources. Nonetheless, it is possible for gerontological nurses to influence the care older people will receive through their advocacy of a reformed and more equitable system of services, par-

ticipation in assessment and management of the health care problems of aging persons in the community and in institutions, and conduct of part of the research essential to understanding the needs of older people. In fulfilling the promises of a caring community to the old among us, we also fulfill those promises to ourselves.

REFERENCES

1. American Nurses' Association: Nursing: a social policy statement, Kansas City, Mo, 1980, The Association.
2. American Nurses' Association: Statement on minimal registered nurse staffing in nursing homes, and Statement on mandatory training for nursing assistants in nursing homes, Kansas City, Mo, 1986, The Association.
3. American Nurses' Association: Standards and scope of gerontological nursing practice, Kansas City, Mo, 1987, The Association.
4. American Nurses' Association: Catastrophic bill signed into law, Capital Update 6(13):1, 1988.
5. Arnold D: The brokerage model of long-term care: a rose by any other name, Home Health Care Serv Q 8(2):23, 1987.
6. Avorn J: Benefit and cost analysis in geriatric care, N Engl J Med 310(20):1294, 1984.
7. Baxter R: Implementation and early operation of the national long-term care channeling demonstration: overview, Princeton, NJ, 1983, Mathematical Policy Research, Inc, Levinson Policy Institute.
8. Brody SJ: Strategic planning: the catastrophic approach, Gerontologist 27(2):131, 1987.
9. Callahan D: Setting limits, New York, 1987, Simon & Schuster.
10. Churchill LR: Should we ration health care by age? J Am Geriatr Soc 36(7):644, 1988.
11. Clark PG: The social allocation of health care resources: ethical dilemmas in age-group competition, Gerontologist 25(2):119, 1985.
12. Cohen D and others: A planning study of alternative home health ventures that improve employment opportunities for the homemaker/home health aide. Final report submitted to the Ford Foundation, 1984.
13. Daniels N: Just health care, Cambridge, 1985, Cambridge Univ. Press.
14. Dawson D, Hendershot G, and Fulton J: Aging in the eighties, functional limitations of individuals age 65 years and over, US Public Health Service Pub No 87-1250, Hyattsville, Md, 1987, National Center for Health Statistics.
15. Diamond T: Social policy and everyday life in nursing homes: a critical ethnography, Soc Sci Med 23(12):1287, 1986.
16. Eastman P: Improving nursing home care, Geriatr Consult 6:7, May/June 1988.
17. Estes CL and Wood JB: The non-profit sector and community-based care for elderly in the US: a disappearing resource, Soc Sci Med 23(12):1261, 1986.
18. Finkelstein MJ: The impact on nursing homes of diagnosis-related groups, Long-Term Care Currents 10(4):15, 1987.
19. Gadow S: Humanities teaching and aging: issues and approaches in medical education. In Spicker SF and Ingman SR, editors: Vitalizing long-term care, the teaching nursing home

and other perspectives, part III, the role of humanities and creative writing, New York, 1984, Springer.

20. Gamroth L: Long-term care resource requirements before and after the prospective payment system, Image 20(1):7, 1988.

21. Gaumer GG and others: Impact of the New York long-term home health care program, Med Care 24(7):641, 1986.

22. Harrington C: Nursing home reform: addressing critical staffing issues, Nurs Outlook 35(5):208, 1987.

23. HCFA says kin can kick in, Washington Report on Medicine and Health 37(19), 1983.

24. Health Care Financing Administration: An overview of long-term care, Health Care Financ Rev 6(3):69, 1985.

25. House Select Committee on Aging: America's elderly at risk, Washington, DC, 1985, US Government Printing Office.

26. Institute of Medicine: Improving the quality of care in nursing homes, Washington, DC, 1986, National Academy Press.

27. Jazwiecki T: Case-mix payment for nursing homes, Long-Term Care Currents 10(4):17, 1987.

28. Kane R and Kane R: Long-term care: can our society meet the needs of its elderly? Ann Rev Pub Health 1:227, 1980.

29. Knapp MT: Filling the gaps in health care: a hospital-based skilled nursing facility, Nurs Manage 17(9):19, 1986.

30. Kovar M: Expenditures for the medical care of elderly people living in the community in 1980, Milbank Q 64(1):100, 1986.

31. Liu K, Manton K, and Liu B: Home care expenses for the disabled elderly, Health Care Financ Rev 7(2):51, 1985.

32. Lubben JE: Models for delivering long term care, Home Health Care Serv Q 8(2):5, 1987.

33. Lynaugh J: Care of the aged: society's mandate to nursing. Paper presented at a Nursing Research Conference on Gerontology, mid-Atlantic Regional Nursing Association, Hershey, Pa, September 30, 1983.

34. Lynaugh J: Is there anything new about this nursing shortage? In McCloskey JC and Grace HK, editors: Current issues in nursing, ed 3, 1989, St Louis, The CV Mosby Co.

35. Mechanic D and Aiken L: A cooperative agenda for medicine and nursing, N Engl J Med 307(12):747, 1982.

36. Meiners MR and Coffey RM: Hospital DRGs and the need for long-term care services: an empirical analysis, Health Serv Res 20(3):359, 1985.

37. Mezey M and Lynaugh J: Facts and issues for nursing in long-term care, Chicago, 1982, American Hospital Assoc.

38. Mezey M, Lynaugh J, and Cartier M: Nursing homes and nursing care: lessons from the teaching nursing home, New York, Springer (in press).

39. Minkler M and Pasick R: Health promotion and the elderly: a critical perspective on the past and future. In Dychtwald K, editor: Wellness and health promotion for the elderly, Rockville, Md, 1986, Aspen Systems Corp.

40. Minkler M and Stone R: The feminization of poverty and older women, Gerontologist 25(4):351, 1985.

41. National Health Policy Forum: Barriers to expanded practice and pay for geriatric nurse practitioners, Issue Brief No 471, Washington, DC, 1987, George Washington University.

42. National League for Nursing: Educational models in long-term care, New York, The League, (in press).

43. Nursing homes: a source book, Series No 937, Washington, DC, 1983, American Health Care Association.

44. Ostrander V: Financing long-term care: no single solution, Nurs Econ 3:349, Nov-Dec 1985.

45. Rivlin AM and Wiener JM: Caring for the disabled elderly, Washington, DC, 1988, Brookings Institution.

46. Roberts KL, LeSage J, and Ellor JR: Quality monitoring in nursing homes, J Gerontol Nurs 13(10):34, 1987.

47. Rossman I: Nursing homes: dim past, bright future, Geriatr Med Today 7(1):23, 1988.

48. Rubenstein LZ and others: The Sepulveda VA geriatric unit: data on four-year outcomes and predictors of improved patient outcomes, J Am Geriatr Soc 32(7):503, 1984.

49. Sheehan NW: Aging in place in public senior housing: past trends and future needs, Home Health Care Serv Q 8(2):55, 1987.

50. Sirrocco A: Nursing and related care homes as reported from the 1986 inventory of long-term care places, US Public Health Service Pub No 88-1250, Hyattsville, Md, 1988, National Center for Health Statistics.

51. Siu AL: The quality of medical care received by older persons, J Am Geriatr Soc 35(12):1084, 1987.

52. Strahan G: Nursing home characteristics, preliminary data from the 1985 national nursing home survey, US Public Health Service Pub No 87-1250, Hyattsville, Md, 1987, National Center for Health Statistics.

53. Strumpf NE: A new age for elderly care, Nurs Health Care 8(8):445, 1987.

54. Tell E, Cohen M, and Wallack S: Life care at home: a new model for financing and delivering long-term care, Inquiry 24:245, Fall 1987.

55. Torrey B, Kinsella K, and Tauber C: An aging world, Washington, DC, 1987, US Government Printing Office.

56. US Senate Special Committee on Aging: Aging America: trends and projections, Washington DC, 1987-1988, US Department of Health and Human Services.

57. Williams TF: Extended care: a physician's perspective. In Vladeck BC and Alfano GJ, editors: Medicare and extended care: issues, problems, and prospects, Owings Mills, Md, 1987, Rand Communications.

CHAPTER 32

Nursing practice in developing countries
The Latin American experience

ALINA A. SOUZA

INTRODUCTION

This chapter analyzes nursing practice and education in Latin America as it exemplifies nursing care in developing countries. Its main purpose is to raise questions concerning alternatives in nursing practice and education that allow the nursing profession to respond most effectively to social and economic conditions.

The historical development of nursing in Latin America is addressed first. The institutionalization of nursing education in the region clearly shows the marked influence of the Nightingale school, and a corresponding adjustment to Latin American social structure and Iberian cultural traditions. Nursing practice is described in terms of its basic features: health care settings, the nursing work force, and actual working conditions.

Finally, issues and trends in nursing practice are discussed, emphasizing the need for a greater integration of nursing into the social and health care systems of Latin American countries. This need calls for members of the nursing profession to rethink, reformulate, and reorganize nursing practice and education in Latin America in order to meet the challenge of better quality nursing care for all.

FEATURES OF NURSING DEVELOPMENT IN LATIN AMERICA

Souza,[15] in her review of the historical development of nursing practice and education in Latin America, distinguished three general periods. The first, covering the colonial period through the end of the nineteenth century, was marked by the organization of nursing under religious control. This was an extension of nursing as practiced in some European countries, primarily Spain and Portugal. The practice was developed by religious sisters and nonprofessionals, mostly women from the lower social classes, some of them previous patients. Nursing was limited to basic functions that involved serving patients' hygienic and spiritual needs in addition to performing housekeeping chores, a function characteristic of the precapitalist organization of health care.[4]

An analysis of Latin American social formation shows its limited autonomy from colonizing European nations. Europe itself had undergone major economic and social change during the eighteenth and nineteenth centuries, making possible the Nightingale reform, among other things. Even after the independence movements that started in the mid eighteenth century in Latin America, major social and economic transformation did not occur. For this reason, even though nursing was an organized occupation, a movement such as the one in Europe (Nightingale reform) did not occur, and nursing remained relatively untouched by European developments.

The second historical period distinguished by Souza was marked by the professional development of nursing. The process began for some Latin American countries during the last quarter of the nineteenth century and lasted until World War II. This period saw the institutionalization of both nursing education and the public health movement.[14] Nursing development was mainly promoted by the state, which took control of health care as part of the secularization process. This process of change has varied for individual Latin American countries and is largely determined by the degree of separation between church and state.[5]

The first Latin American nursing school was established in Argentina in 1886. By the end of the nine-

Table 32-1 Number of nursing schools in Latin America by sponsoring institutions 1886–1939

	Government institutions	Religious congregation	Medical schools	Red Cross	Private hospitals	University	Total
Argentina	3	2	3	2	2	1	13
Brazil	5	2	1	2	1	—	11
Bolivia	—	2	—	—	1	—	3
Chile	5	—	1	—	—	1	7
Columbia	—	2	—	—	1	—	3
Cuba	7	—	—	—	—	—	7
Dominican Republic	1	—	—	1	—	—	2
Ecuador	2	—	—	—	—	—	2
Haiti	—	—	—	1	—	—	1
Mexico	3	—	2	1	—	—	5
Peru	4	—	—	—	1	—	5
Uruguay	1	—	—	—	—	—	1
Venezuela	1	—	—	1	—	—	2

Source: Pan American Health Organization archives.

teenth century there were schools in Argentina, Brazil, Chile, Cuba, and Mexico (see Table 32-1).

These countries were either in the process of secularizing medical care or had strong foreign ties. The programs were based on Nightingale models and their creation was promoted primarily by physicians who had been trained in Europe. During the Third Latin American Congress held in Montevideo, Uruguay, in 1907 Grierson,[8] the founder of the first nursing school in Latin America, presented and received approval for a resolution stating the following:

The physicians of all Latin American countries should work in each one of their own countries for the development of nursing schools, using as a general model the English or North American patterns of education.

The proposition heralded new demands for the secularization and modernization of medical care. This change was part of larger economic and social transformations taking place in Latin America.

The public health movement originating in the United States has had a great influence on Latin American nursing practice.[14] There were more than 20,000 nurses working in public health in the United States in the early twentieth century. Their experience had a significant impact on the health of growing populations in the emerging industrial cities. As Roberts[13] remarked:

Records of the rapid expansion of public health nursing following World War I, convey a sense of sustained drive and enthusiasm which had repercussions in the field of nursing education.

Three important programs can be taken as points of reference for the introduction of this movement into Latin America: the International Red Cross program, the Children's Bureau program of 1921 to 1929, and the Rockefeller Foundation program. These programs promoted the creation of new nursing schools in Argentina, Brazil, Colombia, Costa Rica, Ecuador and Venezuela. At the beginning of World War II the Institute of American Affairs, created to protect areas of strategic interest to the allied countries, also encouraged the organization of public health services and nursing schools in Latin America.[12] By the end of the 1950s the majority of the countries in the region had at least one nursing school.

Under the framework of medical care secularization and modernization, the public health movement of this second historical period was marked by nursing development. Nursing began to fight to acquire social status as a profession, creating national associations as well as specific legislation for nursing practice.

The third broad period of nursing development in Latin America, from World War II to the present, has been marked by the institutionalization of the professionalization process. For the majority of the countries control of nursing education and practice has been exercised by nurses. Social and technical divisions of labor can be seen in the institutionalization of auxiliary personnel training under the leadership of nurses. However, the major development of interest during this period has been the establishment of nursing programs at the university level. Most Latin American countries now have the equivalent of baccalaureate-granting programs (see Table 32-2).

Nevertheless, nursing practice and education in Latin America have continued to follow the dominant trend in hospital practice, which emphasizes greater specialization and reliance on technology.

NURSING PRACTICE

To understand the practice of the nursing profession one must look not only at its historical roots but also at its actual role in the larger health care field, taking into consideration social structure and the division of labor in a given society. An analysis of nursing practice in Latin America should thus include the features and trends of health services, the nursing work force, and working conditions.

Nursing is part of what can be seen as collective work; its aims, together with those of other health care professionals, are to promote and maintain health. It is well known that the specialized work of health care is not solely responsible for the health of a population, yet it is essential to the monitoring and maintenance of health. Nursing possesses specific knowledge and methods that have characterized its practice in terms of providing continuous care and forming liaisons with other professions in the search for comprehensive care.[1] The health care professions are greatly influenced by social issues and agendas. In Latin America economic crises, fueled by decreases in production and increasing unemployment and external debt, are creating a critical social condition with repercussions for health care. Although hospital care continues to evolve, demanding highly trained and specialized personnel, national and international policies have promoted a shift in national health care expenditures from curative to preventive measures and more basic health care. A World Bank report[17] states:

> In order to increase the efficiency of resource utilization and to assure equality of access, it is necessary that governments decrease their expenditures in hospital care and in the development of highly specialized personnel, and make more investments in the training and employment of health personnel at a lower level of care.

Table 32-2   Number of nursing schools in Latin America by sponsoring institution and country, 1988

Country	Total	University	Ministry of Education	Ministry of Health	Other
Argentina	69	12	37	20	—
Bolivia	5	5	—	—	—
Brazil	94	59	2	1	32*
Chile	10	10	—	—	—
Colombia	22	22	—	—	—
Costa Rica	1	1	—	—	—
Cuba	29	1	—	28	—
Dominican Republic	5	5	—	—	—
Ecuador	9	9	—	—	—
El Salvador	3	1	—	2	—
Guatemala	3	—	—	3	—
Haiti	3	—	—	3	—
Honduras	3	2	—	1	—
Mexico	128	104	15	—	9
Nicaragua	4	—	—	4	—
Panama	2	1	—	1	—
Paraguay	3	2	—	1	1
Peru	25	14	—	6	5
Uruguay	1	1	—	—	—
Venezuela	35	3	24	8	—
Total	454	252	78	78	47

Source: PAHOs Archives.
*(State = 3; District = 9; Catholic = 7; Private non Catholic = 13).

Implementation of this policy received support when the Ministries of Health of Latin America established goals for a Ten-Year Health Plan for the Americas. This plan proposed that all populations, including rural communities with less than 2000 inhabitants, were to receive a minimum of health services. A similar goal, that of health care for everyone by the year 2000, was agreed upon by members of the World Health Organization at its 1979 meeting in Alma-Ata (USSR). Such policies advocating increases in health services demand a new approach to the development of nursing human resources and a new ideology for health practice.[10,11]

The nursing work force in Latin America is a complex issue. The number of nurses trained at the baccalaureate level is not known for every country. Although there has been a consistent increase in the last several decades in the number of nurses (the first Pan-American Health Organization [PAHO] census indicated that in 1949 there were a total of 5121 nurses working in hospitals and 1124 in public health services, increasing to a total of 36,807 in the 1960s and an estimated 168,440 in the late 1980s), the ratio of nurses to the general population remains very low (4.05 nurses for every 10,000 people). In addition, the majority of these professionals are in administrative or teaching positions.[9,16]

In Latin America the nursing work force has three basic characteristics: it is highly stratified, female-dominated, and the majority are employed in private hospitals. There are four major categories of nursing workers: nurses with university and nonuniversity degrees; technically trained personnel (training programs require a high school education or below), auxiliary personnel (less than one year of training at below the high school level) and nursing aides (personnel without formal nursing training who are basically trained on the job). According to PAHO data the total number of all types of nursing personnel in the mid-1980s was 3,268,974 (7.86 nurses for every 10,000 people). Although the number of nursing personnel has increased steadily, there has been a decrease in the proportion of trained nurses making up that total. Nursing aides account for the majority of the nursing work force in Latin America.[7]

Male participation is limited in all categories of nursing personnel. There has been a slight increase in the number of male nurses; in Brazil, for instance, 6% of nurses are male.[2] Yet a PAHO study of health personnel found an increase of over 100% in the number of workers employed in the health system in Brazil; the biggest increases were among physicians and aides. There was also a corresponding decrease in salaries for all categories.[7]

As a result of the economic crises faced by most Latin American countries, and their impact on health care systems, nursing practice has become fragmented. The quality of care in a model that demands only quantity is poor, and a risk factor for the client. One need only think about the numbers of untrained nursing personnel in positions of great responsibility in both public and private health care institutions. (In some cases unsupervised nursing aides are found in charge of entire wards.) Most procedures are performed as isolated acts, undertaken without an overall plan and without thought to their integration into a comprehensive program of health care. This is one of the results of the imbalance between professionals and nonprofessionals employed in the health system.[6]

This unfortunate situation has caused nursing care to lose its distinctive focus. In some cases other professionals have begun to assume the supervision and control of nursing work, while nurses have assumed managerial or administrative roles. Nurses attempting to acquire status for the profession have given much of their energy during the last decade to cooperative organizing, following in the footsteps of liberal medical practice, and defining "ideal" models of practice removed from reality.

If it is assumed that actual nursing practice in Latin America adheres strictly to health policies that stress quantity or breadth of care over quality, it can be concluded that nursing care, and health care in general, are deteriorating. In the hospital setting actual working conditions make the organization of nursing care difficult. Shortage of personnel, lack of definition of norms and routines, and lack of equipment and supplies jeopardize safe nursing practice, bringing elements of risk to patients and health care workers. At public health agencies the working conditions are similar, and they are aggravated by the lack of professional identity specific to a technical division of labor.

In summary, the state of nursing practice in Latin America is characterized by:

- Fragmentation and discontinuity of care
- High probability of risk for the patient
- Possibility of iatrogenic developments
- Improvisation of care by untrained support personnel
- Minimal levels of nursing care

- Low satisfaction among clients and nursing personnel

The challenge for nursing in Latin America today is to solve these problems. Two interdependent and complementary strategies are called for: the organization of nursing work processes, and interaction with the larger health care sector with the aim of attaining integrated and comprehensive health care. Only nursing organization can give support to strategic definitions, in order to address issues such as:

- Professionalization of workers who lack specific training
- Rethinking undergraduate and graduate training
- Development of continuing education programs for nurses and auxiliary personnel already in service
- Influencing policy-making
- Improving working conditions
- Reorganization and coordination of nursing services
- Interacting with clients to establish a process of care evaluation

This suggests that nursing in Latin America will need to engage in continuous, constructive, and vigorous debate bringing new dimensions to health policies in order to ensure better quality of life for Latin America's population.

REFERENCES

1. ABEN/INAMPS: Subsidios para a Conceituação de Enfermagem rumo a Reforma Sanitária, Brasilia, 1987, Oficina de Trabalho.
2. Conselho Federal de Enfermagem and Associação Brasileira de Enfermagem: O exercício de Enfermagem nas Instituições de Saúde do Brasil 1982-1983, Rio de Janeiro, 1985, vol 1, Força de Trabalho em Enfermagem.
3. Cueva A: El desarrollo del Capitalismo en America Latina, México, 1978, Siglo Veintauno.
4. Garcia JC: La Medicina en America Latina 1880-1930, Educ Med Salud 17(4):363, 1983.
5. Mariategui JC: Seven interpretative essays on Peruvian reality, Austin, 1971, University of Texas Press.
6. Monfredi M and Souza A: Nursing education in America, Educ Med Salud 20(4):473, 1986.
7. Nogueira RP: Recursos Humanos en Salud en Las Americas, Educ Med Salud 20(3):295, 1986.
8. Oficina Internacional de las Republicas Americanas: Conferencia Sanitária Internacional. 3a. México, D.F., 1907, Washington, DC, 1907, OIRA.
9. Organización Panamericana de Salud: Los Servicio de Salud en Las Americas: Analisis de Indicadores Básicos. Cientific Publication 15:58, 1988.
10. Pan-American Health Organization: Declaracion de Alma-Ata, 13(1):84, 1979.
11. Pan-American Health Organization: Ten-Year Plan for the Americas, Washington, DC, PASB Printing Office.
12. Pan-American Sanitary Bureau: Report of the Director PASB to the Eleventh Pan-American Sanitary Conference, by Surgeon General (Ret.) Hugh Cumming, Washington, DC, 1942, PASB Printing Office.
13. Roberts M: American nursing history and interpretation, New York, 1954, The Macmillan Co.
14. Rosen G: Preventive medicine in the United States, 1900-1975: trends and interpretations, New York, 1975, Science History Publications.
15. Souza AMR: Development of the Pan-American Health Organization nursing advisory services: impact in Latin American nursing education (1940-1980), doctoral dissertation, Columbus, 1982, The Ohio State University.
16. Verderese O: Analisis de La Enfermeria en America latina, Educ Med Salud 13(4):315, 1979.
17. World Bank: Health sector policy paper, March 1975, Washington, DC, The World Bank.

PART FIVE

QUALITY ASSURANCE

Nursing's newest challenge

JOANNE COMI McCLOSKEY
HELEN KENNEDY GRACE

Concerns about the quality of health care are not new, but as the size and cost of the health care industry have grown, it has become imperative to measure and document the quality of the care delivered as well as the competence of the providers. The issues surrounding the documentation and certification of nursing quality are enormously complicated. The authors in this section attempt to sort out these issues that will challenge the profession for at least the next decade.

Whose responsibility is it to assure quality? This is the question that Sliefert asks in her debate chapter. First she defines the components of the quality control process: values clarification, establishment of standards and identification of criteria to measure standards, comparison of standards to practice, actions to change practice, and feedback on results. She then examines the controversy between internal (professional) and external (institutional) control. Responsibility for health care has shifted from the individual practitioner to the health care institutions because professionals have not in the past dealt with issues of quality and cost. Recently, intense competition among health care organizations has influenced the role of institutions in quality control. Sliefert concludes that an effective quality control program requires cooperation from both nursing professionals and health care organizations.

The first three viewpoint chapters discuss the difficult problem of measuring the quality of nursing care. In the first chapter Hodges and Icenhour assert that the measurement of the quality of nursing care is the single most important goal for nursing in this decade. They point out that there are many definitions of quality, but all existing measurement models use the framework of Donabedian: structure, process, and outcome. In the past, nursing has been content to measure structure and process variables, but the new push in the measurement of quality is the measurement of outcomes. Hodges and Icenhour use two patient examples to show that the documentation of only process does not ensure the measurement of outcomes. The problems of outcome measurement are complex for nursing and include the difficult decisions of what to measure and when to measure. Hodges and Icenhour urge the use of a model that integrates structure, process, and outcome measures of nursing care. Both quantitative and qualitative methods should be incorporated, which is now possible because of computer availability. They admit, however, that the methodology for doing this is not well defined. If quality assurance is to be done well, nursing needs to make a strong commitment to the development and testing of integrative methods.

In the next chapter Gamroth and Smith ask whether quality assurance in long-term care is any different than quality assurance in other parts of the health care system. These authors also discuss the many definitions of quality that result in differing measures. They point out that long-term care facilities are both a treatment and living situation, so residents' expectations are different than they would be in acute-care facilities, and outcome measures need to reflect this. In long-term care, the quality of life measures are intertwined with quality of care measures. Using case situations, they discuss the problem of outcomes desired by the patient being in conflict with the standards defined by the regulatory agency. The authors review recent efforts to improve quality in long-term care, including peer review, association efforts, incentive programs, and regulatory effects. The new efforts in nursing are to focus on the measurement of patient outcomes as these relate to process, but the regulatory climate is negative and fearful. According to the authors, quality is not something that can be regulated.

Quality assurance programs in home health are a more recent phenomenon and are not yet mandated as they are in acute or long-term care. In her chapter, Colling first reviews recent developments that have an impact on home care agencies. These include the increase in the aging population, new government legislation, increasing consumer demand, and changes in nursing. According to Colling, there has been an 800% growth in proprietary home health agencies in the past decade. The rapid growth of this segment of the nursing care delivery system has fostered the concern for quality assurance. Colling provides a very useful table that summarizes the individual quality assurance programs in home health. The home setting has some unique characteristics, though, and Colling discusses four issues surrounding the measurement of quality in this setting. Like the previous authors, she urges the measurement of structure, process, and outcome variables and the study of their relationships.

Although the newest challenge in nursing is to measure individual patient outcomes, there are long-standing mechanisms in nursing that are used as indicators of quality. The last three chapters in Part 5 review some of the most common regulatory mechanisms. In their chapter Dvorak and Schowalter describe the functions of the state boards and the national group, the National Council of State Boards of Nursing, that assists them in assuring the competence of nurses. As consumer protection agencies, state boards have three responsibilities: controlling entry into practice, maintaining competent practitioners, and reviewing scope of practice issues. The authors discuss the workings of the organization and point out the issues that concern the profession in this area of regulation. They discuss the many efforts to assure the validity of the licensure examination, and they review ongoing projects. This is a thoughtful, informative chapter that should answer many questions for readers.

Due to the many types of nurses and the many facets of nursing care, nursing uses a variety of credentials to certify competence and quality of its practitioners. The newest and most confusing of these credentials is certification for specialty practice. In their chapter Bulechek and Maas outline three certification models: certification by the professional organization, certification by the state, and certification by the institution. After outlining the goals of certification, they evaluate each model's advantages and disadvantages. They con-

clude that certification for specialty practice best serves the interests of the public when it is conducted by the profession. The largest certification program is conducted by the American Nurses' Association, which has grown tremendously since 1983. Many other nursing organizations, however, also certify specialists, and the multiple efforts cause much confusion. Before a professional model of certification can be established, duplication and lack of coordination among professional organizations must be overcome. Readers will find this chapter an excellent overview on content and issues related to certification.

In the last chapter Kerfoot presents an overview of the numerous regulatory agencies that affect nursing practice and require lengthy and time-consuming documentation of care delivered. She says that the fragmentation of nursing into specialty organizations allows the control of nursing practice to be assumed by a variety of accrediting boards and agencies. Moreover, as the composition of the governing board of the Joint Commission for Accreditation of Healthcare Organizations attests, nursing is underrepresented on these important accreditation organizations. Kerfoot points out that accreditation standards do not necessarily guarantee quality and are very costly to comply with. She says it is time to take an active role in influencing regulatory agencies to develop cost-effective standards. She wants all bedside nurses to be more aware of the regulatory standards and how these relate to their daily practice. "Standards must be a part of the everyday practice of each nurse."

After reviewing the chapters in Part 5, several questions come to mind. How do other countries assure quality? Are there standard indicators of quality that nursing should always measure? What are the best measures of nursing outcomes? Should the measurement of patient outcomes be required and regulated? Do credentials protect the public or the professional? Do they assure quality or even competence? If nursing is successful at measuring patient outcomes and relating these in the practice setting to process and structure criteria, will we need as many credentials and regulatory bodies as we have? Currently we have credentials to accredit our schools, approve our programs, license our nurses, examine our applicants, certify our specialists, review our charting, and evaluate our objectives. But do all these credentials assure quality? Is there a better way? Will this decade's focus on quality create a better system or just add more work and confusion? This is indeed a challenge.

CHAPTER 33

Debate

Quality control

Professional or institutional responsibility?

MAXINE K. SLIEFERT

Historically, quality assurance in health care was linked to professional autonomy, and individuals or groups of professionals determined what constituted "good" practice. This relationship stems from society's expectation that health care professionals will fulfill their obligation to the public for competent practice through self-regulation. Because it has been assumed that high standards of practice have been maintained, sources of external authority have been prevented from interfering in the control and evaluation of professional work. Traditionally, nursing has been granted less autonomy because nurses were believed to be accountable to physicians and the institutions that employed them.[28] Luke and Modrow[28] claim that health care institutions, particularly hospitals, have not been fully accountable for the quality of care provided, nor have quality control activities had much impact on overall institutional performance. Now health care organizations are required to be more accountable for quality control through standards mandated by voluntary agencies (i.e., Joint Commission on Accreditation of Healthcare Organizations) government laws and regulations (e.g., diagnostic-related groups, or DRGs), legal decisions, and increased pressure from consumer interest groups. Such rules, laws, and policies transfer additional responsibility to the agency's administrative level, thus stimulating conflict between professional autonomy and institutional goals of self-regulation. In addition, intense competition among health care organizations has influenced the institution's role in quality control. Health care organizations have recognized that their strategic and competitive edge will depend on the quality of care provided to the consumer. With the increased emphasis on efficiency, productivity,

cost, and market share, top administrators are taking a more active role in quality control management.

Where should the responsibility for quality control lie? This question cannot be answered easily. The issues are tied to the evolving professionalism of nursing, the organizational structures in which nursing is practiced, and the dynamics of the health care environment. Here, *institution* is defined narrowly as the acute-care hospital setting, because nursing has had the most experience with quality assurance activities in hospital settings, and most nurses are employed in acute-care hospitals. The concept of quality control is discussed, and components of both hospital and nursing quality control programs are identified. Issues associated with quality control mechanisms are presented and the professional and institutional perspectives examined.

QUALITY CONTROL

The term *quality control* is a management term that denotes a management process designed to evaluate and monitor the quality of a product. Originally used in industry, quality control has now been applied to health care and hospitals. Quality control refers to a set of functionally related activities that evaluate, monitor, or regulate the quality of service rendered to the consumer. Both management and clinical processes are included. These quality control activities are commonly referred to as *quality assurance*.

The components of a quality control program, whether carried out by the institution or nursing, are similar. The basic elements are standard setting, comparison of the standard to actual practice, analysis and interpretation of the data, selection and implementation of actions to change practice, and feedback on the results of action. Program elements may vary due to social and organizational contexts, program objectives, and available resources.

The Joint Commission on Accreditation of Healthcare Organizations (JCAHO) has been a strong force in the development of quality control programs in hospitals. Although accreditation by the JCAHO is voluntary, it is generally viewed as mandatory because much of hospital reimbursement from third-party payers is contingent on achievement of JCAHO accreditation. In response to a need for a comprehensive and practical approach to quality assurance in hospitals, the JCAHO developed and implemented a hospital quality assurance standard that became effective on January 1, 1981.[37] The standard requires a well-defined, organized quality assurance program "designed to enhance patient care through the ongoing objective assessment of important aspects of patient care and the correction of identified problems." Interpretive statements regarding the standard specifically identify the development of a written plan to assure comprehensiveness and integration of the overall program and to delegate responsibility for the various activities.[37] The essential components of a sound quality assurance program are defined as (1) identification of important or potential problems, (2) objective assessment of the cause and scope of the problem, (3) implementation of decisions or actions to eliminate the problem, (4) monitoring activities to assure achievement of the desired result, and (5) documentation that substantiates effectiveness of the program.[37] Because achievement of these requirements is critical in determining accreditation status, the quality assurance standard has significant impact on the structure and process of institutional quality control mechanisms.

The components of a nursing quality assurance program were originally developed by Lang[23] and adapted by the American Nurses' Association (ANA) as a model for quality assurance in nursing.[5] The evaluation model is open and circular, indicating a cyclical process that can be entered at any point (see Fig. 33-1). Discussion will begin with clarification of values and proceed clockwise.

Identification of values emphasizes the need to clarify the social, institutional, professional, and individual values, along with the advances in scientific knowledge that influence nursing practice. Examination of these beliefs offers insight into what clients, nurses, and others think is important in nursing care. Consensus among all interested parties regarding what constitutes good nursing care is needed in order to determine the standards and criteria used to judge quality.

The standards and criteria derived from the values describe the level of nursing care considered acceptable. These standards may range from minimal to achievable, excellent, or comprehensive. Standards represent the agreed-upon level of excellence, whereas criteria are specific, measurable statements that reflect the intent of the standard and can be compared to actual nursing practice.[24]

There are three types of standards and criteria in general use—structure, process, and outcome.[24] Each is aimed at a different aspect of patient care. Structure standards describe organizational, financial, and physical attributes of an agency or service and provider characteristics, such as type of educational program and years of experience. For example, a patient classification system is used to determine staffing needs; and all registered nurses must have a minimum of a baccalaureate degree in nursing. Process standards focus on the nature of activities, interventions, and sequence of events in the delivery of nursing care. Process includes nurse performance, the nurse-patient relationship, continuity and timeliness of care, and interactions with other health care professionals. For example, the nurse will systematically collect data about the patient's health status, and the nurse will treat all patients with respect. Outcome standards pertain to the end results of nursing care and measurable changes in the patient's health status. Outcomes include increased health knowledge, improved health status, and patient satisfaction. For example, the patient correctly states the names of all medications, and the patient verbalizes that pain is controlled. All three types of standards and criteria can be used alone or in combination to evaluate the quality of nursing practice. However, experts agree that no one type is sufficient to describe quality of care.

The next component involves the measurement of current nursing practice against the established standards and criteria. There are many methods that could be used to perform the comparison, including concurrent and retrospective audit, direct observation of nurse or patient performance, questionnaire, patient or nurse interview, and knowledge testing. The method selected is dependent on the purpose of the evaluation study and the available instruments and resources. Strengths and weaknesses of nursing

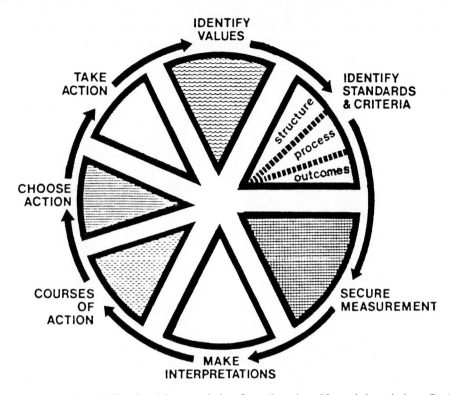

Fig. 33-1 Quality Assurance Model (Reprinted by permission from American Nurses' Association: *Quality assurance workbook*, Kansas City, Mo, 1976, The Association.)

practice should be revealed through this comparison.

Analysis and interpretation of the data follow as the next component of the model. The purpose here is the identification of discrepancies between the established criteria and the current practice. If no variations are discovered, then the remainder of the model is bypassed and one begins again with values clarification. It is unlikely, however, that no discrepancies will be found. Judgments are made about strengths, deficiencies, and other problems in quality.

Suitable courses of action are then considered. Alternatives intended to resolve discrepancies and reward strengths are identified and examined. Decisions may range from simple actions to complex plans entailing many changes. The last two components of the model consist of the selection and implementation of the best actions. Some actions may need to be performed immediately, and others take longer to initiate. The decisions about which action to choose are influenced by the organizational context and available resources. At this point, the cycle is repeated and the actions are reassessed to determine if the expected im-

provements in practice actually occurred or have been maintained.

PROFESSIONAL RESPONSIBILITY

From the professional nursing viewpoint, quality review programs are intended to "judge the quality of services provided by professional nurses and to contribute to the improvement of the delivery of nursing services by the expeditious identification and correction of decision-making problems and service deficiencies."[7] The central focus is the quality of nursing practice, recognizing that quality is related to quantity and cost. "Quality control includes attention to the related quantity of care (utilization) and to cost control so that patients receive only the care they need, provided at the lowest cost compatible with quality."[7] Professional nurses set the standards and criteria, direct the data collection, analyze the data, make the decisions, and implement changes in practice.

There are four major reasons why quality control should be the responsibility of professional nursing:

• Nursing has the right and responsibility to define

and control its own practice (professional autonomy).

- Nursing has a long history of commitment to and participation in self-regulation and serves as a model to other professions in the development of peer review mechanisms.
- Nursing has begun to examine the costs of care as related to the achieved benefits.
- If the institution assumes responsibility and accountability for quality control, the activities and decision making may not be appropriate for professional nursing.

Discussion of each of these points follows.

Professional autonomy

The autonomy of the nursing profession will be eroded if outside authorities are permitted to govern, control, or direct nursing practice. Peplau[31] argues that rapid and significant progress in public accountability will occur if regulation and control of nursing are internal to the profession. Advancement of the profession flows from innovation and refinement of explanations about nursing phenomena and ultimately benefits patients. Quality assurance and other peer review activities are a means by which nursing care is refined and quality enhanced. Nurses possess the knowledge and expertise essential to judge whether standards of practice have been achieved. They know which aspects of practice are important to consider and measure despite the fact that some dimensions of quality are intangible and difficult to quantify. Strengths and weaknesses in practice are more readily identified internally by the profession, and therefore decision making about necessary changes in practice can be more appropriate and timely. Increased outside control of practice would hinder the continued improvement of nursing service through reduction of clinical effectiveness and quality.

History of self-regulation

The nursing profession has been involved with quality control activities since the days of Florence Nightingale. She set standards for patient care and gathered evidence from the hospital wards to support her observations.[30] Since then, nursing has evaluated services continuously, but advances in quality monitoring have been most evident in the last 20 years. The reader is referred to Lang and Clinton[25,26] for an overview of the historical development of quality assurance in nursing.

Under the auspices of various nursing organiza-

tions, nursing has worked diligently to articulate its direct responsibility and accountability to the public. In particular, the ANA has promulgated a definition and scope of nursing practice, a code for nurses, generic and specialty standards of practice, a plan for implementation of practice standards, a quality assurance model, sample sets of outcome criteria, guidelines for review of nursing care at the local level, a statement on peer review in nursing practice, certification for advanced and specialty practice, certification for continuing education programs in nursing, and research guidelines.[1-4,6,7] ANA has actively promoted the participation of individuals and groups at the local level in the development of quality assurance mechanisms through workshops and conferences.[25] In addition, ANA has advocated the use of practice standards for nursing licensure.[25] The National League for Nursing (NLN) has published standards for educational and organized nursing service programs that are used nationally for accreditation purposes.

Professional nursing is a leader in the measurement of quality health care. The development of standards and criteria for nursing practice, models for quality assurance, numerous process and outcome audit tools, and instruments that assess and measure quality across populations are indicators of nursing's significant contribution.* When JCAHO created its quality assurance standards, nursing responded by conducting nursing audits using outcome criteria. Nursing continues to provide leadership in quality measurement through nursing research studies that test and refine instruments[16,18,41] and investigate relationships among the structure, process, and outcome dimensions of nursing care.[26]

Recent developments in nursing that further demonstrate the profession's commitment to increased accountability for practice include unit-based quality assurance programs, quality circles, clinical advancement programs, and self-governance structures. Unit-based quality assurance refers to the performance of quality assurance activities by the professional nursing staff at the nursing unit level.[15] Such a decentralized structure allows nursing staff to deal with immediate practice-related problems or concerns. Staff nurses identify problems, conduct evaluation studies, and institute remedial action. Individuals can see how their personal efforts directly affect the quality of care delivered on the unit. Consequently, enthusiasm for and

---

*References 8, 13, 20, 21, 25, 26, 32, 42, 45.

meaningfulness of the process are enhanced and professional expectations for practice are increased. It also is becoming the norm to monitor performance of individual nurses rather than group practice on a patient care unit.

Quality circles have emerged from industry as another way of dealing with issues in the work environment. A quality circle is a "small group of people from the same work group who meet regularly to identify, analyze, and solve work-related problems."[29] Quality circles are similar to unit-based quality assurance in that staff participate in a problem-solving process. However, quality circles have a broader focus that includes a variety of problems and situations in the work environment not aimed solely at the improvement of patient care.

Clinical advancement programs, commonly known as clinical ladders, have been devised to recognize and reward clinical competence as well as to improve the quality of care. Each level of practice is explicitly defined in terms of clinical practice behaviors. Although the number of levels and types of expected behaviors vary widely, progression to a higher level indicates increased competence. Advancement is dependent on documented evidence provided by peers and others regarding achievement of the performance criteria. Usually the committee that makes the decision about advancement has staff nurse representation. The critical role played by peer review in the clinical advancement process reinforces nursing's accountability for practice.

The creation of shared-governance structures has also strengthened the autonomy and control of professional nursing within the institution.[33] These structures enable all registered nurses to participate in decision making, regulation of nursing practice, and formulation of institutional policy. A major purpose of shared governance is the monitoring of nursing performance and the application of peer group controls. Staff bylaws describe the structure and function of the peer review problem that fulfills this purpose. Hence, shared governance is a means by which nurses assume direct responsibility and accountability for the quality of care provided.

Each of the foregoing developments incorporates the concept of peer review and demonstrates that nursing is striving to strengthen and improve practice through appropriate collaborative efforts. Health care consumers, institutions, and the nursing profession

benefit from implementation of effective peer review systems.

Cost-effectiveness

Nursing has kept pace with the changes in health care and presently is attempting to demonstrate the cost-effectiveness of nursing care.[34,36,39,40] Research results show the differences nursing structure and process can make in patient care outcomes, such as length of stay, physical health status, and patient satisfaction with nursing care received.[9-12,14,19,45] The predominant mode of care delivery has shifted from functional or team assignment to primary or total-care nursing to provide more explicit accountability for the quality of patient care. Studies of all-R.N. and primary nursing delivery systems have consistently shown reduced costs of patient care.[14,19,22] Researchers also have reported increased continuity of care, higher levels of staff and patient satisfaction, and improved physician-nurse communication with primary nursing.[19,38] Two recent developments in nursing care delivery—differentiated practice based on educational preparation and case management—are intended to enhance cost-effectiveness of care delivery and quality of care.[35,45] Patient classification schemes have been devised to objectively quantify the amount of nursing care required by patients so that the costs of nursing care and the number and kinds of staff needed to provide care can be determined.[34,40,44] With these systems, patient care workloads are more equitably and appropriately distributed. Effective allocation and utilization of nursing resources has a positive influence on the quality of nursing care in addition to being cost-effective.[44,45] These examples are evidence that the nursing profession is working toward fiscal accountability for practice while maintaining quality care.

Broader perspective of institution

The institution is concerned with overall quality control of patient services of which nursing is only a part, albeit a large one. Due to the broader focus and involvement of a greater number of disciplines, multidimensional standards and evaluation methods that are inappropriate for nursing might be used to evaluate nursing practice. The emphasis of quality assurance activities could shift from clinical decision making to completion of specific tasks and liability prevention because of the stress on cost containment. Moreover, the persons who determine the standards, collect the data, and make the decisions regarding corrective actions may be nonnurses. Nonnurses lack the necessary knowledge and expertise to make appropriate judgments about nursing practice, especially in the light of increasingly complex patient care problems. Therefore to shift responsibility to institutional administration would lead to a decline in the quality of care.

Quality control in nursing is the right and responsibility of the profession. Nursing has demonstrated full participation in self-regulatory activities and now is a leader in quality assurance mechanisms. There is little evidence to indicate that nursing has abused the privilege of self-regulation. Furthermore, nurse researchers have shown the cost-effectiveness of specific interventions and modes of care delivery. To shift responsibility to hospital administration may reduce professional control over practice, slow advancement of the profession, and change the primary emphasis from quality of care to cost.

INSTITUTIONAL RESPONSIBILITY

From the institutional perspective, the purpose of quality control is the management of professional work to achieve the goals of the organization efficiently, that is, quality care at the lowest cost. This approach is founded in an industrial model of quality control and stimulated by competition for clients and resources in the health care arena. The central focus is management processes because employees directly affect overall institutional performance and productivity. Quality control activities are conducted by institutional administration through strategic plans for quality, standard setting, direction of data collection, data interpretation, and decision making. In most institutions, however, these activities are performed in collaboration with the health professional most affected by them.

There are three major reasons why quality control should be the responsibility of the institution:
- Health care agencies are being held increasingly accountable for the performance of health care professionals.
- Organizational structures facilitate functioning of quality control mechanisms.
- The nursing profession lacks explicit accountability to the public.

These reasons stem from public pressure to bring about change in professional behavior and to provide specific control mechanisms that document perfor-

mance. Each of these points is addressed in the following discussion.

Increased accountability

Responsibility and accountability for health care have been shifted from the individual practitioner to the institutional level because the public has been critical of the way in which professionals have dealt with quality and cost issues. Restrictions through coercive legal decisions and regulations have been levied on professional autonomy in order to better serve the public. The landmark *Darling v. Charleston Community Memorial Hospital* established that hospital governing boards were ultimately responsible for provider performance and assurance of quality care. This legal judgment has been reinforced by numerous others. Federal laws and regulations governing the delivery of health care to Medicare/Medicaid recipients have mushroomed due to spiraling costs. The creation of professional standards review organizations (PSROs) was an attempt to regulate the quality of medical care. Now government has increased accountability for costs by introducing prospective payment mechanisms, that is, diagnosis-related groups. Under this system, institutions are reimbursed a predetermined amount based on the patient's medical diagnosis instead of the actual cost of care delivered.

Increasing institutional accountability is further evidenced by implementation of the JCAHO hospital-wide quality assurance standard. The intent of the standard is to make patient care review processes more objective and systematic. The standard emphasizes the integration and coordination of all quality assurance activities and the importance of targeting problems whose resolution significantly affects patient outcomes. The standard also spans all health care professionals so that communication between health care disciplines will be enhanced and fragmentation of care reduced. The actual impact of the standard is yet to be determined.

Facilitation by organizational structure

The functioning of quality control mechanisms is facilitated by the institutional structure. Because lines of responsibility, authority, and communication are designated, procedures are formalized, and resources provided, quality control is more easily achieved and thus integrated into the institutional framework. Coordination and control of professional practice through codification of standards and quality control procedures ensures systematic, regular performance evaluation, uniform data collection, reporting of results, and application of sanctions—both positive and negative. The resulting documentation of quality control activities can be used to demonstrate public accountability, enhance productivity, and justify distribution of resources.

Nursing's lack of accountability

Nursing, as a profession, lacks explicit accountability to the public for the quality of care provided.[28] Because most nurses are employed within institutions, they have been more directly accountable to the institution and physician than to the patient. In addition, accountability for performance has been modified by group or unit practice within agencies. With group practice, responsibility for the quality of care delivered is spread over a group of nurses so that individual accountability is difficult to determine. It must be noted, however, that nursing is moving toward more explicit accountability with the adoption of the primary nursing care, total care, and case management modes of care delivery.

Based on this discussion, one might conclude that quality control should be an institutional responsibility. Various regulating bodies are holding agencies more accountable for the quality of care delivered, organizational structures provide a framework that expedites quality control mechanisms, and nursing lacks explicit accountability to the public. Institutions may be in a better position to respond to the pressures for improved quality control, because quality is an organizational concern requiring integration of multiple disciplines and organizational functions.

CONCLUSIONS

To argue that responsibility for quality control lies with the profession or the institution is not logical, for in reality the obligation is a shared one. It is neither a professional nor an institutional responsibility exclusively. Currently, accountability for quality of health care is a combination of miscellaneous professional, private, and public mechanisms that have evolved along separate pathways.[27] This has resulted in jurisdictional confusion and competition for turf. However, the goal of a nursing quality assurance program is congruent with the goal of the institution to provide quality patient care. It is not a matter of who or where,

but how the joint responsibility will be fulfilled to achieve an acceptable level of nursing care at a reasonable cost. An effective quality control program requires commitment and cooperation from both nursing professionals and health care organizations. The challenge is to design control mechanisms that accommodate the needs of both the nursing profession and institutions.

Hallett[17] claims that the professions that succeed in the future will be those that blend professional and administrative knowledge. Nursing has grown up in a bureaucratic structure (the hospital) as an integral part of it. Nurses serve as managers and administrators who understand the problems unique to the profession and merge nursing knowledge with their administrative expertise. Nurse managers and administrators hold key positions within the institutional structure that allow them to facilitate the development and advancement of nursing quality control mechanisms. As long as a balance between professional and institutional jurisdictions is maintained, professional nursing and institutions will benefit from quality control activities. Thus the nursing profession seems to be well on the way to fulfilling Hallett's prescription for future success.

REFERENCES

1. American Nurses' Association: The development of ANA certification, Kansas City, Mo, 1973, The Association.
2. American Nurses' Association: Standards of nursing practice, Kansas City, Mo, 1973, The Association.
3. American Nurses' Association: A plan for implementation of the standards of nursing practice, Kansas City, Mo, 1975, The Association.
4. American Nurses' Association: Code for nurses with interpretive statements, Kansas City, Mo, 1976, The Association.
5. American Nurses' Association: Guidelines for review of nursing care at the local level, Kansas City, Mo, 1977, The Association.
6. American Nurses' Association: Nursing: a social policy statement, Kansas City, Mo, 1980, The Association.
7. American Nurses' Association: Peer review in nursing practice, Kansas City, Mo, 1983, The Association.
8. Beyers M, editor: Quality assurance, Nurs Clin North Am 23(3):613, 1988.
9. Brooten D and others: A randomized clinical trial of early hospital discharge and home follow-up of very low birth weight infants, N Engl J Med 315(15):934, 1986.
10. Crabtree M: Application of cost-benefit analysis to clinical nursing practice: a comparison of individual and group pre-operative teaching, J Nurs Admin 8(12):11, 1978.
11. Devine EC and Cook TD: A meta-analytic analysis of effects of psychoeducational interventions on length of postsurgical hospital stay, Nurs Res 32(5):267, 1983.
12. Devine EC and others: Clinical and financial effects of psychoeducational care provided by staff nurses to adult surgical pa-

tients in the post-DRG environment, Am J Public Health 78:1293, 1988.

13. Duke University Hospital Nursing Services: Guidelines for nursing care: process and outcome, Philadelphia, 1983, JB Lippincott.

14. Fagin CM: The economic value of nursing research, Am J Nurs 82(12):1844, 1982.

15. Formella N and Schroeder P: The unit-based system. In Schroeder P and Maibusch R, editors: Nursing quality assurance: a unit-based approach, Rockville, Md, 1984, Aspen Systems Corp.

16. Fox R and Ventura M: Internal psychometric characteristics of the Quality Patient Care Scale, Nurs Res 33(2):112, 1984.

17. Hallet J: Challenge of looking at tomorrow through today's eyes. Paper presented at the American Nurses' Association Convention, June 1984.

18. Hinshaw AS and Atwood JR: A patient satisfaction instrument: precision by replication, Nurs Res 31(3):170, 1982.

19. Hinshaw AS, Scofield R, and Atwood JR: Staff, patient and cost outcomes of all-registered nurse staffing, J Nurs Adm 11(11,12):30, 1981.

20. Horn B and Swain MA: Criterion measures for nursing care quality, NTIS No PB-287 499/3GA, Hyattsville, Md, 1978, National Center for Health Services Research.

21. Jelinek R and others: A methodology for monitoring quality of nursing care, DHEW Publication No 76-25, Washington, DC, 1974, US Government Printing Office.

22. Jones K: Study documents effects of primary nursing on renal transplant patients, Hospitals 49(24):85, 1975.

23. Lang NM: A model for quality assurance in nursing. Doctoral dissertation, Marquette University, 1974.

24. Lang NM: Quality assurance review in nursing, Am J Maternal-Child Nurs 1(2):77, 1976.

25. Lang NM and Clinton JF: Assessment and assurance of the quality of nursing care: a selected overview, Eval Health Professions 6(2):211, 1983.

26. Lang NM and Clinton JF: Assessment of quality nursing care. In Werley HH and Fitzpatrick J, editors: Annual review of nursing research, vol 2, New York, 1984, Springer.

27. Lohr K, Yordy K, and Thier S: Current issues in quality of care, Health Affairs 7(1):5, 1988.

28. Luke R and Modrow R: Professionalism, accountability, and peer review. In Luke R, Krueger J, and Modrow R, editors: Organization and change in health care quality assurance, Rockville, Md, 1983, Aspen Systems Corp.

29. Maser M: Mount Sinai invests in quality circles, Health Serv Manager 15(2):12, 1982.

30. Nightingale F: Notes on matters affecting the health, efficiency, and hospital administration of the British army, London, 1858, Harrison & Sons.

31. Peplau H: Internal vs. external regulation, NJ Nurse 14(1):13, 1984.

32. Phaneuf M: The nursing audit: self-regulation in nursing practice, New York, 1976, Appleton-Century-Crofts.

33. Porter-O'Grady T and Finnigan S: Shared governance for nursing, Rockville, Md, 1984, Aspen Systems Corp.

34. Prescott P and Phillips C: Gauging nursing intensity to bring costs to light, Nurs Health Care 9(1):17, 1988.

35. Primm P: Differentiated practice for ADN- and BSN-prepared nurses, J Prof Nurs 3(4):218, 1987.

36. Shaffer F, editor: Costing out nursing: pricing our product, New York, 1985, National League for Nursing.

37. Shanahan M: The quality assurance standard of the JCAH: a rational approach to patient care evaluation. In Luke R, Krueger J, and Modrow R, editors: Organization and change in health care quality assurance, Rockville, Md, 1983, Aspen Systems Corp.

38. Shukla R: Structure vs. people in primary nursing: an inquiry, Nurs Res 30(4):236, 1981.

39. Sovie M, Tarcinale M, and VanPutte A: Amalgam of nursing acuity, DRGs and costs, Nurs Manage 16(3):22, 1985.

40. Thompson JD and Diers D: Management of nursing intensity, Nurs Clin North Am 23(3):473, 1988.

41. Ventura M and others: Correlations of two quality of nursing care measures, Res Nurs Health 5:37, 1982.

42. Wandelt M and Ager J: Quality patient care scale, New York, 1974, Appleton-Century-Crofts.

43. Wandelt M and Stewart D: Slater nursing competencies rating scale, New York, 1975, Appleton-Century-Crofts.

44. Young J and others: Factors affecting nurse staffing in acute care hospitals: a review and critique of the literature, DHEW Publication HRA No 81-10, Washington, DC, 1981, US Government Printing Office.

45. Zander K: Nursing case management: strategic management of cost and quality outcomes, J Nurs Adm 18(5):23, 1988.

CHAPTER 34

Viewpoints

Measuring the quality of nursing care

LINDA C. HODGES
MARY LOUISE ICENHOUR

Measuring the quality of nursing care may be the single most important goal of the nursing profession in the 1980s. Certainly all indicators point to the fact that quality will be the new buzzword in health care as we face the 1990s. A renewed emphasis on the measurement of quality in contemporary health care can be attributed to a focus on quality directives instituted by the American business community. This interest, reflected in best-selling nonfiction titles on quality measurement from the corporate world, illustrates a new appreciation for the economic power of quality in the marketplace.

The health care industry, like other sectors of the business community, has shown an increased interest in quality measurement. Now that the shock of diagnosis related groups (DRGs) has lessened and health care professionals have successfully responded to that particular system of reimbursement, efforts to measure the quality of care, particularly as it relates to cost, have reemerged as a national outgrowth of rapid change. Other factors also have contributed to a renewed interest in quality health care. Principal among these are consumer demands, health professionals' concerns about the impact of shorter hospital stays on patient outcomes, and third-party payer demands for a greater return on dollars spent for health care services delivered.

Consumer demand for quality health care can be attributed to an increase in knowledge of services that meet a degree of excellence. The increased cost of health care also has affected consumer interest in quality services. As more Americans graduate from high schools and universities including health education in diploma or degree requirements, and as the public in general becomes more informed about health through the media, the mystique of medicine is disappearing. Patients are asking questions about professional credentials and hospital ratings. Increased numbers are also seeking second opinions. As third-party payers increase copayments, the cost of health care is felt on a personal level. As with other goods and services, the consumer is now approaching health care with demands for quality at a reasonable price.

The quality of care is also a major concern for health professionals. As a result of DRGs, patients are in the hospital less time and often return to their homes in need of nursing care. The quality of discharge planning as a component of hospital nursing care has received increased emphasis as professional nurses attempt to bridge the gap between the care received in the hospital and the care needed in the home. For example, the length of stay in maternal-infant units is now so short that the notion of waiting to teach the new mother to care for her baby during the taking-in phase has become passé. The concept of quality nursing care as it was known before DRGs and the current nursing shortage has had to be reconceptualized to fit with the rapidly changing health care delivery system.

Third-party payers are also demanding and reemphasizing quality health care services. The cost of health care during the 1980s has escalated at an unprecedented rate. Currently 12% of the gross national product is spent on health care. Businesses are finding that a greater portion of profits must be allocated to employee health insurance plans, and insurance companies are having difficulty meeting payment schedules while at the same time they are increasing insurance premiums. The largest third-party payer, the federal government, continues to struggle with increasing demands for Medicare- and Medicaid-funded health care programs in the wake of a growing federal deficit. As health care costs continue to rise with no ceiling in sight, consumers, businesses, insurance companies, and the federal government increasingly will put pressure on providers to deliver quality health care services at affordable prices. Methods for measuring quality care as it relates to cost must be established to answer cost-accounting questions of major third-party payers. Since nursing represents a major cost center, there is an urgent need to develop measurement tools and systems to demonstrate the cost-effectiveness of quality nursing care as related to positive patient outcomes, the product line of hospitals.

Although the business community has led the way toward quality measurement, the concern for quality has become the central focus of health care management at the close of the decade. Beckham states that "the 1980s will go down in history as the decade when quality comes out of the closet."[1] Consumers, health care providers, and third-party payers will demand a full accounting of dollars spent for care received.

Cyclical nature of the health care system

Quality is one of four basic concepts underlying any health care system. These four factors are cost, equity, access, and quality. One of these factors tends to dominate the U.S. health care system and thus health care policy at any one time. For example, access to health care was the dominant theme in the Johnson era, more health care legislature was passed than at any other time in history.[17] The advent of Medicare and Medicaid programs provided access to the system and increased the use of health care services. As services expanded and demand increased, so did cost. With rising costs, the focus shifted from access to cost containment, as pressures grew in the health care system in the late 1970s and early 1980s to reduce the price tag for health care.

The passage of federal law 98-21, which instituted the system for prospective payment, was an outcome of the public's growing concern about health care costs.[8] This system of payment, based on time-limited utilization of services for specific medical diagnoses, rewards hospitals discharging patients early. The move to early discharge has helped to refocus the health care system on the issue of quality health care delivery. There is a growing concern among all segments of the health care industry that quality may be sacrificed in an effort to contain costs. The quality theme is expected to extend well into the 1990s as health poli-

cymakers strive to meet the nation's health care needs in the belief that quality care as an expectation is possible. The ability to deliver quality care at a reasonable cost will be the measure of success in the future.

Quality defined

The concept of quality is viewed by different people in different ways. *Webster's* defines quality as "a degree of excellence; a peculiar and essential character."[4] As applied to quality of care, several definitions are found in the literature. Lang and Clinton[16] suggest that quality assessment is the identification and measurement of a certain level of quality of care. Quality assurance in nursing implies that a level of quality can be defined and measured, and that the public can be assured of that level of care.

In Donabedian's seminal work on quality measurement,[10] quality of care is regarded as "the management by a physician or any other health care practitioner of a clearly definable episode of illness for any given patient." DeGeynt[6] argues that quality is defined primarily as the "degree of conformity with present standards" and is focused on patient care as opposed to medical or health care.[6] Consumer satisfaction is viewed by McMillan[18] as an essential component in the measurement of quality of health care. Universally, the measurement of quality examines the attainment of predetermined norms and standards of health care.

QUALITY CARE MEASUREMENT MODELS

Several authors have proposed models for the measurement of quality of care.[10,14] The best known was originated by Donabedian and remains the framework for most research in quality measurement. Donabedian posits that quality of health care can be measured in three ways: as structure, process, and outcome. The structural aspects include institutions (physical facilities, equipment, etc.), programs, and health care providers. The level of quality is determined by relating available resources to any and all of the patient's or the community's health needs. A predetermined standard for numbers and attributes of structural components is needed for quality to be judged as present. DeGeynt[6] argues that using the structure method alone to measure quality narrows considerably the meaning of the concept and the extent to which it can be measured.

The process method is the broad view of all activities that go on between health care providers and patients. A judgment of the quality of these activities may be made by either direct observation or an overview of recorded information that allows the evaluator to reconstruct activities occurring between the patient and the practitioner. A review of the patient's chart is the measure most commonly used in quality assurance programs. Coyne and Killien[5] state that quality assurance is a process that involves evaluating the quality of patient care provided in a particular setting, through establishing standards for care and implementing mechanisms for ensuring that the standards are met. The process method allows evaluation of quality measures of nursing care and care provided by other health care practitioners as well.

The third approach to quality measurement, and one that is suggested as the new directive, is the outcome measurement approach. Donabedian refers to outcome as that part of quality measurement indicating a change in a patient's current or future health status that can be attributed to antecedent health care. In his definition *outcome* in its broadest sense means the improvement of social, psychological, and physical health status. He suggests that outcome measures can also measure various patient attitudes toward health care, including patient satisfaction, patient knowledge of the health care regimen, and any health care behavioral change in the patient. Using this approach it is theoretically possible to measure the exact implications of nursing care: its effectiveness, quality, and the time previously allocated for care.

Recent health services research has shown a renewed interest in the outcome method for quality measurement. Williamson[21] suggests this method has the greatest potential for measuring the implications of health care and the patient's health status after care has been delivered. Starfield[20] has developed an outcome model of quality measurement that addresses the levels of the patient's health status after discharge. She uses a health status profile of seven categories of patient functioning to indicate the effectiveness of previous care. Brook and colleagues also believe that measurement of the process method alone is a narrow approach and that does not measure the care delivered as effectively as do outcome measures.[3]

RESEARCH IN QUALITY OUTCOMES

Donabedian has reviewed the past 20 years of quality studies and suggests that there are two new directions in research studying quality outcomes of care. The first group of studies examine "favorable adverse outcomes," noting mortality and case fatality as quality judgments in and of themselves. An example of such a study would be one conducted at a large university medical center in which institutional differences are noted in the risk of postsurgical fatality. The second grouping of outcome studies identifies adverse outcomes as tools to assess antecedent processes of care.[9] Williamson's studies[21] illustrate this approach, which consists of specifying criteria one expects to achieve and whether or not the outcomes have actually been met. If they have not, the antecedent process and structure of care are carefully examined, especially for those groups of patients who appear to be more vulnerable to substandard care.

The identification of criteria for quality remains difficult because frequently such criteria are value based. It has been suggested that all quality criteria are derived from patient and provider values and perceptions of quality. An accepted model of quality frequently is developed in which these values are integrated with actual organization practice as to what and how care is delivered. Goals of care based on both patient and provider expectations of quality are advantageous, since critical components of care such as health education, patient individuality, and staffing needs are integrated.[19]

Hemenway analyzes the use of outcomes measures from an economic perspective. He posits that although process measurement of care results in measuring levels of performance, process attributes are not proxy measures of outcomes. He quotes Feldstein, stating that "although outcome measures are difficult to determine it would allow more flexibility for the health care professional to achieve outcomes rather than identifying those process measures which may or may not bring about desired outcomes.[14]

The fact that process measures cannot be used to predict outcome is well illustrated in Icenhour's research findings.[15] In a study of quality of care outcomes in ambulatory surgery it was found that although all surgical patients were taught either at the time of discharge or during their ambulatory surgical stay, few patients achieved learning outcomes as established in the outcome quality criteria. The following patient examples from her study illustrate the difference in measuring process versus outcome criteria of quality.

John W., a 37-year old employed postal worker, is discharged after a tumor excision on his back. It was documented (process measures) that both the patient and his wife received instruction on dressing changes. No determination was made at the time of discharge from ambulatory surgery that they knew or understood sterile dressing changes (outcome measures). During a postoperative interview one week later, it was found that the patient's dressings were never changed and that he was being treated for a staphylococcus wound infection.

Mary P is a 57-year old housewife who had surgery on her foot; she required crutches to walk after her discharge from ambulatory surgery. Documentation mentioned only that the patient was issued crutches at the time of discharge (process measure). After discharge she fell while incorrectly using her crutches, injuring her right wrist. Both the physician's office and the surgery center believed the other had taught her crutch walking. No attempt had been made by either to determine her proficiency in the use of crutches (outcome measure).

In this study, process methods alone determined that the patients received quality patient instructions; however, when outcome quality criteria were implemented few patients were found to have achieved the level of patient learning that would have enabled them to carry out compliant, safe, surgical care on their own after discharge. Therefore measuring outcomes of care according to predetermined quality criteria has a greater potential to more accurately identify areas of nonquality health care interventions.

Although individual writers hold slightly different views about quality, there are several commonalities that emerge from a review of their approaches:

1. Quality can be measured
2. Quality measures a standard or a degree of excellence
3. Excellence needs to be determined by validating standards of care or by measurement of professional conduct when caring for patients

These statements represent a beginning point in the consideration of quality measurement in health care. The debatable issue, in our view, is the question of what to measure and, more important, at what point in the health care delivery system quality should be measured. The underlying question for professional nursing is, when in the nursing management of patients will measurement be most effective, most accurate, and measure patient satisfaction, while at the same time indicating what nursing interventions are the most cost effective and providing the greatest opportunity to deliver quality nursing care?

It is our view that the outcome of nursing care should be the primary focus of quality measurement in nursing practice and that outcome should be measured at the conclusion of care in any setting or health care institution. We believe that measurement of antecedent care is the most informative measure and has the greatest potential to influence future nursing care and the accountability of professional practice. It is also consistent with new quality measurement directives from such accreditation bodies as the Joint Commission on Accreditation of Healthcare Organizations (JCAHO). In addition, the measurement of nursing care outcomes vis-à-vis cost is needed to firmly establish the value of nursing care in the health care delivery system. These data can be used to establish a desired staff mix and to justify the use of advanced nursing role practitioners such as clinical nurse specialists, nurse-midwives, and nurse-anesthetists.

The major thrust of quality measurement in nursing in the past has been a measurement of process or an analysis of the degree of compliance with nursing care standards evidenced during a specific episode of patient care. In this model, most institutions have developed standards of nursing practice as related to DRGs or standards related to frequently performed nursing activities such as medication administration or postoperative care.[13] A system for monitoring compliance with the standards, usually through randomized chart audits, is the most commonly used method in quality assurance programs. A standard for patient education regarding self-medication might include the question, Was the patient taught the nature of the medication and how to properly self administer? If the documentation for patient teaching is appropriate, the assumption is that quality nursing care has been delivered. If there is no follow-up on self-medication following discharge, one cannot determine whether the time spent teaching the patient (cost of nursing service) indeed resulted in appropriate self-medication. Therefore measuring only the structural and process aspects of quality of care, when outcomes can be determined only after discharge, falls far short as a measurement of quality. In other words, efficiency does not always guarantee effectiveness.

MEASURING QUALITY CARE

In a recent presentation to members of the American Association of Colleges of Nursing, Diers[7] described a model for quality care measurement (Figure 34-1). In this model,[12] services rendered in the health care delivery system result in products such as X-rays, lab test results, hours of patient care delivered, and meals served. These products or intermediate outputs

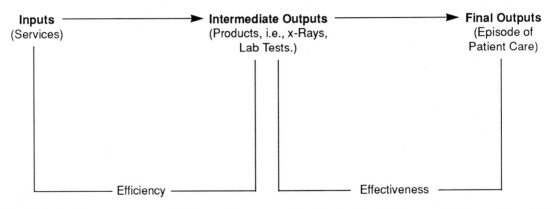

Fig. 34-1 Quality as a measure of efficiency of resource utilization (cost) and outcome effectiveness (benefits).

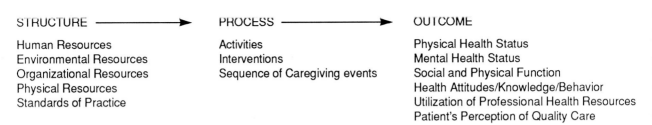

Fig. 34-2 Donabedian's model of quality care measurement.

delivered over a given episode of patient care result in a final output or outcome. When comparing the cost of producing products to final outcomes, a measure of quality of care can be determined based on cost. Diers maintains that data-based arguments in nursing are necessary to relate efficiency to effectiveness and that a comparison of these will be the basis for determining quality in the future. Therefore, unlike past measures of quality that emphasized one component of Donabedian's model (Figure 34-2) over another, the future of quality measurement will seek an integrative approach using cost efficiency of nursing care.

This model (Figure 34-1) of measurement of quality of nursing care views nursing services of a specific type (staff mix and model, i.e., primary care, modular care) as an input that results in a product (patient care hours delivered in compliance with predetermined standards).

It provides a means for analyzing the efficiency or productivity of the nursing unit with respect to care for a specific patient during a given hospital stay. If measurement stops here, as with many quality assurance programs, the most critical question remains unanswered: Did efficient utilization of services delivered according to standards result in quality patient outcomes? By focusing on outcomes as compared to in-

puts (structure and process), the questions become (1) How effective is the utilization of services delivered according to standards? and (2) Comparing the quality of outcome, was the cost efficiency of services within an acceptable range? An integrative model has the potential to address all pertinent issues of nursing care while simultaneously using new aspects of measurement such as computers and cost accounting.

A SYSTEMATIC MEASURE OF QUALITY NURSING CARE

With the aid of new computer technology, nursing has a golden opportunity to demonstrate to the consumer the cost-effectiveness of professional nursing care. In an effort to establish costs for health care services, pressure is being brought to bear on the health care industry to design systems for costing out nursing services. In conjunction with this push from the consumer sector, the JCAHO is refocusing accreditation criteria from a primary emphasis on management and equipment to determining if patient outcomes meet established standards. Effective quality assurance programs in successful health care institutions of the future must be designed to include comprehensive database systems that not only incorporate structure and

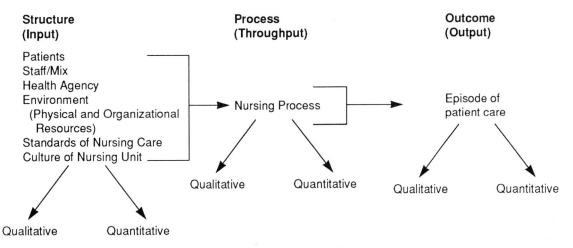

Fig. 34-3 A systematic integrative approach to quality nursing care management.

process variables but also relate them to measurable patient outcomes. To survive in the competitive arena of today's health care delivery systems, these outcomes must be analyzed for cost-effectiveness.

A systematic integrative model for quality care measurement such as that delineated in Figure 34-3 will determine quality of outcomes based on antecedents (structural elements and process). In such a model, aspects of structure or inputs into the nursing care system include elements of the setting in which the nursing care is given such as available equipment and supplies, staff mix, standards set for patient care, characteristics of the patients themselves, and cultural norms of the nursing unit. According to Donabedian,[11] the culture within an organization is the most crucial factor associated with quality care. Therefore the professionalism of the nursing staff should be a consideration in research designs to measure structure.

The process elements measured in such a systemic approach would address the interactions among the nurse, the patient, and the patient's environment. Timely nursing interventions must be determined for nursing diagnoses. The complexity of interventions delivered at an appropriate time in the episode of care delivery must be addressed, as well as the way the care is delivered (the art of nursing). Standards of care developed today are written to elicit objective data. The more subtle subjective aspects of the nursing process that are equally important are, however, more difficult to determine. These aspects relate to the judgments made and attitudes underpinning nursing actions. To date the most comprehensive nursing study exemplifying research into this area of the nursing process is Benner's work on the expert practitioner.[2]

The third component of a systematic model for quality care measurement and the primary focus is outcome. This aspect of quality of care is highly valued by the consumer but often in the past has been neglected as a major measure in quality assurance programs. Arguments have concerned the difficulty of equating outcomes with care delivered given the limited control of variables including genetic makeup, social and environmental factors, and attitudes governing behavior such as adherence to prescribed self-care regimens. Also, research methodologies used to determine outcomes following discharge, such as longitudinal studies that often include time-consuming interviews and content analysis, are costly to conduct.

When considering past nursing research on the assessment and assurance of quality nursing care, Lang and Clinton[16] found many studies that could be categorized as either fitting with the concept of structure, process, or outcome. There remain relatively few studies that approach the measurement of quality from a comprehensive perspective relating outcome to structure and process. Clearly the methodology for research in the field is not as yet well defined. Consideration of quantitative measures alone is too narrow. Identification of the number of professional nurses on a given unit does not provide information about the qualitative aspects such as attitude and commitment to excellence in patient care delivery. There is a need to design research methods that include both quantitative and qualitative dimensions. These methods must cut across all aspects of quality care measurement: structure, process, and outcome. Additionally, studies must be designed to determine the cost-effectiveness of the quality care measure. Therefore a model such as that described in Figure 34-3 would fit the requirements of measurement using the relative components of health care.

MEANS TO A METHOD

As we face the task of defining an acceptable measure of nursing care quality that can be delivered in a cost-effective manner, the development of technology and professional standards will serve the profession well. In addition, we now have a greater number of doctorally prepared nurses with skills in both quantitative and qualitative research methodology. These researchers will provide the designs needed to integrate structure, process, and outcome with appropriate research methods.

The developments in information processing as applied to the health care field now allow comprehensive documentation of nursing care delivery. New software packages are being developed to integrate data on patient care outcomes with those of process and structure. The cost aspects are also being programmed into the directives for analysis. Research projects designed by nursing Ph.D.s employed in hospital settings are addressing the efficiency of staff mix and other resource inputs against compliance of nursing standards and patient care outcomes. We are on the threshold of a new era in the development of quality assurance programs with dollar signs attached.

SUMMARY

As we move toward the 1990s there is a great need for nursing to make a strong commitment to the measurement of the quality of nursing care. Indeed, our future as a profession may depend on our ability to statistically demonstrate professional nursing's value to society. This will mean that nursing education and service must work together to address the issue by educating those nurse researchers who have the knowledge and skills to design measurement tools capable of delineating the comprehensive nature of quality nursing care provided by the practitioner in the field. The use of an integrative model focused on outcome will be able to prove the cost benefits of professional nursing care. Patients recover with fewer complications, need less pain medications, and are more satisfied with their health care when they are cared for by professional nurses. For the first time the technology is available for quantifying patient outcomes according to a rigorous research-based model. Now is the time to make research into the cost-effectiveness of quality nursing care a national priority.

REFERENCES

1. Beckham DJ: The quality revolution: how to meet the challenge, Health Care Competition Week, November 2, 1987.
2. Benner P: From novice to expert, Mento Park, Calif, 1984, Addison Wesley.
3. Brook KR *and others:* Quality of medical care assessment using outcome measures: an overview of the method, Santa Monica, Calif, 1976, Rand Corp.
4. Buralnick DB, editor: Webster's new world dictionary, ed 2, New York, 1980, Simon & Schuster.
5. Coyne C and Killien M: A system for unit based management of quality of nursing care, J Nurs Adm 17(1):26, 1987.
6. DeGeynt W: Five approaches for assessing the quality of care, Hospital Administration 15(1):21, 1970.
7. Diers D: Examining options for leadership: how we should respond. Proceedings of the American Association of Colleges of Nursing's summer seminar, Wyoming, June 1988.
8. Dobson A *and others:* The future of medicine policy reform: priority for research and determination, Health Care Financing Review (suppl):1, 1986.
9. Donabedian A: The epidemiology of quality, Inquiry 22(suppl):282, 1988.
10. Donabedian A: The definition of quality and approaches to its assessment, Ann Arbor, Mich, 1980, Health Administration Press.
11. Donabedian A: The quality of medical care, Science 200(4344):856, 1978.
12. Fetter RB and Frieman JL: Product line management in hospitals, Academy of Management Review, 11(12):41, 1986.
13. Harrington P and Kaniecki N: Standards and Q.A.-A common sense approach, Nursing Management 19(1):24, 1988.
14. Hemenway D: Quality assessment from an economic perspective, Evaluation and the Health Professions 6(4):379, 1983.
15. Icenhour ML: Quality interpersonal care: a study of ambulatory surgery, patients perspectives. AORN J, 47(6):1414, 1988.
16. Lang NM and Clinton JF: Assessment and the assurance of the quality of nursing care, Evaluation and the Health Professions, 6(2):211, 1983.
17. Litman T: Government and health: the political aspects of health care—a sociopolitical overview. In Litman T and Robins LS, editors: Health politics and policy, New York, 1984, John Wiley & Sons, Inc.
18. McMillan JR: Measuring consumers satisfaction to improve quality of care, Health Progress, 3:54, 1987.
19. O'Brian N and others: A managerial perspective in controlling the quality of patient care, Dimensions, p 22, May 1987.
20. Starfield BH: Measurement of options: a proposed scheme, Milbank Memorial Fund Quarterly 52:39, 1974.
21. Williamson JW: Assessing and improving health care outcomes: the health accounting approach to quality assurance, Cambridge, Mass, 1978, Ballinger Publishing Co.

CHAPTER 35

Quality assurance in long-term care

LUCIA GAMROTH
JOY SMITH

Is quality assurance in long-term care (LTC) different from quality assurance in any segment of the health care system? The purpose of this chapter is to explore the answer to that question, to look at different quality assurance efforts, and to draw some conclusions about the essence of a quality program. Although LTC covers an entire spectrum of services across different settings, it is limited in this discussion to long-term care facilities licensed and certified as intermediate or skilled facilities.

Sliefert, in this volume (see Chapter 33), defines the basic elements of quality assurance as "standard setting, comparison of standard to actual practice, analysis and interpretation of the data, selection and implementation of actions to change practice, and feedback on the results of the action." The process of quality assurance in LTC incorporates those elements and is essentially the same as it is in any organization. The differences and difficulties exist within the elements of the process.

Antecedent to the measurement and assurance of quality is the definition of quality. Quality of LTC has been defined as patient or resident satisfaction, safety, prevention of poor outcomes, communication and coordination of care, and medical and nursing services that meet recognized standards of care. Others[4] would include "accessibility and continuity of care or cost-effectiveness." Residents have defined the elements of quality as the ability to make choices, to exercise control over their lives, and to be treated with dignity by staff with positive, caring attitudes.[13] According to Kurowski and Shaughnessy,[9] "The many definitions (and resulting measures) of the quality of long-term care demonstrate its complexity and multidimensionality."

Several phenomena have contributed to the complexity of this issue, including the concept of the home, in addition to the treatment center, as an LTC facility; the nature of chronic illness and disability; the development of public policy and the regulatory process; and the failure of nursing homes to assure adequate quality.

HOME ENVIRONMENT

LTC facilities, in general, are both treatment and living situations in which health care and social support are provided to persons for a period of months or years. The National Citizens' Coalition for Nursing Home Reform (NCCNHR),[13] in a survey of nursing home residents, identified as critical to quality care the ability to make choices and to exercise control over such things as diet, sleeping and rising times, activities, and visits with friends. That is quite a different expectation than exists in acute care facilities. "Many aspects of nursing home life that affect a resident's perceptions of quality of life—and therefore, sense of well-being—are intimately intertwined with quality of care,"[6] and the distinction between quality of life and quality of care becomes blurred. An institution can assure quality of care but it cannot assure quality of life. Even assuring quality of care, however, has its difficulties.

NATURE OF CHRONIC ILLNESS

LTC residents typically have multiple diagnoses and interacting conditions for which there are no easy classification schemes or predictable outcomes. For example, if a patient is admitted with a hip pinning, the treatment would be fairly predictable. However, the hip wound may be infected and draining, the person may be diabetic and have a cardiac condition as well.

Chronic conditions generally require restorative or maintenance services with an emphasis on attaining small improvements or preventing undue decline rather than on the intensive efforts of acute medicine that usually aim for cures, remissions, or other substantial improvements.[6]

A look at structure, process, and outcome criteria as defined by Donabedian[2] illustrates some of the difficulties in determining criteria for quality assurance.

Structural criteria

Structural criteria refer to the capacity of the facility to provide good quality care; they include human, organizational, and supply resources. Staffing ratios, policies and procedures, required consultants, and life safety codes are all examples of structural criteria. Structural criteria are easily measured and consequently have provided the basis for regulatory review until very recently. The problem with structural criteria is that they measure the capacity to provide quality care but do not measure the care actually given or the outcomes of the care. Consequently, facilities could be in compliance with all the structural criteria and, at the same time, have very poor resident outcomes. Conversely, a facility could demonstrate excellent resident outcomes and be cited for paperwork deficiencies. Providers have objected to this approach for years and only recently have efforts of regulatory agencies shifted to a process-and-outcome approach to evaluating quality of care.

Process criteria

Process criteria refer to the procedures or interventions that constitute the service provided. An example of the difficulty in determining process criteria is illustrated in the treatment of a skin condition. There are many approaches to the treatment of skin conditions, and what works for one patient may not work for another. This is due to many factors, such as nutrition, mobility, and cardiac status, in addition to an individual's immune response and cooperation with the treatment protocol. So although process criteria are important, they are very difficult to agree upon and to measure with any validity. More needs to be done to describe effective interventions and to document the relationship of interventions to outcomes.

Outcome criteria

Outcome evaluation in patient care has received a great deal of attention recently as the most appropriate way to approach the concept of quality. Kane[8] discusses the difficulty of using death, disability, and discharge as outcome criteria. Death rates in LTC are not good outcome indicators because many people spend their last days in LTC facilities and many come there for terminal care. Disability as an indicator must also be evaluated because many residents are disabled on admission. Discharge for the short-term resident is a realistic goal but may be inappropriate for the long-term resident.

Kane goes on to discuss the varied needs of a heterogeneous population for emotional well-being and social interaction. Although it is reasonable for staff to address some needs that are short term or are related to the patient's condition, it cannot provide for long-standing deficits.

Conceptually, attaining appropriate outcome represents the ultimate validation of the effectiveness of the care process. However, it is extremely difficult to specify appropriate outcomes of care and to empirically demonstrate their relationship to the process of care.[9]

WHO DECIDES?

Although process and outcome criteria may be the best indicators of quality, there remains one critical question. Who determines the desirable and appropriate intervention or outcome? Is it the resident, the professional staff, or the regulatory agency? The following are examples of such dilemmas.

A. The facility dining room seats approximately 50 residents and guests for dinner. Knowing when dinner is served, residents come to the dining room when they wish. They enjoy a glass of wine and a salad at their table (the table they have chosen to sit at for many months or years). The entree is served individually, followed by a dessert and beverage of their choice. The surveyor cites deficiencies in the following areas: (1) the time between the first course and main course is too long, (2) salt and sugar are readily available to persons at the table, and (3) the entree is not served on a tray.

In this instance, the resident knows when the hot food will be served and chooses to come to the dining room a bit early. The presence of salt and sugar is appropriate to a homelike atmosphere, as is the individual serving of entrees. The surveyor is afraid that someone who should not have salt and sugar may easily get them and, further, that without trays there may be improper identification of resident and kind of diet.

For most persons the choices by the resident and staff are appropriate. The surveyor, however, feels bound to cite this in a survey as a "potential hazard to residents," even though no adverse patient outcomes were cited on the survey. Who has made the quality decision?

B. In another situation, the facility staff has developed expertise in dealing with the wandering resident. The facility has a "code 10" procedure to locate wanderers that involves every staff person in the facility. The facility and grounds are combed within a matter of seconds to minutes. In addition, high-risk wanderers wear an alarm on the arm or leg that is triggered by a person exiting through a designated door. The code program has been effective for three years and the alarm system has been in place for the last year. Residents are allowed to wander, which gives them a sense of freedom. There are no high-risk residents at the time of the survey who need an alarm device. The facility is cited for inadequate precautions for the wandering residents. Who has made the quality decision?

C. Another example relates to the use of restraints and siderails. Nurses in LTC can all tell stories of how a resident untied a restraint and, because the siderails were up, crawled over the end of the bed at night to go to the bathroom. Research studies have shown that although the incidence of falls is higher without than with the use of restraints, the incidence of serious injury remains the same.[10] And yet, if the state regulatory system requires reporting all falls as potential patient abuse, there is not much incentive to decrease the use of restraints. Whose safety is at stake?

There are many examples of these dilemmas. But the point is that values and interpretations of situations will differ according to particular perspectives. The resident and staff deal with these situations each day and are in the best position to evaluate what is appropriate. The surveyor, coming in as an outsider, certainly needs to raise questions but must have the capability to determine what is reasonable and logical without fear of reprisal from some other regulatory body. Quality often requires the balancing of conflicting goals and values, such as patient safety and patient independence, and those goals must be evaluated with reference to one another.

Quality assurance in LTC is in its infancy. A great deal of study needs to be undertaken to determine appropriate process and outcome criteria. Balancing a homelike atmosphere and personal choices with quality nursing care for individual patients as well as for the total group requires continual evaluation.

The discussion to this point has focused on two ways that LTC is different: (1) home environment and (2) the difficulties of defining and measuring appropriate structural, process, and outcome criteria for a very heterogeneous population in LTC. Despite the difficulties, significant efforts have been made to measure and assure quality.

QUALITY ASSURANCE EFFORTS
Peer review

In 1985 the Joint Commission for the Accreditation of Health Care Organizations (JCAHCO) published a guide to quality assurance in LTC; it has since sponsored several workshops on the subject. The Commission's 1988 LTC standards manual[17] includes revised standards for quality assurance (QA). JCAHCO is currently working on the development of outcome measures as a part of an "agenda for change" initiative.

Association efforts

In 1982 the American Health Care Association published *Quest for Quality*,[1] one of the first overall views of quality assurance purposes and tools specific to nursing homes. *Quest for Quality* provides the basis for QA programs in many nursing homes across the country. "In January 1988, Washington State Health Care Association (WSHCA) began implementation of the first industry driven, third-party administered, Quality Validation Program in the nation."[1] All members of WSHCA are required to participate in the program administered by JCAHCO, to validate the quality of provider services, assist facilities with identified problems, and establish an index of quality for overall performance.

Incentive programs

Several states have developed quality measurement programs based on outcome measures. New York has developed a program to meet the state's review requirements; entitled Sentinal Health Events (SHE) it identified undesirable or unexpected outcomes.[12] If the incidence of a particular outcome exceeds the norm of the facilities in the state, a second level of review is triggered that looks at process related to a given outcome. The purpose of the second level of review is to determine whether or not the poor outcome is related to poor care. The issues that the surveyor attempts to resolve include whether a problem should be cited as an isolated problem requiring corrections or whether it is part of a wider pattern of poor patient care in the facility.

Illinois has initiated a program called Quality Incentive Program (QUIP).[5] QUIP identifies problem areas in a facility and provides a financial incentive if the facility shows improvement in those areas. The quality incentive standards are designed to be higher than those for the licensure, certification, and inspection of care surveys. The standards are targeted at those aspects of a facility's care and services that can have the greatest impact on a resident's health, sense of well-being, and quality of life.

Regulatory efforts

Regulatory efforts at assuring quality have been relatively ineffective, for reasons that are best understood in the context of history. Vladeck, in his book *Unloving Care*,[14] and the Institute of Medicine (IOM) study[6] provide excellent historical accounts of the development of LTC public policy and regulatory changes. The growth of nursing homes in this country resulted from the authorization in 1935 of Social Security and the Old-Age Assistance program. In 1950 amendments to the Social Security Act specified a requirement for state licensure of participating facilities but did not define any standards for care.

Nearly 30 years after the program began the Public Health Service issued the Nursing Home Standards Guide which was a combined effort of the Public Health Service, the states, and providers of care. Medicare and Medicaid were enacted in 1965, and amendments passed in 1967 authorized the Department of Health, Education, and Welfare (HEW) to develop standards and to withhold payments from skilled nursing homes not meeting the standards.

The Senate created a Special Committee on Aging and held congressional hearings throughout the 1960s on nursing home problems. The hearings resulted in a series of reports on the deficiencies of the federal regulatory efforts.

In 1972 Congress passed legislation giving federal funding to state surveys and certification activities and directed HEW to develop a single set of standards for Medicare-Medicaid-participating providers. In 1974 the final rules were promulgated for the certification of skilled and intermediate care facilities; they are presently known as the Skilled Nursing Facility (SNF) Conditions of Participation and Intermediate Care Facility (ICF) Standards.

Several unsuccessful attempts have been made to revise the 1974 conditions and standards. Opposition to proposed changes in the regulations finally led the Health Care Financing Administration (HCFA) and Congress to postpone virtually all changes in the regulations until a committee appointed by IOM studied the issues and reported its recommendations for change.

The regulations are again being rewritten, this time to emphasize resident outcomes and mandated quality assessment and assurance programs. This is happening because of major legislative reform (the Omnibus Budget Reconciliation Act (OBRA) of 1987) that has grown out of the IOM study of 1986.[3] This legislation is the culmination of much controversy and debate about the care of our elderly in nursing homes in this country.

PaCS

Concurrently, HCFA has developed a modified survey instrument called Patient Care and Services (PaCS) that is based primarily on direct patient assessments and outcome-oriented indicators of care. "State and/or federal surveyors now perform an on-site, in-depth review of the care provided to a sample of patients and observe and interview them regarding their treatment."[3] The PaCS survey process represents a shift away from structural criteria to outcome criteria.

Even with the PaCS survey process, the pressure on the regulatory agency at the federal and state levels during the last 10 years has swung the pendulum to the extreme of overenforcement or safety at all costs. This phenomenon has created nightmares for facilities that have provided good patient care, whose employees describe "respect for others" as the principle of their practice, and that have a record of remarkable outcomes for their residents. Yet annual surveys cite the facilities for such things as "salt and sugar freely accessible to the residents at their dinner table" or "dinners served without trays." There is something wrong with this system.

Although there is a new survey process that focuses on process and outcomes and a new law that focuses on quality assessment and assurance, a regulatory climate exists that is negative and fearful. Negativism and fear will never provide a quality product.

QUALITY SERVICE

Quality of care in LTC has improved over the years. Many changes have taken place because of new knowledge of the care needs and illnesses of the older population. Medical and nursing advances in care of the elderly have brought about many changes in the medical treatment and nursing care of these persons. The professional preparation of nursing home administrators has increased; 14% held baccalaureate degrees in the 1960s as compared to 75% in recent years. Approximately 30% to 40% of those with baccalaurate degrees also have master's degrees.

Despite all the advances and the improvements in regulation and training, there remain the horror stories of abuse, neglect, and understaffing, and a certain margin of poor quality homes. Why?

The reason is that quality cannot be regulated. Quality relates to excellence, and a commitment to excellence does not grow out of regulations and laws. It grows out of a philosophy of caring that pervades the staff at every level and is evidenced in interactions among staff, residents, facility, and community. It reflects a pride in who we are as long-term care providers, in the richness of elderly persons' lives and what they have to contribute to our society, and in our personal lives.

Striving for excellence assumes basic administrative components. It assumes good management and communication. It assumes educated, properly prepared staff who keep abreast of the new discoveries in their practice fields. It assumes an honest, open approach to new ideas, to challenges from within and without. It assumes shared responsibility for quality on the part of every staff person and every member of the board of directors. And it assumes adequate funding to provide the necessary services. The responsiblity for quality grows out of a respect for the dignity of the people we serve, the people we work with, and the community we represent. It is a positive, creative forward movement.

The characteristics described here are the charac-

teristics of facilities that excel in their services to the elderly, that already meet the quality standards defined by the NCCNHR, and that will not be significantly affected by the OBRA regulations of 1987.

REFERENCES

1. American Health Care Association: Quest for quality, 1982.
2. Donabedian A: Explorations in quality assessment and monitoring: the definitions of quality and approaches to its assessment, vol 1; The criteria and standards of quality, vol 2, Ann Arbor, Mich, 1980, Health Administration Press.
3. Grimaldi PL, Micheletti JA, and Shlala TJ: Quality assurance in a PaCS and case-mix environment, QRB 13(5):170, 1987.
4. Herbelin K: Components of a quality assessment and assurance program: a primer for nursing home providers and staff. Contemporary Longterm Care 14(5):70, May 1988.
5. Illinois Administrative Code, Chapter I, Subchapter d, paragraphs 140.525-140.528, 1985. Illinois Department of Public Aid, Springfield.
6. Institute of Medicine: Improving the quality of care in nursing homes, Washington, DC, 1986, National Academy Press.
7. Joint Commission for the Accreditation of Health Care Organizations: Long term care standards, Chicago, 1988, The Commission.
8. Kane RA and Kane RL: Long-term care: principles, programs and policies, New York, 1987, Springer Publishing Co.
9. Kurowski BD and Shaughessy PW: The measurement and assurance of quality. In Vogel RJ and Palmer HC, editors: Long-term care: perspectives from research and demonstration, Rockville, Md, 1985, Aspen Publications.
10. Mitchell-Pederson L *and others*: Let's untie the elderly, OAHA Quarterly 21(10):10, 1985.
11. Moore V: Providers launch quality validation, Provider 13(7):7, July 1987.
12. Schneider D: Sentinel health events: a process- and outcome-based quality assurance system, unpublished manuscript.
13. Spalding J: A consumer perspective on quality care: the resident's point of view, Washington, DC, 1986, National Citizens' Coalition for Nursing Home Reform.
14. Vladeck BC: Unloving care: the nursing home tragedy, New York, 1980, Basic Books Inc.

CHAPTER 36

Quality assurance in home health care

JOYCE COLLING

Quality assurance programs in home health care are a recent phenomenon and as yet are not mandated by the federal government as they are in other health care settings. Considerable strides have been made over the past 15 years in the design and use of quality assurance programs in settings other than home health care, but very recent literature is less clear about what constitutes an effective quality assurance program and has called for a more careful appraisal of the reliability and validity of these programs. Further, even though well-developed programs may be available in other settings, the parameters that constitute quality may not be useful in home health without thoughtful modification because some of the characteristics of providers and recipients of care are unique to home health care settings. It is likely, however, that in an environment of increasing consumer demands for high-quality care and greater constraints on the cost of care, pressure for quality assurance programs in home health care settings will intensify. In addition, quality and reimbursement are likely to be linked. Caution and careful testing must be exercised in developing and adopting quality assurance programs in home health. Such programs must be sensitive quality care indicators and must accurately reflect the benchmarks of excellence important to the health and well-being of care recipients. They should not be inordinately burdensome to care providers who are often involved in data collection, and their achievement should not be outside the financial capabilities of agencies.

This chapter reviews recent changes in health care that have had a profound effect on some health agencies and the state of quality assurance in home health care. A particular focus is on issues to resolve or consider in applying knowledge about quality assurance from other settings and for other populations to home health care settings and populations.

HEALTH CARE SYSTEM CHANGES THAT HAVE INFLUENCED HOME HEALTH CARE AND QUALITY ASSURANCE

Several recent social changes and major pieces of legislation have had a significant effect on the health care system in general. First, there is an ever-increasing number of people aged 65 and older. Those 85 years and older are the fastest growing segment of society and are the most likely to need frequent episodic or continuing care for multiple chronic medical problems and functional disabilities.

Second, recent Medicare legislation has created an incentive for the proliferation of home health agencies because it provides limited reimbursement for eligible posthospital patients. Home health agencies now number about 10,000, and in the past decade there has been an 800% increase in the number of proprietary agencies that are Medicare-certified.[16] In addition, the limit on the number of home health and skilled nursing visits that can be provided was lifted in 1981 for eligible Medicare beneficiaries. At the same time, Congress authorized the Health Care Financing Administration (HCFA) to permit states to waive eligibility requirements for Medicaid coverage of home health care if the care is a substitute for nursing home care. However, a review of some of these programs suggests that they are not a substitute for nursing but instead are reaching persons who would otherwise receive no care.[23] In any case, both of these actions have served to increase the demand for home health care services.

A third factor that has had a profound influence on health care delivery has been legislation mandating a prospective payment system for medical care. This has decreased the length of hospital stays still further and has shifted a greater number of acute and chronically ill patients into home health care agencies.

The rising demand for high quality health care by

numerous consumer groups in the past two decades is a fourth factor that has affected health care delivery. Consumers want high quality technical care and also care that is accessible and provided in a manner that conveys respect and dignity for the individual.[10] They are becoming increasingly vocal and sophisticated in stating what they want and are demanding a role in policy-making groups where decisions about the future of health care are shaped. Initial efforts in response to these demands for quality control have occurred mainly through regulation, certification, and licensure at both the institutional and individual levels for various categories of health care workers.[12] These actions, however, fall far short of achieving the current objectives of active consumer groups.

Fifth, the Omnibus Budget Reconciliation Act of 1986 (OBRA) includes mandatory discharge planning and a uniform needs assessment. Further, Congress has ordered the Department of Health and Human Services to study the development of a quality review and assurance strategy and to report back in two years. General criteria are to be developed that may be used in establishing priorities for the allocation of funds and personnel and for reviewing and assuring quality of care.

Finally, during this same period of time nursing has experienced dramatic changes that have had an impact on home health care. These changes include a rapid decline in the number of graduates from diploma-granting programs, a large increase in graduates prepared at the associate degree (AD) level, and relatively little change in the percentage of graduates from 4-year baccalaureate programs. Traditionally baccalaureate nurses were the only nurses specifically prepared to function in nonhospital settings. Now, however, many diploma and AD nurses are employed in home health where an increasing amount of high-technology nursing is carried out with considerable independent judgment expected of the nurse. For instance, the physical features of home environments as well as family members require attention if the identified patient is to receive maximum benefit from the prescribed treatment. Often the nurse is responsible for supervising other health care workers and for coordinating care across disciplines involved in providing comprehensive care to a specific client. New regulations have also increased the need to document care in more detail in order to ensure payment by third-party payers. At the same time, nurses are being asked to see more patients per day in order to maintain a

cost-effective organization. These changes have caused many home health nurses to complain that they are being asked to do more in less time with fewer resources and to question whether safe and effective patient care is being maintained.

STATUS OF QUALITY ASSURANCE IN HOME HEALTH CARE

The structure-process-outcome framework for determining quality proposed by Donabedian more than a decade ago has been widely applied in different areas of health care.[17] Early efforts at measuring quality relied mainly on structural variables, which are relatively easy and inexpensive to measure. Unfortunately, although adequate resources may be necessary ingredients for quality care, they are not sufficient to ensure quality. That is, adequate resources are probably necessary for quality care, but they do not guarantee that the resources will be used to achieve quality care. More recently process variables—procedures, activities, and services carried out on behalf of clients—have been widely used, but again, procedures or activities alone cannot predict that the client will progress satisfactorily and certainly predict nothing about client satisfaction with the care received.

The final aspect of the quality triad proposed by Donabedian is outcome measures. They focus on the consequences of care activities. Outcomes are particularly difficult to measure reliably because they can be influenced by many factors, including contextual differences, individual differences (genetic, physical, social, economic, and psychological), and the specific and interactive contributions of all health care professionals engaged in the client's care.[9]

Building on the less-than-satisfactory results of previous attempts to measure quality, the most recent quality assurance programs have recognized that the combined components of structure, process, and outcome are important to measure quality. The American Nurses' Association's Standards of Home Health Nursing Practice have recognized this combined approach to measuring quality. They define quality assurances as the "estimation of the degree of excellence in the alteration of the health status of consumers, attained through provider's performance or diagnostic, therapeutic, prognostic or other health care activities."[2] This definition places considerable emphasis on the skills used by the practitioner to work toward a positive health outcome, but recognizes that the outcome of a positive alteration in the recipient's health status is the goal of therapeutic activity. It also recognizes that quality assurance is broader in scope than what nursing alone contributes.

Table 36-1 describes a number of individually focused quality assurance programs in home health care. As the table shows, few of the early programs were developed with outside funding to support the time-consuming pilot-testing and evaluation necessary to ensure reliability and validity. There is remarkable dedication and creativity involved in developing these early models of quality assurance in home care. They serve as guides for future development. Notably, the more recent examples cited in the table are federally funded programs that are more likely to achieve the goals of reliable and valid measures of quality.

ISSUES OF QUALITY ASSURANCE IN HOME HEALTH CARE

Four major issues to resolve or consider in developing quality assurance programs for home care are contextual factors, multidisciplinary care delivery models, individual differences, and approaches to measurement of quality care. It is unlikely that small independent efforts, no matter how dedicated and creative, can effectively untangle the interrelationships among these areas. Well-designed, well-funded, multisite studies are needed that combine the best thinking of informed consumers, methodological experts, and expert clinicians from diverse health care disciplines.

Multiple contextual factors

Developing useful quality assurance measures in home care is complicated by the fact that each home in which the care is delivered poses differing and multiple contextual factors that can have a bearing on the outcomes of client care. For instance, treating an elderly client's stasis ulcers in a home environment in which the hygiene, nutritional conditions, and opportunities for adequate rest and sleep are poor may yield a different outcome than if the home environment is optimal for healing to occur. In addition, a number of other factors about the client's family situation may have a negative or positive bearing on how well the client responds to care provided by agency personnel. These factors include how supportive the family is in allowing the client to assume the sick role and what competing psychological or physical stressors may be present among other family members.

Multidisciplinary care delivery models

Although the vast majority of home care is delivered by nurses, a number of other health care workers may also contribute care to an individual home care client. Other services can include physical therapy, occupational therapy, social work, medicine, homemaker services, and personal care services. Thus process variables may be a major component of a quality assurance program, and it is not too difficult to determine the specific contribution of each health care worker. The client's satisfaction, however, is not assessed using this perspective, nor does it take into account the interaction and coordination among the several health care workers that may be crucial in determining the overall outcomes of care in a comprehensive quality assurance program.

Accounting for individual differences among clients

One of the most difficult problems to overcome in developing reliable and valid quality assurance measures for home care is that of accounting for individual differences. Although there is some homogeneity among children and younger adult clients, one of the most distinctive characteristics of elderly persons is their *heterogeneity*. As people age, they tend to become less like others who are the same chronological age, which makes the development and testing of measurement instruments difficult to standardize. This problem is an important consideration because the majority of home care clients are elderly. Further, about two thirds of the elderly population have multiple chronic disease or disability problems, which, although they may not be the cause of the home care referral, must be taken into account when developing a plan of care and in assessing the potential for a specified outcome. Knowledge about gerontology and geriatrics is clearly essential to accurately assess and evaluate care. Unfortunately many disciplines, nursing included, do not currently include this content in their curricula.[1]

Measurement limitations

A number of quality assurance projects have developed and tested instruments for use in institutional settings such as hospitals and nursing homes. However, use of these instruments without careful testing for modifications needed to account for the unique characteristics of home care is questionable. Specific areas of knowledge gleaned from previous research or

Table 36-1 Summary of individually focused quality assurance programs in home health care

Year	Author/source	Agency	Key aspects of program
1977	Vincent and Price[20]	Cleveland VNA	Focused on mental health patients; social behavior, employment, medication compliance, and hospital readmission used as outcome measures
1977	Daubert[6]	New Haven, Conn, VNA	Developed patient classification system by prognosis; focused on process and outcome measures
1979	Decker and others[7]	Minnesota Dept. of Health	Based on medical diagnoses with functional and other criteria as subsets of outcome criteria
1980	Legge & Reilly[14]	Atlanta VNA	Focused on cancer patients, using functional status as one outcome measure
1983	Barkauskas[4]	—	Focused on mother and infants using behavior, satisfaction, and physical status as outcome measure
1983	Visiting Nurse and Homecare, Inc.[21]	Hartford Conn, VNA and Home Care	Multidimensional outcome-oriented instrument; Focused on self-management
1984	Visiting Nurse Association of Municipal Detroit.[22]	Detroit VNA	Outcome measures based on nursing diagnoses
1984	Ansak and Zawadski[3]	San Francisco	Focused on elderly clients; Functional and cognitive status, institutionalization, health, and cost were outcome measures
1985	Gould[8]	Philadelphia, United Home Health Services	Used nursing diagnoses as focus of outcome criteria
1985	Miller and others[15]	—	Focused on elderly clients; ADL, IADL,* mental status, number of nursing home days and hospital days were measured
1986	Brouton and others[5]	—	Focused on low birth weight infants; standardized physical and mental growth outcome measures were used
1986	Kline and others[11]	Georgia Dept. of Human Resources	Focused on process measures
1986	Lalonde[13]	Home Care Assn. of Washington	Federally funded study in progress; developing a number of outcome-oriented scales
1986	Simmons[18]	Omaha Visiting Nurse Association	Federally funded project; outcome criteria developed based on nursing diagnoses
1986	Sorgen[19]	Alberta, Canada	Funded study completed in 1988; focused on key structural, process and outcome criteria; A classification system was developed

*ADL, activities of daily living; IADL, instrumental activities of daily living.

quality assurance model development that can be useful in the development of home care quality assurance programs include the following:

- Structural, process, or outcome measures of quality alone are not sufficient.
- Measures that capture relationships, particularly among process, outcome, and even structural components, are more likely to yield useful results.
- Given the cost constraints on health care services and the potential for rationing of care, it may be necessary to determine points at which increases in services result in diminishing outcomes of patient status.
- Knowledge from gerontology and geriatrics is needed to define positive outcomes of maintaining current levels of functioning, rather than recognizing only improvement in function or cure.
- Multivariate techniques should be used that allow one to evaluate all criteria and to determine what combinations of criteria best predict quality of care.
- Computerization of systems of care monitoring allows easier manipulation of variables.

CONCLUSIONS

Quality assurance (QA) in home care is currently less developed than in other settings, and few programs have been tested for reliability and validity. Progress in developing effective QA in home care can build on the mistakes and progress made in other settings. Because of the unique characteristics of home care, QA measures developed for other settings and populations cannot automatically be adopted for the home setting. Finally, the need to develop effective QA in home care is increasing as a greater number of clients receive a wide variety of complex health care services in the privacy of their homes that in the past were carried out in institutions. This creates the potential for less-than-optimal outcomes if quality is not monitored carefully. The need is even more urgent because QA and reimbursement are likely to be linked in some way in the near future.

REFERENCES

1. American Nurses' Association: Gerontological nursing curriculum: survey analysis and recommendations, Kansas City, Mo, 1986; The Association.
2. American Nurses' Association: Standards of home health nursing practice, Kansas City, Mo, 1986, The Association.
3. Ansak M and Zawadski RT: On lok CCODDA: a consolidated model. In: Zawadski, RT (Ed.) Community-based systems of long term care, Philadelphia, Haworth Press, 1984.
4. Barkauskas VH: Effectiveness of public health home visits to primiparous mothers and their infants, Am J Public Health 73(5):573, 1983.
5. Brouton D and others: A randomized clinical trial of early hospital discharge and home follow-up of very-low-birth-weight infants, N Engl J Med 15:934, 1986.
6. Daubert EA: Patient classification system and outcome criteria, Nurs Outlook 27:450, 1979.
7. Decker F and others: Using patient outcomes to evaluate community health nursing, Nurs Outlook 27(4):278, 1979.
8. Gould EJ: Standardized home health nursing plans: a quality assurance tool, QRB 11:334, 1985.
9. Horn BJ and Swain MA: An approach to development of criterion measures for quality patient care. In Issues in evaluation research, Kansas City, Mo: American Nurses Association, 1976.
10. Kelman HR: Evaluation of health care quality by consumers. Int J Health Serv 6(3):431, 1976.
11. Kline MM, Tracy ML, and Davis SL: Quality assurance in public health, Nursing and Health Care 1(4):192, 1986.
12. Kurowski BD and Shaughnessy PW. The measurement and assurance of quality. In Vogel RJ and Palmer HC, editors: Long-term care: perspectives from research and demonstrations, Rockville, Md, 1985, Aspen Systems Corp.
13. Lalonde B: Quality assurance manual of the home care association of Washington, Edmonds, Wash, 1986, Home Care Association of Washington.
14. Legge JS and Reilly BJ: Assessing the outcomes of cancer patients in a home nursing program, Cancer Nurs 3(5):357, 1980.
15. Miller LS, Clark ML, and Clark WF: The comparative evaluation of California's multi-purpose senior services project, Home Health Care Services Quarterly 6(3):49, 1985.
16. Mor V and Spector W: Achieving continuity of care, Generations 4(3):47, 1988.
17. Schneider D: Sentinel health events: A process- and outcome-based quality assurance system. Paper presented at Oregon Health Sciences University, Portland, May, 1986.
18. Simmons DA: Implementation of nursing diagnosis in a community health setting. In Hurley ME, editor: Classification of nursing diagnosis: proceedings of the sixth conference, St. Louis, 1986, The CV Mosby Co.
19. Sorgen LM: The development of a home care quality assurance program in Alberta, Home Health Services Quarterly 7:13, 1986.
20. Vincent P and Price JR: Evaluation of a VNA mental health project, Nurs Res 26(5):361, 1977.
21. Visiting Nurse and Home Care, Inc: Guidelines: self-management outcome criteria, Plainville, Conn, 1983.
22. Visiting Nurse Association of Metropolitan Detroit: Guide for the development of the nursing care plan, Detroit, 1984.
23. Waldo DR, Levit KR, and Lazenby H: National health expenditures, Health Care Financing Review 9(1):1, 1986.

CHAPTER 37

The role of the National Council of State Boards of Nursing in consumer protection

EILEEN McQUAID DVORAK
JOYCE M. SCHOWALTER

Regulatory agencies exist to implement the laws enacted by the duly elected representatives of the government. Boards of nursing, like boards of medicine, pharmacy, or dentistry, are the regulatory entities that administer the practice acts for various professions that are enacted by the state legislatures. These state boards have the responsibility of assuring the public that the practitioners in a specific profession are competent to give health care. The National Council of State Boards of Nursing exists to assist state boards of nursing in assuring the competence of nurses. In this chapter, competence is defined as having the requisite or adequate ability or quality to function as a nurse.

The chapter first reviews the state boards or legal agencies as consumer protection agencies and then reviews the role of the National Council as a consumer protection organization.

BOARDS OF NURSING: CONSUMER PROTECTION AGENCIES

The credentialing (licensing and registering) of health workers was begun in order to protect the public from dishonest and incompetent practitioners. For nursing in the United States, consumer protection by a state agency began 80 years ago when, on March 3, 1903, the governor of North Carolina signed into law the first nurse practice act. The states of New Jersey and New York and the Commonwealth of Virginia enacted similar practice acts within the following two months. By 1923 all contiguous states and the District of Columbia had nurse practice acts.

With the enactment of these laws the state legislatures created administrative agencies, frequently boards of nursing, to implement the laws through the performance of specific functions. Commonly the

functions included the licensing of beginning nurses, restricting the use of certain titles, approving schools of nursing, and disciplining licensees. In recent years some legislatures have added responsibilities, including licensing for advanced or specialty nursing practice and requiring continuing education or evidence of continuing competence on renewal of licensure.

Some legislatures, such as Minnesota, have made explicit in law the policy of the state as it pertains to the regulation of occupations:

The legislature finds that the interests of the people of the state are served by the regulation of certain occupations. The legislature further finds:

(1) that it is desirable for boards composed primarily of members of the occupations so regulated to be charged with formulating the policies and standards governing the occupation;
(2) that economical and efficient administration of the regulation activities can be achieved through the provision of administrative services by departments of state government; and
(3) that procedural fairness in the disciplining of persons regulated by the boards requires a separation of the investigative and prosecutorial functions from the board's judicial responsibility.*

Although it is recognized that licensees benefit from the existence of boards of nursing, the public is the primary beneficiary. The public has a right to expect the state to ensure that those who practice in areas that affect public health and safety are minimally competent to practice. In the exercise of the police power reserved to the states by the United States Constitution, the state board of nursing exercises its respon-

---

*From Minnesota Statutes, Section 214.001, Subdivision 1, 1988.

sibility to so assure the public of competent nurses through the creation of licensure and relicensure requirements and grounds for denial or removal of a license.

In the recent past, criticisms were levied at licensing boards with the claim that they served to protect the practitioner rather than the public and that this would be rectified in part by changing the administrative structure within which boards operate. Indeed, functions of the boards of nursing have not changed even when administrative structures have changed. Boards of nursing continue to have three major responsibilities: (1) controlling entry into practice, (2) maintaining competent practitioners, and (3) reviewing practice acts for interpretation of scope or questions raised about legislative intent, or reviewing legislative issues that affect the delivery of care to the public.

Controlling entry into practice consists of a combination of activities associated with reviewing the candidates for admission to practice as nurses. This controlling responsibility includes the approval of educational programs for nurses and use of a standardized examination that is administered nationally to determine competency for professional or practical level of nursing practice at the point of entry.

Maintaining competent practitioners includes members of boards of nursing reviewing of nurses' practice and considering disciplinary action. According to a study now being conducted, this review has involved the extensive use of resources. In addition, of course, maintaining competence may also entail continuing education, peer review, or other forms of continuing competence measurements.

The third major responsibility is responding to questions about whether or not particular nursing activities fall within the scope of practice as defined by the law. In addition, it means monitoring legislative actions under consideration and often involves testifying as to the impact of any changes on the delivery of care by nurses.

NATIONAL COUNCIL OF STATE BOARDS OF NURSING AS A CONSUMER PROTECTION ORGANIZATION

The structure of the National Council of State Boards of Nursing is based on the belief that boards of nursing should have an equal voice in policy decisions and in establishing the direction taken by the National Council to assist state boards in protecting the public interest.

History, purposes, membership

The National Council was formed to provide an organization through which boards of nursing act and counsel together on matters of common interest and concern affecting the public health, safety, and welfare, including the development of licensing examinations in nursing.[13]

Historically the genesis of the National Council of State Boards of Nursing can be traced back as far as August 1912, when participants at a conference on state registration laws voted to create a committee that would arrange an annual conference for persons involved with state boards to meet during the convention of the American Nurses' Association. The resulting Committee of State Boards of Nursing worked to promote uniform standards, to improve methods and procedures of member boards, and to approve basic nursing education programs preparing nurses for licensure.[9] The major activity of providing the licensure examinations for use by boards of nursing began in the 1940s.

From that point on, the Committee of State Boards of Nursing evolved through various structural changes within the American Nurses' Association until the vote in 1978 that established the National Council of State Boards of Nursing, Inc., as a separate, autonomous organization.

The National Council is composed of 61 boards of nursing in the United States and the territories of American Samoa, Guam, the Northern Marianna Islands, and the Virgin Islands. The boards or legally constituted bodies with similar legislated responsibilities meet to discuss matters of common interest concerning the public's need for competent nursing care. The broadly stated purpose of the National Council, therefore, is to provide a forum for dialog on major common concerns of state boards of nursing and to provide central resources for use by state boards of nursing.

The concepts of consumer protection as a major focus for both state boards of nursing and the National Council is expressed by Mildred S. Schmidt,[18] National Council president from 1979 to 1981:

Each board of nursing is accountable to the people of the state for protecting the public health, safety, and welfare with respect to the practice of nursing . . . each board of nursing is responsible for administering a licensing examination for the titles stipulated in its nurse practice act. When a delegate votes on a matter affecting the licensing examination, such as a revision of the test, that delegate is casting a vote for the respective member board which, in turn, has responsibility to the people of the state for the licensing examination.

The National Council provides services and products to the state boards of nursing as it assists them in ensuring the competence of nurses. The products are the licensure examinations, which are based on national standards and are derived from analyses of current nursing practice. The examinations used by boards of nursing help assure the public that the licensure candidates who successfully complete the examinations demonstrate the level of competence necessary to give safe, effective nursing care.

Other services are reflected in the statement of functions contained in the National Council bylaws.*

1. Develop, establish policy and procedure, and regulate the use of the licensing examinations for nursing;
2. Identify and promote desirable and reasonable uniformity in standards and expected outcomes in nursing education and practice; as they relate to the protection of the public health, safety and welfare;
3. Assess trends and issues affecting nursing education and nursing practice as they affect the licensure of nurses;
4. Identify mechanisms for measuring the continuing competence of licensed nurses and assist in efforts to promote the same;
5. Collect, analyze and disseminate data and statistics relating to the licensure of nurses;
6. Conduct studies and research pertinent to the purposes of the Council;
7. Provide consultative services for Council members, groups, agencies and individuals concerned with the protection of the health and welfare of the public;
8. Plan and promote educational programs for its members;
9. Promote and facilitate effective communications with related organizations, groups, and individuals.

---

*From National Council of State Boards of Nursing: Bylaws, revised 1988, Chicago, p. 1-2.

Major functions

The state boards, as consumer protection agencies, have three major functions as detailed earlier. The major functions are controlling entry, maintaining competent practitioners, and reviewing the scope of practice issues that affect the delivery of health care. The National Council's stated objectives relate to these three major functions.

Controlling entry into practice. The approval of nursing programs or nursing schools has been a mandate to boards of nursing by state legislatures since the enactment of the original nurse practice acts. In fact, the title given to the first staff person of a board of nursing in New York was "inspector of schools." These staff titles varied according to states, then and now.

The primary assistance given to state boards by the National Council is in the form of guidelines, such as those generated by the Model Nursing Practice Act and the Model Nursing Administrative Rules and Regulations.

In the Model Nursing Practice Act, the section on approval of nursing education programs suggests guidelines for establishing standards for nursing education programs. The Model Administrative Rules give specific directions for establishing the purpose of the standards, standards for program approvals, periodic evaluation standards, and conditions for the denial or withdrawal of approvals.

Since 1981 questions have been raised with regard to the need for approval of nursing education programs by state boards of nursing. Challenges to the approval process were made in Arizona, North Carolina, and Wyoming. The two major questions concerned the need for state approval when voluntary accreditation is received, and the placement of the responsibility for program approval as a state board function as opposed to a higher-education agency function. Legislative study committees examined the questions and reported that the state boards of nursing should maintain the approval process. The state boards of nursing in Arizona, North Carolina, and Wyoming retained approval authority. Since that time several boards of nursing have developed ways to conduct joint approval visits and survey mechanisms with the National League for Nursing.

Boards of nursing use the National Council examination as part of the assessment system to determine if the person who wishes to practice nursing is capable of giving safe and effective nursing care. The examination, formerly known as the State Board Test Pool Examination, was renamed the National Council Licensure Examination (NCLEX) to reflect the purpose and ownership of the licensing examinations. The development of the licensing examination for registered nursing and for practical or vocational nursing is an important responsibility of the National Council. Performing that responsibility entails maintaining the currency, validity, and reliability of the measurement.

The validity of the examinations was established through the results of ongoing studies of entry-level performance. One study, *Critical Requirements for Safe/Effective Nursing Practice*,[6] established a comprehensive behavioral definition of nursing practice. As a result of this study 49 categories of critical behavior were identified from 11,173 critical incidents of nursing behavior. From these categories the behaviors in the registered nurse examination test plan were determined. An update study entitled *Registered Nurse Performance Update Study* verified that the behaviors contained in the registered nurse examination test plan were in fact performed by entry-level registered nurses.[5]

In 1986 *The Study of Nursing Practice and Role Delineation and Job Analysis of Entry-Level Performance of Registered Nurses* was conducted by Kane and colleagues[7] under contract to the National Council of State Boards of Nursing. The primary purpose of this study was to determine the performance levels of entry-level registered nurses to identify whether or not the licensing examination was continuing to measure the knowledge, skills, and abilities necessary for entry-level practice. The study identified 222 activities, and entry-level nurses were asked to rate whether or not they performed these activities, how frequently, and how critical they deemed the performance of the activity. The National Council used the results of this study in revising the test plan for the registered nurse licensure examination.

In 1983 a study of practical nurse performance was conducted by Ference[4] for the National Council of State Boards of Nursing. In this particular study, activities performed and not performed by licensed practical or vocational nurses at entry level into practice were identified. This study and subsequent updates form the basis for the test plan for the practical/vocational nurse licensure examination.

Ongoing development of the licensing examinations demands the incorporation of developments from the field of psychometrics. These developments include criterion-referenced passing scores, test equating, and ethnicity-gender bias studies.

In a criterion-referenced approach, a candidate's test performance is compared to a consistent standard or criterion judged by experts in the nursing profession to represent acceptable nursing competence. The standard is set at the point that distinguishes the competent from the incompetent by a technique known as the Angoff method. Judges who are experts in the nursing profession determine the point by assessing how the minimally competent candidate would respond to each test question in an examination.

The protection of the public derives from the fact that the criterion or standard is consistent and represents a cut point distinguishing those who may safely practice from those who may not. Changes in the standard for any reason other than correlation with valid nursing practice would violate the trust the public has in state boards and the trust the state boards have in the National Council.

In order to apply the same standard of minimal competency to subsequent administrations of the examination, a psychometric technique known as test equating is employed. Test equating, essentially, is the process of producing comparable information from different administrations of the examination. In the case of NCLEX, this is accomplished by including common subsets of items in each administration of the examination. Test equating, thus, assures the public that each candidate is evaluated according to a standard that remains the same from examination to examination. Ethnicity-gender bias studies were initiated in early 1988.

Because such steps are taken to maintain the currency, validity, and reliability of the licensure examinations, the consumer can be assured that the beginning nursing practitioners who pass the examinations have given objective evidence that they are competent to provide nursing care. This assurance pertains to nurses educated in the United States or in foreign countries. All who wish to practice nursing must give evidence of competence to do so. Foreign-educated nurses have had difficulty in providing such evidence by means of the licensing examination. One form of assistance, instituted in 1978, is the use of a screening test to help foreign-educated nurses determine their probabilities of success in taking the licensing examinations. The screening test is prepared and administered worldwide by the Commission on Graduates of Foreign Nursing Schools. A majority of state boards of nursing require success on this test as a requirement for admission to the licensing examinations.

In addition to the development of the examination, the National Council is also responsible for assuring the consumer that the security and integrity of the examinations are maintained. This is accomplished by establishing rigorous standards for the test service and for each state board of nursing to maintain for all phases of examination administration. Lack of security might result in candidates obtaining advance information about the examinations and in the subsequent licensure of candidates who are not competent to give nursing care.

In addition to providing the examinations for use in licensing candidates, the National Council provides other forms of licensing assistance to the state boards. The Model Nursing Practice Act[10] and Model Nursing Administration Rules[11] were developed in 1988 to serve as guidelines for implementing changes in licensing requirements or procedures.

Ongoing projects conducted by the National Council include projects related to the computerized administration of the licensing examinations. Currently the National Council is conducting a self-funded study on computerized adaptive testing. The concept underlying this testing is the identification of a person's ability level on the basis of items calibrated according to Rasch. One hoped-for result is that fewer questions will be needed to make more accurate predictions of individual's competency level. The public will thus benefit from speedier and more precise examination results. The final report of this project is expected in August 1990.

Another project, undertaken with funding from the W.K. Kellogg Foundation, is the computerized clinical simulation testing project conducted in conjunction with the National Board of Medical Examiners. Its intent is to develop simulations that can give a totally uncued examination for licensure and that will test different aspects of judgment not currently capable of being tested in paper and pencil mode. Again, greater speed and accuracy of results translate into increased public confidence in the capabilities of the nursing graduate. The expected date of completion of this feasibility study is August 1991.

Maintaining competent practitioners. State boards of nursing act to ensure that licensed nurses continue to be capable of delivering care in a safe, effective and ethical manner. Any indication of a nurse's lack of fitness or ability to deliver such care can result in dis-ciplinary action by the state board or equivalent state agency. To assist state boards of nursing in this major function the National Council offers guidelines for discipline, maintains a disciplinary data bank, and provides educational forums.

Through the Model Nursing Practice Act and the Model Nursing Administrative Rules, the National Council has assisted states by suggested requirements for reporting unsafe or unethical practice. The Model Nursing Practice Act, for example, lists broad categories of grounds for disciplinary action.

Since 1980 the National Council has maintained a disciplinary data bank for use by the state boards of nursing. In effect, each state board of nursing sends a record of disciplinary action taken against licensees to the National Council. The information is tabulated and a monthly compilation is distributed to all state boards of nursing. This service helps in ensuring that a person licensed in more than one state who is found to be practicing in an unsafe manner also will be reviewed in the other states where he or she is licensed.

With the advent of a national practitioner data bank mandated by the federal government, there is continued support to ensure that persons licensed in any profession related to health care will be reviewed before they are granted a license in another jurisdiction.

Educational programs are offered by the National Council on matters of interest to the state boards of nursing. Discipline, with all its ramifications, continues as a major topic of concern for the state boards. The protection of the consumer from the incompetent nursing practitioner is the rationale for the emphasis on disciplinary functions of the state boards of nursing.

Information exchange. Through various surveys, publications, consultations, and workshops the National Council provides state boards of nursing with data on such subjects as credentialing, personnel utilization, federal and state regulatory legislation, and test development.

Since 1982 the National Council has obtained extensive data from each state board of nursing to generate comparison data for use by state boards of nursing and others interested in trend analysis. The data include information about board structure, powers and duties, educational programs, qualifications for licensure, licensing examination information and statistics, and disciplinary actions. These are the basis for a legal data bank serving the state boards of nursing in researching issues pertaining to nurse licensure and the protection of the public.

Another comprehensive study, a comparative analysis of the operations of state boards of nursing, is in the final stages of analysis and will be prepared for distribution in the near future. This particular study supports the continuation of the major responsibilities of boards of nursing—controlling entry, maintaining competent practitioners, and responding to questions on scope of practice and other legislative issues.

As another form of information exchange, *Issues*, a quarterly publication, addresses topics of interest to and about boards of nursing. Books and videotapes about the licensing examinations have been produced to assist candidates and schools of nursing and to minimize any interference with the assessment of candidates' nursing knowledge.

SUMMARY

In summary, the role of the National Council of State Boards of Nursing is to assist state boards of nursing in ensuring nursing competence. Boards of nursing are regulatory agencies specifically designated to implement a portion of the state's mandate to protect its citizens. Through the periodic evaluation of a nurse's competence, that is, on initial licensure, relicensure, and if warranted, on receipt of a complaint of incompetence, boards of nursing operate as consumer protection agencies.

The National Council assists the states in performing legislated activities that provide a direct form of quality control. The development of an evaluation system for entry into nursing practice and the provision of guidelines, resource data, and an information exchange system enable the National Council of State Boards of Nursing to claim its role as a consumer protection organization.

REFERENCES

1. American Nurses' Association: Facts about nursing 1980-1981, New York, 1981, American Journal of Nursing Co.
2. Developing, constructing and scoring the National Council licensure examination, Issues 4:1, 1983.
3. Public Health Service: Developments in health manpower licensure, Washington, DC, 1973, Pub No (HRA) 74-3101.
4. Ference H: Practical nurse role delineation and validation study for the national council licensure examination for practical nurses, Monterey, Calif, 1983, CTB/McGraw-Hill Book Co.
5. Holmes S and Sanders L: Registered nurse performance update study, Chicago, 1984, National Council of State Boards of Nursing.
6. Jacobs A et al: Critical requirements for safe/effective nursing practice, Kansas City, 1978, American Nurses' Association.
7. Kane M and others: The study of nursing practice and role delineation and job analysis of entry level performance of registered nurses, Chicago, 1986, National Council of State Boards of Nursing.
8. Malone G, Fondiller S, and Heidorn D: From an idea to an organization, Chicago, 1983, National Council of State Boards of Nursing.
9. Minnesota Statutes, Section 214.001, Subdivision 1, 1988.
10. The model nursing practice act, Chicago, 1988, National Council of State Boards of Nursing.
11. The model nursing administrative rules, Chicago, 1988, National Council of State Boards of Nursing.
12. National Council of State Boards of Nursing: Bylaws, revised 1988, Chicago, The Council.
13. National Council of State Boards of Nursing Resolution: Book of reports, Chicago, 1983, The Council.
14. Public Health Service: Credentialing health manpower, Washington, DC, 1977, US Department of Health, Education, and Welfare No (OS) 77-50057.
15. Report of the Committee. In The study of credentialing in nursing: a new approach, I, Kansas City, Mo, 1979, American Nurses' Association.
16. Report on licensure and related health personnel credentialing, Washington, DC, 1971, US Department of Health, Education, and Welfare No (HSM) 72-11.
17. Rowland M, Keefe H, and Peterson A: Sunset review: three states reports, Issues 2:3, 1981.
18. Schmidt M: To whom is the NCSBN accountable? Issues 1:1, 1980.
19. Shimberg B and Roederer D: Occupational licensing: questions a legislator should ask, Lexington, Ky, The Council of State Governments, 1978.
20. Waddle F: Licensure: achievements and limitations. In The study of credentialing: a new approach—II: staff working papers. Kansas City, Mo, 1979, American Nurses' Association.

CHAPTER 38

Nursing certification

A matter for the professional organization

GLORIA M. BULECHEK
MERIDEAN L. MAAS

How to grant credentials to professionals to assure that they are qualified to provide specialized services to consumers is a subject fraught with misunderstanding and vested interests. The controversy has produced a number of views of how professionals should be awarded credentials for specialized practice and who should do it. The nursing profession has experienced this conflict. Several models have evolved for granting credentials to nurses who practice a nursing specialty.

The dominant models for certification of registered nurses for specialty practice are: (1) certification by the professional organization—a statement issued by a professional organization declaring that a nurse has met predetermined qualifications to practice a specialty; (2) certification by the state—a legal endorsement by a state board of nursing certifying that a nurse has met the legal requirements for specialty practice; and (3) certification by an institution—a statement issued by an academic or health service agency recognizing that a nurse has completed the requirements of a program of study for specialty practice.[10] The ambiguous status of nursing certification is confusing both to nurses and to the public. The American Nurses' Association (ANA) and a number of specialty nursing organizations have developed national programs of certification. State certification of the nursing specialties has been a trend in nursing practice law since the mid-1970s.[7] Many nurses are recognized as specialists on the basis of local certification by an academic or service institution. Debate has continued among members of the nursing profession and other interested parties over which of these models best serves the profession's and the public's interests. Certification for entry into specialty practice was one component of *The Study of Credentialing in Nursing: A New Approach.*[2]

The purpose of this chapter is to clarify the status and functions of nursing certification. A rationale is presented for the view that certification for specialty nursing practice best serves the interests of the public and the profession when it is conducted by the profession. This rationale is based on the concept of a profession, the norms for autonomy and accountability of a profession, and the expectation that professions serve the best interests of their clients. Goals of certification for the profession and the public are discussed. The current status of certification in nursing is described, and the advantages and disadvantages of each of the dominant models for meeting the goals are weighed.

SELF-REGULATION OF PROFESSION

Professions evolve in society because their knowledge and services function to meet societal needs.[21] Autonomy is given to professionals so that important work will be done effectively by experts who in turn are competent judges of the needed expertise.[24] It is because of specialized knowledge that professionals are judged competent to define the standards used to assure safe and effective practice. However, society demands accountability of a profession to assure that the profession and its members use authority in the client's best interest. In 1980 ANA outlined in *Nursing: A Social Policy Statement* the specific mechanisms of the nursing profession's "social contract" with society whereby nursing's responsibility for self-regulation is met and the authority for nursing practice is gained. There are a number of ways that professions demonstrate accountability. The definitions of standards for entry into the profession, codes of ethical conduct, standards for practice, and standards for research to define and expand the knowledge base of the profession are some of these mechanisms. Professional peers collectively establish standards for safe and effective practice and use them to evaluate the qualifications and practice of members to hold them accountable.[21]

Acountability for the knowledge that is possessed and used by members to deliver quality services to clients is a critical obligation of a profession. Changes in the society, in technology, in the values and demands of consumers, and in the growth of knowledge require that the profession develop systems to assure that the appropriate knowledge is held by members to deliver specific services. With rapid social change, the threat of obsolescence increases. Universal competence by members of a profession is not possible. To an increasing degree the knowledge base of professions is highly complex and specialized. The professional's commitment is to a lifetime of learning.[25]

Certification by a professional organization is the model that has been used most commonly to inform the public of the truth of claims to the possession of knowledge for specialized practice. Certification by the professional organization is the process used by the medical profession and most health professions. A number of sociopolitical, economic, educational, and health care trends have influenced the development of certification for specialty nursing practice in such a way that there is little consensus about which model of certification best serves the profession's and public's interests.[26] However, there appears to be agreement about the goals that a certification model should strive to meet.

GOALS OF NURSING CERTIFICATION

The appropriate model for certification to practice a nursing specialty must be based on the assumption that both the status of the nurse specialist and the public will be enhanced.[29] More specifically, the goals of a model for certification are to enhance (1) consumer access to health care, (2) consumer and provider protection, and (3) consumer and provider benefit over cost.

Consumer access to quality health care

Certification of nursing specialists offers an alternative to consumers for quality health care. Specialization in maternal-child care, gerontology, adult health, and other areas of nursing is the result of societal pressures for an expanded nurse role in health care and of advances in health care technology and knowledge. To assure that consumers have access to this alternative for health care, a stable, standardized, and credible system for nursing certification must be established. The system should define the appropriate specialty areas of nursing practice, determine the number of specialties, and define the standards and educational qualifications for each area of practice. The system also should provide for orderly translation of new nursing knowledge into the practice of qualified specialists and clearly communicate these credentials to consumers.

Consumer and provider protection

The public needs to be protected from the possible effects of nurses' self-interests and from the vested interests of other organizations and groups. Restriction of qualified individuals from specialty practice, standard setting by persons who lack nursing expertise, and nonuniversally applied standards are some of the possible adverse effects on consumers. Nursing certification procedures should include mechanisms for public input within a structure that can respond quickly to rapid changes in healthcare knowledge, technology, and values. Conversely, nurses need to be assured that they will have autonomy and legal sanction to practice their specialties.

Consumer and provider benefit over cost

There are a number of economic concerns about the appropriate model for nursing certification. The system for certification should minimize costs to both the consumer and provider while maximizing benefits. To minimize costs, overlapping certification processes, limited geographic mobility of practitioners, and inflexible certification processes should be avoided.

CURRENT SITUATION

A description of the current situation for each of the dominant models and a discussion of the advantages and disadvantages of each model for attaining the desired goals will clarify the direction of certification for specialty practice.

Certification by professional organizations

Certification in nursing by professional organizations was begun in 1945 by the American Association of Nurse Anesthetists. The explosion of knowledge and technology during the past 2 decades has been accompanied by a proliferation of specialty organizations, many of whom offer certification. The purpose of certification by professional organizations is (1) protection of the public and (2) recognition of the expert practitioner. Table 38-1 lists the certification programs in nursing. The 20 certifying organizations and their eligibility requirements appear in Collins[9] and Fickeissen.[13] The two major eligibility requirements are experience and education. The educational requirement varies from a short-term continuing education program to a formal academic program granting a master's degree. The dominant process of certification is a multiple-choice exam often conducted by a national testing organization. Most often the certification is for a finite period of time and a renewal process is designated. Renewal requirements include work experience and continuing education requirements. Each organization awards a specific title of certification, designated by appropriate initials. The nurse adds the initials to her name and R.N. designation.

The largest certification program is conducted by ANA, accounting for about 40% of the nation's 150,000 certified nurses.[22] Table 38-2 lists the 17 programs offered by ANA, the certificate designation, and the number of nurses certified in 1983 and 1988. Three of the clinical programs require master's preparation, and the certified specialist (C.S.) title is reserved for these programs. The advanced nursing administration program also requires master's preparation. Programs requiring a B.S.N. include community health nurse, all of the nurse-practitioner programs, and nursing administration. Two additional practice areas, general nursing and school nurse, were given for the first time in October 1988. In 1989 a new offering was introduced for clinical specialists in gerontological nursing, and the offerings for high-risk perinatal nurse and maternal-child nurse were merged into a perinatal nurse offering. The ANA program has had tremendous growth between 1983 and 1988, as Table 38-2 illustrates. In 1983 the largest proportion of certificates was in the nurse-practitioner programs; in 1988 it was in the nurse generalist programs.

Certification for critical care nursing is conducted by the American Association of Critical Care Nurses. AACN began certification in 1976, and by 1988 there were approximately 25,000 C.C.R.N.s. Eligibility requirements include an R.N. license and 1 year of experience in critical care. Another sizable program is

conducted by the Council on Certification of Nurse-Anesthetists, which has certified more than 18,000 nurses. Candidates must have a current R.N. license and be a graduate of an approved nurse-anesthetist program. Certification for nurse-anesthetists and nurse-midwives is necessary for entry into practice in the specialty. Certification of midwives is conducted by the American College of Nurse-Midwives, which has certified approximately 2500 specialists.

The professional organization model of certification offers many advantages. It fosters responsibility in demonstrating professional accountability. The model enables the profession to use its expertise to determine universal standards, evaluate those competent to practice a specialty, and communicate an orderly, credible, and standardized system of certification to consumers. The profession is best equipped to identify the appropriate areas of specialization and set the qualification for entry into specialty practice. Furthermore, the professional model is more flexible, as opposed to the governmental body model, and can respond to new knowledge and changes in practice without the need to revise statutes or governmental rules. This model is less subject to the influence of powerful vested interest groups, such as medicine and hospitals. The system of granting credentials is supported by the practitioners and professional organization and thus is less costly to taxpayers and consumers. Because the system is voluntary rather than mandatory for the practitioner, geographic mobility of the practitioner is facilitated.

The disadvantages of the professional organization model include public distrust of professional use of autonomy and accountability. There is increasing concern about the restriction of free trade by professional organizations involved in certification. There is also concern about lack of control of economic return and status because of vested self-interests. Raymond and Ketchum[28] illustrate through a task analysis study that the areas of specialty practice in nursing are not currently defined according to knowledge and skills performed but appear to be designated by the social, economic, and political context within which nursing is practiced. There are multiple routes for entry into specialty practice. Educational requirements vary from R.N. preparation (A.D.N., Diploma, or B.S.N.) to master's preparation. Required experience varies from completion of an accredited program to 2 years of supervised practice. Raymond[27] has determined that there is a positive relationship between amount of ed-

Table 38-1 Certification programs in nursing*

Certifying organization	Certification programs	Certification designation
American Nurses' Association	Pediatric Nurse Practitioner	
	Adult Nurse Practitioner	
	Family Nurse Practitioner	
	School Nurse Practitioner	
	Gerontological Nurse Practitioner	
	General Nursing Practice	
	Medical-Surgical Nurse	R.N.,C.
	Gerontological Nurse	
	Psychiatric and Mental Health Nurse	
	Community Health Nurse	
	School Nurse	
	Maternal-Child Health Nurse	
	High-Risk Perinatal Nurse	
	Child and Adolescent Nurse	
	Nursing Administration	R.N.,C.N.A.
	Nursing Administration, Advanced	R.N.,C.N.A.A.
	Clinical Specialist in Medical-Surgical Nursing	
	Clinical Specialist in Adult Psychiatric M.H. Nursing	R.N., C.S.
	Clinical Spec. in Child & Adol. Psych. M.H. Nursing	
NAACOG Certification Corporation	Inpatient Obstetric Nurse	
	Neonatal Intensive Care Nurse	
	Low-risk Neonatal Nurse	R.N.C.
	Neonatal Nurse Clinician/Practitioner	
	OB/GYN Nurse Practitioner	
Others:	Emergency Nurse	C.E.N.
These programs are typically	Operating Room Nurse	C.N.O.R.
offered by a particular	Critical Care Nurse	C.C.R.N.
specialty society or a	Neuroscience Nurse	C.N.R.N.
board affiliated with that	Nurse Anesthetist	C.R.N.A.
specialty organization	Post-Anesthesia Nurse	C.P.A.N.
	Urological Nurse	C.U.R.N.
	Oncology Nurse	O.C.N.
	Enterostomal Therapy Nurse	E.T.
	Gastrointestinal Clinician	C.G.C.
	Hemodialysis Nurse	C.H.N.
	Intravenous Therapy Nurse	C.R.N.I.
	Infection Control Practitioner	C.I.C.
	Nutrition Support Nurse	C.N.S.N.
	Rehabilitation Nurse	C.R.R.N.
	Occupational Health Nurse	C.O.H.N.
	School Nurse	C.S.N.
	Pediatric Nurse Practitioner/Associate	C.P.N.P./A.
	Nurse Midwife	C.N.M.

*Source: Raymond MR and Ketchum EL: Certification in nursing. Paper presented at the annual meeting of the American Educational Research Association, New Orleans, April 1988.

Table 38-2   American Nurses' Association certification programs*

Specialty area	Certification designation	Number certified through May 1, 1983	Number certified through January 1, 1988
Nurse generalist	R.N.,C. (Registered Nurse, Certified)		
1. Maternal-Child Health		59	497
2. Child and Adolescent		173	967
3. High-Risk Perinatal		45	587
4. Medical-Surgical		971	9051
5. Psychiatric and Mental Health		1389	10,225
6. Community Health		482	2730
7. Gerontological		785	5831
	Total	3904	29,888
Nurse-practitioner	R.N.,C. (Registered Nurse, Certified)		
8. Pediatric Nurse Practitioner		687	1415
9. Family Nurse Practitioner		3173	5588
10. Adult Nurse Practitioner		3042	4601
11. School Nurse Practitioner		364	467
12. Gerontological Nurse Practitioner		218	922
	Total	7484	12,993
Nurse specialist	R.N.,C.S. (Registered Nurse, Certified Specialist		
13. Clinical Specialist in Medical-Surgical Nursing		247	775
14. Clinical Specialist in Adult Psychiatric and Mental Health Nursing		1179	3118
15. Clinical Specialist in Child and Adolescent Psychiatric and Mental Health Nursing		108	354
	Total	1534	4247
Nurse administrator	R.N.,C.N.A. (Registered Nurse Certified in Nursing Administration)		
16. Nursing Administration		1700	7501
17. Nursing Administration, Advanced	R.N.,C.N.A.A. (Registered Nurse, Certified in Nursing Administration, Advanced)	528	1267
	Total	2228	8768
	Grand total	15,150	55,896

*Source: American Nurses' Association 1983 certification catalog and The American Nurse, September 1988.

ucation and performance on nursing certification exams.

The current major problem of certification by professional organizations is duplication and lack of coordination. Some specialists, including pediatric nurse-practitioners and maternal-child health nurses, could seek certification from more than one professional organization. It is unlikely that an individual would do this because of eligibility requirements and cost. Fees for professional certification are in the $100 to $300 range. Some of the organizations have a reduced fee for members, and other organizations open certification to members only. In essence, many individual nurses are forced to choose a professional organization to support. Some nurses, believing that ANA is the one professional organization that represents all nurses, seek certification there. Others find that a specialty organization is more responsive to their continuing education needs and brings them together with other health professionals who have similar interests and concerns. Another cadre of nurses takes the "why bother at all" position in view of the current certification situation. A 1979 survey by Edari[11] of certified nurses revealed that little employer support was given for seeking certification, and few nurses received salary increases, job security, or promotion after achieving certification.

In 1987 Collins[9] reported that for the most part employers still do not recognize certification, although some hospitals demand certification of nurses in critical care or emergency care so that the institution can be accredited as a trauma center.

Certification by the state

State certification for nursing specialty groups appeared around 1975. Nurse-midwives and nurse-anesthetists, as well as other nurse-practitioners, began seeking legal endorsement for specialty practice in addition to the basic license as a registered nurse. These nurses were leading the way with the expanded role of nursing and were encountering opposition to the practice of their specialties. The scope of function for these specialists has been incorporated into a state certification movement that had resulted in legal endorsement for advanced nursing practice in 39 states and territories by 1982.[7] The rules and regulations for state certification are promulgated in each state. La Bar[20] reviewed these state regulations, noting that they are frequently revised. Several states have mandated that national certification (by a professional organization) is required for state certification. In other states national certification is one option for demonstrating competence in the field. Other options include an education program, a continuing education requirement, or a state examination.

The trend toward an additional license for specialty practice is not supported by ANA. ANA's historical position has been that the purpose of state licensure is to protect the health and welfare of the public through legal standards that are recognized as minimum standards to provide safe and effective nursing practice. Principle 6 in the ANA publication *The Nursing Practice Act: Suggested State Legislation* relates to the question of legal regulation of advanced practice:

The nursing practice act should provide for the legal regulation of nursing without reference to a specialized area of practice. It is the function of the professional association to establish the scope and desirable qualifications required for each area of practice, and to certify individuals as competent to engage in specific areas of nursing practice. It is also the function of the professional association to upgrade practice above the minimum standards set by law. The law should not provide for identifying clinical specialists in nursing or require certification or other recognition for practice beyond the minimum qualifications established for the legal regulation of nursing.

In summary, ANA's position has been that specialty practice should be recognized through voluntary national mechanisms rather than state statute.

The advantages of the state model are public recognition of specialty practice and public sanction of those who are certified. There is control of those who identify themselves as qualified to perform specialist activities. Consumers and practitioners tend to recognize certification by a governmental body as indicating superior position and as providing tighter controls on performance. Nurse-practitioners see state certification as a way to gain legal sanction for the expansion of their scope of practice, especially in areas of diagnosis and prescription writing. The advantages of obtaining additional legal recognition are related to several areas of concern: (1) establishing requirements that only persons holding such additional recognition be allowed to practice in the given area; (2) reimbursement by third-party payers; and (3) the availability and cost of malpractice insurance.[35]

State certification for specialty practice presents several disadvantages. The intent to give nurse-practitioners legal authority to practice in what has traditionally been medical diagnosis, treatment, and prescription writing can end in limitations to nursing practice if the legal regulations that are promulgated give the physician authority over that practice.[19] The policy of mandating or recognizing certification is, in effect, surrender of the state's authority for establishing the standards for protecting the health and welfare of the public to a professional organization. When that professional organization restricts its certification mechanism only to members, the state is in effect requiring membership in a specific organization in order to practice a profession.[35]

The rules and regulations regarding specialty practice are difficult to amend and are subject to powerful lobbies. Employers often resist new licensure attempts. A state agency, typically the board of nursing, must regulate the certification process, and traditionally these agencies have had few economic resources. Overseeing of individual practice typically does not occur unless a complaint is filed. Finally, there is a great deal of diversity among states in the naming of specialties and the qualifications for specialty practice.

Certification by institutions

Many nurses have been awarded certificates to practice a specialty by institutions after the successful completion of advanced educational programs. Nurses enroll in specialty programs sponsored by schools of nursing, medicine, or health science colleges and universities, independent commercial groups, and hospitals. These programs focus on specific content that is defined according to the needs and structure of the specific institution. Specialty areas may be defined by age groups (e.g., child, adult, elderly), diseases (e.g., cardiac, renal, pulmonary), or special skills (e.g., midwifery, anesthesia, critical care).[14] The programs vary in length from a few weeks to 2 years, and there is little state or professional control over methods and content.

The nurse-practitioner movement was launched in the 1970s largely through certificate programs and the support of the Division of Nursing, Department of Health, Education, and Welfare. A three-part series of articles in *Nursing Outlook* in 1983 traced the evolution of this movement. The distinguishing criterion for inclusion in the survey as a nurse-practitioner program was because the program prepared nurses for expanded roles in the provision of primary care. In 1973 there were 86 certificate programs and 45 master's programs preparing nurse-practitioners; by 1977 there were 117 certificate and 61 master's programs; in 1980 there were 83 certificate programs and 112 master's programs. Thus during the decade of the 1970s, certificate programs were the predominant type of educational preparation for nurse-practitioners. However, by 1980 the number of master's programs exceeded the number of certificate programs. During the decade the total estimated number of graduates from certificate programs was 12,568, and the estimated number of graduates from the master's programs was 5586. By 1981, however, the number of graduates from the two types of programs was almost equal.[32] Thus the trend in nurse-practitioner education is toward master's preparation and away from certificate preparation.

Hospitals have become increasingly concerned about the specialty knowledge and skill performance of their nurse employees. This concern is greatest in complex, tertiary care centers in which each new specialty unit and each new piece of equipment require additional technological skills in monitoring and intervention. Orientation and continuing education needs in these situations have taken the form of competency-based testing. In essence, the institution is certifying that a nurse is competent to perform certain activities. The standards for this type of certification are unique to each institution although the Joint Commission for Accreditation of Healthcare Organizations (JCAHO) reviews these activities during an accreditation visit.

The advantages of the institutional model of nursing certification arise primarily from the solutions of immediate problems. Nurses who practice in specific organizations or who attend a practitioner program in an educational institution find institutional certification convenient in the short term. Likewise, health care organizations are assured of a supply of nurse specialists to provide needed services. Consumers tend to view academic and health care agencies as organizations that have the expertise and resources required to prepare nursing specialists and to provide surveillance over their practice.

The wide variability in standards among these certification programs is a major disadvantage of the institutional model. Programs appear to be shaped by local needs and resources and are fragmented. Furthermore, institutional certification programs are vulnerable to the competing vested interests of powerful lobbies. Nonuniversally applied standards, the lack of control by professionals with the needed expertise, and lack of interorganizational and interstate practitioner mobility promote satisfaction with lower standards. Clearly these are weak controls to assure accountability. Self-regulation and colleague control by professionals are inhibited, and governmental regulation is diluted, if not absent altogether. In addition to these disadvantages, the cost-benefit ratio for the institutional model of certification is questionable. The duplication of expensive structures and processes places stress on institutional costs that are already burdensome. Another cost that is often overlooked is the increased liability of institutions for litigations brought by former students who have not been certified for specialty practice by the professional organization. These costs are likely to be passed on to the consumer.

Table 38-3 Advantages and disadvantages of models according to goals of certification

Goals/Model	Professional		State		Institution	
	Advantages	Disadvantages	Advantages	Disadvantages	Advantages	Disadvantages
Access to health care	possess needed expertise to define standards; standardized specialty areas; standardized qualifications; national standards established	potential restriction of trade to those qualified	public recognition and sanction	nonstandardized specialty areas; nonstandardized qualifications restrict development of new methods, skills	public views/academic health care institutions as experts; supply of specialists	public disenchantment with academe; fragmented, confusion to public; nonstandardized specialty areas; nonstandardized qualifications
Consumer and provider protection	combat vested interests of powerful competing groups; universal standards; responsive to new knowledge/values	potentially self-serving; public distrust of professional autonomy	legal control	restricts title—not practice; discipline not communicated to other states; nonuniversally applied standards difficult to amend; subject to powerful lobbies; lack expertise	surveillance of practitioners	may make do with lower standards; subject to competing vested interests; fewer controls; nonuniversally applied standards; inhibits professional self-regulation
Consumer and provider benefit over cost	interstate and interagency mobile practitioners; self-supported by practitioners; voluntary rather than mandatory	current duplication of certification by organizations		dependent on professional organizations; need for repeated costly update; cost of maintaining boards; lack of practitioner mobility	convenient for practitioner	redundant costs of system passed on to consumer; lack of practitioner mobility

Finally, the institutional model is further weakened by the generally accepted belief that education that does not lead to a recognized academic degree lacks credibility and status among consumers and professionals because it may not meet universally recognized standards.

VIEWPOINT

The advantages and disadvantages of the three models of certification for specialty nursing practice are summarized in Table 38-3 according to the desired goals of certification. The preference for a specific model is a matter of judgment. We believe that the advantages associated with the professional organization model hold high value for both the public and the profession, and thus we prefer this model. Attainment of the desired goals of certification is enhanced through professional expertise, development of a standardized system, and geographic mobility of practitioners. The profession is aware of the major problem with this model, the duplication of service, and is working to correct the situation. We believe that it is essential for the profession to assume responsibility for self-regulation of specialized nursing practice.

The advantage of public recognition of specialty practice associated with the state model holds high value for many nurses. We believe that this is a time-limited advantage that has great potential for creating problems for both the public and the practitioner. It is forcing encodement of rules and regulations for specialized practice that are likely to be outdated in a few years. Each time the rules are updated, the specialty will be subject to the influence of vested interest groups that have traditionally tried to control nursing practice. Even the names of areas of specialization are likely to change as nursing theory develops. What is a prudent direction for the future now that a majority of the states have adopted this model? We believe that it would be best to proceed with all due speed to implement the ANA entry-into-practice recommendations and then to move to incorporte the expanded role of the nurse into the state practice acts, eliminating the need for state certification. It should also be recognized that state certification is dependent upon certification by the professional organization for establishing competence in the field. It is time for nurses to end the division of loyalties for these two models and unite in developing a certification system that will both enhance the public's access to specialized nursing care and recognize the practitioner.

The usefulness of the third model, institutional certification, also appears to be time limited. The educational trend for specialty practice is clearly toward the master's degree program. This is in keeping with the definition of specialization in the ANA's *Nursing: A Social Policy Statement*. This document establishes two criteria for the specialist: (1) a master's degree, and (2) certification by the professional organization. We lend our support to this definition in the belief that this direction is in the best interest of both the public and the profession.

REFERENCES

1. American Nurses' Association: The study of credentialing in nursing: a new approach, vol 1, Pub No G-136, 1979, The Association.
2. American Nurses' Association: The study of credentialing in nursing: a new approach, vol 7, Pub No G-138, 1979, The Association.
3. American Nurses' Association: Take the extra step: become a certified nurse, Kansas City, Mo, 1983, The Association.
4. American Nurses' Association: The nursing practice act: suggested state legislation, Kansas City, Mo, 1981, The Association.
5. American Nurses' Association: National registry of certified nurses in advanced practice, American Nurses' Association Pub No CR-23, 1987.
6. Aydelotte M: Professional nursing: the drive for governance. In Chaska N, editor: The nursing profession: a time to speak, New York, 1983, McGraw-Hill Book Co.
7. Bullough B: State certification of the nursing specialties: a new trend in nursing practice law, Pediatr Nurs 8(3):121, 1982.
8. Bullough B: Prescribing authority for nurses, Nurs Econ 1(2):122, 1983.
9. Collins HL: Certification: is the payoff worth the price? RN, July 1987, pp. 36-44.
10. Dunkley PH: The ANA certification program, Nurs Clin North Am 9(3):485, 1974.
11. Edari RS: A profile of the certified nurse. In The study of credentialing in nursing: a new approach, vol 2, Kansas City, Mo, 1979, The Association.
12. Ellis B: AHA looks at nurse credentialing, Hospitals 53(17):87, 1979.
13. Fickeissen JL: Getting certified, Am J Nurs 85(3):265, 1985.
14. Hinsvark IG: Educational preparation for the changed role of the nurse. In The study of credentialing in nursing: a new approach, vol 2, Kansas City, Mo, 1979, The Association.
15. Hinsvark IG: Credentialing in nursing. In McCloskey JC and Grace HK, editors: Current issues in nursing, ed 2, 1981, Boston, Blackwell Scientific Publications.
16. Jacobs JA: Legal aspects of voluntary credentialing programs. In The study of credentialing in nursing: a new approach, vol 2, Kansas City, Mo, 1979, The Association.
17. Jacox A: Collective action and control of practice by professionals, Nurs Forum 10:242, 1971.
18. Jones F: Certification for specialization. In McCloskey JC and Grace HK, editors: Current issues in nursing, ed 2, Boston, 1981, Blackwell Scientific Publications.

19. Kelly LS: Licensure laws in transition, Nurs Outlook 30(6):375, 1982.
20. LaBar C: The regulation of advanced nursing practice as provided for in nursing practice acts and administrative rules, American Nurses' Association Pub No D-76, 1983.
21. Maas M and Jacox A: Guidelines for nurse autonomy/patient welfare, New York, 1977, Appleton-Century-Crofts.
22. McCarthy P: ANA is the leader in certification for RNs, The American Nurse, Sept 1988, p. 11.
23. Mauksch I: Certification: assurance of quality, Am Nurse 10(3):4, 1978.
24. Merton R: The search for professional status, Am J Nurs 60:662, 1960.
25. Moore WE: The professional: roles and rules, New York, 1970, Russell Sage Foundation.
26. Passarelli A: Credentialing in nursing: background issues. In The study of credentialing in nursing: a new approach, vol 2, Kansas City, Mo, 1979, The Association.
27. Raymond MR: The relationship between educational preparation and performance on nursing certification examinations, J Nurs Educ 27(1):6, 1988.
28. Raymond MR and Ketchum EL: Certification in nursing. Paper presented at the annual meeting of the American Educational Research Association, New Orleans, April 1988.
29. Sammons LN: Control of credentialing for advanced practice: analysis using a Lewinian model, Adv Nurs Sci 5(4):13, 1983.
30. Sullivan S: Why certify? Heart Lung 10(5):217, 1981.
31. Sullivan S: Is certification necessary for specialty practice? Focus on Critical Care 10(3):37, 1983.
32. Sultz HA and others: A decade of change for nurse practitioners, Nurs Outlook, parts 1-3, 31:137-142, 216-219, 266-269, 1983.
33. Task force on credentialing asks for "commitment" from nursing groups, Am J Nurs 80:2125, 1980.
34. US Department of Health, Education and Welfare: Report on licensure and related health personnel credentialing, DHEW Pub No HSM, 72:11, Washington, DC, 1971.
35. Waddle F: Licensure: achievements and limitations. In The study of credentialing in nursing: a new approach, vol 2, Kansas City, Mo, The Association.
36. Weitzel E: In pursuit of ANA certification in gerontological nursing, J Gerontol Nurs 6(3):136, 1980.

CHAPTER 39

Standards of regulatory agencies

Blue print for quality or bureaucratic morass?

KARLENE KERFOOT

INTRODUCTION

Regulation is a fact of life, one that is not likely to change in the near future. A large percentage of the bedside nurse's time is spent documenting and performing tasks to satisfy the needs of many organizations, such as insurance companies, the Joint Commission for Accreditation of Healthcare Organizations (JCAHO), and Medicare. In addition, our litigious climate requires more extensive documentation to defend against potential lawsuits. It is not unusual to have 2 or more hours of a nurse's 8-hour shift involved in documentation to meet the regulatory agencies' requirements and also to communicate within the organization. Bedside computers can speed up the process of documentation, but the fact remains that exorbitant amounts of valuable nursing time are spent satisfying the requirements from regulatory agencies.

Nurses choose nursing because they want to take care of patients. Spending hours writing about what one has just finished doing to satisfy the needs of external regulatory agencies does not lead to job satisfaction or necessarily to excellence in the quality of nursing care. Many nurses feel they are not allowed to do what they came into nursing to do, namely, take care of patients. Bureaucratic regulations that do not appear from the nurse's perspective to guarantee quality have been a major source of dissatisfaction for nurses.[15] It is time for nurses, working through professional nursing organizations, to become more involved in influencing the regulatory agencies to be concerned about the quality of nursing care and not just the process of documentation. For too long process has been emphasized at the expense of outcome. The profession of nursing must work with regulatory agencies to define the appropriate achievable outcomes for patients and the methods for attaining them.

WHO CONTROLS THE PRACTICE OF NURSING?

It is a widely shared view that professionals should control their own practice. However, there are many agencies that direct and control a portion of the practice of nursing. For example, state boards of nursing determine the curriculum requirements, standards for licensure, and the scope of nursing practice. Regulatory agencies, such as JCAHO and Medicare, develop standards for the practice of nursing, as do professional nursing organizations, which also write position papers on the subject. For example, the American Nurses' Association (ANA) published *Nursing: A Social Policy Statement*,[2] which described various aspects of nursing practice; the ANA has also published standards for clinical specialties. Regulatory agencies have clout. If their standards are not met, a sanction is imposed. Medicare, for example, can decide that a facility is no longer safe. The facility will lose its Medicare-provider status, and notices to that effect will be published in local newspapers. Professional nursing organizations do not have such clout. The only way they can be influential is by convincing the regulatory agencies to adopt their professional standards.

The fragmentation of nursing into many specialty organizations allows the control of nursing practice to be assumed by a variety of accrediting boards and agencies. To be influential in the development of standards for practice, the specialty nursing organizations will have to join with the larger nursing organizations to present one clear voice for nursing. The only clear solution for the future is for nursing organizations to organize under one umbrella organization or federation to be truly influential.

DO ACCREDITING STANDARDS GUARANTEE QUALITY?

It is difficult to state that the standards of accrediting and regulatory agencies actually do maintain quality. The problem lies in the fact that there is no consensus about what determines quality in health care. Patients, for example, may define quality nursing care as nurses who smile at them and are able to spend time with them. The patient is generally not aware that nurses perform surveillance activities when they interact with patients; patients therefore cannot judge the quality of those surveillance activities. Physicians might judge the quality of nursing care on the basis of how quickly they are alerted to abnormal lab results. Physicians often are unaware of the amount and quality of patient teaching provided by nurses and therefore cannot judge this aspect of nursing care. The hospital administrator might look for cost-effectiveness and the hospital legal staff for the absence of litigation. The problem is that many different consumers define quality in a wide variety of ways. The old adage of "not documented, not done" does not guarantee quality. Because a definition of quality in health care has not been agreed on, quality is difficult to define and therefore measure.

Recently a *Wall Street Journal* article[3] called attention to the issue of accreditation and quality. As a result of an investigation, the author charged, "The joint commission allows dangers to health and safety to go uncorrected for weeks, months and even years. Sloppy, irresponsible hospitals have little to fear from the commission. Punishment in recent years has been nearly nonexistent. Although the law requires federal officials to monitor the commission, their efforts are disorganized, weak and ineffective." The Chairman of the House Ways and Means Committee, Representative Fortney "Pete" Stark, has asked the General Accounting Office to investigate the quality of accreditation performed by the JCAHO.[14]

At present the 22-member governing board of JCAHO is composed of representatives from the American Medical Association, American Hospital Association, American College of Physicians, American College of Surgeons, and the American Dental Association.[12] One nurse currently serves as one of the representatives from the American Hospital Association. No representation from professional nursing organizations is present on the board of JCAHO, perhaps at least partly because JCAHO was founded by physicians. Consequently, the voice of professional nursing is not as loud as it should be. This situation may continue until professional nursing organizations develop a more unified voice for nursing.

THE COST OF REGULATORY STANDARDS

Regulatory standards most certainly have increased the cost of health care. At a time when there is much concern about a nursing shortage, many full-time positions have been created for nurses to do nothing but meet regulatory standards.[1] Utilization review, quality assurance, and other mandatory programs have created an expensive system requiring many registered nurses. Some public regulatory bodies are beginning to mandate that certain nurses have credentials from private organizations such as the ANA and other certifying bodies.[6] JCAHO has announced an "Agenda for Change" to measure a health care facility's actual performance.[11] Extensive computerization of information will be necessary to demonstrate compliance. Unfortunately, hospitals are not reimbursed for the cost of this agenda for change. This is one more program mandated by outside regulatory agencies that cuts into the profits of hospitals and, consequently, the money available to nurses for compensation. Traditionally, hospitals have depended on patients with private insurance to pay for these additional programs. With more patients on capitated and prospective payment systems, there is no one to pay these extra costs. Consequently, many hospitals are in serious financial trouble, partly because of expensive regulatory standards.

The profession of nursing has not critiqued new standards in an organized, effective way. The cost of health care has risen in part due to these standards. We must take an active role in influencing agencies to develop cost-effective standards that truly measure quality.

THE STAFF NURSE AND REGULATORY STANDARDS

Unfortunately, it is unusual for a staff nurse to be conversant about JCAHO, Medicare, and other regulations. The nursing staff often becomes aware of the standards just before anticipated visits by regulatory agencies. Because the standards direct and guide practice, every nurse should be knowledgeable about them and how they are implemented in daily practice. In a professional model, the professional measures the quality against standards. In a technical or industrial model, the manager measures practice against standards. With nursing's move to professional autonomy, it is imperative that each staff nurse be knowledgeable about the JCAHO and Medicare standards and be able to measure outcomes against these standards.

The bedside nurse needs to be more than an assembly-line worker or a cog in a wheel. Nurses need to be given total control over the clinical aspects of patient care. This involves peer review, the careful auditing of compliance to standards, and the development of action plans to meet these standards. Although traditionally these tasks have been thought to belong to management, it is imperative that the staff nurse be given this kind of responsibility as a professional.[7,8] Determining compliance with regulatory standards must be part of the job of every staff nurse.

The accrediting standards are not standards of excellence. They are merely standards of minimal, optimal, and achievable outcomes. Any viable organization would not be content to settle for the level implied in accreditation standards. An organization should go beyond the minimum to achieve standards of excellence. For example, a quality assurance program as prescribed by the JCAHO is the beginning. However, if a quality assurance program is combined with nursing research, it will provide solutions to problems that are not available in a quality assurance program. The Quality Assurance Model Utilizing Research,[10] developed for a grant application and decribed by Watson, Bilechek, and McCloskey,[16] is an example of a model that goes beyond mandated standards to provide answers to nursing care problems. Nurses can and must take the standards and incorporate them into a usable system that makes sense for them, for their patient care, and for their institutions.

Nurses have a choice of being proactive or reactive to the standards of regulatory agencies.[13] It behooves each nurse to take a proactive approach and determine an action plan that will best meet the standards and also the goal of quality care. Standards must be a part of the everyday practice of each nurse.

Nurses must get involved to influence the development of standards. At no time in our history has the profession of nursing been under greater assault from a wider variety of groups to define its practice. The American Medical Association's proposal for registered care technicians is an example of another profession trying to impinge on the practice of nursing. At the same time, as competition between professions worsens because of the shrinking health care dollar, it will be necessary for nursing to protect itself through organized professional action. Nursing practice and the legislation and regulation that define this practice have undergone dramatic changes in the past few years,[5] and new standards are evolving constantly.[4] Professional nursing *must* influence these changes. Accreditation standards are not what they should be. With thought, research, and extensive discussions, nurses can work to influence accreditation standards that will better delineate the quality of care the professional should provide.

Quality is everyone's concern. We have only begun to address the issue in a way that makes sense. It will take many qualified clinicians working with regulatory agencies to reach an agreement on the best and most economical way to determine quality outcomes. We have the expertise to do this. We need the structure. The time is now for professional nursing organizations to provide a united front about what quality nursing care must be.

REFERENCES

1. Adams R: The impact of utilization review on nursing, J Nurs Admin 17(9):44, 1987.
2. American Nurses' Association: Nursing: a social policy statement, Kansas City, Mo, 1980, The Association.
3. Bogdanich W: Prized by hospitals, accreditation hides perils patients face, Wall Street Journal 222:A1, October 12, 1988.
4. Davis N: New JCAH chapter requires the RN circulator, AORN J 46(2):173, 1987.
5. Greenlaw J: Definition and regulation of nursing practice: an historical survey, Law, Medicine & Health Care 13(3):117, 1985.
6. Hutton E: Regulation of advanced nursing practice: a commentary, Nursing Economics 3(1):21, 1985.
7. Kerfoot K: "Managing" professionals: the ultimate contradiction for nurse managers, Nursing Economics 6(6):321, 1988.
8. Kerfoot K: Retention: what's it all about? Nursing Economics 6(1):42, 1988.
9. Kerfoot K: Regulatory agencies: an impetus for change. In Johnson M, editor: Series on nursing administration—changing organizational structures, vol 2, Redwood City, Calif, Addison-Wesley, 1989.
10. McCloskey J, Watson C, and Bulechek G: Quality assurance model using research (QAMUR). Department of Health and Human Service Public Health Service (DHHSPHS) Grant #1-42-6004-813-A1. College of Nursing, University of Iowa Hospitals and Clinics, Iowa City, 1987.

11. O'Leary D: The Joint Commission looks to the future, JAMA 258(7):951, 1987.
12. Roberts J, Coale J, and Redman R: A history of the Joint Commission on Accreditation of Hospitals, JAMA 258(7)936, 1987.
13. Thompson T: A proactive approach to accrediting standards, Rehabilitation Nursing 11(5):8, 1986.
14. Tokarski C: Rep. Stark requests inquiry into JCAHO procedures, Modern Healthcare 18(46):6, 1988.
15. Department of Health and Human Services (USDHHS): Secretary's commission on nursing, Final Report, vol 1, Washington, DC, 1988.
16. Watson C, Bulechek G, and McCloskey J: QAMUR: a quality assurance model using research, Journal of Nursing Quality Assurance 2(1):21, 1987.

PART SIX

GOVERNANCE

Under pressure for change

JOANNE COMI McCLOSKEY
HELEN KENNEDY GRACE

As the health care system changes, governance of nursing education and practice is under considerable pressure to change. Although the opportunities for long-lasting change within the nursing profession are perhaps greater than ever before, the resistance to change, both from without and within, constitutes a formidable obstacle. Part 6 provides an overview of some of the facets of governance in the nursing profession during this time of rapid and dramatic change.

This section opens with a debate chapter by Sweeney and Witt, which asks, "Does nursing have the power to change the health care system?" After singling out critical elements related to power, the authors first argue that nursing is relatively powerless in creating change within the health care system. This premise is supported by observations that in the face of a nursing shortage and a shift from institutional to home care, the proposed solution has been to find substitutes for nurses, either registered care technologists in the hospital or family and friends in the home and community. Further factors inhibiting the exercise of nursing power are (1) the inability to use the power of the collective number of nurses, (2) a lack of financial independence, (3) a value system that focuses on nurturing rather than on power and competition, (4) the inability to wield power in institutional settings in which nursing is the main provider of care, and (5) the tendency for nurses to function as small aggregates rather than as a cohesive group.

Drawing upon the same conceptualization of power, the authors argue that nurses do have the power to change the system by (1) setting the direction for the profession themselves rather than letting it be set by others, (2) demonstrating the ability to provide affordable health care services to an aging population and those segments of the population that are currently underserved, (3) using the direct relationship with patients as a source of power, (4) using the caring ideology of the nursing profession as a means of garnering support, (5) reaffirming the nurse's position of centrality in coordinating health care services, and (6) divorcing the definitions of nursing practice from institutional settings through movement into community-based practices.

Moving to some specific governance issues in nursing, O'Connor and Gibson speak to factors underlying increased unionization as a means of gaining power within the health care delivery system. They observe that although unionization in general is declining, the trend is in the opposite direction in the health care field. They account for this difference by noting the impact of changed payment systems that have shifted control of health care decision making from physicians to hospital administrations and the business concerns that are now pushing health care. This change has resulted in greater reliance on unions in the health care field to protect the interests of the worker. Other factors include the changing characteristics of patients, the increased technology in hospital settings, and the movement of patient care from tertiary settings to the community. These factors, coupled with characteristics of a profession composed primarily of women, who in many instances are single parents or supporters of elderly parents, have resulted in increased concerns for support systems that will allow nurses to meet their multiple responsibilities. The collective bargaining process is seen as a positive force in counteracting the tendency of management to make decisions based solely on business concerns. As collective bargaining in nursing becomes increasingly sophisticated, part of the process concerning quality patient care is being addressed. The authors argue that this trend of increased unionization is likely to continue because of the nursing shortage, the decline in numbers and diversity of students entering nursing, and the change in regulations that now allows for the formation of unions composed only of nurses, in contrast to previous regulations that required a mix of health professionals to be part of a bargaining unit.

One way for nurses to gain increased independence in their practice is through providing direct nursing services to individuals without an intermediary. Lundeen discusses the evolving definition of a nursing center and its initial strong association with academic settings. The current definition makes the concept more inclusive and allows for a variety of arrangements for providing direct nursing services to individuals. She then mentions a number of key issues that need to be addressed for nursing centers to thrive: (1) direct client access to professional nursing services, (2) collaborative practice models that are operating from bases of equal power and mutual respect, (3) emphasis on health promotion and health education services, the traditional activities of nursing, (4) direct reimbursement, and (5) use of nursing centers for student learning and faculty research and practice. Addressing some of the governance issues, Lundeen concludes that "long term health policy goals must continue to include a redefinition of health provider roles and a more equal allocation of professional power and decision making so as to facilitate the development of collaborative, holistic delivery provider models."

Turning to the perspective of nursing administration, O'Grady points to the radical restructuring of traditional services and environments and cautions that nursing must respond in a positive fashion to these changing conditions. Shifts in the economic structure resulting in an emphasis on constrained resources and the retooling of the entire health care industry have important implications for nursing. Decision making within hospital settings is shifting to the front-line managers. Nursing must assure that these managers of patient care have the necessary background for their newly defined managerial role. Also, as health care shifts from an institutional to a community base, new models for the organization of nursing care must evolve. With the relationships increasingly driven by service providers, O'Grady poses a number of provocative questions that nursing has to answer. He challenges nursing leadership to adapt to and direct changes within the nursing field.

In providing direction during this time of change, nursing organizations have a critical role to play. Hegyvary presents a succinct overview of the types of nursing organizations and the role that they play vis-à-vis the profession. Given an overall function for nursing organizations as "obtaining and maintaining power," she categorizes four types of structures: (1) the multipurpose organizations representing nursing as a whole, (2) clinical specialty organizations promoting the identify and interests of nurses in specialty organizations, (3) functional specialty organizations representing nursing education and administration, and (4) developing alliances. Noting a decline in membership in multipurpose organizations and an increase in membership in specialty groups, Hegyvary predicts that in the future, there will be an increase in the alliances formed between organizations as a way of addressing issues related to the total field.

Turning to academic governance issues, Ostmoe and Sparks first address the issue of change in the composition and characteristics of faculty within nursing education programs. In 1982 the authors were concerned about the underemphasis on scholarly work as part of the expectations for nurse faculty members in contrast to the expectations held for faculty in other areas of the university. Noting a number of indicators, such as nearly doubling the number of doctorally prepared faculty and increases in numbers of doctoral programs, the authors conclude that this situation has changed considerably in a very short span of time. Ironically, as nursing has increased its emphasis on scholarly productivity, the concerns of the broader university have shifted to undergraduate instruction as a matter of prime concern. With a decrease in student enrollment and an increased emphasis on faculty practice, the authors argue that the components of a faculty member's role should be seen as interactive rather than as mutually exclusive. Scholarship should underpin all areas of faculty functioning, so that faculty promotion and tenure are based on scholarly teaching, scholarly practice, and scholarly service.

Turning to governance issues on a worldwide scale, Ohlson addresses the structure and function of the International Council of Nurses (ICN) and of nursing within the World Health Organization (WHO). Composed of national nursing organizations from 100 countries, the ICN provides a forum for addressing the interests, needs, and concerns of nursing throughout the world. WHO, as an intergovernmental agency, is primarily concerned with helping governments strengthen basic health service in their countries. Nursing within WHO is primarily concerned with the participation of nursing in the delivery of health care services throughout the world.

Returning to the debate question that sets the frame for Part 6, the ability of nursing to build organizational structures that lend cohesion to the profession and unite nurses in a common voice is critical if the power of nursing to promote change within the system is to be realized.

CHAPTER 40

Debate

Does nursing have the power to change the health care system?

SANDRA S. SWEENEY
KAREN E. WITT

This chapter asks, "Does nursing have the power to change the health care system?" The question is neither new nor original, but the issues have become increasingly important to the profession, given the dramatic changes that have taken place in health care organizations and delivery of services thoughout the industry. This is particularly true for the more drastic changes that have occurred during the past 5 years. While some are writing of the current crises confronting the profession of nursing,[20] others note the unparalleled opportunities such changes can bring if nurses mobilize and capitalize on the challenges being placed before them.[12,21,28,37]

The turmoil and chaos surrounding the American health care delivery system today have sparked a renewed interest in the concept of power, particularly by nurses who are concerned not only about their own or their profession's interests but also about the quality of care received by consumers. This chapter analyzes both the positive and the negative implications of using power to change the health care system and suggests obstacles nurses can expect to confront should they demand change. Power is conceptually defined, and actual and potential relationships that exist between the concept of power and the profession of nursing are illustrated.

The framework used to organize and structure the debate was selected from the seminal work published by Berle.[8] Berle considers power to be a "universal experience and a human attribute of man with five discernible natural laws."[8] The laws of power are as follows:

1. Power invariably fills any vacuum in human organization.
2. Power is invariably personal.
3. Power is invariably based on a system of ideals or a philosophy.
4. Power is exercised through, and depends on, institutions.
5. Power is invariably confronted with, and acts in the presence of, a field of responsibility.

Laws, by definition, allow generalizations while also providing a structure for logical reasoning. Berle's[8] laws seemed to provide an appropriate framework for the question raised in this chapter. Each law will be briefly restated followed by an amplification of the law and the argument in which power and its relationship to the profession of nursing is debated relative to our contemporary health care delivery system. The literature on power is replete with definitions, none of which seemed inclusive enough for the purposes of this debate.

Therefore, we synthesized the following conceptual definition of power for use in this chapter:

Power is an ability to employ effort toward attaining specific ends. It exists as either a stimulus, state, or response and is situationally specific. Power is experienced internally or externally and is consciously or unconsciously employed in symmetrical or asymmetrical equations. It emerges in a specific form and is constrained at microcosmic or macrocosmic levels. Power emerges, can be used or diffused, has sustenance requirements, is subject to challenge, possesses limitations, and may be either won or lost by election, expiration, resignation, or expulsion. Power is a universal attribute of humans and is governed by five invariant natural laws.

NURSING DOES NOT HAVE THE POWER TO CHANGE THE HEALTH CARE SYSTEM

To repeat Berle's first law: "Power invariably fills any vacuum in human organization. As between chaos and power, the latter always prevails."[8] The health care industry has enjoyed several decades of public-supported expansion and substantial freedom in self-governance but now finds itself facing radical change. Impending changes are occurring in access, finance, organizational ownership, management, payment systems, and limited hospital stays. In addition, there are movements by consumers to encourage, it not mandate, agencies at local, state, and national levels to impose more prescriptive, not restrictive, policies to improve and protect the rights of all citizens to affordable, quality health care. The possibility of enforced changes is creating a chaotic situation at best while simultaneously producing even larger numbers of individuals whose health care needs remain unmet.

Berle maintains, "when a vacuum occurs at any level of the power structure, the immediate result is to throw power downward to the next lower institutional echelon."[8] The changes in health care delivery in the United States during the past 5 years, combined with the increasing plight of the homeless, greater numbers of uninsured and underinsured, the increasing needs of a chronically ill and aging population, and shortened hospital stays might lead one to think that nursing has accumulated unprecedented power by now; but nursing's services have not been demanded by those in positions to recognize how valuable nurses can be to an organization. Indeed, instead of delegating power downward from hospital administrators and physicians to competent nurses, the medical profession has proposed instead a new category of health provider, the registered care technologist (RCT), who is supposed to replace nurses at the bedside and provide effective, efficient quality care after only a 9-month course of instruction![1] While the American Medical Association (AMA) has been busy formalizing the RCT proposal, there has also been a slow but steady trend toward shifting the responsibility for caring for individuals who need close monitoring from institutions to homes or day-care facilities; this is also a move-ment away from care given by professional nurses toward family members or other less prepared health care workers. If nurses have the power to change or influence health care, why have they not emerged with a new mantle of power?

Lynaugh and Fagin[28] list five paradoxes—characteristics of the profession—that pose dilemmas nurses have had to face thoughout history. One of the dilemmas is that our society has systematically undervalued care, particularly the care given by nurses. Now, especially, with prospective payment systems, increased acuity levels, earlier discharges, increased technology, improved pharmaceutical agents, and longer life spans, the assumption that nurses can substitute for family members or servants is being reversed to suggest that family members and servants can substitute for nurses. Nursing will not be able to reverse this trend until it can document its efficiency and effectiveness in dollars and cents. Although there may be a general unwillingness of health care policymakers to think of quality nursing care in terms of a monetary value, nursing's inability to document its relative merit is also largely responsible for contributing to the profession's weak power base when issues of health care are addressed and policies formulated. Reverby[38] concurs with the problems contemporary nursing faces in attempting to care for a society that refuses to value caring.

Nurses cannot hope to change the health care delivery system in this country until they are entitled to receive monetary compensation for their services, particularly in the realm of third-party reimbursement. At present, thousands of nurses are providing care to hundreds of thousands of American citizens in need of professional services. However, the nursing care being provided is either unreimbursed or, worse, being paid to a health care organization or physician! Even when armed with statistical estimates of their cost-effectiveness, nurses have been unable to marshall the support necessary to achieve (1) recognition of the financial worth of their work, and (2) the right to receive direct payment for their services. Andrews[5] states, "Conservative estimates suggest even if non-physician providers undertook the readily delegable portions of adult primary and pediatric primary care, between one-half billion and one billion dollars would be saved annually, cutting 19 to 49 percent of the total primary care provider bill," and further, "an examination of 58 different health care tasks indicated that the costs averaged $8.13 when the tasks were performed by a nurse practitioner and $16.48 when performed by a physician."[5] Nurses must find mechanisms through which existing reimbursement systems can be revised. They must unite their economic capacity with their professional capabilities if they are to wield the power necessary to change the health care system.

Finally, I believe nurses must be able to overcome their own conflicts and divisions, beginning with the problem of what level of educational preparation should be required for entry into practice, before there is any hope of coalescing power and influencing change in areas outside the profession. Currently, the entry into practice issue is perceived by many nurses and others as a major source of division. Even though people understand the history behind the current controversy, they remain polarized over the proposed solutions. The education for beginning practice issue is further confounded by issues of gender and a history of being an oppressed group.[28,39] Unless and until the philosophical and practice components of nursing's constituencies are able to focus their energies on combating the problem in the health care system instead of fighting with each other, nursing will never succeed in garnering the power it needs to effect change in a health care system already too accustomed to male control and physician domination.

Berle's second law suggests power "is invariably personal; that there is no such thing as class power, elite power, or group power; although classes, elites, and groups may be the processes of organization by which power is lodged in individuals."[8] Nurses and nursing are in double jeopardy when it comes to describing potential power bases using this law. First of all, nurses have rarely, if ever, found a common interest that they as individuals or collectively through the processes of organization have fought to preserve, protect, or alter. It may be argued that various speciality groups of nurses have been somewhat successful in effecting change; however, as a group or class of professionals, nurses have not used their collectivity to pursue either institutional or professional goals or objectives. At present, there seems to be a unified and organized reaction among nurses and their organizations to vehemently oppose the registered care technologist proposal being advanced by the American Medical Association.[2] If this effort is successful, it may provide the impetus nursing needs to formulate future

policies and agendas that have the potential to enlist the broad-based support from among its membership and ensure the power that accompanies strength in numbers.

This debate is about the present, however, not the future. If nurses are to effectively implement the law of power described above, they must first recognize the need to develop personal power. May[30] argues one's denial "of the importance of power commits oneself to continued helplessness . . . and manifests itself in depression and self-hatred as one's psychological growth is thwarted by an unwillingness to exert influence and affirm one's own worth." How can nurses who care and are concerned about the needs of the unserved patient-clients fully express their concerns when faced with the possible loss of their jobs? How can nurses confront hospital administrators and refuse to stay at home "on-call" for $1.50 an hour when policies are implemented by their head nurses or supervisors? How can individual professional nurses fight for quality care when they are unable or unwilling to unite to openly express their outrage and concern or to enlist the public's awareness to arouse support for change? Perhaps it is because many nurses lack personal power, the power one invests in oneself—self-esteem, self-respect, and self-confidence. Nurses do not seem to possess the personal power needed to go forward, and without it, they will not have the ability to know when to lead or when to follow, both essential strategies in the appropriate utilization of power.

Nurses either have not developed or have not been able to sustain a keen sense of their individual responsibilities as professionals, which further impedes their ability to attain personal and professional goals. Nurses cannot expect to wield power until they join a professional organization or group in which their individual and collective agendas can be put into motion. Although many nurses talk of our collective numbers—the largest group of health professionals in the United States—those numbers become unimportant when legislators, physicians, and corporations are quick to note that the American Nurses' Association (ANA) currently represents only about 10% of all nurses in America.[4] Organizations are composed of individuals, but without their support, it is difficult, if not impossible, for organizations to make their members see the potential power in numbers.

Another obstacle for nurses and their organizations in their quest for a strong power base is a tendency to fight battles reactively rather than proactively. Nurses need to anticipate and propose changes that will work to their benefit rather than to resist change. Nurses have a long history of accommodation, particularly in relation to external forces, such as coping with the revolving cycle of shortages, accepting temporary staff nurses from external agencies, accepting one-time bonuses in lieu of annual salary increases, and accepting decisions made and enforced by nonnursing personnel. This process of accommodation is typical of a group that perceives itself to be powerless and helpless. "Individuals who do not perceive themselves to be in control of material, social or intellectual resources are generally found to act passively and believe that luck or chance controls their fate."[23] If nurses expect to possess power and be able to actualize it as individuals and through groups and organizations, they must be prepared to identify and follow a new group of individuals who will lead them into proactive postures.

Nurses who want themselves, their group, and the profession to have power must also be willing to pay the price; that is, there must be a commitment to finance such efforts. Nurses do not readily part with their hard-earned money and usually want to be informed of exactly how funds have been spent.[42] When nursing has an established financial foundation, it will then be able to represent individuals and organizations and to promote and actualize its programs and agendas.

"Power is based on a system of ideals or a philosophy. Two ingredients of power are inseparable . . . an idea system, a philosophy . . . and . . . an institutional structure transmitting the will of the power holder," states the third law of power.[8] Nursing's system of ideals and philosophical premises can be traced to the beginning of civilization, but they have become more closely aligned within an occupational structure since the Florence Nightingale era. A typical dictionary definition of nursing today continues to suggest nursing means to suckle, take care of, nourish, foster, or to serve as a nurse.[43] Although nurses do take care of others in need, nourish when necessary, foster independence when possible, and serve client-publics as part of their functions, such descriptors fail to convey a unique set of ideals or philosophical posture conducive to establishing a strong competitive power base in today's health care arena.

Nurses have a long history of struggling to legitimize themselves and the work they do to the societies they serve. Whether nurses have served well in either military or civilian sectors, their contributions have frequently gone unrecognized, if not unnoticed. Recent struggles have involved nursing's attempts to move from occupational to professional status, from hospital-based programs of education to university settings, from dependent to independent or interdependent practice opportunities, and from modalities of trial and error to sophisticated methodologies including the formulation of conceptual or theoretical models. Each of these changes, however, has been greeted with distrust, misgiving, and suspicion both from within and without the nursing community. Thus our diversity and lack of agreement in identifying common ideals and philosophical postures has prevented the profession from being able to develop the power necessary to effect change in many of the institutions in which nurses function.

It has been suggested by Norris[34] that the nursing community has agreed on four phenomena unique to the discipline: nursing, patient, health, and environment. If this were indeed true, then nursing would have a framework on which to begin structuring a system of ideals, a philosophy, and a common will among its membership. However, in reality, it seems only a small number of nurses actually accept or are even aware that these concepts exist, let alone subscribe to the belief that they are the foundation of nursing's theory and practice. The issue is further confounded when one analyzes the increasing number of conceptual/theoretical models published for and by nurses relative to the discipline. Each theory has its own terminology, definitions, framework, and philosophical message and its relationship to nursing theory and practice. These diverse positions may provide academicians with an opportunity to discuss, debate, and verify the relative merits of each contribution, but they do little to stimulate or convince the greater majority of practicing nurses that there is any relationship between the theoretical conceptions of nursing and the daily work world encountered by staff nurses.

Ideologies speak with one voice and espouse a common philosophy. As long as nurse academicians and theorists continue to speak a language unaccepted, impractical, and difficult to apply by practitioners, it will be impossible for the profession as a whole to champion a united cause. Nursing needs to address the concerns, contexts, and interests of both academic and practicing nurses if there is to be any hope of establishing common bonds and shared ideals. As long as nurses remain a group of health care providers who cannot extend their historical traditions of caring and nurturing and consolidate their existing estranged positions, they will continue to be powerless in both the academic and health care institutional environments.

Nursing must determine who or what institution will identify and communicate its ideals, philosophy, and structure. Organizations espousing nursing's interests now number close to 50, and all lack sufficient membership to truly represent the profession as a whole. Unions are attempting to organize and represent the profession, but many question whether agreement is possible given the professional-union dichotomy in purposes, objectives, and philosophies. Individual nurses cannot be expected to operate alone without the collective support of colleagues and leaders. There are those who speak of the opportunities available to nurses now,[35,37] but who will lead, coalesce, and unite the community of nurses to make the opportunities a reality?

Berle's fourth law states: "Power is exercised through and depends on institutions. Power is invariably organized and transmitted through institutions."[8] The profession of nursing has been closely associated with hospitals since its immigration from England. Although in Britain, Florence Nightingale may have insisted on separating nursing education from formalized institutions such as hospitals, such divisions did not accompany the establishment of educational programs in the United States. Whether the affiliations nursing education established with hospitals are to blame for many of our current problems, the fact remains that relatively few nurses have achieved success either as independent practitioners or as pioneers in entrepreneurial enterprises. The vast majority of nurses continue to work within hospitals or institutions closely affiliated with hospital-based centers of control. Harriman suggests:

Organizational policies award power to individuals who can exert influence upward and outward in the organization. This power is based on achieving credibility and creating dependency through the control of resources of supply, information and knowledge. The more critical one's activities are to the organization's success and survival, the more dependent other elements of the organization and the more power is generated.[16]

If Harriman is correct, then one can only deduce that nurses employed in hospitals and related institutions are unable to exert influence within the organization, lack credibility, are not able to create situ-

ations requiring dependency on their work by others, and do not have control over critical resources such as supply, knowledge, or information! Assuming this scenario to be correct, how realistic is it for nurses to expect to exert influence on institutional policy-making?

Until the arrival of home health care, the only service patients received in hospitals that could not have been offered almost equally well on the outside was nursing care. Logic suggests, therefore, that professional nurses would command significant organizational power within hospital-based complexes. But the fact remains that they have not nor do they now. One explanation for this is offered by Reverby, who implies that the endorsement and utilization of scientific management theory and its techniques by nurses during the middle of this century led to the unanticipated consequence of dividing patient care into many individualized tasks. It became easy, therefore, to delegate specific responsibilities to others, many of whom were relatively untrained workers earning wages substantially lower than those earned by professional nurses. "Nurses found themselves often doing the same work as nurse aides or licensed practical nurses and trying desperately to define and justify what the differences were between their skills.[38]

Task differentiation and subsequent rationalization of what constitutes professional nursing services have prompted hospital administrators to continue to hire individuals with meager nursing preparation as substitutes for registered nurses. Administrators can do this as long as they are able to meet their specific regulatory agencies' minimum requirements regarding supervision by professional nurses. The continued diffusion of tasks among so many categories of workers undermines nursing's ability to effectively influence institutional policy because it remains unable to demonstrate its unique contributions to the organization's mission.

Hickson and others proposed a strategic contingencies theory, with a hypothesis that three variables governed a subunit's power within an organization: (1) centrality—the degree of interdependence and indispensability; (2) substitutability—the possibility of easy replacement by others; and (3) coping with uncertainty—the ability to handle inevitable and unpredictable occurrences.[19] It is difficult to argue that nursing care should not be central to most care-providing institutions, such as hospitals, nursing homes, and public health and home health agencies. It is not difficult, however, to see that nursing has been unable to make others realize the centrality of its services. Nurses are hard pressed to define their area of expertise, demonstrate significant findings to support their knowledge base or clinical practice, and determine who among the more than 2.5 million individuals engaged in the practice of nursing are considered to be the professionals.[13]

The next assault on nursing's credibility and status within health care institutions may very well come from physicians. Given the projected oversupply of physicians, there is reason to suspect physicians may attempt to resume responsibility for tasks previously delegated to nurses, or at the very least attempt to further restrict nurses from initiating independent interventions they now provide patient-clients under their care. Nurses will have to determine what they want their roles and responsibilities to be if they expect to escape what Ginzberg calls the "rising protectionism of the medical profession."[13]

The credibility of professional nursing has also been diminished by nurses who reject graduate study in favor of the more "attractive," "exciting," and, most important, "lucrative" areas of business administration, psychology, counseling, and so forth. This disregard for the need to study advanced nursing suggests to nurses and others that there is nothing to be gained professionally, personally, or monetarily from further preparation in one's chosen profession. Indeed, nurses are frequently encouraged not to pursue graduate study in nursing by the very people who have benefited most by hiring less prepared individuals to replace nurses at the beside, who seem to have the view that a nurse is a nurse is a nurse! Such views diminish even further the idea that nurses should develop areas of specialization and place a low value on furthering one's education. As long as nurses willingly succumb to such advice and perceive success as being possible only outside the profession of nursing, they will not be able to convey a sense of the importance of nursing because they themselves do not see its importance. A professional whose practice boundaries are being threatened externally and who cannot envision a potential future internally will be unable to project a credible image, garner power, or earn respect from either constituency.

"Power is invariably confronted with and acts in the presence of a field of responsibility."[8] A field of responsibility is further defined by Berle as "aggregates made up of tiny or great power organisms to whom the powerholder is responsible."[8] Given this context, it will be difficult for nursing to ever create a cohesive field of responsibility, because the profession is composed of large numbers of relatively small aggregates, each perceiving itself as unique and somewhat removed from the larger population of registered nurses, which now numbers more than 1.5 million individuals. The field of responsibility, rather than addressing the common needs and rights of nurses generally, is more frequently perceived as belonging to specialty practice areas, special interests groups, or those having particular educational credentials. This wide diversity only serves to dilute and diminish the paramenters within which a field of responsibility can exist and survive.

Nursing's early endeavors to reach consensus on what constituted its field of responsibility consisted of attempts to create formal organizations that would represent and speak for the emerging profession. The leaders of the time, Robb, Nutting, Dock, Wald, and Stewart, believed that power would accompany strength of purpose and courage of convictions when large numbers of nurses attempted to achieve common goals and objectives. Today, however, the contemporary organizations that have evolved from those early efforts no longer possess the memberships necessary to justify any claim to speak for professional nursing. Indeed, the overwhelming lack of participation by nurses in their professional organizations is frequently used by opposing groups to refute agendas for change proposed by nursing's leadership.

"Nursing's power base originates at the bedside."[24] Practice, then, should define nursing's field of responsibility. Although this may seem ideal, practicing nurses must identify and document nursing's role and field of responsibility as opposed to the responsibilities ascribed to them by other health care professionals. Thus practicing nurses must be immune to the dictates of others if they are to formulate their own paramenters of practice. This may not be feasible given the overwhelming workloads being managed by most nurses in today's health care institutions. Nurses are actively engaged in determining parameters of practice as evidenced by the National Implementation Project[32] and the Nursing Knowledge Project.[14] Whether or not the findings of these efforts will be accepted and endorsed by practicing nurses, however, remains open to question.

If nursing's field of responsibility is to emanate from practice, then the way nurses view power in the workplace and in relation to one another will have to undergo change and modification. Although the number of studies exploring the concept of power and nurses in hospital organizations is limited, findings by Heineken suggest nurse executives and staff nurses hold quite different perspectives regarding at least two areas of power: "(1) the power that is associated with political abilities and (2) the power that is needed to maintain control and autonomy. . . . Nurse executives scored significantly higher than nurses holding lower level positions on both dimensions."[17] Findings such as these have significant consequences for nursing practice. For example, these findings suggest executives will attempt to cultivate political alliances, use power to influence decisions, have a higher and different span of influence, and be perceived as the institution's leaders and role models for nursing. Staff nurses, on the other hand, will not have political interests; will have fewer power connections with which to use their influence, establish strong working relationships among their peers, other health care workers, and their patient-clients; and will be perceived as the followers and implementors of policy-level decision making.[17] These differences in perceptions of power, control, and autonomy must be resolved if both clusters of nurses are going to arrive at some measure of agreement regarding a common field of responsibility. Further, if these discrepancies reflect one community of nurses, imagine how much greater they must be in the total aggregate!

Studies such as Heineken's, however, do carry a message and a vision for the future of nursing that must not be overlooked. The findings deserve careful analysis because they may hold the key to defining nursing's field of responsibility. The responses of nurses to these findings, however, must come from the total community to implement new directions and recommendations. Continued fragmentation will not breed success.

NURSING DOES HAVE THE POWER TO CHANGE THE HEALTH CARE SYSTEM

There is no doubt that the profession of nursing has the power to change the health care system! Nursing has always had the power to effect change but perhaps has hesitated to challenge existing systems in institutions designed to provide primarily acute and medically dictated care. Now, however, we would argue that nurses not only have an opportunity to change health care delivery services, but they have a professional responsibility to do so. Berle clearly states as his first law of power: "Power invariably fills any vacuum in human organization. As between chaos and power, the latter always prevails."[8]

One of the most disturbing realities confronting American society today concerns the organization, distribution, availability, and access of health care services to individuals in need. It is, indeed, a contradiction to recognize that although this country's "health care system may now be capable of providing quality health care to all segments of our society, that we are no longer sure we can afford to do so."[15] This dilemma has resulted, we believe, from the vacuum and chaos that resulted from the introduction of diagnosis-related group (DRG) categorizations that formed the foundation for the prospective reimbursement payment system initiated in 1983. Berle maintains that whenever chaos and power coexist power will always prevail; to date, the drastic effects this revolutionary change has had for the delivery of nursing care seem to suggest that nursing lacks the power to make a difference in health care. However, before nurses can effect change, they must be knowledgeable, informed, and willing to assume the risks incumbent with any initiative designed to challenge existing conditions.

When the diagnosis-related group–prospective payment system was first initiated, hospital administrators were quick to bemoan the catastrophic effects the system would have on the state of hospital finances. Nurses were summoned to many meetings in which the deleterious effects of the impending policies were discussed and strategies delineating how various components of nursing service departments would be expected to respond were carefully outlined. Cutbacks would have to be made in staffing levels, full-time employees would have to reduce their employment status to .5 or .8 time, and ancillary personnel would be severely reduced or, in some cases, eliminated from the workforce. Nurses at all levels of the organization complied with the mandates, simultaneously complaining about being overworked, underpaid, forced to care for more patients than could possibly be managed with any measure of safety, and becoming more and more disenchanted with their ability to function in a professional capacity. This scenario, one of my colleagues suggested, is hardly the portrait of a profession with power.

Why, if nursing has power, does such exploitation occur? It occurs, we will argue, because rather than pursue the power inherent in knowledge, it is easier to embrace the powerlessness of compliance; rather than challenge the "facts" being presented, it is easier to accept administrative dictates; and rather than pursue common goals, objectives, and perhaps avenues of accommodation that would work to nursing's advantage, it is easier to adopt a reactive posture and expect solutions to come from the organization's hierarchy rather than from within the professional complement of nurses. It is conceivable that professional nurses could have responded to the preceding situation in an entirely different manner. For example, if a committee of nurses charged with maintaining quality assurance and/or patient care standards in the nursing service department had obtained, analyzed, and evaluated the policy statements generated by the Health Care Financing Administration regarding prospective payment, it might have been able to counteract the dictates made by hospital administrators, enlist the assistance of physicians, and propose alternative strategies that would have met the intent of the policy changes but not at the expense of patient care.

One example of nursing's failure to capitalize on these policy changes occurred in the area of patient discharge. While nurses were lamenting the numerous instances in which patients in poor condition were being discharged too early, it was Ralph Nader who pushed for the addition of an advocacy clause that would guarantee patients the right of appeal and the right to a hearing if they felt they were being discharged too soon. Well-informed nurses could have served the patients equally well, but even today many nurses remain unaware of such provisions in the policy. In this instance, therefore, power remained with hospital administrators.

Today nurses have more opportunities than ever to capitalize on the chaos in the health care system in the United States. The prospective payment system remains in effect for many facilities, and similar systems will probably soon be initiated by other paying agencies, such as private insurance companies and health maintenance organizations. Nurses must become informed on all aspects and consequences of such payment systems if they expect to improve the quality of care being provided consumers. Nursing must continue to develop and improve data-base systems that clearly document its role in delivering quality, cost-effective care. Although progress has been made in this area, more needs to be done.

The next decade will present other opportunities to nurses to exercise their influence and power. There will be a continued decline in mortality rates, continued increases in the morbidity rates, and the number of aging Americans will continue to expand at an exponential rate, as will the projected costs of health care.[12] Nurses have the knowledge, skills, and abilities to manage and cope with these potential problems and patient populations.

Nurses need to initiate and implement creative strategies if they are to assume a major role in caring for these segments of the population. Nurses need to become familiar with economic concepts such as supply and demand, production functions, product lines, and product-line management; in addition they must learn to cost out their services if they are going to state their case effectively and remain a viable component of the health care system of the future. The potential for chaos exists in many segments of the health care arena, not just in traditional health care delivery settings. At present, many individuals in the greatest need of health care are not able to get it: the homeless, the poor, the disadvantaged, the unemployed, and the elderly. Another group, the uninsured, is also quickly making its presence known. Nurses can serve these publics as well and perhaps even better than other health care providers and should expand efforts to assist these groups in formalized ways through nursing clinics, community health agencies, or other innovative mechanisms and structures.

Nurses comprise the largest single group of health care providers in this country. The educational level of its practitioners continues to increase steadily, and nurses remain the professionals who continue to have the greatest amount of contact with the patient-client. The changes in health care policies to date have not limited the practice of nursing as much as they have endangered traditional opportunities enjoyed by medicine. Fagin reports:

"In the past five years, health care costs have risen at a rate almost three times that of the general inflation rate . . . and . . . according to a report from the Office of Technology Assessment, the increases are due to an intensification of services, expanded availability and use of costly diagnostic and treatment services, and sophisticated technologies.[12]

Physician services were responsible for 20% of all health-related expenditures in 1984, and the rate has continued to grow at approximately 14% each year since.[12]

Costs such as these cannot continue to escalate. Nurses provide an attractive care alternative because of their unique knowledge, skills, and ability to deal with their client-patients' responses to actual and potential health problems. Legislators, unions, and the public at large are beginning to support the idea of nurses having new roles designed to provide necessary health care services. If nurses do not respond and capitalize on the dramatic changes occurring in the health care marketplace, other providers will no doubt manage to fill the vacuum, as can be seen in the recent proposals by physicians to introduce yet another health care provider—the registered care technician.[1] Nurses cannot be content to sit back and watch while other health care providers act.[12] If nurses will accept the opportunities available to them, they will not only assist in bringing order out of chaos, but also will acquire the power necessary to significantly influence and change the health care delivery system of this country.

Berle's second law states: "Power is invariably personal. There is no such thing as class power, elite power, or group power; although classes, elites, and groups may be processes of organization by which power is lodged in individuals."[8] This law mandates that before nurses can use the power they have, they must first recognize and internalize their capacity for holding power as individuals. Historically, however, nurses have been content to invest their power collectively in such organizations as the American Society of Superintendents of Training Schools of Nursing— the forerunner of the National League for Nursing,— and the Nurses' Associated Alumnae of the United States and Canada— better known now as the American Nurses' Association.

Although nurses must maintain a strong sense of professional identity through membership in professional organizations, they must simultaneously promote efforts designed to enhance their individual sense of worth. Feminist authors have described power as having two dimensions: power-over and power-within.[26] Power-over reinforces the traditional forms of power so often described in the organizational literature and encompasses such concepts as bureaucracy, control, vertical lines of authority and decision making descending from above. Nurses have some familiarity with the basic tenents of a power-over dimension. The power-within dimension, however, suggests power can exist on a horizontal plane and recognizes all individuals have some part or role in decision making in encouraging the establishment of cooperative rather than competitive relationships.[26]

Nurses need to appreciate the power they possess as employees. Patrellis noted, "To believe you are powerless is the beginning of your downfall . . . supervisors need to feel their employees have what it takes to accomplish the organization's objectives . . . your supervisor needs you . . . when you realize mutual dependence exists, and you can provide what is needed . . . you have power."[36] Nurses are professionals who are frequently employed by organizations. The proximity of the professional nurse to the patient-client in most health care organizations is an enviable one and can be useful as a source of power. In brief, the success of those institutions whose primary mission is patient care, is dependent upon the quality of the nursing services rendered. Rather than lamenting a salaried employee status, nurses need to find ways to channel their unique and important contributions into strategies designed to improve relationships with hospital administrators and governing boards, increase the opportunities for interdependent working relationships with other employee health care providers, strive to achieve win-win situations, and ultimately enjoy the benefits that consistently accrue with outstanding levels of performance.[36]

Nurses can further cultivate and enhance their personal power by developing a sense of their ability to communicate using nonverbal behavior and dress. Power is, indeed, communicated by one's nonverbal behavior, whether it results from illlusion, perception, or one's self-confidence, dress, or mannerisms.[25] Lamar illustrates the power of nonverbal behavior when she gives the following negative example:

Ms. A., the Vice President or Director of Nursing arrives to an administrative committee meeting 10 minutes late wearing a well-worn and slightly snug white uniform. She is carrying a stack of file folders, each filled with paper. The meeting has already begun and she pulls up a chair to the table. She offers her usual apologies as she shuffles papers in an attempt to find the material being discussed and that which she is expected to present.[25]

Who among us has not worked with such an individual, and what lasting impressions have we formed of this person's capabilities? Certainly the image of power is not paramount in such individuals. Therefore, nurses should be aware of what Lamar identifies as impression management as one means of increasing an individual's personal power.[36]

Another component of personal power is the ability

to analyze and tend to the language individuals use to communicate with others in the workplace. Language is the means by which humans communicate and interpret ideas, emotions, and experiences.

"Words captivate and compel, or hobble and bag. . . . Words rich in meaning generate excitement, and the use of metaphors can give added meaning to work. . . . nurses need to give added attention to the use and subtleties of language, to the need to develop strong linguistic skills, to remain sensitive to the values implicit in varying lexicons, and to appreciate the discretions often "implied" in verbal and written forms of communication if they expect to strengthen their overall ability to improve their performance and acquire power."[18]

Communication is highly valued as an integral element of the nursing process. Nurses focus on the need to develop excellent communication skills, but as Henry and LeClair note: "While communication is widely discussed in nursing . . . language and the recognition that words have different meanings for different people" is frequently neglected.[18] Nurses work with different kinds of people on a daily basis: patients, and their families, colleagues, and other health professionals—and may need to use different words with different people, recognizing that the words selected may also have different meanings for different people. Quality care, for example, might "mean timely and courteous service to clients; holistic assessment and family education to nurses; and an appropriate per case cost and reimbursement to finance officers."[18] Developing their language use and analysis skills in the workplace could lead to an increase in power and influence.

Finally, if nurses are to utilize personal power, they must distinguish between using personal power as a form of self-aggrandizement and using personal power to achieve the goals of the organization. Booth argues quite persuasively that individuals who must achieve personal goals at the expense of others will find themselves consistently involved in tenuous situations, rendered powerless, and displaced within a given period of time.[9] Power accrues, however, when individuals use personal power to achieve the goals of the organization. These individuals derive satisfaction from seeing others achieve; they reward talent and eventually build teams in which power is shared. Thus the group gains influence and is able to foster reciprocal loyalties and relationships between the organization and employee groups.

Nurses must, therefore, endorse attempts to promote the cultivation of personal power, keeping in mind the need to articulate personal power with professional and organizational goals. Once individual nurses recognize our sense of professional identity and accept, maintain, and defend our common interests, particularly in relation to our workplace, then we will indeed demonstrate our power to change the conditions under which we presently practice.

The third law of power identified by Berle states: "Power is invariably based upon a system of ideals or a philosophy."[8] Throughout it's history nursing has been guided by concepts that have exemplified its ideals and philosophical foundations. Concepts such as caring, health, nursing, environment, and individuality have remained dominant concerns among nurses who perceive their task as assisting patient-clients to attain, maintain, or regain health through the "diagnosis and treatment of human responses to actual or potential health problems."[34] Indeed, although these concepts can be gleaned from the early writings of Nightingale, they are present in the published works of contemporary nurse theorists.

Ideologies serve to communicate visions, doctrines, ideas, manners, or a set of characteristics subscribed to by individuals, groups, or programs. Ideologies often draw individuals and groups together whenever there is consensus about an issue or the need to appear united in order to achieve definite goals. They can form a basis upon which individuals or groups structure their thinking or attempt to convince others to share in particular views of life or specific cultural norms. Rokeach suggests there are three major ideological belief systems: (1) descriptive-existential, (2) evaluative, and (3) prescriptive-proscriptive. Descriptive-existential beliefs are those capable of being either true or false; evaluative beliefs offer judgments regarding the goodness or badness of an object or topic; and prescriptive-proscriptive beliefs are those that judge the degree of desirability or undesireability of the means or ends of specific actions.[40] Ideologies often incorporate personal, social, and moral aspects of one's visions, doctrines, ideas, programs, or agendas.

Nurses have generally not subscribed to the descriptive-existential belief system, perhaps because of the difficulties in establishing the rightness or wrongness of specific actions in a fluid profession such as nursing. Nurses have, however, utilized both the evaluative and prescriptive-proscriptive belief systems in conceptualizing and operationalizing their ideological and philosophical positions. Nursing has evolved from early perceptions describing it as "woman's work" to recognition as a professional discipline.

Although nursing's basic ideologies, as outlined in the concepts stated above, have remained remarkably intact throughout the professionalization journey, numerous internal disagreements have served to distract nurses, diverting their efforts from the profession as a whole toward more specialized group constituencies. Although nurses themselves may have understood the issues being debated and the need to resolve their differences internally, other groups such as consumers, physicians, and other health care providers have become increasingly confused about what nurses view as their visions, doctrines, and missions of caring.

Recently, the AMA proposed introducing the registered care technologist into the health care system. These individuals would be prepared to function in acute-care facilities after having received a minimum of 9 months of instructional and practical preparation.[1] Nurses have focused on such issues as the minimum educational preparation necessary to practice professional nursing, entry into practice, licensure requirements, titling, and appropriate roles and responsibilities; the AMA proposal, however, presents a clear challenge to nursing's evaluative and prescriptive-proscriptive belief systems. Nurses from all constituencies have been quick to respond to the proposal, describing it as poorly conceived, and a most undesirable means of solving the problem of providing quality care.

There is no doubt that the caring ideology espoused by nurses embodies power! The need to maintain quality care has emerged as a focal point in arguing against the AMA proposal. Nurses everywhere are being urged by their individual organizations to renew their commitment to the profession first and to individual specialized concerns second. "Professional bonding," based upon a set of mutual ideals, has become a reality as evidenced by the united stand taken at a recent summit meeting by nurses representing 46 national nursing organizations, all of whom endorsed a position opposing the AMA proposal.[2] Now is the time for nurses and the profession to reach a new consensus regarding the direction the profession should take and the methods by which success can be achieved. Only by reaffirming nursing's basic ideologies can nurses realize their potential in providing care, while simultaneously experiencing a sense of completeness that comes from fulfilling work. The power inherent in ideologies can be used by nurses to display their talents to consumers, physicians, and other health care providers.

"Power is exercised through, and depends on institutions," states Berle's fourth invarient law of power.[8] *Institutions* refer to a set of established practices or systems and organizations with a particular purpose. Institutions have two facets: (1) they have organized patterns of roles, the behaviors of which are often enforced by using positive and negative sanctions; and (2) there are patterned habits of thought learned by individuals assigned to perform the roles deemed necessary for the institutions effective and efficient functioning.[11]

Nurses have historically practiced their profession within a variety of institutional structures, although hospitals, clinics, physician's offices, and schools have been the key locations. Unfortunately, structure often dictates function, and institutions such as those listed above have tended to dictate the roles and functions to nursing within parameters largely influenced and dominated by the intrinsic medical establishment. Added to these restrictions were those imposed by legal definitions of what constituted nursing care and the requirement in some instances that nurses be supervised by a physician, dentist, or podiatrist! Even today, many of these institutions continue to ignore the independent functions and professional services nursing is capable of providing consumers.

Nursing has begun to initiate actions designed to modify, if not replace, some of the traditional structures that have prevented nursing from becoming an institution in its own right, responsible for determining its own parameters of practice. Many state nursing associations have obtained legislative support to revise state nurse practice acts to reflect an enlightened perspective of nursing practice using definitions of professional nursing such as the one suggested by the ANA. It is highly likely that the changing health care delivery scene will facilitate more of these efforts and will enlarge significantly nursing's power to serve patient-client populations in ever-expanding roles.

Bakalis maintains that power must combine with purpose in a harmonious relationship to achieve effective action and that institutions, no less than people, must possess the right combination of both in order to operate effectively.[6] Nursing has published a very clear statement of purpose in "The Social Policy Statement"[3] Keeping that purpose in focus, nurses must combine their strong sense of professional identity with their knowledge of the organizations in which they work in order to exercise their power through the use of organizational processes. Hickson and others proposed three variables that when blended together govern the power a subunit has within any single organization: centrality, substitutability, and coping with uncertainty. Centrality refers to the extent to which a subunit's activities connect with other organizational units and the degree to which other units operations would be affected should the subunit stop functioning. Substitutability refers to how easily members of any given subunit can be replaced either from within or from outside the organization; and coping with uncertainty is defined as the ability of a subunit to respond effectively and efficiently to anticipated or, more often, unanticipated events that may confont the organization. The theory argues that the more a subunit can remain central, reduce its vulnerability to substitutability, and constructively cope with uncertainty, the more power it will accrue relative to other subunits in the organization.[19]

If Hickson and others[19] are correct, then their theory offers a framework easily adapted to those institutional structures most frequently encountered by nurses in their work situations. In most health care institutions, nurses are not just a central component of the organization but the primary element of most services provided patient-client consumers. Perhaps it is time to recognize this important position and to develop strategies that illustrate how crucial the delivery of nursing care really is in meeting institutional objectives. It was interesting to note that specific positions such as discharge planners, utilization reviewers, and admission workers were viewed as holding a central place in many health care institutions and were in fact recommended as choice positions for "social workers" seeking to accrue strategic organizational power.[10] Nurses might do well to reclaim these functions, which, when combined with the roles and responsibilities already ascribed to nurses, should ensure both a central role in the organization and the power that accompanies it.

A second source of power evolves around the notion of substitutability: the vulnerability to replacement by someone from within or without the institution.[19] Nurses have long suffered from the perception that a nurse is a nurse is a nurse. Hospitals and other care organizations continue to hire, assign, and even promote nurses without demanding appropriate educational and experiential credentials. The designated float nurse or float pool provides another example of

how nurses have been viewed as easily substituted commodities within organizational structures. Perhaps nurses should consider the notion of substitutability in a new light and rather than be victimized by it, replace it with nurse-designated categories of substitutability to ensure safe practice. For example, perhaps critical care nurses could be cross-leveled with emergency room nurses, labor room and delivery nurses with operating room nurses, and intermediate level surgical or medical nurses with their staff nurse counterparts. Perhaps it is time to rebel against nurses being supplied by external employment agencies and insist on personnel who are loyal to the nurses within the institution. If substitutability is managed properly and purposely, it can provide nurses with immeasurable power.

Coping with uncertainty, the third variable in strategies for developing organization power,[19] should not pose any problems for the average nurse working in most health care delivery systems today, because nurses are known to be masters of adaptation and improvisation, especially in using resources creativity. However, nursing's responses to uncertainty have tended to be more reactive than anticipative in most instances. A slight philosophical adjustment by most nurses would enable them to garner increased organizational power by adopting proactive anticipatory postures designed to improve their own services by enhancing the organization as a whole as it too copes with an ever-changing health care arena.

Nurses have a comprehensive awareness of all aspects of the increasingly complex health care industry, as well as its strengths and weaknesses. They are also aware of the needs and concerns of clients, have the capability of using leverage to better shape and improve the system, and therefore must resign themselves to fighting to maintain principles of care with those forces that threaten to undermine and dilute the quality of nursing care.[27] A new health paradigm is materializing in this country in which the emphasis is shifting rapidly from the cell to society, from illness care to wellness care, from institutional care to home care, from physician care to team care, from individual-focused care to group-centered care, from specialty knowledge to general knowledge, and from holistic to humanistic care.[29]

Changing opportunities such as these are giving the profession of nursing new challenges and new possibilities for work within institutional structures. Now is the time for nurses to solidify their posture of centrality, identify acceptable surrogates for substituta-bility, and demonstrate their ability to anticipate and cope with uncertainty. Once nurses assume more re-sponsibility for practice and believe that they are in-dispensable resources for health care institutions, they will acquire and solidify the power bases required not only to effect change in health care institutions, but also to become a force actively engaged in deter-mining the structure and functions such organiza-tions will have relative to the delivery of health care.

Berle's fifth and last law of power states: "Power is invariably confronted with, and acts in the presence of, a field of responsibility."[8] A field of responsibility implies, by definition, the power to perform tasks or duties and to fulfill obligations to those individuals who expect and trust they will receive quality care. Acceptance of a field of responsibility signifies accep-tance of a commitment to being fully accountable to one's designated duties and obligations.

Nursing's field of responsibility has been histori-cally defined by Nightingale as manipulation of the patient's environment, attending to the patient's needs, and observing the patient's condition in order to assist restorative processes.[33] The ANA definition of nursing's field of responsibility suggests "nursing is the diagnosis and treatment of human responses to actual or potential health problems."[3] Finally, contem-porary nurse models such as one proposed by Loomis and Wood extend the ANA's definition to include four major categories specifying groups of actual or poten-tial health problems, designate six categories of human responses, and stipulate how nurse's clinical decisions evolve from the data being assessed within four pro-totypes of care-giving situations.[27] If these three def-initions are merged, the result provides individuals and the profession with a clear notion of what constitutes nursing's field of responsibility.

The one variable not included in the preceding de-lineation of nursing's field of responsibility is that of setting. Unfortunately, nursing has traditionally al-lowed its field of responsibility to be defined within organizational settings and has, therefore, found its field of responsibility often being defined by hospital administrators, physicians, and even unions rather than by the nurses themselves. Adopting and sub-scribing to a field of responsibility independent from organization contexts permits nurses to perform professionally, with commitment, and assuming full accountability for their role in providing care. Nurses must divorce their responsibilities from settings if they wish to accumulate the power to perform nursing tasks and duties independently or even interdependently with other health care professionals.

Naisbitt suggests the new health paradigm is shift-ing from medically administered care to self-care and from institutional help to ambulatory or home-based assistance. This transition to a self-help/self-care par-adigm features prevention, wellness, and the need to assume personal responsibility for one's health.[31] This paradigm shift also opens new settings and new op-portunities for the practice of nursing. With a clearly defined field of responsibility such as the one proposed above, there is no reason why nurses cannot enlarge the scope of their responsibilities and fully meet the challenges always available to those who seek and ac-cept them.

Nurses now have an opportunity to respond to changing health needs and populations; indeed, nurses have already indicated how they would change health care delivery in this country. Nurses maintain they would establish programs in which nurses assume pri-mary responsibility for well maternity clinics and birthing centers; they would also establish and main-tain managed-care programs for the mentally im-paired, the developmentally disabled, the physically disabled, and the frail elderly. Nurses suggest a re-newed emphasis on promoting health and would in-stitute rigorous programs in school systems, where problems could be screened early and programs could be designed to foster healthy life styles. Nurses feel they can better serve their clients in home nursing situations if they assume full responsibility for refer-ring their patient-clients to needed services, because physicians rarely know the available options. Nurses have proposed a multitiered system of healthcare in which they could serve in a variety of roles; nurse-practitioners would assess clients, treat them when appropriate, and refer them to the medical community when necessary; nurses would reestablish the control of home care in the tradition of Wald; and obviously nurses would lobby, finance, and work collectively to alter the legislative statutes currently preventing many of these changes from occurring.[21] These changes are possible given a clear statement and collective en-dorsement of a field of responsibility.

The acceptance of a field of responsibility would provide not only a strong sense of personal and profes-sional identity, but also the motivation to support their common interests. Berle states:

Members of a group must realize that their interest is common . . . and they must be willing to accept, maintain, and defend that common interest . . . or risk being divided against each other to the detriment of their common interests . . . let members ask themselves when they conceive of the existence of any they, whether they consider themselves within it . . . the they many times never becomes a we . . . and when an individual speaks of we he/she thinks of himself/herself as a member of an organizational body with common attributes.[8]

The diversity of opinion that seems to pervade so many issues in nursing today might not assume the same level of prominence if nurses agreed on the basic parameters that form the boundaries of a field of responsibility.

A field of responsibility is also based on scientific knowledge and a scientifically based practice theory.[45] Knowledge is frequently recognized as one source of power. Nurses can now identify the major phenomena unique to their field of responsibility and have made rapid advances in recent years in clarifying their concepts and verifying assessment and intervention modalities by conducting sound programs of research. These efforts not only must continue, but also must enlist the support of all nurses if they are to find their way from the research laboratory or journal into practice.

Nurses must continue their education beyond the baccalaureate degree and pursue graduate study at both the master's and doctoral levels. The state of nursing's knowledge is rapidly advancing primarily because of the increased sophistication of research being conducted. Advanced study provides nurses with the processes by which they can organize and communicate their nursing knowledge to other health care professionals to effect change in the delivery of care. Advanced educational preparation provides nurses with specialized knowledge and skills that structure and improve the delivery of quality nursing care while simultaneously documenting its cost-effectiveness. The additional preparation provided by advanced training allows nurses to develop a philosophy and set of beliefs that can withstand the assaults on care dictated by institutional administrators, finance officers, and physicians; and the addition of graduate-level degrees offers the credibility associated with exacting and difficult work that is voluntary rather than work that is mandatory for entry-level positions. Finally, those nurses who complete graduate study have the security of knowing they are at least as well, if not better, prepared in their chosen field of study as many

of their colleagues in other health related professions. What power and confidence! If nurses sought graduate study as the norm rather than the exception, there would be increases in salaries, responsibilities, roles, credibility, and accountability—and nurses would have a major role in establishing institutional policies. In fact, we have often wondered if the advice given to nurses not to pursue graduate work in nursing may not be just another ploy to prevent nurses from gaining full control of their work environments.

Given the power of knowledge and its role in guiding practice, nursing could determine how, where, and when it might extend its field of responsibility beyond existing boundaries and settings. Nursing has the ability and resources to offer comprehensive health care in conjunction with other health care providers. Nursing can respond to the challenges coming before it and will continue to change accordingly, but it must do so with vision, purpose, and a field of responsibility if it is to be successful.

SUMMARY

This chapter has considered the question, "Does nursing have the power to change the health care delivery system? Power is a perceptual entity, and although power is perceptual so also is perception power. How one perceives power, then, is a delicate portion of all interactions and is a crucial component of how one receives, transmits, integrates, and reacts in any given situation.

Willman notes a new generation of nurses is emerging: nurses who are creative rather than conforming; initiating rather than reacting; assertive rather than passive; change agents, not retardants; political activists, not victims; and independent, not dependent.[44] Today a new set of career opportunities is available in nursing. The future belongs to the visionary—to those who can create new configurations to respond to new demands and who have the courage to follow their vision.[41] Perhaps the time has come for nurses to cease their discussions and concern for power and instead direct their energies toward assuming enlarged roles in a rapidly changing health care environment. Perhaps returning to traditional values of caring, humanity, and recapturing the spirit of nursing will ultimately provide more power than is currently imaginable. Nursing has an opportunity to institutionalize itself as an integral component of the health care system when so many health care providers are voicing concern over and competing for resources. Nursing's primary resources are the aggregate of nurses themselves combined with their patient-clients.

Nursing has previously demonstrated its ability to make a significant difference in health care; there is no reason why it should not do so in the future. However, nurses must keep in perspective and balance the role of power and its related concepts, for as Benner notes:

When power, status, autonomy, and wealth are preferred characteristics . . . [used to select or define a profession] . . . who can understand wanting to be a nurse? Only those who have participated in the triumph of the human spirit in circumstances as extreme as birth and death. Only those who have the courage to master the technology now used for cure and the virtuosity to provide care that makes the modern cures accessible, safe, humane, and healing.[7]

Need we say more? We think not.

REFERENCES

1. Am J Nurs: "News" 88(8):1131, 1988.
2. Am J Nurs: "News" 88(12):1716, 1988.
3. American Nurses' Association: Nursing: a social policy statement, Kansas City, Mo, 1980, The Association.
4. American Nurses' Association: personal communication, Kansas City, Mo, 1989.
5. Andrews L: Health care providers: the future marketplace and regulations, J Prof Nurs 2(1):51, 1986.
6. Bakalis MJ: Power and purpose, Phi Delta Kappan 65(1):7, 1983.
7. Benner P: Taken from Vital Signs Calendar, Menlo Park, Calif. 1989, Addison-Wesley Co., Inc.
8. Berle AA: Power, New York, 1969, Harcourt, Brace, and World.
9. Booth RZ: Power: a negative or positive force in relationships? Nurs Admin Quart 7(4):10, 1983.
10. Chernesky RH and Territo T: Sources of organizational power for women in the health care field, Soc Work Health Care 12(4)93, 1987.
11. Dugger WM: Power: an institutional framework of analysis, J Econ Issues 14(4):897, 1980.
12. Fagin CM: Opening the door on nursing's cost advantage, Nurs and Health Care 7(7):353, 1986.
13. Ginzberg E. The economics of health care and the future of nursing, J Nurs Admin 11(3):31, 32, 1981.
14. Gorman S and Clark N: Power and effective nursing practice, Nurs Outlook 34(3):129, 1986.
15. Gunn IP: Nursing innovations help reach traditional goals, Nurs and Health Care 7(7):359, 1986.
16. Harriman A: Women/men/management, New York, 1985, Prager Publishers.
17. Heineken J: Power-conflicting views, J Nurs Admin 15(11):36, 1985.
18. Henry B and LeClair H: Language, leadership, and power, J Nurs Admin 17(1):19, 1987.
19. Hickson D and others: A strategic contingencies theory of organizational power, Admin Sci Quart 16:216, 1971.
20. Holcombe B: Nurses fight back, Ms. 16(12):72, June 1988.
21. Huey FL: How nurses would change V.S. health care, Amer J Nurs 52:1482, 1988.
22. Kalish BJ: The promise of power, Nurs Outlook 22(1):42, 1978.
23. Kipnis D: The powerholders, Chicago, 1976, Univ of Chicago Press.
24. Kuhn R: Gaining power through practice, Heart and Lung 14(b):22A, 1985.
25. Lamar EK: Communicating personal power through non-verbal behavior, J Nurs Admin 15(1):41, 1985.
26. Lind A, Wilburn S, and Pate E: Power from within: feminism and the ethical decision-making process in nursing, Nurs Admin Quart April 1986, p. 50.
27. Loomis ME and Wood DJ: Cure: the potential outcome of nursing care, Image 15(1):4, 1983.
28. Lynaugh JE and Fagin CM: Nursing comes of age, Image 20(4):184, 1988.
29. McCormick KA: Preparing nurses for the technologic future, Nurs and Health Care 4(7):379, 1983.
30. May R: Power and innocence: a search for the sources of violence, New York, 1982, WW Norton & Co.
31. Naisbitt J: Megatrends, New York, 1982, Warner Books.
32. National Implementation Project. De Back, V. The nation's nurses: A credible profession doing an incredible job. No date.
33. Nightingale F: Notes on nursing, New York, 1969, Dover Publications.
34. Norris CM: Nursing theory: state of the art; projections for the future. Paper presented at the University of Wisconsin-Eau Claire, April 8, 1983.
35. Ostrander VR: Consumers look to nurses for affordable quality care, Nurs and Health Care 7(7):369, 1986.
36. Patrellis AJ: Your power as an employee, Supervisory Management 30(4):37, April 1985.
37. Peck SB: Nursing: on the cutting edge of opportunity, Nurs and Health Care 7(7):365, 1986.
38. Reverby S: Ordered to care: the dilemma of American nursing 1850-1945, New York, 1987, Cambridge Univ Press.
39. Roberts SJ: Oppressed group behavior: implications for nursing, Adv in Nurs Sci 5(4):21, 1983.
40. Rokeach M: The nature of human values, New York, 1973, The Free Press.
41. Smith G: The new health care economy: opportunities for nurse entrepreneurs, Nurs Outlook 35(4):182, 1987.
42. Sweeney SS: An analysis of selected exchange relations and transactions between a college of nursing and a selected public—its alumni, doctoral dissertation, Iowa City, 1982, University of Iowa.
43. Webster's Ninth New Collegiate Dictionary, Springfield, Mass, 1985, Merriam-Webster Inc.
44. Willman MD: Change and power. In Stevens KR, editor: Power and influence, New York, 1983, John Wiley & Sons.
45. Wooldridge PJ and others: Behavioral science and nursing theory, St. Louis, 1983, The CV Mosby Co.

CHAPTER 41

Viewpoints

Why are we seeing more unionization?

KAREN S. O'CONNOR
JULIA FRY GIBSON

Nurses have been effectively addressing professional and economic issues through collective bargaining for more than 40 years. However, the majority of nurses have only general knowledge about the process or its achievements. In spite of nurses' relative lack of awareness, unionization in health care is increasing at a time when union strength in other sectors is generally declining. Nurses are contributing significantly to this expansion of collective bargaining.

This trend in the health care industry is the opposite of trends in other economic sectors. In other industries, unions lose most of the representation elections. Yet in health care, unions win approximately 50%. Although the total proportion of unionized workers in the United States has dropped to 17% of the total workforce, the proportion of unionized health care workers (including nurses) has risen 6% since 1980 to approximately 20%. In 1987 the number of registered nurses (R.N.s) covered by collective bargaining agreements had grown to approximately 239,000. Although a number of different unions represent R.N.s, the majority are represented by the state constituents of the American Nurses' Association.

Nurses' growing awareness of and participation in collective bargaining is indisputable. Thus the question to be analyzed is not "whether" but "why." This analysis must consider the impact of today's dynamic economic and political environment on health care, consumers, individual practitioners and the nursing profession. Understanding these factors leads to the conclusion that nurses will continue to seek out collective bargaining in ever-increasing numbers.

This conclusion has far-reaching implications for the profession. Nursing historically has been reticent to question the system in which it practices. Such reticence is rapidly crumbling as the profession strives to meet the increased demand for nursing services and moves into a leadership role in the health care industry. The mechanisms chosen by nursing to meet these challenges will ultimately determine its success.

Success or failure will have direct, immediate consequences for patients and clients. Nursing's commitment to quality patient care is indisputable. Indeed, it is this commitment that leads nurses to choose collective bargaining. Nurses have always known that working conditions and their ability to provide quality of care are inextricably intertwined. And collective bargaining has proved to be an effective tool for shaping a workplace that supports practice.

ENVIRONMENT

Health care in America has changed profoundly since the introduction in 1983 of Medicare's prospective payment system (PPS). Cost-containment was a growing concern throughout the 1970s, but despite various initiatives, costs continued to spiral. The theory of PPS was radical: prospective fixed pricing rather than unlimited retroactive billing. Competition was to be introduced into the system with resultant savings to consumers. Health care providers began focusing on marketing a product to a customer rather than on delivering needed care to a patient. Hospitals shifted their efforts toward pleasing the payers. Many believe this has resulted in a major power shift from physicians to hospital administrators, insurers, and other reimbursing entities.

Although health care has always been a business, the ramifications of being a competitive business are becoming increasingly clear. The for-profit sector in health care has become prominent. Shareholders who expect dividends of necessity affect the mission of such entities. Although the not-for-profit institution technically does not derive profit, many factors are driving even that sector to maximize revenue over expenses. Corporate restructuring is common as facilities seek to expand their market and limit financial losses and tax consequences. Health care managers and workers alike are now accustomed to discussing competition, productivity, and marketing.

Corporate restructuring has simultaneously produced trends toward centralization and decentralization. Centralization of institutional control has emerged most prominently in multifacility chains, whether profit or not-for-profit. Centralized control moves the locus of decision making farther away from the bedside. The result is decision makers with little direct contact with the bedside or the nurses responsible for providing care. Decentralization has been prescribed as a cure, yet it carries problems of its own. Although decentralization moves the locus of decision making nearer to the bedside, it also creates opportunities for inconsistent policies and inconsistent execution of policies within a single institution. Corporate restructuring has implications far beyond financial concerns.

Concurrent with these developments, theories of human resource management have become increasingly important over the past decade. The goal of human resource management is to create a "positive" labor relations or personnel environment. This is accomplished through extensive company communication with employees, pay structures with fewer job classifications and wage grades, and extensive (internal) dispute-resolution systems. Some observers have described human resource management as seeking to coopt unionization by providing unorganized workers with most of the benefits provided by a union. In fact, these techniques have become prominent in health care at a time when health care employees have increasingly sought out unionization.

CONSUMER CHARACTERISTICS AND SOCIETAL DEMAND

Demographic and societal changes are placing increasing demands on nursing. America is "graying" because of the increased proportion of older people. Older people typically require more nursing care. The need for more care is compounded by the shortened length of stay mandated by PPS. Patients are hospi-

talized for the most acute stages of illness and then discharged to recover at home.

Advances in health care technology have supported two separate but related trends: more complex and technologically advanced care and simpler, more mobile, less tertiary-centered care. Both trends result in a broader spectrum of care being delivered across the lifespan.

Demand for nursing care is high in today's acute-care settings. The advances supporting more complex care are turning hospitals into a conglomerate of special care units. In 1972 hospitals employed an average of 50 nurses for every 100 patients; by 1986 that average had risen to 91 nurses for every 100 patients.

Refinements in management of both chronic and recovery phases of acute illness are increasing the demand for nursing care in the home. Likewise, long-term care facilities now provide a broader range of services in addition to traditional custodial services. Nonetheless, it should be noted that despite the expansions of demand in these arenas, approximately two thirds of all nurses continue to practice in acute-care settings.

CHANGING NATURE OF THE PRACTITIONER

The aggregate characteristics of the profession and the demographic profile of individual nurses are changing and reflect societal changes.

Nursing remains predominantly female. Approximately 97% of employed R.N.s are women. Historically, many nurses have chosen to continue working even after the birth of children. However, that trend is even more pronounced as the proportion of nurses who continue to work after having children parallels the increasing proportion of working mothers in the general population. More practitioners are likely than ever before to be single heads of households or have income coequal in importance to their spouses. The average age of practicing nurses is now approximately 39 years. Although no clear data are available, the average number of years worked is probably increasing.

These demographic changes mean that individual nurses have a broad range of economic issues to consider. Child care has emerged as a high priority issue. Concerns are being expressed about not only starting salaries, but also salaries for nurses with 15 to 20 years experience. Elder or respite care is becoming an issue for nurses with aging parents. Pension and retirement issues are gaining increased attention. It is obvious that today's practitioner is necessarily concerned about the economic return from work.

GROWING AUTONOMY OF THE PROFESSION

The basic components of professionalism have been described as autonomy, a specialized body of knowledge, service orientation, a code of ethical conduct and standards of practice, and a professional association. Of these, autonomy appears to be the key to professional status. Autonomy has been defined as practitioners' right to exercise some control over actions and standards. According to Pointer,[1] the true essence of professionalism is "control over both the performance of professional tasks and the immediate environment in which such tasks are performed."[1] Autonomy is also the key to nursing's ability to deliver quality patient care.

Nursing now employs a variety of sophisticated strategies to regulate and promote autonomous professional practice. Nurses are increasingly successful in managing institutional politics (within organizations) as well as traditional politics (external to organizations). Coalitions with a wide variety of health care and consumer groups are being used to move legislative and regulatory initiatives vitally important to the nursing profession. All of these mechanisms have some impact on the workplace. Nurses are also turning now to collective bargaining to directly shape the workplace and control their practice.

WHY UNIONIZATION?
Historical perspective of employment

Nurses' decision to seek collective bargaining is complex. To fully understand the choice, it is important to recall the traditions of nursing and nurses' experiences as employees in health care.

Nursing's traditions are firmly rooted in its religious and military antecedents as well as its ethos of service. Loyalty and obedience were historically emphasized. The role has been characterized in the past as that of mother-surrogate. Nurses believed that the client's or patient's needs were superior to their own and precluded concern about economic and working conditions.

Since the late 1930s the vast majority of nurses have been employees in health care institutions. Employers also emphasized loyalty and obedience. The implicit quid pro quo was that the employer would then attend to the needs of the nurse. However, this quid pro quo went largely unfulfilled. Congress enacted the Social Security Act in 1935, yet it took another 30 years for unemployment insurance programs to be mandated in all sectors of health care. The Fair Labor Standards Act was adopted in 1938 to, among other things, set a ceiling on hours of work and a minimum wage level. Amendments to cover health care workers were not adopted until 1966.

In addition, the workplace poses special challenges to most nurses. They must function simultaneously as independently licensed professionals and as employees subject to the direction of an employer. Individual practitioners have a legal obligation to those in their care. Failure to fulfill that obligation may result in administrative action affecting their license or a civil lawsuit alleging negligence. Conflicts arise regularly between nurses and employers over business decisions that adversely affect the delivery of care.

The collective bargaining process

Collective bargaining as a process must also be considered when analyzing why nurses are choosing unionization. The Labor-Management Relations Act defines collective bargaining as "the performance of a mutual obligation of the employer and the representatives of the employees to meet at reasonable times and confer in good faith with respect to wages, hours, and other terms and conditions of employment, or the negotiation of any agreement or any question arising there under. . . ." The fundamental terms of employment about which labor and management bargain are (1) the price of labor; (2) rules that define how labor is to be utilized, including hours, job practices, and job classifications; (3) individual job rights; (4) union and management rights in bargaining relationships; and (5) methods of enforcement, interpretation, and administration of the agreement, including resolution of grievances.

Within this legal framework, nurses, through their elected representatives, can compel employers to discuss and reach a legally enforceable agreement on the above subjects. Issues such as orientation for new nurses, floating, and nursing practice committees are subject to bargaining. Additionally, the parties can agree to bargain beyond the scope of mandatory subjects and include their agreements in the contract.

Conflicts between the employer and nurses are settled through the contractual grievance procedure ending in arbitration by a neutral third party. Principles of equity and due process are at the heart of the process.

According to Stern,[2] once nurses gain bargaining power, "the virtually supreme decision-making authority of management regarding employment policies and practice must now be shared." The collective bargaining process puts into place a defined means for nurses' input.

Collective bargaining delivers

As stated previously, nurses have been using collective bargaining for more than 40 years to address practice and economic issues. An analysis of those achievements is the final element in understanding why nurses choose collective bargaining.

Collective bargaining was originally developed in industrial settings and only addressed salaries and benefits. The principles of collective bargaining also have application for professionals. White-collar professionals (including physicians) engage in collective bargaining and are disproving stereotypes about the process and what it achieves.

Initial contracts in any industry tend to be somewhat general. However, as the contract is renegotiated over time, the provisions become increasingly sophisticated and imbued with the nuances of a particular workplace. Collective bargaining contracts for nurses reflect both the characteristics of nursing and the health care industry.

Contracts negotiated by the state nurses' associations (SNAs) initially focused on salaries, benefits, and working conditions. SNA leaders knew that salary and benefits affected recruitment and retention. They also knew that, as a profession of practice, working conditions directly affected the delivery of care. Over time SNA contracts began to address increasingly complex work and practice issues.

Today SNA contracts are forcing improvements in the workplace that support nursing practice and benefit patient care. Contractually mandated nursing practice committees are almost universal in SNA contracts. These committees provide for ongoing communication and problem solving relating to employment and professional issues between the nurses and management. SNAs have also negotiated for improved orientation for new nurses and nurses required to float. Other contracts have eliminated floating entirely.

Other improvements include input into patient classification systems that determine staffing levels; in-house per diem pools providing flexible scheduling and compensation while maintaining a nursing staff knowledgeable about the facility; diversion of ambulances and admissions if staffing falls below agreed upon levels; and elimination or limitations on nonnursing activities, which keep nurses away from the bedside.

Nurses know that working conditions are inextricably linked with standards of care. Collective bargaining creates the power base and provides a legally enforceable mechanism to address employment conditions that prevent nurses from delivering high-quality nursing care.

FUTURE DEMANDS
The nursing shortage

Today's nurses are facing a critical shortage, which is placing increasing demands on the profession. However, unlike past shortages, the current shortage has been precipitated by a rapidly increasing *demand* for specialized nursing services. At least two contributing factors have been identified: advances in technology requiring delivery of increasingly complex care and a rapidly aging population producing growing long-term care needs.

Evidence of the tremendous strain that the current shortage is placing on the existing work force fills the nursing and nonnursing literature. Nurses report a lack of adequate orientation for new graduates, floating of experienced nurses to unfamiliar clinical areas, and many hours of mandatory overtime. Patient caseloads or assignments allow nurses to respond only to the most basic or urgent needs of patients and families.

The seeds of tomorrow

There are fewer women in the 18 to 24 age bracket, but available career opportunities for these women have expanded dramatically. Nursing is no longer one of few options available to young women, and nursing school enrollments have dropped significantly. A recent study documented that, for the first time, more female college freshmen planned a career in medicine than in nursing. Another study demonstrated that today's college freshman is more interested in a career that pays well rather than one with meaningful social value. All indicators project that the shortage will continue for some time, fueled by ever-increasing demands for complex nursing care, a shrinking pool of qualified applicants and recruits, poor working conditions, and changes in the health care industry.

The changing legal environment

By the time this publication goes to press, the National Labor Relations Board (NLRB) will have issued an administrative ruling that will sanction bargaining units composed only of R.N.s. Although R.N.s have historically organized by themselves, NLRB procedures between 1984 and 1988 did not allow formation of units composed solely of R.N.s. Only all-professional bargaining units composed of R.N.s and other health care professionals employed by a facility were accepted by the NLRB. Although organizing efforts continued during this period, they were hampered considerably by the difficulties of organizing larger groups of diverse professionals with divergent workplace and practice concerns. The new rule will dramatically decrease procedural delays before elections and, consequently, will result in an increased number of union victories.

The NLRB's acknowledgment that R.N.s are a discrete professional group that organizes around and bargains over nursing practice issues demonstrates that collective bargaining has been recognized as a tool uniquely suited and responsive to nurses' concerns. The confluence of this historic ruling, the nursing shortage, the general expansion of unionism in health care, and collective bargaining's record of achievements guarantees that more nurses will turn to collective bargaining as a mechanism for controlling their practice environment and assuring quality nursing care.

CHALLENGES FOR THE PROFESSION

Nursing faces many challenges on the eve of the twenty-first century. Retaining experienced nurses in the work force is an issue of pressing concern. Recruiting new applicants will be crucial. Success in meeting these challenges requires attention to economic incentives to practice nursing and efforts reinforcing nursing's right to control the implementation of practice in the workplace.

Nursing's success in meeting these challenges ultimately hinges on its ability to demonstrate and document the effect of nursing care in improving patient outcomes. This documentation will provide a method for responding to pressures in the economic and political environment. It will establish a clear and redefined definition of nursing practice that is critical to nursing's efforts to control the implementation of practice in the workplace.

Collective bargaining enables the profession to effectively control the practice environment. Control of the work environment is crucial to the practice of nursing. The legal framework provides a reliable mechanism for adapting the workplace to the changing demands of practice. By controlling their practice environment, nurses can alleviate situations that prevent them from delivering high-quality nursing care.

The benefits derived from collective bargaining provide an unequivocal answer to the question, "Why more unionization among nurses?" Collective bargaining has contributed substantially to nursing's evolution as a profession in the past and will continue to increase nursing's power in meeting present and future challenges. It serves a useful and necessary function in the dynamic political and economic environment that surrounds professional nursing practice.

To improve the environment for nursing, nurses will turn increasingly to collective bargaining, demonstrating their commitment to improving practice where they work. And, as a result, patient care will benefit.

REFERENCES

1. Pointer DD: Hospitals and professionals: a changing relationship, Hospitals 50:20, 1976.
2. Stern EM: Collective bargaining: a means of conflict resolution, Nurs Admin Quart, Winter 1982.

BIBLIOGRAPHY

AFL-CIO Committee on the Evolution of Work. *The changing situation of workers and their unions.* Washington, D.C.: AFL-CIO, 1985.

Are unions going the way of dinosaurs? Creative evolution may keep them alive. *Government Employee Relations Report*, May 27, 1985, 759.

Flanagan, Lyndia. *Braving new frontiers: ANA's economic and general welfare program, 1946–1986.* Kansas City, Missouri: American Nurses' Association, 1986.

Flanagan, Lyndia. *Collective Bargaining and the Nursing Profession.* Kansas City, Missouri: American Nurses' Association, 1983.

Freeman, Richard B. and James L. Medoff. *What do unions do?* New York: Basic Books, Inc. Publishers, 1984.

Industrial Union Department (AFL-CIO). *The inside game: winning with workplace strategies.* Washington, D.C.: The Department, 1986.

Lehr, Richard I. and David J. Middlebrooks. *The new unionism—*

a blueprint for the future. New York: Executive Enterprises Publications Company, Inc. 1987.

Unions focus on statistics in support of NLRB's proposed Health Care Unit rules. *Daily Labor Report*, Oct. 26, 1987, A-11–A-14.

Unions today: new tactics to tackle tough times—A BNA special report.

Washington, D.C.: The Bureau of National Affairs, Inc., 1985.

Unions seek ways to address nursing shortage in bargaining. *Labor Relations Week*, April 27, 1988, 401–402.

Work & family: a changing dynamic—a BNA Special Report. Washington, D.C.: The Bureau of National Affairs, 1986.

CHAPTER 42

Nursing centers

Models for autonomous nursing practice

SALLY PECK LUNDEEN

During the past decade there has been growing interest among the professional nursing community in the development of innovative practice models known as "nursing centers." Also described in the literature as "nurse-managed centers," various models have been documented since the First Biennial Conference for Nurse-Managed Centers was held in Milwaukee in 1982.

Most nurses active in this "new" movement agree that nursing centers have existed in the United States for at least a century. Familiar nursing practice models that fit the definitions of extant nursing centers include the Nurse's Settlement at Henry Street[21] and the Frontier Nursing Service.[4] These are classic examples of practice settings developed and managed by nurses long before the current movement. This proud historical tradition has set the stage for the models reported in the more recent literature.[11]

The first effort to develop a consensus definition of a nursing center was undertaken by Fehring, Schulte, and Riesch at the Second Biennial Conference for Nurse-Managed Centers in 1984. With the help of a Delphi survey, the following definition was established by the participants of that conference:

Nurse-Managed Centers are organizations which provide direct access to professional nurses who offer holistic, client-centered health services for reimbursement. With the use of nursing models of health, professional nurses in Nurse-Managed Centers diagnose and treat human responses to potential and actual health problems. Examples of professional nursing services include health education, health promotion and health-related research. Services are targeted to individuals and groups whose health needs are not being met (e.g., the poor, women, the elderly and minorities). An effective referral system and collaboration with other health care professionals are an integral part of Nurse-Managed Centers. As models of professional nursing practice and research, Nurse-Managed Centers are ideal sites for faculty

practice and research. They are administered by a professional nurse.[9]

This definition was an expansion of one proposed at the First Biennial Conference in 1982, where nurse-managed centers were defined simply as settings "in which care was nurse-managed and which had potential for student learning, faculty practice, and nursing research."[17] This definition may reflect the fact that the majority of the participants at this conference (and the second conference as well) were faculty at academic institutions sponsoring nursing centers.

Limiting the conceptualization of nursing centers to the confines of academia did not do justice to the variety of models being developed, however. There are descriptions in the literature of solo nurses establishing nursing clinics, neighborhood health centers operating on a nursing-center model, and an increasing number of community health nurses and nurse-practitioners operating in a variety of innovative settings not directly affiliated with any academic setting. The difficulties seemed to be in identifying these settings and fostering a support network.

The emphasis on academically based nursing centers has diminished somewhat over the years. Five years after the initial survey, an American Nurses' Association (ANA) task force was appointed to review and refine the 1984 definition. The deliberations of this group (most of whom were involved in the initial Delphi process) resulted in the following definition:

Nursing centers—sometimes referred to as community nursing organizations, nurse-managed centers, nursing clinics, and community nursing centers—are organizations that give the client direct access to professional nursing services. Using nursing models of health, professional nurses in these centers diagnose and treat human responses to actual and potential health problems, and promote health and optimal functioning among target populations and communities. The service provided in these centers are holistic and client centered, and are reimbursed at a reasonable fee level. Accountability and responsibility for client care and professional practice remain with the professional nurse. Overall accountability and responsibility remain with the nurse executive.

Nursing Centers are not limited to any particular organizational configuration. Nursing centers may be freestanding businesses or may be affiliated with universities or other service institutions such as home health agencies and hospitals. The primary characteristic of the organization is responsiveness to the health needs of the population.[1]

Although there are many similarities in these two definitions, the differences indicate the more inclusive conceptualization of nursing centers that evolved during this developmental period.

It is not difficult to determine why there has been a proliferation of nursing centers during the past decade. It is, in fact, difficult to be unaware of the rapid and profound changes that have characterized the health care marketplace during this period. The issues of cost containment and competition, a shift away from the emphasis on acute institutionalization, and the proliferation of health maintenance organizations (HMOs), preferred provider organizations (PPOs), and other alternative payment structures all have heralded the need to develop alternative models for health care delivery. The nursing centers movement is one developmental trend that deserves serious study and consideration by policymakers concerned with both the cost and the quality of health care delivery.

Several issues outlined in the previous definitions require careful examination to highlight key issues that must be addressed by nursing centers in order to survive in today's marketplace. Such a discussion is meant to provoke continued discussion and debate on the form(s) these organizations may take in the future and their potential place in the health care delivery system.

DIRECT CLIENT ACCESS TO PROFESSIONAL NURSING SERVICES

Regardless of the mission or the program of services offered by any particular nursing center, all centers should provide consumers direct access to professional nursing services. This implies that nursing centers must be viewed either as an additional, adjunct option in the healthcare spectrum or as an alternative provider choice for the consumer. In either case direct access very clearly dictates that there need be no mandatory referral or directive from any other health care provider for a consumer to seek the services of a professional nurse through a nursing center.

This emphasis on direct consumer access to nursing services reflects a significant change from most current delivery models. Many home care agencies still require a physician's order for a patient to be able to access the services of a professional nurse. Third-party payers frequently require a physician's order or the signature of a supervising physician to provide a client access to professional nursing services. Such mandated control by one professional group over consumer access to another professional group must no longer be tolerated by either nurses or consumers.

In the current cost-conscious environment, consumer's direct access to any service that promotes health and avoids or delays the use of more costly, high-tech care alternatives should be welcomed by payers and clients alike. Nursing centers have both the opportunity and the responsibility to document the positive impact that increased access to professional nurses can have on different population groups. In addition to improved marketing to alert more consumers to the availability of nursing-center services, we must conduct the necessary research to document the outcomes, in both human and fiscal terms, of services provided at nursing-center sites.

COLLABORATIVE PRACTICE MODELS

It is important to state that the direct access to professional nursing services does not imply, as some may fear, that nurses are interested in usurping the roles of the physician or of any other health provider. There is a specific and unique body of knowledge and expertise nurses can offer the public that is independent from the supervision or direction of any other professional group. Nursing centers provide excellent opportunities for nurses to develop and expand their maximum practice potential as independent health care professionals.

On the other hand, nurses must recognize the need for collaborative and interdisciplinary practice models.[13] It is inappropriate for nurses to engage in long-term conflicts with medicine, social work, or psychology over the establishment of separate-but-equal nursing service models in the primary care arena. Ultimately, consumers stand to gain the most from organizational models that incorporate the unique skills of many health and health-related disciplines into collaborative models. These models may be developed as "one-stop shops" with multiple services available under one roof, or as "service networks" with elaboratively developed contractual or referral relationships. In either case, these models should recognize the interdependence of all health professionals in pursuing the goal of comprehensive, holistic client care.

Professional nursing must take a leadership role in advocating such collaborative practice models. Realistically, however, we also must recognize that truly collaborative, interdisciplinary practice models are possible only for disciplines that are operating from bases of equal power and mutual respect. Independence must therefore precede interdependence. It is imperative that nurses be prepared to compete to prove that they can provide professional services designed to promote and maintain health. Nursing centers offer an excellent venue through which to demonstrate independent nursing practice models as the basis for developing the innovative collaborative practice models of the future.

EMPHASIS ON HEALTH-PROMOTION AND HEALTH-EDUCATION SERVICES

Nursing services provided through nursing centers focus on health-promotion and health-education activities. This attention to basic prevention and education is a key factor in understanding the potential of nursing centers as an important organizational structure in future health care delivery. It is now known that the great majority of all health problems can be traced to lifestyle issues. The reduction of most current morbidity rates will be made possible not through medical cures or high-technology intervention but through education and lifestyle-modification efforts. It is also apparent that the long-term-care issues that face the United States because of its growing elderly population call for solutions that require health professionals to provide home-based support and care to forestall institutionalization.

Early screening, health-education and health-promotion services, supportive and caring supervision, and monitoring and follow-up activities have been directly linked to improved health care status in a variety of populations. These are nursing activities. Caring and teaching, case finding and long-term follow-up have been the work of nurses for the past century and longer. Many people now recognize the importance of the traditional activities of nursing to the health status of consumers. In the past decade many health professionals have shown a new or renewed interest in home-based care; primary prevention, education, and counseling services; and public health approaches to the improvement of health status. It is important that we speak out clearly about the expert role nurses have played for years in community-based care delivery, and that we continue to exercise leadership in the evaluation and development of the delivery systems of the future.

Nurses have understood for decades that care is as important as cure. It is critical that we now retain our rights to offer services to consumers within the traditional nursing framework. To do this we must document our nursing interventions and our practice delivery structures. We must simultaneously prepare to collaborate as well as compete for our place in the delivery systems that are emerging. Nursing centers are logical agencies within which to develop and provide community-based nursing services and achieve greater sophistication in health care politics, fiscal management, and multidisciplinary program design.

DIRECT REIMBURSEMENT

Services provided by nurses through nursing centers must be reimbursed. Currently many nursing centers are underwritten by private foundation grants, federal grants, or funds allocated by schools of nursing. Although client fees and some reimbursement from third-party payers are collected in nursing-center sites, in very few of the academically sponsored institutions do these constitute more than a small percentage of the total budget. Although hard data are not available for freestanding centers, direct reimbursement from third-party payers, including Medicare and Medicaid, is difficult for most nurse providers.

The issues of direct reimbursement established in Titles XIX and XX must be addressed by professional nurses in many arenas. The current attempt to pilot direct reimbursement for nursing services under Medicare Part B will proceed through the development of four demonstration sites subject to the Community Nursing and Ambulatory Care Act, which was authorized by Congress in late 1987. ANA has been identified as the Health Care Financing Administration (HCFA) subcontractor to develop selection criteria for the selection of the pilot Community Nursing Organization (CNO) sites. These projects will not begin until 1990.

Although this is an important step toward direct reimbursement for nursing services, other proactive agendas must be developed. The actual costs of these services must be determined by nurse administrators and providers. Clients should be educated to both the short- and long-term worth of nursing services. Employers must be presented with the option to contract with professional nurses to provide health education and primary care services to their clients. Municipalities and county and state governments should be approached by nurses for block grant monies or contracts directed at the comprehensive health care needs of their neediest citizens. HMO plans and private insurers should be encouraged to include nursing centers on their members' lists of approved provider organizations.

Only recently have cost issues forced the reassessment of the physician-dominated, institutionally based system that dominates this nation's current system of care. A restructuring of the financing mechanisms for prevention and wellness services and capitation for ambulatory and acute care has been a keystone of health maintenance organization plans since the 1970s. We must argue (and present well-documented evidence) that the reimbursement of nurses for nursing services will be a cost-saving policy rather than an additional health care expense. Nurses will have to develop greater sophistication in policy and economic matters if nursing centers are to successfully lobby for an adequate piece of the health care dollar. It is time that nurses lobby for recognition as autonomous professionals eligible for direct reimbursement capitation within the health care financing structures of today and with an equal say in the development of the financing structures of tomorrow. Nursing centers offer a unique opportunity to demonstrate the effectiveness of nursing interventions.

AGENCIES FOR LEARNING
The nursing center as a site for student learning

Nursing centers have exceptional potential as sites for clinical education experiences. Such learning experiences are as appropriate for nursing masters and doctoral students as they are for baccalaureate and RN continuation students. Not only do students benefit from the opportunity to work in autonomous nursing practice settings, but they are able to enhance the quality of services provided to nursing-center clients. Freestanding and academically based nursing centers should be used to educate students.

Nursing centers offer nurse-educators the opportunity to provide nursing students with excellent role models for autonomous nursing practice. Since most nursing centers are community based, they are in the forefront of testing methods of reaching and serving the populations that are emerging as the clients of the future: homebound elderly and chronically ill clients, the homeless, AIDS patients and their caretakers, disadvantaged children and families, substance abusers, and the victims of domestic violence and abuse. The nursing leaders of tomorrow must be faced today with this picture of reality to prepare for the challenges ahead. Nursing centers provide the opportunity to confront these challenges in an environment directed by innovative, risk-taking professional nurses.

The nursing center as a site for faculty practice

The ability of nursing educators to engage in clinical practice while fulfilling their obligations as teachers and active researchers has been questioned by some. These multiple roles are demanding and sometimes can seem fragmented, thus making difficult their optimal integration in the service of the profession, consumers, students, and even the individual nurse. The professional literature contains numerous examples of models proposed to resolve this multiplicity of roles.* Perhaps one of the most exciting challenges facing academic nursing centers is the opportunity and responsibility to test models that facilitate the integration of education, service, and research.

Nearly a decade ago Mausch[15] challenged all nursing educators with the "professional imperative" to continue to remain active practitioners of nursing. She thoughtfully enumerated the reasons that nursing has found itself in the awkward position of offering students few clinical role models among nursing faculty. According to Mausch this situation graphically illustrates "nursing's great paradox: [that it is] a profession committed to the delivery of a practice and yet a profession that least rewards those who deliver that practice." This disengagement of nurse-educators from clinical practice roles reduces the profession's ability to make credible contributions to policy decisions af-

---

*References 3, 5-8, 10, 14, 16, 18-20, 22.

fecting the delivery of health care. As Mausch pointedly observes, "Other health professionals . . . cannot understand how a profession can claim the right to decision making in an arena where its leaders and experts do not participate in the delivery of the very services they claim to promote."[15]

Nursing centers provide unique opportunities for faculty to engage in clinical activities. Since by definition and design nursing centers are controlled by nurses, the ability to develop and test innovative nursing interventions for targeted populations can be maximized in these settings. Implementation of programs and plans of care based on the most current research findings, and without the concommitant interdisciplinary conflicts inherent in many other clinical settings, should also be encouraged.

Pragmatic organizational support can also be built into many nursing centers, thereby increasing faculty incentives to engage in clinical practice. These incentives include close proximity to teaching sites, work load credit for clinical practice, additional financial remuneration, access to populations for scholarly research activities, and the opportunity to work directly with students in a clinical capacity.

Despite the opportunities afforded by academic nursing centers to bridge the gap between service and practice, full advantage has not yet been taken of these centers by many nursing educators. In a survey of all National League for Nursing accredited baccalaureate nursing programs, Barger reported that 51 schools of nursing were operating a nursing center at the time of the study.[2] She found that there was not necessarily a relationship between the presence of an academically based nursing center and positive administration policies regarding faculty practice. It appears that this is an area in which greater development is necessary.

The nursing center as a site for continuing education

A potential benefit of nursing centers that is frequently overlooked is the opportunity they can afford nurses for a unique continuing-education experience. With the current shift in emphasis from cure to care, and the shift in care delivery sites from acute-care settings to community agencies and homes, nursing centers should be explored as settings with exceptional continuing-education potential.

Most nursing centers are community based; many are free standing or are located in public health or nontraditional practice settings. Sites include housing complexes, church basements, social service agencies, vehicles, homes, schools, and various other locations that provide direct access to nursing services. Professional nurses whose experience has been primarily in acute-care settings and who are interested in learning more about community-based modalities or in preparing for a possible career shift to primary or even long-term care could be provided with exceptional learning experiences at a community nursing-center site.

Developing on-site continuing-education courses for acute-care nurses could also strengthen nursing-center staffs. The inclusion of experienced acute-care colleagues as active participants in planning and providing services for nursing-center clients, side by side with faculty and students, would afford another unique opportunity for nurses to bridge the gap between service and education.

Nursing centers as sites for research

Nursing centers provide excellent opportunities to conduct nursing research in many different areas, including (1) the effects of specific nursing interventions on various populations; (2) the effectiveness—in both human and fiscal terms—of various nursing practice models; (3) the characteristics of various population groups utilizing nursing services; (4) the most effective teaching methods and learning experiences for students of nursing practice; and (5) the testing of nursing theories, in addition to many other topics of vital interest to the nursing profession.

Although nursing centers are by no means the only sites where such studies can be conducted, they make possible the gathering of inordinately rich data on nursing activities in settings free from the complications and competing agendas present in settings not under the control of professional nurses. A further advantage of many nursing-center sites is that they are able to link nurse-educators, nurse-scientists, and experienced nurse clinicians and administrators into research teams, providing an optimal context in which to develop research programs that will have important and lasting effects on the nursing profession.

Research on the development and impact of the centers themselves is an important aspect of current nursing research. The U.S. Public Health Service's Division of Nursing recognized a number of years ago the potential for nursing centers as innovative service-delivery organizations.[12] In 1986 funds were allocated through a new category of special projects grants for the development and evaluation of selected centers. The data from these initial projects should offer the profession additional insight into the potential for nursing centers' long-term impact on the organizational structure of the health care delivery system and the health status of various population groups.

SUMMARY

Nursing centers are organizations operated and administered by nurses that provide consumers direct access to nursing care. They emphasize health education, health promotion, and support services. These functions, which focus on the care of clients, comprise the special expertise that nurses bring to a comprehensive health care environment. Nursing centers highlight the need to continue to struggle for direct reimbursement by consumers and third-party payers.

Although nursing centers may be promoted as innovative and autonomous practice models grounded in the rich tradition of public health nursing, a case is made for caution in touting centers merely as separate-but-equal delivery structures that can compete with medicine. Long-term health policy goals must continue to redefine health provider roles and to include a more equal allocation of professional power and decision making, so as to facilitate the development of collaborative, holistic models of health care delivery.

Nursing centers are valuable for students and professinal nurses interested in community-based continuing-education opportunities. They also offer an optimal setting for faculty practice and nursing research programs. Nursing centers provide settings in which the service-education dichotomy can be addressed in unique ways, and they show great potential for long-range policy impact on the health care models of the future.

REFERENCES

1. American Nurses' Association: The nursing center: concept and design, Kansas City, Mo, 1987, The Association.
2. Barger SE: Academic nursing centers: a demographic profile, J Prof Nurs 2:246, 1986.
3. Bellinger K and Sanders DH: Faculty practice policy, J Nurs Educ 24(5):214, 1985.
4. Breckenridge M: Wide neighborhoods: a story of the Frontier Nursing Service, Lexington, 1981, University of Kentucky Press.
5. Diers D: Faculty practice: models, methods and madness. In National League for Nursing Pub No 15-1831, New York, 1981, NLN.
6. Diers D: Preparation of practitioners, clinical specialists, and clinicians, J Prof Nurs 1:41, 1985.
7. Dinsmore VK and Pollow RL: Credit-for-faculty practice model: a proposal, Nursing and Health Care 2:17, 1981.
8. Duffy DM and Halloran CS: Meeting the challenges of multiple academic roles through a nursing center practice model, J Nurs Educ 25(2):55, 1986.
9. Fehring RJ, Schulte J, and Riesch SK: Toward a definition of nurse-managed centers, Journal of Community Health Nursing 3(2):59, 1986.
10. Free T and Mills BC: Faculty practice in primary care, Nurs Outlook 33(4):192, 1985.
11. Glass L: The historic origins of nursing centers. Paper presented at the Fourth Biennial Conference on Nurse-Managed Centers, Milwaukee, May 27, 1988.
12. Henry OM: Demonstration centers for nursing practice, education, and research. In Mezey MD and McGivern DO, editors: Nurse, nurse practitioners: the evolution of primary care, Boston, 1986, Little, Brown & Co, Inc.
13. Lundeen SP: An interdisciplinary nurse-managed center: the Erie Family Health Center. In Mezey MD and McGivern DO, editors: Nurse, nurse practitioners: the evolution of primary care, Boston, 1986, Little, Brown & Co, Inc.
14. MacPhail J: Promoting collaboration/unification models for nursing education and service. In National League for Nursing Pub No 15-1831, New York, 1981, NLN.
15. Mauksch IG: Faculty practice: a professional imperative, Nurse Educator 3:21, 1981.
16. Ossler CC and others: Establishment of a nursing clinic for faculty and student clinical practice, Nurs Outlook p402, 1982.
17. Riesch S: Survey of nursing centers. Paper presented at the First Biennial Conference on Nurse-Managed Centers, Milwaukee, June 10, 1982.
18. Rodgers MW and Peake-Godin H: Implementing faculty practice in an atomosphere of retrenchment, J Nurs Educ 27(2):87, 1985.
19. Royle J and Crooks D: Clinical practice: a dilemma for nurse educators, Nursing papers 18(4):27, 1986.
20. Spero J: Faculty practice as one component of the faculty role. In National League for Nursing Pub No 15-1831, New York, 1981, NLN.
21. Wald LD: The nurse's settlement in New York, Am J Nurs 2:8;567, 1902.
22. Williamson JA: Faculty practice in a nursing center: an integrated model. In National League for Nursing Pub No 15-1831, 1981, NLN.

CHAPTER 43

Decentralization of nursing practice

TIMOTHY PORTER-O'GRADY

Health care is dramatically affected by the major cultural and social changes occurring in the world community.[5] Although economics appears to be the focus of these changes, they are much broader in scope and impact. The rush of technological advances, sophisticated communication processes, complex information systems, and the formation of an extensive global community all have contributed to the changing world within which we must live.

The health care delivery system is adapting to the impact of these major social, cultural, and economic changes. It is responding to new paradigms for which there are no existing scripts. Executives in the health care system are struggling to find appropriate placements, work processes, and structures for their institutions that will meet the health care needs of the community. It is in this context that nursing struggles both to seek its identity and to perform its work in a coordinated and integrated fashion. The abilities to render patient care services and to determine nursing's market and appropriate service framework are directly affected by the greater social and health care system changes. The role of nursing is to sort out these changes, responding to the essential needs of the nursing organization and identifying newer frameworks applicable to the direction of health care. There is no area of nursing practice unaffected by these major changes. Because of their scope, radical reallocation of resources and restructuring of traditional services and environments will be necessary for nursing to respond to the changing conditions.

ECONOMIC FORCES

It has become clear that the basic economic underpinnings of the U.S. financial system are in need of dramatic structural adjustment. Deficit spending, a negative balance of trade, the mounting national debt, and other serious financial concerns all have a dramatic impact on the economic health of our society. In health care this impact is evident in the ways health care services are paid for.[3] Over the past two decades access to services has been increased through the building of a health care delivery system providing all Americans the opportunity to obtain basic health care services. However, in the last decade, as the cost of those health care services has accelerated by some 15% per year (about 9% to 10% above the gross national product index), major adjustments have been made to compensate for the increased cost.[3] In the early 1980s entirely new approaches to the payment of health care services demanded an emphasis on curtailing resources and on retooling the health care delivery system to make it more productive and competitive in the marketplace. This sensitivity to the increase in health care costs has focused on the mechanisms and modes of delivering services. The current structuring of health care also has been the subject of close examination. The search for broader-based structures that allow a wider range of health care services, increased market share, and enhanced positioning within the community has had an impact on the way in which health care services are delivered.[6]

Nursing practice, in turn, has been dramatically affected. The focus on cost has encouraged nursing organizations to look carefully at the relationship between staffing levels and services provided. The methodologies of nursing service delivery also have been questioned. Examining delivery mechanisms and their costs is an integral element of organizational review in determining productivity and financial efficacy.

DECISION-MAKING STRUCTURES

Looking at decision-making systems and organizational structures has also been an important part of the health care system in transition. Structuring the organization in a way that allows decision making to occur at the lowest management levels results in the greatest degree of control. Controlling services and costs has been emphasized as part of the strategy for dealing with economic downsizing. Nurses have deeply felt the impact of downsizing and delimiting expenditures. The role of the front-line manager in nursing has been defined and enhanced to ensure that control exists at the operational level of the organization. Along with this expectation has come increasing accountability for performance and a willingness on the part of the organization to allow accountability to be widely shared at the clinical levels. However, along with enhanced accountability has come the need to ensure the competence of the front-line manager to undertake the demanding roles of resource manager and systems manager within a more defined practice framework in the nursing organization.[8]

DECENTRALIZED SERVICES

Decentralization to date is only a small part of the long-term process of disseminating health care services to better respond to the marketplace. The marketplace has become one of the key driving forces influencing the provision of health care services. Sensitivity to the marketplace, to the consumer, and to the payers has become a focus for leadership in the health care delivery system. Bringing services to the market has become a new imperative for health services.[1] Decentralizing services to individual communities has established a new direction for health care, and therefore continued efforts in community-based decentralization have become a major part of the health care leadership role. Beyond decentralization is the need in most organizations to extend services over a broad base so they no longer are institutionally fixed. The institution or hospital is now dedicated to highly intensive critical-care services for ill persons. Further, the hospital has become a multiservice health care corporation, moving into broader areas of service, some non-health related, to ensure continued economic support for its health services base. Essentially this means moving a number of services out of the hospital setting into the community and providing services in a way not previously considered or even conceived by the health care institution.

FUTURE ORGANIZATION OF NURSING

The nursing organization of the future will provide leadership in the alternative structuring of health care services. Only now is nursing addressing ways in which nurses can take the lead providing health care services other than those traditionally defined by others in the institution. A problem exists, however, in that most nurses are prepared for institutional practice. In fact, the majority of nurses in the United States practice in institutional settings. Yet the profession has begun to retool. In order to provide services in different formats in a community-based system, nursing practice models and framework also will have to change. The nurse who is successful in a community-based practice needs a different set of skills, abilities, and resources than the nurse who is successful in institutional practice. This is not to suggest that the institutional nurse will play a less significant role in the delivery of health care services. What it does suggest, however, is that a greater number of nurses will be needed to provide community-based services, and that they will therefore be expected to possess the requisite skills to practice in a framework significantly different from traditional institutional nursing practice.

Structural changes in the health care organization are evident through the increasing "lateralization" of health care systems. In the industrial model, representative of an age that is quickly passing, health care institutions are very hierarchical in design; that is, they are essentially top-down structures and are integrated along a vertical continuum. In these systems control is maintained at the "top" and work unfolded at the bottom. The assumption is that the worker does not share an obligation in control decisions affecting the work such as mission, policy, or direction of the enterprise. However, as we prepare for changed organizational systems representing newer social values, there is increasing attention to the creation of multilateral organizational systems. Multilateral organizations are defined more by their relationship to other organizational components than by their vertical structure. Each organizational entity parallels other organizational components, and their success depends on their ability to promote communication, integration, and the negotiation and sharing of work arrangements based on mutually determined outcomes and system goals. Organizations are therefore moving into a social system in which the relationship of one component to others in the organization will be of primary value to the structure. The abilities to negotiate, position, relate, seek mutual opportunities, and facilitate outcomes are the earmark of a successful organization.[4] See Fig. 43-1.

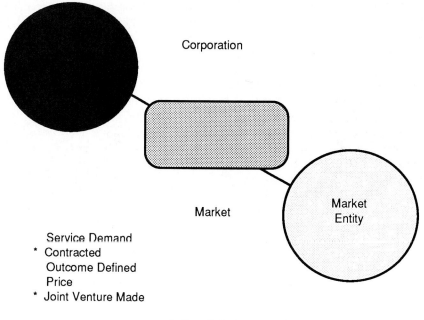

Fig. 43-1 Market entity.

In such a system the nursing leadership will use skills in negotiation and collaborative practice by establishing relationships between the service provider (the nurse) and others. The nature of the relationship will be determined by the needs of the community served. Those needs will define the framework within which services are provided. Clearly the nursing practice leadership of tomorrow will need to develop negotiating, business, structural, practice, and functional skills to operate within diverse community contexts. Creative health maintenance organizations and preferred provider systems are the initial environments in which much of this activity will unfold. However, even they are subject to change: their dynamic interactions and interconnections with other services, facilities, groups, and professionals will provide the relational junctures leading to unique service arrangements.

THE NURSING ROLE IN HEALTH SERVICES OF THE FUTURE

Within the context of this radical organizational transformation and change, the leader in nursing management and practice will have to ask some signif-

icant questions regarding changes in the nurse's role:

1. How does the practicing nurse fit into this radical reorganization and restructuring of health care?
2. What is the role the nurse will play in a highly decentralized organization?
3. What are the skills essential to a professional operating in a multilateral, multiservice institutional system?
4. How does the internal organizational structure of the nursing service interface with broader organizational changes leading to a greater community focus?
5. What preparation is required, and what roles must be adopted, for effective nursing practice in a broad-based multilateral health care system?
6. Who are the new players in a changing health care system with whom the nurse must negotiate, collaborate, and integrate the clinical provision of nursing care services?
7. What recipient groups are indicated by changing demographics, and what specific services will those groups require for their health care needs to be satisfactorily addressed?

Clearly if nursing is to answer these questions in a positive, productive manner, and to respond appropriately to increasing demands for nursing services, restructuring and reorganizing are key. Because the corporate health care organization is undergoing broader decentralization, and because the corporate units are assuming more responsibility for their individual contributions to the organization, nurses must define those contributions and provide systems and structures within which service outcomes are pursued. The nursing organization also must determine in what areas it will be competitive, its frames of reference in relation to service, its marketability, what it contributes to the service system, and the outcomes of nursing care in terms of its contribution not only to the organization but also to the health care of the community. In other words, nursing must be able to articulate and validate its contribution to itself and to the society it serves.[2]

THE NEED FOR NURSING LEADERSHIP

Clear leadership is called for in establishing new organizational systems. Models for restructuring that provide corporate integrity and independence of the nursing organization will have to be considered. Building the corporate nursing service organization is consistent with the restructuring of hospitals and health care systems into corporate units. The nursing organization will be one of many corporate units working to meet the goals and objectives of the organizational system. What may often occur in the future is that the system leadership itself will define the mission and provide the direction for the corporate organization. After the mission and objectives are defined the corporate units will decide on ways they will functionally carry out the mission and meet the objectives of the system. Within that context each corporate unit will define its own area of service provision, competitive marketplace, framework for service, and structure for meeting the demand for services. The corporate units will be required to negotiate with one other. They will need to find ways to provide support and the skills, resources, and personnel necessary to assist each corporate unit in fulfilling its goals and mission. From this conception emerges a self-sustaining, self-directed corporate nursing service (see Fig. 43-2).

If the corporate nursing service is to remain self-sustaining and self-directed, it must be structured in such a way as to obtain support and sustain its activities without guidance from or economic dependence on the prevailing corporate health system. The following conditions will have to be met:

1. Nursing practice must be defined in concrete terms. The nature of nursing practice, its contributions to the organization, how it can be measured and validated, and its relationship to outcomes all will have to be clearly articulated.
2. Nursing's contribution to the profitability or revenue margin of the institution must be clearly identified. The value of nursing practice must be ascertained so that costs and revenues can be identified.
3. The breadth and depth of nursing practice must be identified within the context of the organization's mission. Therefore nursing practice must begin to reflect the mission and values of the organization as exemplified by a defined quality of care.
4. Nursing's relationship to and value in the marketplace depends on consumer perceptions of nursing's contributions as definable and measurable, leading consumers to invest in nursing services.
5. The practice framework, roles, and skills of the nurse must be articulated in the context of the needs, demands, and community calls for nursing practice. Nurses must make an appropriate and viable clinical response to the marketplace, assuring the consumer that health care needs can best be met by the quality and range of services provided by nurses.

CREATING NEW STRUCTURES FOR NURSING

If the nursing service corporation is to be successful, it must be able to manage its own activities and be self-sustaining and self-directed. Further, if it is to represent the interests of nursing as they are traditionally defined, it must evidence a distinctly nursing set of values. Also, because it is a professional organization, it must show evidence of shared governance strategies that perpetuate the professional values and organizational system directed at meeting the health care needs of consumers.[7]

At the corporate levels of the organization, the executive staff must reflect the values of the professional staff. Leadership must guide the nursing organization

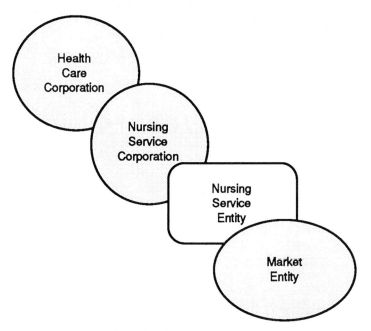

Fig. 43-2 Service structure.

according to the system's goals and the corporate mission and objectives. Because the role of the executive in new organizational models is no longer determined through status or position alone, the value of the role must be identified through its relationships and linkages with other roles of the organization. The role of the nurse executive in the corporate nursing organization provides a link between the external and the internal organizational system. The external system is identified as the hospital or health care system, the internal system as the nursing organizational structure. This corporate linkage is exemplified by the nurse executive's role at the board and administrative levels, the highest levels of corporate decision making in the system. Through participation at the policy level the nurse executive brings to bear the constraints and resources associated with the nursing organization on the collective decision-making process. Through this cross-referencing role the nurse executive articulates professional nursing roles and services and defines how they fit into the organization's mission and the requirements of the health care system.

Finally, the nurse executive represents the staff and its corporate posture to the executive and administrative levels of the organization, and represents the organization's imperatives to the professional staff, providing a framework for corporate, collective, and professional decision making. The nurse executive also is responsible for assessing and monitoring the community environment that affects the nature and direction of corporate decision making. In this position the visionary nurse executive alerts the professional staff to both the constraints and opportunities in the greater health care environment having an impact on the decisions of the corporate nursing organization. The nurse executive does not operate outside the decisional framework of the nursing corporate organization, but this person does have an obligation to ensure that adequate and appropriate information is available for effective decision making. Through the leadership of the nurse executive, in conjunction with the collective efforts of the clinical staff, the integrity and drive of the new corporate organization are facilitated. Shared governance, through the contribution of different roles to a common endeavor, provides the "glue" and energy that motivates and moves the system toward success. Indeed, it provides the vehicle for assuring the value and viability of nursing well into the twenty-first century.

REFERENCES

1. Arnold D, Capella L, and Sumrall D: Organization, culture, and the market concept, Journal of Healthcare Marketing, p 18, March 1987.

2. Aydelotte M: Nursing's preferred future, Nurs Outlook p 114, May-June 1987.
3. Davis CK, Poul PD, and Gross MS: The changing health care environment, Top Health Care Financ 1, Winter 1987.
4. Drucker P: The coming of the organization, Harvard Business Review, p 45, Jan-Feb 1988.
5. Gilder G: Revitalization of everything: the law of the microcosm, Harvard Business Review, p 49, March-April 1988.
6. Jaeger J, Kaluzny A, and Maguder-Habib K: A new perspective on multi-institutional systems management, Health Care Manage Rev, p 9, Fall 1987.
7. Peterson M and Allen D: Shared governance: a strategy for transforming organizations, parts 1 and 2, J Nurs Adm, p 9, Jan-Feb 1986.
8. Porter-O'Grady T: Creative nursing administration: participative management into the twenty-first century, 1986, Aspen Publishers.

CHAPTER 44

A guide to nursing organizations

What they are and how to choose them

SUE THOMAS HEGYVARY

Humans and most other forms of life exhibit a consistent tendency to organize themselves. Types of organizations vary with regard to their purpose. The most basic type of organization exists to promote survival and protect the group from external threats.

As human societies developed over time, population subgroups began to perform specialized functions. Practitioners of a particular trade found it desirable and sometimes necessary to organize themselves for various reasons—a sense of identity and social support, the delineation of standards, and control of the trade. This focus of human organization continued to develop in sophistication in industrialized societies.

The development of occupations and professions has been accompanied by the continued evolution of trade associations. This chapter explores the formation of professional organizations in nursing and the continuing development of four types of nursing organizations: multipurpose, clinical specialty, and functional specialty organizations, as well as the recently formed interorganizational alliances. This discussion contrasts existing organizations and projects aspects of the future of nursing organizations. The overall picture is of a diversity of personal and professional choices. A more extensive review of these topics may be found in a recent publication of the American Academy of Nursing.[6]

THE FORMATION OF PROFESSIONAL ORGANIZATIONS

In previous decades the literature on professional organizations has centered on the development of standards of practice and alliance, control, and promotion of practitioners in a particular trade or profession. A predominant focus was the delineation of characteristics of occupations and professions and of the appropriate activities of the professional organization. That focus has shifted in recent years. Hall[5] notes the shift toward emphasizing linkages among occupational groups and between the organization and other parts of the social structure. He concludes that "obtaining and maintaining power in the broader social context . . . would be the major activity or goal for a professional organization." Hall states further:

The professional organization would appear to be the only source of power for establishing nurses as a profession and supporting its members as paid professionals. It would appear that the empowerment of nursing as a profession and of nurses as individuals can only come about through the actions of the professional organizations.[5]

Although it is clear that professional organizations need to serve the purposes of self-regulation, representation, and organizational development,[10] the current trend is to focus less on structure and definitive static purposes. Increasingly, professional organizations are concerned about interorganizational linkages and changing activities in response to changing environments. This discussion of the past, present, and future of nursing organizations reflects that changing focus.

Studies of the development of formal organizations cite three major themes, the first of which is differentiation. Lawrence and Lorsch[7] note that as groups become larger they tend to differentiate into specified parts. The result is increasing differences within the organization, both in the orientation toward goals and in the formal status of subunits within the structure.[7]

The development of specialized subunits gives rise to the second theme in organizations, the need for integration. Integration refers to the processes and methods used to increase collaboration among functional departments in working toward common goals. The nature and extent of integration presents the third theme, that of interdependence among units. The integration of differentiated units requires linkages based on the type and extent of interdependence.

The issue of interdependence is of more than academic concern in nursing. Because of the very large number of nursing organizations, their overlapping memberships, and their parallel attention to issues of common concern, their activities certainly influence each other. When the views and goals of nursing organizations are shared and jointly promoted, the result can be the increased strength of the profession. An example is the response of organized nursing to the American Medical Association's intent to create three new categories of care givers. When the interests and activities of nursing organizations are in conflict, however, the perception both within and outside nursing may be of trouble within the profession. An example of an issue generating considerable conflict is that of entry into practice.

The following description of nursing organizations portrays differentiated units within nursing, not necessarily by rational design. Each of the organizations described below has evolved from other organizations as a response to changes in the organizational environment. Some of those pressures for change, coming both from within and outside organizations, are evident in nursing today. An individual nurse's choice of membership in professional organizations very likely will be based on the historical image, perceived goals and functions, and trends and probable future directions of each organization.

Multipurpose organizations

Two national nursing organizations are categorized as multipurpose organizations. This section describes the American Nurses' Association (ANA) and the National League for Nursing (NLN) as umbrella organizations that serve a variety of functions and constituents.

American Nurses' Association (ANA)

For many nurses the American Nurses' Association is *the* professional organization. It is the only multipurpose organization solely for registered nurses. Its

origins can be traced to 1893, through several other organizations. Its most recent merger was with the National Association of Colored Graduate Nurses in 1950.

ANA activities range from those considered typical of a professional association, such as setting standards for practice, to those considered typical of a labor union, for example, ensuring a collective bargaining program for nurses. The ANA also includes two semiautonomous organizations: the American Academy of Nursing and the American Nurses' Foundation.

The purposes of the ANA as stated in its bylaws are (1) to work for the improvement of health standards and the availability of health care services for all people; (2) to foster high standards of nursing; and (3) to stimulate and promote the professional development of nurses and advance their economic and general welfare. The bylaws of the ANA designate 15 functions related to standards of nursing practice, education and nursing services, code of ethics, credentialing, legislation, health policy, evaluation, research, economic and general welfare, professional leadership, professional development of nurses, affirmative action, collective bargaining, communicating with the membership, consumer advocacy, and representation of the profession.[4]

The ANA's achievements over the decades are remarkable, particularly in view of its internal diversity, combined with increasing professional, social, and political turbulence. Further, in 1985 12.1% of the registered nurses in the country were ANA members, down from a peak of 24.1% in 1970. The ANA has successfully represented the profession in many ways, despite the small percentage of nurses who are members.[2]

The ANA is the only U.S. nursing association with official representation in the International Council of Nurses. Although its approximately 200,000 members do not comprise a majority of the profession, it is still the most visible, active, and comprehensive of all American nursing organizations.

National League for Nursing (NLN)

The National League for Nursing was incorporated in 1952 by a merger of the National League for Nursing Education, the National Organization of Public Health Nurses, and the Association of Collegiate Schools of Nursing. The creation of a second multipurpose organization, in addition to the ANA, was based on a decision made at the 1950 ANA convention.

Because of the perceived need to restructure national organizations, the members voted for the ANA to continue as the membership association for registered nurses. The NLN, as a new multipurpose organization, would include nurses, interested nonnurses, and relevant institutions to strengthen nursing education and service.

Unlike the ANA, then, membership in the NLN is open to both individuals and agencies. The inclusion of nonnurses as members adds a new perspective, as well some controversy about control of the profession. Agency membership includes organizations providing nursing services or nursing educational programs.

The eight designated missions and functions of the NLN include strengthening and supporting nursing services, promoting research for the knowledge base of nursing education and practice, maintaining responsiveness to its membership, promoting public understanding and support of nursing, and exploring new avenues for promoting nursing such as alternative health care settings.[9]

Like the ANA and multipurpose organizations in other professions, the NLN has suffered a decline in membership in recent years. Currently it has approximately 1700 institutional members and 1500 individual members.

Clinical specialty organizations

As specialization in health care has become more pronounced, specialty organizations have gained strength and membership. This trend is evident in both nursing and medicine. Undoubtedly the growth of clinical specialty organizations has contributed to the declining membership of multipurpose organizations such as the ANA and the NLN. Membership in these organizations, however, is overlapping. Many nurses retain membership in the large multipurpose organizations and also express their clinical identity through a specialty organization.

Clinical areas around which specialty organizations have formed include critical care, nephrology, nurse anesthesia, neuroscience, occupational health, nurse midwifery, ophthalmology, plastic and reconstructive surgery, postanesthesia, urology, infection control, operating room, pediatric oncology, rehabilitation, emergency, enterostomal therapy, orthopedics, pediatric associates and nurse-practitioners, school nurses, intravenous therapy, addictions, oncology, obstetrics and gynecology, and public health.

Nursing specialty organizations serve a variety of purposes, differ in organizational structure, and vary greatly in membership size. Some specialty organizations, such as the American Association of Critical Care Nurses, have a large number of members. Others, such as the National Nurses' Society on Addictions, have few members and offer much more limited services to their memberships.

The concern shared by these organizations—that is, promoting the identity and professional interests of nurses in specialty areas—led to the formation in 1981 of the National Federation of Specialty Nursing Organizations (NFSNO). By 1984 the NFSNO reported that it represented 400,000 nurses through its 27 constituent organizations. The nature of representation through this national federation has been very limited, however, as the NFSNO has maintained the role of a voluntary alliance of organizations and does not have the intent of formalizing any control of constituent organizations. Individual nurses are members of the constituent organizations, just as the national federation is comprised of members' organizations.[8]

The NFSNO represents a significant chapter in the history of nursing organizations in the United States. Not only does it present a challenge to the two large multipurpose organizations, it also illustrates changing trends in the profession and in society at large. Nurses have indicated through their membership in specialty organizations that they want to be identified with a clinical specialty area. At the same time, they recognize the necessity of a national alliance of nurses with common interests. Since the mission and goals of the NFSNO parallel some of the functions and activities of the ANA and the NLN, they compete for members as well as to represent the profession. In a later section this chapter further discusses the trend toward national alliances.

Functional specialty organizations

This section differentiates organizations that center on a "functional role" as opposed to a specialty area of practice. The two major examples of this type of national organization are the American Association of Colleges of Nursing (AACN) and the American Organization of Nurse Executives (AONE).

American Association of Colleges of Nursing (AACN)

The American Association of Colleges of Nursing exists to improve the practice of professional nursing through (1) advancing the quality of baccalaureate and graduate programs in nursing, (2) promoting research in nursing, and (3) providing for the development of academic leaders. AACN was established in 1969 in response to the need for a national organization devoted specifically to baccalaureate and graduate education in nursing. Schools of nursing in all 50 states and Puerto Rico are represented by the AACN. In 1986 there were 383 member schools of nursing in senior colleges and universities, and the membership has since continued to grow.

The AACN has an institutional membership and does not provide for individual membership. Its activities focus on all aspects of academic concern and development, including governmental affairs.[1]

American Organization of Nurse Executives (AONE)

Formerly known as the American Society of Nursing Service Administrators, the AONE has grown rapidly to a membership of over 3700 members. Initially one of 156 personal membership groups in the American Hospital Association (AHA), the AONE has continued to distance itself from the umbrella of the AHA. In doing so, it has maintained an alliance with hospital administration but also has positioned itself for more autonomy as a professional nursing organization.

The central purpose of the AONE is to promote safe and effective patient care. Its designated functions center on influencing health care delivery in nursing practice, participating in the formulation of public policy related to health and nursing, promoting nurse-executive practice, supporting nursing research and education, providing information and data for members regarding analysis, and contributing to policy formation and strategic planning at local, state, and national levels.[6]

The AONE is an individual membership organization that continues to grow in size and national influence. Its increasing identity as a professional nursing organization, combined with continued ties to hospital administration, position the AONE as a relatively small but focused and powerful national organization.

Developing alliances among nursing organizations

Several of the nursing organizations mentioned above illustrate the formation of coalitions and alliances that produce new organizations. These coalitions and alliances occur for varying reasons. One reason is the proliferation of organizations with common pur-

poses, so that reason suggests combining forces. Another driving force can be perceived threats, either from other nursing organizations or from forces external to the nursing profession.

In addition to the existing formal alliances (the NFSNO and the alliance of state organizations that now constitute the ANA), there are two existing alliances of nursing organizations; the Tri-Organizational Nursing Council and the Nursing Organization Liaison Forum (NOLF), which are growing in strength.

Tri-Council

The Tri-Council now formally includes four nursing organizations: the ANA, the NLN, the AACN, and the AONE. Organizations such as the American Association of Critical Care Nurses, the American Academy of Nursing, and the National Council of State Boards of Nursing, among others, also may meet with the Tri-Council. Most recently, under the pressure of the national nursing shortage and the proposal of the American Medical Association for three new categories of care givers, the Tri-Council invited all national nursing organizations to participate in a summit meeting. Both the precipitating factors and the success of that meeting illustrate the recognition of the need for national coalitions in response to a changing environment.

The Tri-Council, formed in 1972, emerged as a response of nursing organizations to their multiple interdependencies and the need for a unified nursing approach to issues of mutual and national concern. It is composed of the presidents, presidents-elect or vice presidents, and executive directors of the member organizations. The Tri-Council lacks a formal organization and legitimacy as a single umbrella organization. Its success is based on shared interests and goals and on the mutual consent and benefit of the participants. Given the current pressures and directions in nursing organizations, it appears possible and even likely that the Tri-Council as an interorganizational alliance will continue to grow in strength and perhaps to evolve further as a formal alliance of nursing organizations.[6]

National Organization Liaison Forum (NOLF)

Another example of an organizational alliance has occurred under the auspices of the ANA. The NOLF was formed in 1982 to provide a forum for discussion among nursing organizations and the ANA and to promote concerted action among national nursing organizations. The NOLF currently claims 41 participating organizations.

It is clear that the agenda of the NOLF has many similarities to those of the NFSNO and the Tri-Council. These common agenda and overlapping interests illustrate both the need and the probability of increasing organizational alliances in the future.[3]

The future of nursing organizations: personal and professional choices

This brief overview has presented some of the major nursing organizations; it certainly is not a complete list. Among those not included in the discussion are Sigma Theta Tau, the international honor society of nursing that selects individuals for membership; a number of regional nursing associations, such as the Western Institute on Nursing; and the National Council of State Boards of Nursing.

Individual nurses and institutions have a variety of choices for organizational membership, depending on their interests and desires for affiliation. Nurses tend to join professional organizations for several reasons. It is likely that the two major reasons are to gain a stronger sense of professional identity and to support an organization that represents nurses' personal and professional goals.

It is likely that nursing organizations of the future will represent greater alliances than exist at present. Such alliances, analogous to formalized networks or systems in other sectors of society, may result in greater national control of the nursing profession and in less autonomy for the many individual organizations. At the same time, however, such alliances may be essential for the future of the profession. Individual nurses influence these developments by their membership and participation in national nursing organizations.

REFERENCES

1. American Association of Colleges of Nursing: Bylaws, Washington, DC, 1981, The Association.
2. American Nurses' Association: Facts about nursing, 1984-1985, Kansas City, Mo, 1985, The Association.
3. American Nurses' Association: Operating guidelines: the Nursing Organization Liaison Forum. Unpublished document, Kansas City, Mo, 1984.
4. American Nurses' Association: Staff organization, philosophy, and functions, Kansas City, Mo, 1983, The Association.
5. Hall RH: Organizations: structure and process, ed 3, Englewood Cliffs, NJ, 1982, Prentice-Hall Inc.
6. Hegyvary ST and others: The evolution of nursing professional organizations: alternative models for the future, Kansas City, Mo, 1986, American Academy of Nursing.
7. Lawrence PR and Lorsch JW: Organization and environment: managing differentiation and integration, Cambridge, 1967, Harvard University Press.
8. National Federation of Specialty Nursing Organizations: The first ten years, Washington DC, 1984, The Federation.
9. National League for Nursing: NLN mission and goals, 1983-1985, New York, 1983, The League.
10. Ryan JA: Force of professional control: determinants of member orientation to internal and external program strategies of the American Nurses' Association, Ann Arbor, Mich, 1983, University Microfilms International.

CHAPTER 45

Issues related to promotion and tenure, revisited

PATRICIA M. OSTMOE
RITA KISTING SPARKS

In 1985 Ostmoe argued that the survival of academic nursing as a legitimate discipline in higher education depends on the extent to which promotion and tenure decisions of the future reflect the valuing of the scholarly productivity of faculty.[41] She further noted that the descriptive data from her 1981 study suggested that the academic, educational, and attitudinal profile of nurse faculty did not conform to the usual standards of academia. Ostmoe found, for example, that even at the major research universities included in her study, less than 50% of the tenured or tenure-track nurse faculty held the earned doctorate, only 25% of the faculty respondents reported being primarily interested in research, a mere 20% believed publication should be a very important consideration in the awarding of promotion, and the mean number of lifetime publications of the nursing faculty was 6.5.[40,41]

Data from a number of sources indicate that this faculty profile may be changing. Between 1982 and 1986 the number of doctorally prepared nurse faculty holding appointments in baccalaureate and higher degree programs increased 70.2%, from 1278 to 2176.[37] Similarly, the number of doctoral programs in nursing increased during this same 4-year period, from 25 to 38, and the number of graduates from these programs increased by 81.7%.[37] The National League for Nursing (NLN) criteria for accreditation of baccalaureate and higher degree programs, as revised in 1983, provide further evidence that research and scholarship are perceived to be more important for faculty holding appointments in nursing programs. These criteria require that the faculty of all accredited nursing programs include individuals with research expertise and that faculty endeavors include participation in scholarly activities consistent with the mission(s) of the parent institution and the goals of the program.[36] The

criteria also require that a majority of faculty members teaching graduate courses hold earned doctorates. In addition, schools of nursing, even those located in comprehensive universities whose primary mission is teaching, now require the earned doctorate and scholarly activity for the awarding of tenure.[52]

Another indicator of increased scholarship among nurses can be seen in the proliferation of nursing journals in recent years. Brandon and Hill's list[9,10] of selected nursing books and journals identified 48 journals in 1982 and 69 in 1988. These authors noted that they encountered difficulties in choosing journals to be included in the 1988 list because of the large number of new nursing journals that had appeared within the previous two years.[9]

The nursing community's growing appreciation of and changing values concerning the importance of research was also reflected in the successful efforts of nurse leaders, many of them academics, to assure the establishment in 1986 of a National Center for Nursing Research within the National Institutes of Health. The center's mission is consistent with the increase in doctoral programs in nursing. That is, the research emphasis at the Center for Nursing Research is on basic and clinical nursing research, training, and other programs in patient care research.

It is more difficult to determine, however, from the findings of empirical studies, if in actuality the profile of nurse faculty has changed. Andreoli and Musser[2] reported in their 1986 literature review of faculty productivity that there were fewer studies of faculty research productivity than of teaching productivity. They concluded that this finding reflects the apparent hierarchy of these two role components in academic nursing.[2] Although this conclusion seems to indicate that nurse faculty may continue to value teaching more than scholarly activity, findings from two empirical studies suggest this value system may be slowly changing. Nieswiadomy[39] found in 1984 that although faculty with 20 or more years of experience reported the largest number of past studies in comparison to younger faculty, they also reported fewer current research studies. Kruger and Washburn[27] also found that all of the nursing program administrators included in their study believed research was a critical factor in tenure and promotion decisions, with teaching performance ranking second (98%).

Hayter[26] also reported that when findings from her 1979 and 1984 studies were compared, some very encouraging trends emerged. She found that nurses were increasingly assuming responsibility for writing articles in their own journals, more nurse authors had doctoral degrees, and in most institutions offering doctoral programs in nursing, scholarly productivity was high.

Most recently Megel, Langston, and Creswell[31] examined the factors associated with the scholarly productivity of 96 leading nurse researchers who held doctorates and were tenured at NLN-accredited schools of nursing. The profile of the productive nurse-faculty researcher that emerged in this study showed these individuals had published slightly fewer than one research article per year for the previous three years. They had a mean career total of 20.9 research articles, journal articles other than research, books or monographs, and chapters in books. Although it is difficult to compare the findings of publication productivity studies because of the different methodologies used, the findings of Megel and colleagues appear to compare quite favorably with those of Creswell and Bean,[14] reported in 1981. The latter found faculty holding appointments at institutions classified in the Carnegie typology as "research universities I and II" and "doctoral-granting institutions I and II" reporting a mean lifetime number of publications of between 5.67 and 8.23. It should be noted, however, that the faculty surveyed to obtain the data for the Creswell and Bean study were not defined as "leading researchers," while those in the Megel, Langston, and Creswell study were.

Scant as the evidence is, our position is that the academic, educational, and attitudinal profile of nurse faculty is changing and is beginning to conform to the usual standards of academia. It is believed doctoral preparation, research, and scholarly activity must continue to receive a primary emphasis in promotion and tenure decisions for nurse faculty. Novice faculty members must be continuously and systematically socialized to the value of scholarship. However, as Ostmoe[40] has noted, academic nursing has been and is still disadvantaged by its late entry into higher education. Just as nursing is beginning to value scholarship, we are witnessing a renewed emphasis on the importance of undergraduate education, academic advising, and public service. In a report published in 1985 by the Association of American Colleges,[3] convincing evidence is presented that the devaluation of the undergraduate degree is the cause of the educational crisis of the 1980s. This report indicates an exaggerated emphasis on research may be at the root of this problem:

Central to the troubles and to the solution are the professors, for the development that overwhelmed the old curriculum and changed the entire nature of higher education was the transformation of the professors from teachers concerned with the characters and minds of their students to professionals, scholars with PhD degrees with an allegiance to academic disciplines stronger than their commitment to teaching or to the life of the institutions where they are employed.

The study group on the conditions of excellence in American higher education,[51] which issued its report in 1984, also emphasized the need for more faculty effort and expertise in delivery of undergraduate instruction. Its recommendations include:

1. Deans and department chairs should assign as many as possible of their finest instructors to classes attracting large numbers of first-year students.
2. Learning technologies should be designed to increase, not reduce, the amount of personal contact between students and faculty on intellectual issues.

These themes are reiterated in other recent reports, such as *Higher Education and the American Resurgence* (1985),[38] *To Secure the Blessings of Liberty* (1986),[45] and *Transforming the State Role in Undergraduate Education* (1986).[46]

The roles and expectations for nurse faculty holding appointments in institutions of higher education are further complicated in the 1980s by declining undergraduate student enrollments and an increasing emphasis on faculty practice. The nursing literature of the late 1980s abounds with articles discussing the nursing shortage, declining undergraduate enrollments in baccalaureate nursing programs, and the establishment of nursing centers. The need for faculty clinical competence and for faculty practice to maintain that competence are recurring themes in the current literature. At the same time, nursing deans are faced with appointing new doctorally prepared nurse faculty who are well socialized to the research and scholarship values of doctoral education. However, many of the new appointees no longer want to spend a significant amount of their time teaching undergraduate students or participating in clinical instruction, serving on school and university committees, engaging in practice, or participating in continuing education programs or other forms of public service.

The purpose of this chapter, therefore, is to briefly discuss the issues related to the relationship—or lack thereof—among scholarly activity, teaching, practice, and public service. It is argued that promotion and tenure reviews of faculty performance in all areas should be conducted within a scholarship framework. The rest of this chapter, therefore, addresses the need for evaluation of scholarly teaching, scholarly practice, and scholarly service.

SCHOLARSHIP AND TEACHING

It is often argued that teaching and scholarship, although not mutually exclusive, are somewhat incompatible because of limits on time. Nieswiadomy[39] found that nurse educators identified lack of time as one of the primary reasons they were not involved in research.[40] Ostmoe also found that time spent in teaching was one of the variables accounting for the variance in publication productivity of nurse faculty. Conversely, a study by Faia[19] using data from 53,034 college and university faculty members showed that even in institutions where research is not strongly emphasized, teaching awards are more likely to go to professors who publish than to those who do not. These data seem to refute the notion that one cannot be both a scholar and an effective teacher.

Nurse faculty are often socialized to the 8-hours-a-day, 40-hours-a-week, every-other-weekend work pattern associated with nursing service. In the past, many nurse faculty were attracted to academia because of the perceived benefits of the academic calendar, including frequent vacation breaks and free weekends and summers. Zanecchia,[53] however, reports that university nurse faculty currently spend approximately 56

hours per week attempting to meet role expectations. If this estimate is accurate, nurse faculty should have sufficient time to be both productive researchers and effective teachers.

Most universities, including research universities, insist that faculty must first and foremost be excellent teachers. Too often, however, because of the difficulties associated with evaluating teacher effectiveness, promotion and tenure decisions are made primarily on the basis of research productivity. As was noted in *Involvement in Learning*, "the true frontiers of knowledge in any academic field are usually explored by but a handful of researchers."[51] The report's authors argue for a broader definition of scholarship and assert that it is "more critical that professors replicate the forms and processes of research to improve the learning experience of students."

How should the teacher operating in a framework of scholarship be expected to teach? It has been suggested that faculty make greater use of active modes of teaching and require that students take greater responsibility for their learning. The teacher with a scholarship orientation is likely to use some of the following teaching strategies[52]:

- Involve students in faculty research projects
- Encourage internships and other forms of carefully monitored experiential learning
- Organize small discussion groups, especially in large classes
- Require in-class presentations and debates
- Develop simulations
- Create opportunities for individual learning projects

Effective teacher-scholars are concerned with improving students' skills in writing and speaking, extending abilities in critical thinking and analysis, and developing capacities to synthesize, imagine and create.[51] Bevis[7] recently postulated that only syntax, context, inquiry, and innovative learning are truly educative. Teacher-scholars in professional nursing programs must be much more than deliverers of knowledge and facts. The effective scholarship-oriented nurse faculty member should demonstrate competence in designing a syllabus reflective of the most current research findings in the discipline. Such faculty should develop examinations and questioning approaches that require students to apply higher-level cognitive abilities, as opposed to merely recalling facts and principles. Lectures, which are continually updated, should have a conceptual focus and should facilitate students' grasp of the essential processes and understandings associated with the discipline of nursing.

Evaluation of these critical skills and attributes of the teacher-scholar cannot be obtained through easily quantifiable and random assessment methods. Reliance on computer-scored student evaluations of teachers, coupled with infrequent peer observation of faculty teaching performance, is inadequate to assess nurse faculty teaching effectiveness. A discussion of the evaluation of teaching effectiveness is beyond the scope of this chapter, but many excellent sources are available, such as Centra's *Determining Faculty Effectiveness.*[11] It should be emphasized, however, that with the growing number of faculty prepared at the doctoral level, declining student enrollments, and tight budgets, tenure decisions no longer involve separating the competent from the incompetent. Rather, these decisions involve fine distinctions among generally competent faculty.[11]

The current emphasis in doctoral programs in nursing and related fields is almost exclusively on the development of substantive knowledge and research skills. The Association of American Colleges' report[3] on the integrity of the college curriculum states, "During the long years of work toward the doctoral degree, the candidate is rarely, if ever, introduced to any of the ingredients that make up the art, the science and the special responsibility of teaching." The nurse teacher-scholar must therefore be nurtured. Peer review committees must find mechanisms to provide formative evaluation to new teacher-scholars in a nonthreatening environment. If such a process is used, the value of utilizing a scholarly approach to teaching will be inculcated in the novice teacher. Such a process should result not only in more effective teaching in undergraduate and graduate nursing programs, but also in an increase in scholarship in its purest sense.

Academic nurse administrators need to consider the indirect message concerning the value of teaching that is communicated when faculty development policies use language that "releases" or "frees" faculty for research and scholarly pursuits. Similarly, undergraduate teaching often appears to be undervalued when doctorally prepared faculty are assigned to teach exclusively in master's and doctoral nursing programs. Deans and department chairs also have a responsibility to ensure that faculty teaching assignments, including clinical assignments, are compatible with faculty members' areas of expertise and research interest. This compatibility and a reemphasis on the value of teaching are essential to ensure the development of the nursing teacher-scholars who will be needed in the twenty-first century.

SCHOLARSHIP AND PRACTICE

In 1987 Lynton and Elman[28] suggested that universities need to be as involved in the dissemination and application of knowledge as they are in its generation, and that universities, in their teaching and professional activities, need to "relate theory to practice, basic research to its applications, and the acquisition of knowledge to its use." Although the authors were promoting the concept of the extended university, faculty practice follows logically from this charge to interpret, disseminate, and apply knowledge.

Faculty practice has been given much attention over the past few years. In 1979 the American Academy of Nursing endorsed the idea of faculty practice as a means of improving the relationship between service and education.[47] Subsequently several nursing leaders developed a "Statement of Belief Regarding Faculty Practice," which endorsed the concept of faculty practice and encouraged the design of models to promote integration of practice into research and teaching.[50]

A review of faculty practice literature reveals many models and strategies for implementation. Frequently mentioned modes of practice are joint appointment, dual appointment, collaboration, unification, affiliation, and private practice.[24] *Translating Commitment to Reality,* the published proceedings of the Third Annual Nursing Faculty Practice Symposium, contains descriptions of a variety of faculty practice models.[20] Nurse-managed centers are becoming a popular phenomenon for combining nursing practice, education, research, and service. In 1986 Barger[5] reported 51 schools operating nursing centers. Davis[15] provides a summary of some of these centers.

Though the concept of faculty practice is valued within the profession, may issues related to implementation have yet to be resolved. Definitions of faculty practice vary; administrative support is more verbal than actual; workloads are heavy, allowing little time for practice; and tenure and promotion guidelines place little weight on faculty practice.*

Faculty practice has been defined in a variety of ways, ranging from any contact of faculty with patients

---

*References 1, 2, 6, 16, 17, 29, 34, 48.

during clinical supervision of students to more formalized contractual arrangements between agencies. However, the definition and criteria espoused by Ford[22] at the First Symposium on Nursing Faculty Practice seem most relevant for this discussion: "Faculty practice refers to those functions performed by faculty within a service setting that have as their principal goal the continued advancement of the nursing care of patients/clients, a goal congruent with the role of an academician in a professional discipline." To be considered faculty practice, activities of faculty members related to the care of patients must be scholarly in orientation with associated scholarship outcomes and must have as their central focus the care of the patients or clients. Included in this definition are the direct or indirect care of clients, involvement in staff development, quality assurance, consultation, clinical advancement, and committee participation. Excluded from this definition are clinical teaching, which has the student as its focus, and routine client care, which is not scholarly in nature.[22] It is a debatable issue whether or not "moonlighting," that is, working for pay evenings, weekends, or vacations outside the academic contractual time frame, is considered faculty practice.

Faculty practice, as with other faculty activities, should flow from the institution's mission and philosophy. However, the literature on faculty practice indicates this is not always so. Anderson and Pierson reported in 1983 that only 37% of the schools included in their study had a written philosophy related to faculty practice. Furthermore, they found "no significant relationship between the amount of hours spent in faculty practice and the existence of a philosophy that incorporated faculty practice."[1] However, they identified administrative support as the greatest facilitator of faculty practice; this finding was significantly higher for the group practicing within a unification model than for the group practicing outside such a model. In 1986 Barger[5] did not find a significant correlation between the existence of a nursing center and administrative policies supportive of faculty practice. Barger and Bridges,[6] in a later study, also found administrative policies to have no significant effect on the extent of faculty practice. Institutional factors that had a significant positive effect on practice were the presence of a doctoral program and the public status of the institution.

Work load was the greatest inhibitor of faculty practice for all faculty respondents in Anderson and Pier-

son's study.[1] The majority of the 212 faculty members indicated that the school did not provide time for faculty practice; 48% of the faculty were moonlighting. This finding was consistent with that of Dickens,[17] who found that the majority of full-time faculty practiced during weekends, summers, or recesses during the academic year. In 1985 Redmen, Cassells, and Jackson[44] found that only 32% of the deans surveyed indicated faculty were provided time during the week for clinical practice. The presence of a nursing center does not seem to make a difference in the hours faculty members can devote to practice, as compared with other types of practice settings.[6]

Teaching, research, and service are the components traditionally recognized in tenure and promotion decisions, and they are usually weighted in the order listed. Most often faculty practice is considered a type of service or an aspect of teaching effectiveness.[1] In general, faculty practice is not perceived as important for tenure and promotion considerations.[42,53,54] The relatively low priority of practice in tenure and promotion considerations has created a dilemma for nursing schools, because they need clinical experts in their teaching ranks. To accommodate the expert clinician some schools have created two tracks, the typical academic tenure track and a clinical, nontenure track.[18,43] Some nursing leaders are concerned that the latter relegates the practitioner faculty member to second-class status.[49] Some schools, such as Rush, do not have tenure for the nursing faculty.[13] This is not a viable option for most schools in a university setting.

Faculty practice should enhance clinical research possibilities. Clinical settings are ripe for generating clinical questions; the faculty have access to clients and the expertise to design and carry out research. Although research on faculty practice is very limited and faculty practice models are relatively new, study results indicate that there does not seem to be a significant relationship between faculty practice and traditional measures of scholarly activity such as research and publication. The faculty respondents in Anderson and Pierson's study[1] were involved in neither research nor professional writing. Furthermore, they ranked enrichment of teaching skills, maintenance of clinical skills, and personal satisfaction as the main reasons for their practice. Research and curriculum aspects were considered least relevant. Chickadonz[12] expressed concern over this finding in 1987, stating, "If impact on curricula and clinical nursing research were not important reasons for faculty practice, one could question seriously the value of the effort expended by both administrators and faculty to achieve faculty practice."

Barger and Bridges's 1987 study[6] of the productivity of practicing versus nonpracticing faculty showed that 44.6% of the 1036 faculty respondents were practicing; 51% of those practicing were engaged in research, while 56% of nonpracticing faculty reported research involvement. The latter finding might be related to the fact that 22.4% of the practicing faculty held doctorates, compared with 38.9% of the nonpracticing faculty. However, there was no relationship between research or publication activity over the previous three years and faculty practice. There was a significant inverse relationship between the earned doctorate and extent of faculty practice. This may have been because faculty members with doctorates were directing their energies toward research and publishing for tenure purposes. Of those practicing, 28% were tenured, compared with 39.6% of the nonpracticing respondents. There was no relationship between the number of contact hours with students and the extent of faculty practice.[6] It is important to note that the definition of faculty practice in the above study included moonlighting. Miller's 1988 research[33] confirmed the lack of relationship between scholarly outcomes of research and publications and faculty practice. If faculty practice does not result in greater scholarly productivity, some might question the necessity of incorporating it into tenure and promotion criteria.

How faculty practice can be incorporated into reappointment, tenure, and promotion guidelines has not been clearly delineated. Many academic institutions do not recognize clinical practice as important in tenure decisions; others require practice without the accompanying rewards.[1,30,53] If faculties decide to include faculty practice within their tenure and promotion guidelines, the question of how to evaluate faculty practice must be resolved. Anderson and Pierson[1] found only 26% of the faculty respondents reported criteria for evaluating the practice component of their teaching positions. Those who did not report criteria suggested a strong need for them. One of the comments on the evaluation process was that it was unfair to judge by the quantity (number of hours) of practice rather than the quality of practice. Nurse faculty also objected to being evaluated by head nurses who were less educated than they.[1]

Scholarly practice could be evaluated in a manner similar to that used by clinical nurse specialists and described by Hamric[25]; that is, according to structure, process, and outcome. Structurally, the number of clients seen and the number and type of research grants received might be included. Scholarly practice as a process might be evaluated by clients, peers, supervisors, or through self-evaluation. This would give an indication of the quality of the practice. A variety of tools are available for consideration and modification in references such as Hamric. Outcomes of scholarly practice would include publications, research reports, or presentations. Outcome measures of the effectiveness of patient care might also be used. Client records also may be useful in documenting client outcomes.

SCHOLARSHIP AND SERVICE

Service is consistently viewed as the least important component of the faculty role by nursing and nonnursing faculty and administrators.[8,21,28,53] Yet those in academia know how vitally important the service role is to the functioning of the institution, to the profession, and to the acceptance of the institution by the community. Studies of the value of service in tenure decisions indicate that quality of service is a significant predictor of tenure achievement, although not as significant as quality of teaching or research,[32] and that those with the highest rates of published research show a statistically greater preference for institutional service than faculty who are less productive.[31] The challenge is to determine what service activities are reportable for tenure and promotion and to evaluate the scholarliness of those service activities. Generally, service includes that given to the community, profession, and institution.

Community service tends to generate the most discussion and disagreement. In 1982 Blai[8] found that the majority of faculty in community colleges and universities who responded to his survey regarding the importance of pay-promotion criteria rated community service as not important for a pay-incentive plan. Zanecchia's 1985 study[53] showed campus service to be the least important of 14 faculty work load activities for tenure and promotion decisions.

To be considered for tenure and promotion, community service activities should be consistent with the mission of the university, related to the curriculum, and requested or needed by the community; they should also be related to the faculty member's professional expertise. The activity should advance the profession of nursing or higher education.[35] Disagreements exist within nursing as well as in the broader university community about specific reportable activities. Using the definition of professional activity as "the application of high-level expertise in an attempt to relate the results of basic research to their utilization," Lyton and Alman[28] have suggested these reportable professional service activities:

1. Directed or contracted research
2. Consultation, technical assistance, policy analysis, technology assessment, and program evaluation
3. Targeted briefing and other didactic activities
4. Informational and explanatory activities for a general audience.[28]

Natapoff and Pennington[35] criticized the finding of Baird and colleagues[4] that nursing faculties report as scholarly activities such as giving a speech to a national group or speaking to a regional or local group. Natapoff and Pennington believe these activities to be service-related and suggest that most other disciplines would as well. They advise nursing faculty to revise their thinking about scholarly activities.[35] Using the framework suggested by the authors, these activities might indeed be considered scholarly service activities. Other professional service activities might include serving as an officer of a professional organization or on local, state, or national committees or task forces. Service on review panels for research activities or publications, presentations to professional groups, inservice education activities, and faculty consulting are other examples of service activities.

Service to the department, school, and university is the responsibility of all faculty members. Yet studies such as Zanecchia's indicate that faculty see such service as low on the list of activities that should be considered in tenure and promotion decisions.[54] This may be because it is difficult to evaluate, not because it is unimportant. The challenge, then, is to be able to evaluate the scholarly nature of committee work and other service activities. If such service is weighted very little in tenure and promotion considerations, some faculty may limit their service activities to allow time for teaching and research.

Teaching continuing-education courses for registered nurses is frequently considered under the service component. Baird and others[4] reported in 1985 that contributing to continuing education was one of the top 10 scholarly activities identified by faculty in NLN-accredited baccalaureate and graduate nursing programs. Zanecchia[53] presented similar findings. In both studies it was considered less important as scholarly work for tenure decisions than were teaching, research, and publishing.

In some schools faculty are reluctant to commit themselves to continuing education, because it is given little recognition by tenure and promotion committees. They prefer to spend their time on activities traditionally recognized as meeting the scholarly activity criteria. Lyton and Alman[28] call for a resurgence and recognition of the scholarly transfer and application of knowledge through extension or outreach programming. They urge that "significant changes in the current system of priorities, values, and incentives are needed if the new categories of scholarly work of the faculty are to be adequately documented, evaluated, and rewarded."

As with practice, whether or not remunerated involvement in continuing education should be considered for tenure and promotion has become an issue. Some believe that if education or practice is scholarly, it should be remunerated and recognized in tenure and promotion decisions. The scholarly nature of the activity should be judged separately from the issue of financial reimbursement.[28] Others believe the activity is not within the faculty role if additional funds are received for it.[35] One might question the message conveyed when offering continuing education programs is viewed as "overload" rather than as incorporated into the faculty member's work load.

It is possible to evaluate scholarship in service activities. The structure, process, and outcome approach again can be utilized. Using self-evaluation as well as those of peers, committee colleagues, and supervisors, the quality and quantity of service activities can be evaluated. Research efforts can arise from service activities, as can publications. To be evaluated, professional service activities must be documented. Documentation should include the purpose of the activity, what was done, for whom, how the outcome was measured, and evaluation of the outcome by clients or contracting persons. Tenure and promotion committees then must determine the value of such activities. Factors to be considered when weighing the merit of activities are (1) the complexity or difficulty of the problem addressed by the work; (2) the use of state-of-the-art knowledge, methodologies, and databases; (3) originality of the work; (4) comprehensive analysis of the problem and possible solutions; and (5) the objectivity of the work.[28]

SUMMARY

It has been suggested that the components of the faculty role should be viewed not as mutually exclusive activities but as interactive processes, with participation in one benefiting the other.[23] The challenge to tenure and promotion committees within nursing schools is to evaluate the scholarliness of teaching, practice, and service. The academic nursing community can benefit from the experiences of our colleagues in disciplines with a long association with higher education. And overemphasis on the importance of research and scholarship should be avoided. The publication-dominated reward system should be seriously reevaluated. "We must create new reward structures which truly reflect and encourage the multiple purposes of higher education and the varied skills and efforts of the faculty."[28]

REFERENCES

1. Anderson ER and Pierson P: An exploratory study of faculty practice: views of those faculty engaged in practice who teach in an NLN-accredited baccalaureate program. West J Nurs Research 5(2):129, 1983.
2. Andreoli KG and Musser LA: Faculty productivity. In Werley HH, Fitzpatrick JJ, and Taunton RL, editors: Annual review of nursing research, vol 4, New York, 1986, Springer Publishing Co.
3. Association of American Colleges: Integrity in the college curriculum: a report to the academic community, Washington, DC, 1985, The Association.
4. Baird SC and others: Defining scholarly activity in nursing education, J Nurs Educ 24(4):143, 1985.
5. Barger SE: Personnel issues in academic nurse managed centers: the pitfalls and the potential, Nurse Educator 11(3):29, 1986.
6. Barger SE and Bridges WC: Nursing faculty practice: institutional and individual facilitators and inhibitors, J Prof Nurs 3(6):338, 1987.
7. Bevis EM and Clayton G: Needed: a new curriculum development design, Nurse Educator 13(4):14, 1988.
8. Blai B: Faculty-ranked importance in the 1970s of pay-promotion criteria, Rep No HE 015-567, Washington, DC, 1982, US Department of Education.
9. Brandon AN and Hill DR: Selected list of nursing books and journals, Nurs Outlook 36(2):92, 1988.
10. Brandon AN and Hill DR: Selected list of nursing books and journals, Nurs Outlook 30(3):186, 1982.
11. Centra JA: Determining faculty effectiveness, San Francisco, 1981, Jossey-Bass, Inc, Publishers.
12. Chickadonz GH: Faculty practice. In Fitzpatrick JJ and Taunton RL, editors: Annual review of nursing research, vol 5, New York, 1987, Springer Publishing Co.
13. Christman LP: Response to institutionalizing practice: historical and future perspectives. In Barnard KE and Smith GR, editors: Faculty practice in action, Kansas City, Mo, 1985, American Academy of Nursing.
14. Creswell JW and Bean JP: Research output, socialization and the Biglan model, Research in Higher Education 15(1):69, 1981.
15. Davis GC: Practice, education and research. In Zanecchia MD, editor: Career guide for nurse educators, Norwalk, Conn, 1988, Appleton & Lange.
16. DeTornyay R: Toward faculty practice, J Nurs Educ 26(4):137, 1987.
17. Dickens MR: Faculty practice and social support, Nursing Leadership 6(4):121, 1983.
18. Fagin CM: Institutionalizing practice: historical and future perspectives. In Barnard KE and Smith GR, editors: Faculty practice in action, Kansas City, Mo, 1985, American Academy of Nursing.
19. Faia MA: Teaching and research: rapport or mesalliance? Research in Higher Education 4(3):235, 1976.
20. Feetham S and Malasanos LJ, editors: Translating commitment to reality, Kansas City, Mo, 1986, American Academy of Nursing.
21. Florestano PS and Hambrick R: Rewarding faculty members for profession related public service, Educational Record 65(1):18, 1984.
22. Ford LC: Organizational perspectives on faculty practice: issues and challenges. In Barnard KE, editor: Structure to outcome: making it work, Kansas City, Mo, 1983, American Academy of Nursing.
23. Gaul AL: Teaching and service. In Zanecchia MD, editor: Career guide for nurse educators, Norwalk, Conn, 1988, Appleton & Lange.
24. Grace HK: Unification, reunification, reconciliation or collaboration: bridging the education/service gap. In McCloskey JC and Grace HK, editors: Current issues in nursing, ed 1, Boston, 1981, Blackwell Scientific Publications, Inc.
25. Hamric AB and Spross J, editors: The clinical nurse specialist in theory and practice, Orlando, Fla, 1983, Grune & Stratton, Inc.
26. Hayter J: Institutional sources of articles published in 13 nursing journals, 1978-1982, Nurs Res 33(6):357, 1984.
27. Kruger S and Washburn J: Tenure and promotion: an update on university nursing faculty, J Nurs Educ 26(5):182, 1987.
28. Lynton EA and Elman SE: New priorities for the university, San Francisco, 1987, Jossey-Bass, Inc, Publishers.
29. Mauksch IG: Faculty practice: a professional imperative, Nurse Educator 5(3):21, 1980.
30. McClure ML: Faculty practice: new definitions, new opportunities. Nurs Outlook 35(4):162, 1987.
31. Megel ME, Langston NF, and Creswell JW: Scholarly productivity: a survey of nursing faculty researchers, J Prof Nurs 4(1):45, 1988.
32. Messmer PR: Factors affecting the granting of academic tenure in schools of nursing, doctoral dissertation, Cincinnati, 1988, University of Cincinnati.
33. Miller V: Relationships between nursing faculty practice and faculty productivity, doctoral dissertation in preparation, Morgantown, West Virginia University.
34. Munroe DJ and others: Establishing an environment for faculty practice: a primary affiliation, J Nurs Educ 26(7):297, 1987.
35. Natapoff JN and Pennington EA: Faculty roles in higher education: teaching, service, and scholarship. In Pennington EA, editor: Understanding the academic role: a handbook for new faculty, New York, 1986, National League for Nursing.
36. National League for Nursing Council of Baccalaureate and

Higher Degree Programs: Criteria for the evaluation of baccalaureate and higher degree programs in nursing, New York, 1983, NLN.

37. National League for Nursing Division of Research: Nursing data review, 1987, New York, 1988, NLN.

38. Newman F: Higher education and the American resurgence, Princeton, NJ, 1985, Carnegie Foundation for the Advancement of Teaching.

39. Nieswiadomy RM: Nurse educators' involvement in research, J Nurs Educ 23(2):23, 1984.

40. Ostmoe PM: Correlates of university nurse faculty publication productivity, J Nurs Educ 25(5):207, 1986.

41. Ostmoe PM: Issues related to promotion and tenure. In McCloskey JC and Grace HK, editors: Current issues in nursing, ed 2, Boston, 1985, Blackwell Scientific Publications, Inc.

42. Parascenzo LK: Nursing faculty clinical practice: myth or reality?, doctoral dissertation, Pittsburgh, 1983, University of Pittsburgh.

43. Petersdorf RG: A report on the establishment, J Med Educ 62(2):126, 1987.

44. Redman BK, Cassells JM, and Jackson SS: Generic baccalaureate nursing programs: a survey of enrollment, administrative structure/funding, faculty teaching/practice roles, and selected curriculum trends, J Prof Nurs 1(6):369, 1985.

45. Report of the National Commission on the Role and Future of State Colleges and Universities: To secure the blessings of liberty, Washington, DC, 1986, American Association of State Colleges and Universities.

46. Report of the Working Party on Effective State Action to Improve Undergraduate Education: Transforming the state role on undergraduate education: time for a different view, Denver, 1986, Education Commission of the States.

47. Resolution on unification of nursing service and nursing education: American Academy of Nursing Newsletter 1:4, Winter 1980.

48. Rosswurm MA: Characteristics of 23 faculty group nurse practices, Nursing and Health Care 2(6):327, 1981.

49. Smith DM: Response: faculty practice from a 25-year perspective. In Barnard KE and Smith GR, editors: Faculty practice in action, Kansas City, Mo, 1985, American Academy of Nursing.

50. Statement of belief regarding faculty practice, Nurse Educator 4(3):5, 1979.

51. Study group on the conditions of excellence in American higher education: Involvement in learning: realizing the potential of American higher education. Washington, DC, 1984, National Institute of Education.

52. Van Ort SR and Putt AM: Teaching in collegiate schools of nursing, Boston, 1985, Little, Brown & Co, Inc.

53. Zanecchia MD: Productivity and workloads. In Zanecchia MD, editor: Career guide for nurse educators, Norwalk, Conn, 1988, Appleton & Lange.

54. Zanecchia MD: Roles and responsibilities. In Zanecchia MD, editor: Career guide for nurse educators, Norwalk, Conn, 1988, Appleton & Lange.

CHAPTER 46

International nursing

The role of the International Council of Nurses and the World Health Organization

VIRGINIA M. OHLSON

The International Council of Nurses (ICN) and the World Health Organization (WHO) play significant roles in nursing and health care worldwide and in promoting the global goal of "Health for All" by the year 2000. Yet in view of questions frequently raised by nursing students and practicing nurses, it seems that some nurses know relatively little about either of these international organizations: "I would like to attend an ICN congress; how can I become a member of the ICN?" or, "I am interested in working with the WHO some day; how do I apply for membership?"

Usually the inquirer is surprised to learn that direct membership in either of these organization is not open to them as individuals. Members of the ICN are national nursing associations; when an individual nurse holds membership in a national nursing association belonging to the ICN, that individual is qualified to participate in many of its activities and programs. Similarly, members of the WHO are countries. Although certain WHO activities are at the government level, opportunities exist for individual health professionals to participate in working assignments in various parts of the world and to utilize many programs and resources of the organization.

This chapter provides a brief description of the ICN and the WHO and their unique roles in international health as they relate to nursing. Being neither a staff worker nor a current member of a committee or board of either organization, I write not from a position of authority but rather as an interested American nurse who, over a period of years, has had the opportunity to participate in numerous activities and programs of the ICN and the WHO. My account is not comprehensive; rather, it is an attempt to share my understanding and perceptions of the efforts of these two international organizations to affect the health care of people in countries around the world.

It is not difficult to discuss the role of the ICN in international health from a nursing perspective, because it is a federation of nursing associations managed by nurses and financed primarily by nurses. The WHO, in contrast, is an organization of many health disciplines; nevertheless, nursing always has had an active role within the WHO and its influence has been felt in numerous ways in all areas of the world.

INTERNATIONAL COUNCIL OF NURSES

The ICN was founded in 1899 as an independent, nongovernmental federation of national nursing associations. It is the oldest international professional organization in the health care field, and the only body representative of the nursing profession worldwide.[15]

Organization and administration

The national nursing associations of 100 countries comprise the 1989 membership of the ICN. In addition, the organization is in contact with nursing bodies or groups of nurses in many countries. Only one national nursing association per country can belong to the ICN. However, as nursing and the conditions under which nurses practice have continued to change, consideration is being given to possible adjustments in the organizational structure that might more appropriately accommodate the ICN's growing relationships with other organizations.

The governing body of the ICN is its Council of National Representatives (CNR), composed of two delegates from each of the member associations. Each member association has one vote in the conduct of

ICN business, regardless of the membership size. Currently the largest national nursing association belonging to the ICN is the United Kingdom's Royal College of Nursing, followed by the nursing associations of the United States, Japan, and Canada. The CNR meets every two years. In the interim periods, program decisions are made by a board of directors elected by the CNR that meets annually or as frequently as necessary. Membership on the board includes a president, three vice-presidents, seven area representatives, and four members at large. Area representatives are elected from the seven ICN areas—Africa, Europe, North America, South and Central America, southeast Asia, the eastern Mediterranean, and the western Pacific. The ICN has only one standing committee, the Professional Services Committee, a very active group vested with responsibility to consider problems and trends in nursing education and practice and to make recommendations to the board for further exploration by the CNR. Ad hoc committees are appointed as needed to deal with matters pertinent to the concerns of the ICN.

The ICN, headquartered in Geneva, Switzerland, employs an international corps of five nurse consultants and other nonnurse professional and support staff. Constance Holleran of the United States has served as the organization's executive director since appointment by the board of directors in 1981.

Purpose and objectives

The purpose of the ICN is the same today as it was at the time of founding: "to provide a medium through which the interests, needs and concerns of member national nurses' associations can be addressed to the advantage of the public and nurses."[3] The ICN's program is based on four objectives[15]:

1. To promote the development of strong nursing associations
2. To assist national nursing associations to improve the standards of nursing and the competence of nurses
3. To assist national nurses associations to improve the status of nurses
4. To serve as the authoritative voice for nurses and nursing internationally

Objective one: the national associations

Promotion of the development of strong national nursing associations is a prime objective of the ICN. All ICN programs and activities are planned by the member associations, their elected representatives (the CNR), and the highly qualified staff persons at headquarters, all of whom have been appointed or approved by ICN's Board of Directors. Collectively, the member associations and their representatives set goals for nursing education, practice, and research and authorize the staff to use resources to assist member associations, singly and collectively, in ways that will enhance or strengthen their development. Staff consultation is provided on request to member associations by telephone, correspondence, or in person as well as through assistance with the implementation of projects pertinent to ICN goals. Manuals, guidelines, and other resource materials are made available to member associations. All aspects of the ICN's programs and activities are directly or indirectly related to the attainment of the organization's prime objective—the development of strong national nursing associations.

Objective two: education and practice

Since 1978 a prime program emphasis of the ICN has reflected the organization's commitment to primary health care and the global goal of health for all by the year 2000—the goal adopted by 134 nations at the WHO/UNICEF conference convened in 1978 at Alma-Ata (USSR). In collaboration with its member associations, the ICN has endeavored to influence and prepare nurses and nursing services to participate more effectively in a primary health care system. Recognizing that nursing has the potential to influence decision making for health at all levels of government, as well as in the society at large, the ICN has committed staff and resources to the sponsoring of numerous workshops on primary health care in all of the seven ICN regions. Workshops have been directed to the national nursing associations' potential for leadership in their countries, with the purpose of strengthening nursing's role in achieving the goal of health for all. Great emphasis has been placed in all workshops on the continuing-education needs of nurses working in primary health care in rural areas. Various government-related agencies have assisted the ICN with the funding of these workshops, including the United Nations International Emergency Children's Fund (UNICEF), the Canadian International Development Agency (CIDA), the Norwegian Development Agency (NORAD), and the Pan American Health Organization (PAHO).

Throughout its lifetime the ICN has maintained an interest in the regulation of nursing education and practice worldwide. High priority has been given to encouraging and assisting nursing associations in their efforts to establish and update nursing standards. Periodically the ICN has conducted studies and seminars related to nursing regulations and standards and published reports on these efforts.[1,5-7,10,14] In recognition of the need for an official statement of position regarding regulatory mechanisms affecting standards for nursing education and practice, an ICN study was conducted under the direction of Styles[11] in 1983 and 1984.

The purpose of the study was twofold: (1) to collect, organize and report data on how nursing currently is regulated worldwide, and (2) to derive guidelines that might be helpful to the ICN in the development of an official position for assisting member associations in the evaluation and development of a regulatory system for nursing.

"Overall findings of the study revealed that the structure of the profession is ill-defined and diverse; educational requirements and legal definitions of nursing are generally inadequate for the complexity and expansion of the nursing role as it is emerging in response to health care needs; and the goals and standards of the profession worldwide are less apparent than one-half century ago, although they may be well crystalized in some countries; the conclusion is inescapable that the welfare of the public, the profession and the practitioner will be better served if greater relevance, rationality, consistency and clarity are brought to bear on the regulatory system.[11]

In response to these findings, the CNR in 1987 adopted an official statement of position on regulation of nursing, guided by twelve "Principles of Professional Regulations" and "Associated Principles and Policy Objectives for Nursing."[11] An opportunity to test the processes set down in these regulatory guidelines has been provided by two nongovernmental philanthropic organizations, the Carnegie Corporation of New York and the Kellogg Foundation of Battle Creek, Michigan. Funding from these two organizations will enable the ICN to work with national nursing associations and ministries of health in selected countries in Africa and South and Central America in beginning efforts to develop and improve nursing regulatory systems in education and practice. No doubt the ICN's "Report on the Regulation of Nursing" will have a high priority on the ICN agenda in coming years as the organization seeks to assist member countries to improve standards for nursing and nurse competence.

Objective three: social and economic welfare of nurses

The ICN gives high priority to assisting national nursing associations in matters relating to the socioeconomic welfare (SEW) of nurses. Major stress is placed on the importance of providing assistance and resources to those associations that are able to initiate and implement SEW programs in their countries. However, since collective bargaining techniques are not applicable for use in some parts of the world, the ICN also must consider a variety of other approaches for improving the socioeconomic status of nurses.

The SEW program of the ICN has four major objectives: (1) to identify information and data about socioeconomic welfare; (2) to provide information, educational programs and consultation on SEW to national nursing associations; (3) to work and communicate with other international organizations in regard to the social and economic welfare of nurses—particularly the International Labor Organization (ILO) and the WHO; and (4) to examine and determine how the present socioeconomic situation affects health services and the lives and working conditions of nurses.[13] Pertinent information about SEW is shared with member associations through a regularly published newsletter, the *Socio-Economic News*. The association's dedication to the socioeconomic status of nurses has had a tremendous influence on the improvement of working conditions of nurses worldwide.

Objective four: a unified voice for nursing

The ICN, composed of 100 member associations representing 1 million nurses, has the unique potential, opportunity, and responsibility to serve as the authoritative voice for nursing and nurses internationally. The extent to which it honors and accepts this responsibility has been demonstrated and documented on many occasions and in various ways. On frequent occasions at the WHO's World Health Assembly, which convenes annually in Geneva, Switzerland, the ICN has presented position statements on issues relevant to health care as well as to nursing. Examples are the ICN's recent statements on infant feeding, nursing in primary health care, and the role of nursing in the WHO. Although the ICN is a nursing organization and the WHO is an interdisciplinary health organization, the high degree of camaraderie and collaboration that exists between these two organizations and their nursing staffs has contributed immeasurably to a unified voice for nursing in the international arena.

The ICN has maintained an active publishing program, issuing books, manuals, monographs, reports, and guidelines relative to nursing education, practice, and research. Its official organ is the *International Nursing Review*, a bimonthly journal published in Switzerland.

The ICN has published (in English, French, and Spanish) numerous statements reflecting the organization's stance on issues related to nursing, health care, and societal matters of concern to the profession. A recent listing of these position statements in the *International Nursing Review* reflects the ICN's broad range of concerns.

Primary emphasis has been placed on the ways in which the ICN carries out its work in relation to its four primary objectives. It is important to recognize the extent to which its staff must interact with numerous other international organizations and agencies—including such organizations as the WHO, the UNICEF, the International Labor Organization, and other governmental and nongovernmental philanthropic agencies—in order to achieve these objectives.

Recognition also should be given to the ICN's work with the International Committee of the Red Cross (ICRC), the International Commission of Health Professionals for Health and Human Rights, and other organizations, in efforts to trace nurses who have disappeared or have been imprisoned because of their work activities.

Blueprint for future action

In view of the ICN's many programs and nursing's pressing needs, the CNR set down a 5-year plan of action (1988 to 1991). Nine priority areas were identified[12]:

- Continue efforts to strengthen the effectiveness of national nurses' associations (NNAs)
- Support the work of NNAs to improve employment conditions for nurses in all settings and to promote the social and economic welfare of all nursing personnel
- Strengthen the ICN and NNAs in ways oriented to promote participation in effective relationships with interdisciplinary, interprofessional, and international government agencies, for the purposes of improving the health of the public
- Review changes and adjustments in the organizational components and relationships of the ICN
- Encourage NNAs to be more active in setting and enforcing standards for nursing education and nursing practice, leadership, and management in their countries
- Assist NNAs and others in bringing about more appropriate regulatory mechanisms for nursing practice, thus making it possible for the knowledge and skills of nurses to be more effectively utilized and recognized within the health system
- Orient NNAs to promote and assist as feasible with health personnel planning and development for nursing in all its areas of practice
- Ensure that the ICN Code for Nurses continues to provide the ethical guidance required by nurses in a rapidly changing world with constant social, technological, genetic and pharmacological advances
- Work with NNAs to encourage and facilitate the development of research in nursing and by nurses and the dissemination of research findings

THE WORLD HEALTH ORGANIZATION

The WHO was established in 1948 as a specialized agency of the United Nations in Geneva, Switzerland, where it is still headquartered. It came into existence as the world was attempting to recover from World War II and as millions were falling victim to poverty and disease.

It was in these troubled times that the constitution of the WHO was formulated. The preamble of that historic document gives evidence of the concern for social justice on which the organization was founded and has firmly stood for more than 40 years. Its succinct statement of beliefs is widely known: "The enjoyment of the highest attainable standard of health is one of the fundamental rights of every human being without distinction of race, religion, political belief, economic or social condition." Article 1 of the WHO constitution states the organization's objective: "The attainment by all people of the highest possible level of health."

Organization and administration

The WHO is an intergovernmental agency. In 1948, there were 56 member countries; by 1988 membership had increased to 166. The highest policy-making body of the WHO is the World Health Assembly (WHA), which is responsible for the execution of WHO policies in collaboration with its employed staff, referred to as the WHO Secretariat. The highest officer in the WHO is the director-general, elected by the WHA on nomination by the executive board. Currently this position is held by Hiroshi Nakajima of Japan. Numerous administrative and technical personnel with diversified knowledge and skills are employed at WHO headquarters in Geneva.

The WHO's program is decentralized into six regional offices: AFRO, the African regional office, in Brazzaville, Congo; PAHO/AMRO, the Pan American Health Organization, which serves as the regional office for the Americas, in Washington, D.C.; EMRO, the eastern Mediterranean regional office, in Alexandria, Egypt; EURO, the European regional office, in Copenhagen, Denmark; SEARO, the Southeast Asian regional office, in New Delhi, India; and WPRO, the western Pacific regional office, in Manila, Philippines.

The WHO's activities are financed by annual contributions from its member countries, and by voluntary contributions from government and private agencies.

Functions of the WHO

The WHO constitution specifies 22 functions, summarized as follows[3]:

1. Coordination of international health work undertaken by national and international groups, both governmental and voluntary, or by scientific and professional groups
2. Assisting governments in strengthening health services through technical assistance, through direct aid as requested, or though providing counseling or personnel support in the development of programs
3. Fostering action in specific fields of particular need such as maternal and child health and welfare, mental health, disease eradication, nutrition, and improvement of water supplies
4. Developing or promoting international agreements and standards including policies and regulations; standards of teaching and training in health, medical, and related fields; standardization of the international nomenclature of diseases and of diagnostic procedures and standards
5. Conducting, encouraging, and supporting studies and research in the field of health, including studies of administration and social techniques for health care.

Although the constitution of the WHO was written over 40 years ago, its 22 statements of functions have not changed. However, the programs necessary for their implementation have changed considerably with increased understanding of the world's health problems. Similarly, the administrative structure of the WHO and the size and nature of the secretariat also have changed as new policies have been formulated by the WHA and new priorities established.

Health for all by the year 2000

Fulop and Roemer[4] describe the ways in which WHO policies and programs have been influenced over time by the variety of social forces operating within the organization and its member countries. Certainly, the changing nature of the WHO membership has influenced program directions. In 1948, 57% of WHO member states were developed countries and 43% were developing countries. By 1978 many new countries had become sovereign states and joined the WHO, considerably changing the nature of its membership. Currently over 75% of the members represent the developing countries. Interestingly, it was not until 1977 that growing concern over the health conditions in many countries resulted in establishing the year 2000 as the target date for reaching the WHO's long-standing objective, "the attainment of the highest possible level of health for all people."[4]

In the following year an international conference on primary health care was convened by the WHO and UNICEF in Alma-Ata, bringing representatives of 134 governments and 67 United Nations organizations and other specialty agencies and nongovernmental organizations. It was at this conference that the now-renowned Declaration of Alma-Ata was formulated, recognizing primary health care as the key to attaining health for all by 2000. The conference declared that the health status of hundreds of millions of people was unacceptable and could only be rectified by a new, equitable approach to health and health care that would close the gap between the world's haves and have-nots. In 1979 the Thirty-Second World Health Assembly endorsed the Declaration of Alma-Ata.[18] In 1981 the WHA established the Global Strategy for Health for All by the Year 2000,[19] and countries were encouraged to formulate their own national policies, strategies, and plans of action for attaining this goal. Since that time the pursuit of health for all has become the central focus for WHO policies and program strategies.

Recognition must be given to Halfdan Mahler, director-general of the WHO for 15 years, who gave leadership to the primary health care approach to the health for all goal from its beginnings in 1977 until his retirement from the WHO in July 1988.

Nursing in the WHO

Where does nursing fit in this complex intergovernmental, interdisciplinary health organization? What is nursing's role in the WHO in this decade, and what will it be by the year 2000? Some understanding of the structure of nursing within the WHO could assist in answering these questions.

Structure for nursing in the WHO

The highest administrative post for nursing in the headquarters of the WHO is the position designated as "chief scientist for nursing." As the chief administrator for nursing in the WHO, the nursing chief reports to the director-general through the assistant director-general, as do other administrative position chiefs. Simultaneously, the nursing chief also holds a position in the Division of Health Manpower and in this role reports to the director of that division. A few other nurses are employed at the WHO headquarters, assigned not to nursing but to other divisions representing specific program areas such as employee health services, immunizations, and maternal and child health.

The chief scientist for nursing is the primary voice for nursing in the organization and in this capacity must interpret the potential, contributions, and needs of nursing within an interdisciplinary context. In carrying out the responsibilities of the office, the chief scientist for nursing maintains contact with numerous international agencies and organizations concerned directly or indirectly with nursing, as well as with nursing personnel in the six WHO regional offices. The administrator reviews program plans and projects of the regions, provides technical assistance as feasible, and participates in conferences and workshops at the request of the regional offices. Possibly the greatest responsibility of the nursing administrator in this interdisciplinary organization is that of communicating, interpreting, stimulating, and planning nursing's contributions to the various areas of the WHO's programs.

Each of the WHO regional offices has its own nursing and other health-related personnel whose responsibilities and programs of work are designed and implemented within the regional areas. The relationship between the WHO headquarters and the regional offices is advisory rather than administrative, since the WHO operates on a decentralized basis that permits autonomy within broad policy guidelines. As a result, nursing may be organized quite differently in each region. The WHO's primary commitment at all levels is to its member countries and to the strengthening of those countries' institutions. Although problems in nursing in the various countries are to some extent quite similar, they differ significantly in degree in various areas of the world. The WHO nurses in the regions deal with a wide range of programs and problems related to nursing practice, education, training, organization, administration, and research. Duties have encompassed such activities as the analyses of nursing needs in a country or area, the design of projects to meet a particular need, the recruitment or assistance with recruitment of personnel for various projects of the organization or a member country, and the evaluation of project outcomes.

Nature of nursing in the WHO

Nursing has had an important role in the WHO from the time of the organization's founding. The programs of nursing have been carried out through (1) long- and short-term projects in many parts of the world with goals and objectives that have varied according to place and time; (2) workshops, conferences, and committees that have enabled the development and dissemination of reports, recommendations, and guidelines; and (3) a wide variety of administrative functions and activities.

Projects have been developed for implementation at the local, regional, and interregional levels. Although some projects have related specifically to nursing, many have been interdisciplinary. In the early years of the WHO, nurses were involved in projects as members of specialized teams concerned with treatment and control of diseases such as malaria, venereal diseases, and tuberculosis, and also with maternal and child health programs. In later years a higher priority was placed on programs of nursing and midwifery education.[19] Although consideration is still given to such projects, prime emphasis in recent years has been on projects particularly relevant to the achievement of the goal of health for all by 2000 through primary health care.

The WHO maintains a system of expert panels, representative of the various disciplines, which function as advisory bodies to the organization. The expert panel in nursing includes representatives of the various specialty areas in nursing and of the geographic regions. The panel does not meet as a group, but from time to time representatives from the panel meet to deliberate and make recommendations on a matter of concern to nursing and the WHO. An example is the actions reflected in the report of the expert committee of 1984, "The Education and Training of Nurse Teachers and Managers with special regard to Primary Health Care."[20] Each time an expert committee on nursing is convened, a report summarizing its deliberations and recommendations is published and made available to governments, professional organizations, educational institutions, and other interested agencies and individuals.

Throughout the years a wide variety of guides, reports, and materials relevant to nursing practice, education, administration, and research have been prepared and disseminated by the WHO headquarters and the regional offices. Numerous statements have been developed and published as summaries and recommendations of conferences or workshops convened to deliberate on some specific aspects of nursing.[16,21-24] Frequently these publications represent the work of an individual or group commissioned by the WHO to conduct a specific study. Many of these publications are available through the headquarters and regional offices; in some of the regional areas bibliographies of studies are available.

As a discipline within the WHO, nursing supports and affirms the programs of the organization and the attainment of its goals. Health care planning and implementation uses the team approach, and within this context nursing must carve out its directions, its functions, and its role.

WHO collaborating centers for nursing development

For many years the WHO has designated a number of health-professional colleges or departments in universities and other health-related agencies and institutions as WHO Collaborating Centers. This designation has been given in recognition of the institution's or agency's potential to participate in the furtherance of WHO goals and objectives. The first nursing centers to be so designated were in Europe. Two of these centers were named in 1980: the Collaborating Center for Nursing Research and Education, located at the Danish Institute for Health and Nursing Research in Copenhagen, and the Collaborating Center for Nurs-

ing associated with the Hospices Civils De Leon, in Lyon, France. The most recent European center to be designated was the Collaborating Center for Primary Health Care Nursing established in 1986 at the Health Center in Maribor, Yugoslavia. For the four years prior to its official designation, the center at Maribor was a participating center connected with the Collaborating Center in Lyon. Subsequently, other institutions in various parts of the world have been designated as WHO Collaborating Centers for Nursing Development—the School of Nursing of Cumberland College of Health Sciences, Lidcombe, Australia; the Rajkumari Amrit Kaur College of Nursing in New Delhi, India; the Nursing Colleges Division of the Ministry of Public Health in Bangkok, Thailand; and the College of Nursing of Yonsei University, Seoul, Korea. Three of the subsequently designated WHO Collaborating Centers for Nursing Development are located in the United States: the College of Nursing of the University of Illinois at Chicago (1986); the School of Nursing of the University of Pennsylvania, Philadelphia (1988); and the School of Nursing of the University of Texas Medical Branch at Galveston (1988). In addition to these 10 centers, 3 other university schools of nursing are in the process of designation: the Universidade de São Paula Escola de Enfermagem de Ribeirao Preto, São Paulo, Brazil; the Universidad Nacional de Colombia, Bogota, Colombia; and the University of Manchester in the United Kingdom.

In April 1988 the first general annual meeting of the Global Network of the WHO Collaborating Centers for Nursing Development was convened in Maribor, Yugoslavia. Representatives of the designated and potential collaborating centers were in attendance. It was a historic meeting. The work of the network is facilitated by the WHO, although the network itself is not a component part of the WHO. The College of Nursing of the University of Illinois at Chicago currently functions as the secretariat for the network. Being newly organized, the network can best be described in terms of its future promise rather than its history of past accomplishments. The premises underlying the organization are that networking can be a most effective instrument of technical cooperation and that network members will support one another through information sharing, exchange of materials and expertise, and the mobilization of resources. It is expected that member centers will participate in identifying common goals of high priority, and will plan collaborative action toward their realization. Achievement of these goals should strengthen the capacity of each center to move forward with its particular primary health care mission.[2] Special recognition should be given to Amelia Maglacas, who served as WHO's chief nurse scientist from 1976 to 1989, for her untiring efforts to bring nursing institutions the world over into the WHO network of Collaborating Centers.

In these few pages I have attempted to describe the role of the ICN and the WHO in relation to nursing internationally. Much more could be said of the many ways in which the nurse leaders of these two organizations work collaboratively in their office headquarters in Geneva and in the many regions and countries of the world. Nurses in these two organizations are few in number, yet their accomplishments on behalf of nurses and for nursing and health care are far-reaching and impressive. In their crucial positions the WHO and ICN nurses are influencing directions for nursing and patterns of health care delivery all over the world. Individually and collectively, we too have a role in the global endeavor.

REFERENCES

1. Bridges D: A history of the International Council of Nurses, 1899-1964, Philadelphia, 1965, Lippincott.
2. Duxbury M: The global network of World Health Organization collaborating centers for nursing development, unpublished, 1988.
3. Freeman R: Nursing in the World Health Organization, Geneva, 1965, WHO.
4. Fulop T and Romer M: International development of health manpower policy, Geneva, 1982, WHO.
5. International Council of Nurses: Nursing legislation: report on survey of nursing legislation, London, 1960, ICN.
6. International Council of Nurses: Principles of legislation for nursing education and practice: a guide to assist national nursing associations, New York, 1969, S Karger.
7. International Council of Nurses: Report on an international seminar on nursing legislation, Warsaw, Poland, 1970, Geneva, 1971, ICN.
8. International Council of Nurses: Report of the Professional Services Committee, Geneva, 1973, ICN.
9. International Council of Nurses: ICN adopts definition of nursing, Int Nurs Rev 22(6):184, 1975.
10. International Council of Nurses: Nursing legislation in Latin America the last half of the 20th century, Geneva, 1975, ICN.
11. International Council of Nurses: Report on the regulation of nursing: report on the present, a position for the future, Geneva, 1986, ICN.
12. International Council of Nurses: Nursing's priorities set at New Zealand, Int Nurs Rev 34(6):276, 1987.
13. International Council of Nurses: Report of the Social Economic Welfare Committee, Council of Nurse Representatives, Auckland, Geneva, 1987, ICN.
14. Mussalem H: Succeeding together: group action by nurses, Geneva, 1983, ICN.
15. Quinn S: What about me? caring for the carers, Geneva, 1981, ICN.
16. Storey M and others: Guidelines for regulatory changes in nursing education and practice to promote primary health care, Geneva, 1988, WHO.
17. World Health Organization: Constitution of the World Health Organization, Geneva, 1948, WHO.
18. World Health Organization: Alma-Ata, 1978: primary health care, Geneva, 1978, WHO.
19. World Health Organization: Global strategies for health for all by the year 2000, Geneva, 1981, WHO.
20. World Health Organization: Education and training of nurse teachers and managers with special regard to primary health care, Tech Rep 708, Geneva, 1984, WHO.
21. World Health Organization: Division of Health Manpower Development: Nursing in support of the goal of health for all by the year 2000, Geneva, 1982, WHO.
22. World Health Organization, Regional Office for Europe: Postbasic and Graduate Education for Nurses, Copenhagen, Denmark, 1988, WHO.
23. World Health Organization and University of North Carolina: Health manpower for primary health care: the experience of the nurse practitioner, University of North Carolina, Chapel Hill, NC, 1987.
24. World Health Organization and Pan American Health Organization: Meeting on planning for change in nursing development, Washington, DC, 1987, PAHO.

PART SEVEN

GOVERNMENT INTERVENTION

Influence on nursing

JOANNE COMI McCLOSKEY
HELEN KENNEDY GRACE

One crucial factor in determining whether nurses gain greater independence is willingness of the government to reimburse for nursing services and thus to recognize the contributions of nurses to the provision of health services. To gain such recognition, nurses first need to be aware of the issues affecting reimbursement.

In the opening chapter of Part 7, Langford provides a comprehensive overview of issues related to reimbursement for long-term care services. Noting the increase in cost of long-term care, she points to two difference approaches to controlling health care costs: (1) using competitive forces, and (2) relying on increased regulation. With this as a framework, and noting the projected increases in numbers of elderly and the anticipated increase in cost of care for elderly, she sees the lack of a coherent policy for the funding of long-term care as a major problem. Factors contributing to this lack of coherent policy are the scope of long-term care, the complexity of the funding sources, the difficulties in defining an appropriate case mix, the difficulties in measuring quality of care, and the scarcity of health professionals providing long-term care. Strategies for controlling costs of care are limiting payments to nursing homes, controlling the bed supply, and developing incentive systems for cost control and quality of care. Approaches to increasing the efficiency of the system identified include careful patient assessment, case management, payments by social/HMOs to families for care of elderly members, and financing of health care through home equity conversions. Risk pooling to provide reimbursement for health care services for the elderly is being addressed through insurance companies and life care communities. One

major gap in coverage of health care services for the elderly is under Medicare, which does not cover long-term care services. The current system of payment for long-term care continues to favor institutional care for the treatment of illness, giving limited attention to the nature of the comprehensive needs of the elderly for a range of services, including social and health services. With the projected increase in numbers of elderly, the impending bankruptcy of the Medicaid system in the 1990s, and the increased cost of care for the elderly, it is unlikely that a more coherent public policy for long-term care will develop in the immediate future.

In the first viewpoint chapter of Part 7, Davis discusses the impact Medicare and Medicaid legislation have had on health care delivery systems and nursing in the United States. Medicare payments nearly doubled between 1981 and 1985, and the program is now in danger of more reductions to protect its basic solvency. Davis predicts a reform of the program in the late 1990s that will likely require increased contributions from wealthier beneficiaries. Significant changes in the delivery of care have occurred since the change to prospective payment. Between 1980 and 1986 approximately, inpatient hospital days declined 27%, with a corresponding increase of 85% in home care agencies, a 39% increase in skilled nursing facilities, and a 516% growth in ambulatory surgical centers, which were virtually unknown before 1980. This is the era of managed care, says Davis, with a new emphasis on productivity.

More emphasis will be given to increasing quality and access and decreasing cost. It is now recognized that nurses play an enormous role in helping patients recuperate from illness, and Davis predicts that we will continue to see awareness of the importance of nursing in the 1990s. Nursing, however, must respond. Nursing departments must restructure to become more efficient and productive. Nurses must change their expectations about how and where health care services are provided.

One factor that is crucial in establishing nurses as recognized providers of health care services is the clarity of the scope of nursing practice presented to the public. Clarity about the contributions of nursing to the provision of health care services can best be achieved through a coherent body of knowledge validated through the research process. Establishment of the National Center for Nursing Research (NCNR) in 1986 constituted a major advance in providing a recognized structure for development of nursing knowledge. Hinshaw provides a succinct overview of the mission of the National Center for Nursing Research and the way in which this mission is being translated into programs directed toward building a body of knowledge for the practice of nursing and guiding the process by which this knowledge base is generated and tested. With a focus on three areas of research, (1) health promotion/disease prevention, (2) acute and chronic illness, and (3) nursing systems, NCNR is fostering depth of knowledge in areas that will make a major contribution to clarification of the scope and focus of nursing practice. The establishment of a national research agenda with an emphasis on career development for nursing researchers, support for programs of research development for individual researchers, and an encouragement of collaborative research both within nursing and with scientists from other fields will undoubtedly contribute substantially to increased visibility of nursing, a factor critical to achieving increased recognition.

Turning to the issues related to reimbursement, Streff and Netzer speak from the perspective of nurses who have been successful in achieving enactment of legislation providing third-party reimbursement for certified psychiatric clinical specialists in Massachusetts. One of the most important factors in achieving this goal was in addressing the issue of scope of practice of the nurses to receive reimbursement and issues related to accountability and responsibility to patients and third-party payers. Stressing the importance of patience, perseverance, and vigilance, the nonlegislative strategies of attending meetings of insurers to gain

an understanding of their perspectives and of joining with community action groups to gain consumer report are described. A clearly stated fact sheet describing scope of practice, cost analysis, and the projected impact of the bill, effective lobbying on the part of nursing groups, and the selection of key sponsors are factors contributing to the success of this effort. Noting that an initial attempt to achieve support for all services of nurses as advocated by the American Nurses' Association was a total failure, the authors instead address a strategy of gaining recognition of the contribution of particular specialty groups on an individual basis to clarify the scope of nursing practice to be reimbursed. Most easily understood is the nurse's role in assessment, diagnosis, and treatment. The role of nursing in teaching disease prevention and in working with individuals to promote self-help is most difficult to clarify to legislators.

Moving to an entirely different context, Ngcongco and Pfau describe the impact of government intervention on health services in Botswana. After achieving independence in 1966, the country of Botswana systematically developed national health policies to ensure the availability of health services to all of the population. With a commitment to rural development and social justice as a framework, a primary health care system has been developed.

The major thrust of government intervention has been to mobilize and manage local and international resources for health care; to create balance between services for rural and urban populations; to achieve collaboration among governmental health services, traditional healers, midwives, mission endeavors, and private sector providers; to develop particular programs directed toward high priority problems; and to emphasize community participation. With this system in place, the current emphasis is on manpower development, improvement of the planning structure, and enhancement of the physical infrastructure of community clinics and other health facilities.

Looking ahead, the authors note that future priorities need to include the strengthening of manpower management and that increased attention needs to be focused on the providers of health services. In contrast to the U.S. experience, in which so much of the decision-making about health care is in the hands of the providers, there is concern in Botswana about an overemphasis on community health needs and an underemphasis on the needs of providers.

Although the papers in this section are somewhat limited in scope, the critical influence of governmental policies on nursing and the importance of nurses being engaged in shaping public policy are vital issues to be addressed.

CHAPTER 47

Debate

Controlling health care expenditures
Strategies for cost containment in long-term care

ANITA M. LANGFORD

The control of health care expenditures is a problem that attracts an increasing amount of attention from legislators and policymakers, providers and users of the health care system, and, of course, from those who have to pay for health care. There are good reasons for this attention. In 1982 expenditures for health care accounted for more than 10.5% of the gross national product, an increase from 7.9% in 1972.[9] In 1982 total national expenditures for health care were $322 billion, and in that year 15% of the federal tax dollar went to health care, up from 1% in 1965.[9] The cost of medical care in the United States rose more than twice as fast as all other costs in 1982. Alternative solutions to the problem of cost containment have been proposed. Two basic approaches to controlling cost are (1) introducing competitive forces into the system, and (2) direct economic regulation.[28,31]

Strategies that seek to utilize competitive forces are:

1. Increasing consumer choices through education and development of alternatives
2. Increasing consumer cost sharing
3. Changing tax treatment of insurance and medical care
4. Controlling terms of insurance[21,31]

Historically, direct government regulation has been the solution when a program that affects a large number of people is on shaky economic grounds. These regulatory efforts to contain costs usually encompass three general areas:

1. Controls on reimbursement
2. Controls on the supply of facilities
3. Controls on utilization[31]

This chapter will describe the characteristics of long-term care and the long-term care industry, discuss the impact of demographic projections on long-term care, and describe existing and alternative strategies for cost containment in long-term care based on approaches utilizing competitive forces and direct economic regulation. Sources of financing of long-term care and the current lack of a cohesive, comprehensive national health policy that includes long-term care will also be discussed.

Long-term care is an integral part of the health care continuum. It is a unique part of the system, not always well defined, and subject to a great deal of regulation in terms of reimbursement and quality assessment. Kane and Kane define long-term care as "a range of services that addresses the health, personal care, and social needs of individuals who lack some capacity for self-care."[18] Although the population in need of long-term care includes persons of all ages, most long-term care is delivered to elderly people in a variety of settings.

The United States is spending more than 3% of its gross national product on health services for the elderly. In 1984 an estimated $120 billion was spent for personal health care for those over 65 years of age, a per capita expenditure of $4200. Two thirds of this was for institutional care, including $54 billion for hospital care and $25 billion for nursing home care.[32] Since the 1965 enactment of Medicare and Medicaid, the rate of spending for medical care has been rising more rapidly for persons 65 and older than for younger persons. This rapid rate is attributable to increases in the number of services provided and to increases in the costs of those services.[32]

In any discussion of cost containment in long-term care, it is important to understand some of the characteristics that set long-term care apart from other kinds of health care. The first such characteristic is the scope of long-term care and includes types of services and modalities of service. Types of services range from sophisticated nursing and medical services to more basic supportive and maintenance care, including functional, emotional, and social support. Preventive and rehabilitative services that focus on maintaining function and dealing with chronic illness are also included. Facilities for providing care include nursing homes, hospices, hospital swing beds, rehabilitation hospitals, chronic care centers, day-care programs, home health agencies, geriatric outpatient centers, foster care programs, and residential communities.[33] An expanded range of services can be found in additional settings, such as group homes, foster homes, congregate care homes, retirement communities, respite care, sheltered workshops, senior citizen centers, protective services, and monitoring services.[16] The many types of care and modalities makes integration and coordination of services an important factor to consider in designing cost-containment strategies.

The second unique characteristic of long-term care is its funding sources. Approximately 50% of nursing home expenditures are funded by Medicaid.[20] States vary in the methodology for Medicaid payment, some using case-mix systems, in which patient conditions or health problems are considered to have a major influence on nursing care requirements, staffing requirements, and costs; others using facility-specific rates for an individual facility, usually based on costs; and still others using class rates, a system in which facilities are classified into class or peer groups by such characteristics as size, location, ownership, occupancy rates, and other factors.[1,33,35]

A third characteristic of long-term care is the complexity of measuring case mix because of the diverse nature of medical care, functional and psychosocial needs, and the interaction of these in a single patient. Because case mix often drives resource consumption, it is essential in any discussion of cost containment.

Another characteristic of long-term care is the difficulty in measuring quality of care. The degenerative nature of many long-term care problems makes recovery impossible, so outcomes are difficult to measure. The long-term care setting is concerned with the total patient, the quality of life, and combinations of the medical, functional, and psychosocial needs of patients. In addition, patient needs change over time and require different levels of care, so outcomes are not so easily attributed to specific providers.[23]

The relative scarcity of physicians and licensed nurses as providers of care and the preponderance of other health care workers, such as aides, social workers, and therapists is another characteristic of long-term care. This makes a coordinated interdisciplinary team approach to care essential. These characteristics of long-term care make it a unique segment of the health care system and one that must be examined separately from the acute-care system in discussing cost containment.

Two major forces make clear the pressing need to examine the cost-effectiveness of current approaches in the delivery of long-term care. The first is the rapid growth in the elderly population, and the second is the inception of the prospective payment system by Medicare.

Longevity is increasing, numbers of the elderly are increasing, and the proportion of the elderly in the general population is increasing. In 1900 only 25% of the population in the United States survived the age of 65, but by 1985 approximately 70% survived.[3] This dramatic shift in mortality has been attributed to improvements in living conditions, sanitation, nutrition, and medical breakthroughs. In 1900 4.1% of the population was 65 years of age and older, in contrast to 11.6% of the total in 1982. By the year 2020 this age group is projected to double and account for 17.3% of the population. Most elderly persons live in a household with a spouse present; in 1981, 36% of the females and almost three quarters of the males lived with a spouse. In 1981 approximately 39% of the women lived alone compared to 14% of the men.[3]

The population segment that is growing most rapidly and will more than double between now and 2010 to 6.5 million persons is the group older than 85 years.[16] The central issue of increasing longevity is how many of the additional years will be fully functional years as opposed to years of compromised function; present data, though weak, suggest that for each functional year added to age 65 by increased longevity, about 3.5 years of compromised function are added.[3] Throughout human history, men and women did not age; they died. The current trend is new, and it raises many issues about health care, quality of life, and the need for a clearly formulated national health policy that integrates long-term care into a comprehensive approach to health.

The second force driving the need to examine the

cost-effectiveness of care is the advent of prospective payment for acute care under Medicare. The payment plan under the diagnosis-related group (DRG) system has and will continue to shorten length of stay, and patients will be discharged needing more intense care.[20] Efforts to contain cost by this method did not take into account the spillover effect that such incentives for early discharge would have on both resource requirements and length of stay in components of the system such as home health services and nursing homes.[11] The cost-effectiveness of such measures remains to be seen.

GROWTH AND SCOPE OF THE LONG-TERM CARE INDUSTRY

Long-term care is a multibillion-dollar service enterprise,[19] involving government agencies at the federal, state, and local levels as well as private for-profit and nonprofit organizations. It is financed through public and private sources. The absence of a national strategy for long-term care has caused inequities in financing and some gaps in access and equity in the long-term care delivery system. Most policymakers favor a mixture of privately and publicly funded models for delivery to respond to the enormous need for comprehensive long-term care for an increasingly older population.

The long-term care industry is composed of agencies providing a variety of services in institutions and in the community. The institutional settings include nursing homes, chronic care hospitals, rehabilitative hospitals, and state mental hospitals. The community settings include home health services, adult day care, foster care, and a large amount of uncompensated informal care.

Nursing homes are the most frequently utilized agencies and the most expensive kind of service provided. Nursing home care is one of the fastest growing sectors in the health care industry, with expenditures increasing from $2.1 billion in 1965 to $35.2 billion in 1985[16,20]; it is the third largest segment in the health care industry, following hospital and physician services.[16] The number of nursing home residents is expected to increase by 54% by the year 2000 and by 132% by 2030.[20]

Expenditures in 1980 for nursing homes accounted for 63% of all formal long-term care payments (other expenditures were for hospital days for patients awaiting nursing home placement and community-based care).[23] Payments to nursing homes represent the largest commitment of public funds to long-term care. For this reason, proposals to contain costs often focus on limiting the rate of expenditures in nursing homes.

Sources of reimbursement for nursing home costs are primarily from public funds, with Medicaid paying 51.3%, Medicare paying 2.2%, Veteran's Administration paying 1.8%, other public monies .1%, private insurance .6%, business .6%, and consumers themselves 43.4%.[23] Expenditures on nursing home services constitute approximately 44% of Medicaid outlays.[7] Occupancy rates in nursing homes since 1965 have been more than 92%.[23] A substantial number of residents enter nursing homes as private patients and then deplete their resources and convert to Medicaid.

Nursing homes treat a heterogeneous population with a range of services, for whom expected outcomes vary. There is evidence for three major groups of nursing home admissions, including (1) 40% to 50% of admissions who stay longer than 90 days and who stay an average length of approximately 2.5 years, (2) 30% to 40% of admissions who stay less than 90 days for rehabilitation and are discharged, and (3) 10% to 15% of patients who die within 90 days.[25] Shorter-stay patients are more likely to be married, to be bedridden, and to be diagnosed with hip fractures, whereas longer-stay patients are more likely to have a diagnosis of chronic brain syndrome, mental status impairment, and to be wheelchair bound.[23,25]

Other types of institutional care settings include the chronic care hospital, rehabilitative hospitals, and state mental hospitals. To establish new sources of revenue many acute-care hospitals are establishing "swing beds" to provide nursing home care in otherwise nonoccupied beds.

Though institutional long-term care programs consume most long-term care dollars, 71% of the long-term care population resides in the community and receives services there. In 1980 only 26.5% of all government long-term care spending was devoted to in-home services, adult day care, and foster care, the rest having gone to nursing homes.[16]

Another segment of long-term care involves services and care that are not compensated but are given to the aged by "traditional caregivers"—family, friends, and neighbors. The Health Care Finances Administration estimates that this care comprises 60% to 80% of all long-term care, and most of the caregivers are women, usually wives, daughters, or daughters-in-law.[16,29] If this source of care were reduced due to increased participation of women in the workforce and reduced family size, there might be a tremendous increase in expenditures for formal provision of care.

COST CONTAINMENT IN LONG-TERM CARE

Strategies for cost containment in long-term care can be targeted at (1) current policies to limit payment for nursing home care, (2) increasing efficiencies by creating alternatives to nursing home care, (3) increasing family responsibility, (4) shifting a greater portion of the financing of long-term care to the private sector, and (5) Medicare reform.

Limiting payment to nursing homes

Total expenditures on nursing homes are related to the number of people eligible for Medicaid, the admission rate, the days of service per admission, and the cost of care per day. Therefore states may control costs through eligibility policy, control of utilization, and policy on reimbursement.[23]

Eligibility policy controls cost by defining the numbers of people who may participate in a program through establishment of criteria that may be based on financial status, age, physical condition, and other factors. Costs may be lowered by reducing the numbers of persons eligible for Medicaid payment for nursing home occupancy.

Forms of utilization control are preadmission screening and certificate of need policies. Preadmission screening attempts to insure appropriate level of care placement according to a patient's need. In 1977 the Congressional Budget Office concluded that levels of care for 10% to 20% of skilled patients and 20% to 40% of intermediate patients were higher than needed.[6] More recent data suggest that nursing home patients are sicker since the advent of the prospective payment system of Medicare.[23] Preadmission screening programs include several components: client intake, determination of Medicaid eligibility, client assessment, and recommendation for placement. Although such programs are effective in assessing appropriate placement and, therefore, appropriate use of funds, they also add administrative costs to overall expenditures.

Certificate of need programs are based on the notion that there is a strong relationship between Medicaid spending on nursing home care per resident and the bed per population ratio. Therefore regulators in the Medicaid program believe that controlling the bed supply is necessary to control expenses. If more beds are opened, it is believed they will be filled with people who are eligible but who are currently cared for in the community.[23] The disadvantage of this approach is that it may hamper access to nursing home care to those who need it.

Reimbursement policy affects expenditures for Medicaid by direct payment for services and by influencing the willingness of nursing homes to take Medicaid patients. There are diverse payment systems across states providing different incentives for cost control and quality care. It is assumed that payment rates related to costs will enhance quality of care and access of medical assistance patients to nursing homes[38]; however, this system does not provide incentives for efficiency. On the other hand, flat rates will encourage nursing homes to improve efficiency or decrease quality of care. The medical assistance incentive system is moderated by proportion of private-pay patients in nursing homes. Because of the difference in rates paid by private patients and Medicaid, nursing homes may be selective in their admission practices and may be reluctant to take medical assistance patients who need a greater intensity of services, for example, patients with dementia of the Alzheimer's type.[23] To address this concern, several states have implemented reimbursement systems based on patient needs for care and services to reflect the intensity of resource utilization.[23] These provide an incentive for nursing homes to accept more patients with greater health care needs. The disadvantages are twofold: (1) the system adds administrative costs to implement, and (2) once admitted into the system, there is not an incentive to improve the patient's functional status because reimbursement rates would be lowered.

Increasing efficiencies in long-term care

Many types of services exist in the community to provide long-term care to people in their homes. Examples of such services are homemaker services, meals on wheels, and home health aides to provide personal care. Adult day-care centers and respite care programs permit care to be given out of the home but in the community. These services are provided by a variety of agencies and have varied eligibility criteria, which often causes confusion among the elderly when they attempt to negotiate their way through such an array of services.

The planning assumption includes the belief that

home and community-based services are substitutes for institutional long-term care and therefore are sources of cost savings. A number of demonstrations have tested this hypothesis by investigating several factors: the effect of more comprehensive service, comprehensive patient assessment, care planning, and case management.[23] The cost implications of these demonstrations were not favorable. The Government Accounting Office (GAO) noted that several factors make the cost-effectiveness of these methods difficult to assess, one of them being the difficulty in targeting people most at risk for institutional placement. If people at high risk cannot be accurately targeted for use of services as substitutes for nursing home placement, then new services based on assessment and need identification are likely to be added for populations that formerly received no formal services instead of substituting for nursing home services.[15,23]

Other studies have compared foster home, home care, and nursing home patients and found that the patients in the two community settings had made significantly greater improvement in activities of daily living (ADL) and mobility, expressed greater well-being, experienced similar kinds and amounts of morbidity, and cost Medicaid less than the nursing home patients. However, patients in the nursing homes were the most disabled, a fact that suggests that placement settings were not substitutable.[2]

More recently, the National Long-Term Care Demonstration was established to evaluate the consequences of expanding home and community services to older people at risk for institutionalization.[23] The National Channeling Demonstration is testing two models, both of which add case management to services covered by Medicaid. Case management includes client outreach and screening, service needs assessment, care planning, arranging for services, monitoring of care, and reassessment.[26] One of the two models also expands the range of covered services, reduces eligibility requirements, and creates a pool of funds for community services. In both models the average cost of providing services must be kept to 60% of average state rate for intermediate care facility (ICF) care.

In contrast to the past policy bias toward nursing home care, many states in recent years have been using waiver authority under Section 2176 of the Omnibus Budget Reconciliation Act of 1980 to develop home- and community-based alternatives. This authorizes the Department of Health and Human Services to waive existing statutory requirements to finance, through the Medicaid program, noninstitutional home- and community-based services and to direct these services to Medicaid-eligible persons who would otherwise be institutionalized.[7,23]

The assessment and case management function are the core of these new approaches to long-term care. The assessment function includes determination of level of care, determination of suitability for community care, and development of a plan of care. The case management function provides for the coordination and appropriate utilization of services. There is a great deal of variety in these waivered state programs that will add to knowledge of new and more efficient models of long-term care delivery.

One other alternative to traditional models is the social/health maintenance organization (HMO), a managed system of health and long-term care focusing on elderly populations. The social/HMO provides a full range of services, including acute inpatient, ambulatory, rehabilitative, nursing home, home health, and personal care services. It operates under a fixed budget and can be financed by premiums from Medicare, Medicaid, and the enrollees.[23]

There is still much debate on the issue of cost-effectiveness of increased home- and community-based services that centers around issues of targeting at-risk populations, increasing management efficiency, and intervention strategy development.[13] Much research is yet needed in this area.

Increasing family responsibility

In the strictest sense, policy initiatives that encourage family care are not completely private because they are related to government policy, but they do transfer some responsibilities for care to private individuals.

Despite the common belief and fear that the family is disintegrating and abandoning its elders, the data indicate that many long-term care services are being provided in the community by family and friends.[4,24] Data also indicate that 60% to 88% of all disabled and impaired people are helped by family in significant ways.[5] Two broad kinds of policies that encourage family responsibility are those that make it easier for families to keep their members at home and those that increase family financial liability.[23]

Policies that encourage care at home by family are those providing for (1) direct services at home, (2) payments to families, and (3) tax incentives. Provision of direct care services at home has been discussed in the section exploring home and community alternatives to nursing home care. Although such services, both in and out of the home, would alleviate the stress of the care giver, they may become as or more expensive than nursing home care. Targeting appropriate populations for such services to include only those people who would otherwise require nursing home care is an issue in this model. Factors that influence selection are medical, functional, and social disabilities and family values attached to keeping family members at home.

Making direct financial payments to families has raised a number of complex problems, for example, administrative implementation, deciding on what amounts to pay or what care is worth, and determining how much care is being given.[5] Tax incentives would allow care givers of disabled persons to take a tax credit or claim a tax deduction. The disadvantages of such tax incentive programs are several. The financial gain is too limited to make a difference in the family's decision to institutionalize when such decisions are usually based on deteriorating health rather than financial conditions.[23] Family care givers themselves indicate a preference for service and social supports rather than financial incentives. Additionally, many low-income people do not itemize taxes or even pay taxes and so would not utilize such a policy.

The second broad area of increasing family responsibility includes policies that increase family financial liability, that is, force immediate family members to pay for care of elders. Such policies would be expensive to administer and would be likely to cause social divisiveness in families. In addition, most families who would be affected have low incomes and/or children in college or are about to retire themselves.[23,24]

Another more promising source of funds is private savings. Two methods for promoting this are long-term care individual retirement accounts (IRAs) and home equity conversions.[17,24] There are, however, problems with both of these plans. IRAs would be a new tax expenditure and, as such, would be unlikely to find support among taxpayers today.[24]

The home equity conversion is essentially the reverse of a conventional mortage loan. A paid-for home is sold to a bank or financial institution in return for either a life-long annuity and the right to live in the house or a loan that would be repaid only after the owner moves or dies. In both cases the owner receives monthly checks, including principal and interest, from the bank. Three fourths of households headed by the elderly live in houses that are owned or occupied by the head of the household, and the average amount of equity in a house is $50,000.[17] It has been suggested that such a loan may be used to supplement low incomes, pay for home health care, or pay for premiums for private nursing home insurance. Some problems associated with this method are lack of public awareness of financial risks associated with serious chronic illness, state banking regulations that sometimes preclude reverse mortgage loans, and concerns that the aged may lose eligibility for public assistance if home equity (which is now exempted from countable assets) is converted.[17]

Risk pooling

Another method for financing long-term care is to pool the risk and finances for a large number of people. This is typically done in indemnity plans commonly used to pay for acute care and also done in the HMO model. Most people think of this type of pooling as being funded privately by contributions of participants, but in long-term care it may be funded by some federal and state dollars as well.

Many insurers are interested in developing long-term care indemnity plans.[36] More than 20 companies offer long-term care insurance. In the past insurers have been reluctant to market long-term care insurance for several reasons. One is a belief that young people find it too unpleasant to think of nursing home care; another is that there is much confusion among the elderly themselves about what Medicare covers.[10] The former reason focuses on the possibility that people with a greater than average risk of needing long-term care will buy policies but others will not, thus concentrating the risk. A related fear that average life expectancy with concomitant disability will continue to rise indefinitely. Because the underlying principle of insurance is to provide a broad base to delete risk, these new plans might have to be mandatory, such as compulsory coverage under a public program or mandated employer-based coverage of younger persons.

Other factors that create obstacles to effective long-term care insurance plans are the heterogeneity of the population needing long-term care with respect to medical needs and financial and family resources; organizational and administrative complexity in providing coordination of medical, nursing, and social services; excessive orientation to technological solutions rather than to continuity of care; and the fear of uninsurable risks.[34] In addition to these factors, there is uncertainty about public demand for long-term care insurance. For example, a much-publicized survey conducted for the American Association of Retired Persons in 1984 found that 79% of its members thought Medicare covered all nursing home expenses.[34] Other surveys have revealed much different results. The point, however, is that there is still a great deal of confusion about long-term care, which has been one possible reason for a limited demand for insurance. In 1987 Indiana passed legislation to relax Medicaid eligibility requirements for those who have private insurance for long-term care.

Life care communities, another form of risk pooling, have existed for a while, and they do provide full insurance for long-term care. Their typically high entry fees, however, make them available only to an upper-middle-class population.

The social/HMO is another model that is based on the principle of risk pooling. It attempts to extend the HMO acute-care financing and delivery model to include long-term care management. It may be financed by either private or public funds and has several essential features. First, a sponsoring agency takes responsibility for creating a system with a full range of services. Second, the enrollment must include able-bodied as well as disabled elders. Third, the system is paid on a "prepaid capitation basis" by both individual funds and third parties. Fourth, the system takes responsibility for meeting its own budget.[2,24] Its major strengths are its ability to pool financial risk in a system with built-in controls on utilization plus the consideration of cost-effectiveness as an important criterion for decision making. The social/HMO is able to insure a range of long-term services because it includes three key concepts: (1) integration of acute- and chronic-care systems, (2) provision of a system of managed care of clients, and (3) incentives for efficiency in providing services.[12]

Medicare

Any discussion of cost containment in health care for the elderly is incomplete without some mention of Medicare. The Medicare program was started in 1965 and has been effective in promoting the health of the elderly. It was designed to provide health insurance to most persons aged 65 and over and to disabled persons under 65 who meet certain criteria. Medicare is federally administered and financed for all persons eligible for Social Security without regard to income. Part A of Medicare is the Hospital Insurance program, which is financed with Social Security trust funds and covers inpatient hospitalization, limited skilled nursing care, and medically necessary home care. There are deductibles and copayments. Part B of Medicare, the Supplementary Medical Insurance program, covers physician services, outpatient therapy, medical equipment, and home health visits. This supplementary program is voluntary and is financed through federal revenues and premiums paid by enrollees.[27]

Medicare does not cover long-term care services, out-of-institution drugs, dental care, eyeglasses, hearing aids, and other services. In 1981 almost three quarters of Medicare expenditures were for hospital care, one quarter for physician services, less than 1% for nursing home care, and less than 1% for home health care. Because of Medicare's limited coverage of long-term care, Medicaid has become the primary payer for nursing home services.

In looking at the future of Medicare three major issues emerge: (1) problems in the current system relating to beneficiaries, (2) the system of paying providers, and (3) the financing of the Medicare system, especially in the light of future needs.

Beneficiaries are directly affected by a number of factors, the first of which is the cost-sharing arrangement for Medicare, which involves premiums and copayments. Over the past 20 years the proportion of copayments has increased, but the proportion of costs paid through premiums has decreased. The net effect is that the sick, and often the poor, pay much more than the healthy, an effect that is inconsistent with principles of insurance. These payments are also unpredictable and are usually paid by persons on a fixed income. Additionally, when premiums for Medicare increase, the low-income elderly are affected disproportionately.[27]

Another factor affecting beneficiaries is the lack of coverage for long-term care and chronic illness, for extended home health care, for mental health services, and for care in outpatient settings. Several concerns about providing more of these types of coverage are (1) that some nursing home costs represent room and board rather than medical care, and there is a belief that other funds should pay for room and board; (2) that nursing home coverage would be used excessively and inappropriately; and (3) that the increased coverage could result in more use of services and, therefore, greater expenditures.[27]

Beneficiaries are directly affected by the lack of incentives to seek early care, to participate in screening programs, and to utilize other preventive strategies. The deductibles allowed for physician care and for annual physical examinations may prevent beneficiaries from seeking early or preventive care. Beneficiaries must also deal with the administrative complexity of the Medicare system, which leaves many with an incorrect understanding of coverages and of how to use the system.

The second major issue that arises in a discussion of Medicare concerns providers, particularly physician providers. The fee-for-service method of charging at "customary, prevailing and reasonable" rates perpetuates high fees and utilization of high-technology services. Specialists receive different fees for the same services when rendered by primary care practitioners. Some reforms that may address these concerns are (1) "managed care" systems, (2) payment of physicians according to a relative-value scale adjusted by a dollar-value multiplier,[14] (3) establishment of an annual target budget for total physician expenditures, and (4) requirements that all physicians accept Medicare's fee as payment in full.[27,37]

The third major issue is how to finance the Medicare system. The funds for Medicare come from Social Security trust funds (payroll tax), federal general revenues, and premiums paid by enrollees. There is general agreement that Medicare benefits are not adequate to protect the elderly financially, but the outlays of this system are projected to increase 12% annually from 1987 to 1992.[8] Part A, hospital insurance, funded by payroll taxes, will start to spend more than the revenues it receives by 1995 and may be entirely depleted by 2002.[8,19] Among the options for keeping this fund solvent are (1) increasing the payroll tax, (2) reducing expenditures, (3) limiting benefits, or (4) finding additional revenue sources. Part B, the Supplementary Medical Insurance program, is more sound because of its flexible and adjustable funding sources, namely, general tax revenues (75%) and premiums (25%).[8]

The two ways in which Medicare expenditures and revenues can be brought into balance are clear but complex. These are, simply, to reduce expenditures and/or increase revenues. Methods for reducing expenditures include (1) reducing the number of people covered by increasing the age for eligibility, (2) eliminating some benefits, (3) increasing cost sharing with higher deductibles and premiums, (4) reducing utili-

zation of services, and (5) reducing provider payments. Revenue sources that may provide additional income include increases in payroll tax, other federal trust funds, general tax revenues, specific taxes such as on alcohol and cigarettes, and an increase in premiums.[8]

There are advantages and disadvantages to each of these alternatives. One proposal to insure the future solvency of Medicare focuses on the creation of a new Medicare trust fund. Such a fund would both merge current revenues for Parts A and B and add new revenue sources; the Part B premium would be replaced by a premium for the entire Medicare program that would fluctuate with beneficiary income.[8]

The major issue of whether to include comprehensive long-term care benefits in the package has drawn a number of suggestions for financing long-term care, such as an increase in the payroll tax, the payment of income-related premiums, raising the threshold for Social Security taxes to $75,000, and lowering the threshold for inheritance taxes.[8] The issue is complex and likely to be a major public policy issue in the future.

CONCLUSION

Cost containment in health care appears to be a worthy yet elusive goal. Evaluations of current policies and methods for controlling expenditures have produced a variety of results. Future innovations in health care policy need to recognize the dynamic interrelationships between the acute- and long-term care systems, Medicare, Medicaid, and private pay financing. Financing and delivery systems for health care that cut across these dimensions will be needed.

Because health care services are so varied, a number of strategies to contain costs are necessary. Strategies associated with both direct regulation and competition as forces to regulate the health care market need to be explored, with the recognition that funding will continue to come from both public and private sources.

Efforts toward establishment of a national policy on long-term care are essential. Such a policy should emphasize patient autonomy and responsibility, be available to all Americans, encourage support from the family, include a comprehensive continuum of coordinated care, include preventive care, involve a broad mixture of public and private enterprise, and have adequate and responsible financing through multiple sources.

REFERENCES

1. Birnbaum and others: Public pricing of nursing home care, Cambridge Mass, 1981, Abt Books.
2. Braun KL and Rose CL: Geriatric patient outcomes and costs in three settings: nursing home, foster family, and own home, J Am Geriatr Soc 35(5):387, 1987.
3. Brody JA, Brock DB, and Williams TF: Trends in the health of the elderly population, Annu Rev Public Health, 8:211, 1987.
4. Brody RM: "Women in the middle" and family help to older people, Gerontologist 21(5):471, 1981.
5. Callahan JJ and others: Responsibility of families for their severely disabled elders, Health Care Financing Review 1(3):29, Winter 1980.
6. Congressional Budget Office: Long-term care for the elderly and disabled, Washington, DC, 1977, US Government Printing Office.
7. Curtis R: The role of state governments in assuring access to care, Inquiry 23:277, Fall 1986.
8. Davis K: Medicare financing and beneficiary income, Inquiry 24:309, 1987.
9. Estes CL and Lee PR: Social, political, and economic background of long term care policy. In Harrington C, Newcomer RS, and Estes CL, editors: Long term care of the elderly—public policy issues, Calif, 1985, Sage Publications.
10. Firshein J: Long-term care insurers confront difficult dilemma, Hospitals April 20, 1986, p. 89.
11. Gamroth SL: Long-term care resource requirements before and after the prospective payment system, Image 20(1):7, 1988.
12. Greenberg JN and others: The social/health maintenance organization and long term care, Generations IX(4):51, Summer 1985.
13. Greene VL: Nursing home admission risk and the cost-effectiveness of community-based long-term care: a framework for analysis, Health Serv Res 22(5):655, 1987.
14. Hadley J: How should Medicare pay physicians? Milbank Mem Fund Q 62:279, 1984.
15. Hughes SL and others: Impact of long-term home care on hospital and nursing home use and cost, Health Serv Res 22(1):20, 1987.
16. Isaacs JC and Tames S: Long-term care: in search of a national policy, New York, 1986, National Health Council, Inc.
17. Jacobs B and Weissert W: Using home equity to finance long-term care, J Health Polit Policy Law 12(1):77, 1987.
18. Kane RA and Kane RL: Long-term care: a field in search of values. In Kane RA and Kane RL, editors: Values and long-term care, Lexington, Mass, 1982, Heath.
19. Klees B and Warfield C: Actuarial status of the HI ahd SMI trust funds, Social Security Bulletin 50:11, 1987.
20. Kramer AM, Shaughnessy PW, and Pettigrew ML: Cost-effectiveness implications based on a comparison of nursing home and home health case mix, Health Serv Res 20(4):387, 1985.
21. Langwell K and Moore S: What is competition? Hyattsville, Md, 1982, US Department of Health and Human Services.
22. Larson E and Carniglia-Lowensen J: State case mix systems for reimbursing long-term care for the elderly, Nurs Economics 5(2):77, 1987.
23. Lave JR: Cost containment policies in long-term care, Inquiry 22:7, Spring 1985.
24. Leutz W: Long-term care for the elderly: public dreams and private realities, Inquiry 23:134, 1986.
25. Liu K and Manton KG: The characteristics and utilization pattern of an admission cohort of nursing home patients (11), Gerontologist 24(1):70, 1984.
26. Mathematic Policy Research: The planning and implementation of channeling: early experiences of the national long-term care demonstration, Princeton, NJ, 1983, MPR.
27. Muse DN and Sawyer D: The Medicare and Medicaid data book, 1981, Washignton, DC, 1982, US Health Care Financing Administration.
28. Newcomer RJ and Bogaert-Tullis MP: Medicaid cost containment trials and innovations. In Harrington C, Newcomer RJ, and Estes CL, editors: Long term care of the elderly—public policy issues, Beverly Hills, Calif, 1985, Sage Publications.
29. Paringer L: Forgotten costs of informal long term care, Generations 9(4):55, Summer 1985.
30. Paringer L: Medicaid policy changes in long term care: a framework for impact assessment. In Harrington C, Newcomer RJ, and Estes CL, editors: Long term care of the elderly—public policy issues, Beverly Hills, Calif, 1985, Sage Publications.
31. Reitz JA and Horn SD: Controlling health care expenditures: strategies for cost containment. In McCloskey JC and Grace HK, editors: Current issues in nursing, ed 2, Boston, 1985, Blackwell Scientific Publications, Inc.
32. Rice DP: Introduction—long-term care, Generations 9(4):5, Summer 1985.
33. Shaughnessy PW: Long-term care research and public policy, Health Serv Res 20(4):489, 1985.
34. Somers A: Insurance for long-term care: some definitions, problems, and guidelines for action, N Engl J Med 17(1):23, 1983.
35. Swan JH and Harrington C: Institutional long term care services. In Harington C, Newcomer RJ, and Estes CL, editors: Long term care of the elderly—public policy issues, Beverly Hills, Calif, 1985, Sage Publications.
36. Tresnowski BR: Long-term care insurance: the private sector leads the way, Inquiry 22:215, Fall 1985.
37. Vladeck BC: Reforming Medicare provider payment, J Health Polit Policy Law 10(3):513, 1985.
38. Vladeck B: Unloving care, New York, 1980, Basic Books.

CHAPTER 48

Viewpoints

Financing of health care and its impact on nursing

CAROLYNE KAHLE DAVIS

With the advent of Medicare and Medicaid in 1965, the federal government embarked on a significant subsidy of health care. Today 31 million Americans are enrolled in Medicare, a program for the eldery, disabled, and those with end-stage renal disease, and 21 million indigent qualify for Medicaid. It is easy to see why a significant proportion of health care services are now paid for by these programs. The initial thrust of the program during the 1970s was concern for access to care, but this focus has changed to one of concern for escalating costs. By the 1980s it was apparent that structural changes in both payment and delivery of services needed to occur. To understand the impact of fiscal policy on the delivery system and on nursing, we must first have a basic understanding of Medicare and Medicaid.

Medicare, as envisioned in its original legislation in 1965, was to assist people over the age of 65 to pay for their acute-care illnesses. Additional coverage was provided later that recognized the unique needs of disabled individuals as well as people with end-stage renal disease. For more than 2 decades the decisions about which services would be covered reflected almost totally payment for care received in hospitals as well as payments to physicians. During the early 1980s it was recognized that many ambulatory-type services not previously provided by Medicare should be covered so that there would be attractive alternatives to expensive inpatient hospitalization. For example, ambulatory surgery was approved in 1981, and now almost 40% of a hospital's surgical interventions are done in same-day surgery facilities that cater to am-

bulatory care procedures. As more elderly citizens receive care for their acute health needs, their lifespans have been lengthened until now the average life expectancy is 75 years. Indeed, we now have 3.3 million Americans over the age of 85 and 45,000 over the age of 100.[1] Projections are for these latter two groups to grow considerably over the next 2 decades.

As our elderly live longer, they suffer from more chronic diseases that require different therapeutic care. Many more people now need skilled nursing home care or continued therapeutic support in the home with or without community support services. Medicare has been under constant pressure to expand its coverage of these services. Congress introduced legislation annually to expand home care programs and nursing home care, but until the Medicare Catastrophic Illness Protection Act of 1988, little legislation was ever successful. With the passage of this landmark legislation, Congress did indeed expand both home care and skilled nursing home services to further protect the elderly from devastating financial problems brought on by their chronic care needs.

At the same time, the enormous growth in Medicare outlays has put the Health Insurance Trust Fund in danger of bankruptcy by 2005 unless the payroll contribution to Medicare is increased by 16% or outlays reduced by 14%. Increasing payroll taxes is not viewed as a popular move by either the administration or Congress. So the Medicare program's $99 billion fiscal year 1990 budget is in danger of further reductions to protect the basic solvency of the program. Clearly, neither alternative of payroll tax increases or decreased outlays alone will solve the long-range solvency of Medicare. A reform of the entire Medicare program will undoubtedly occur in the late 1990s that will probably require increased contributions by wealthier beneficiaries.

Despite the above-mentioned concern, the public sector share of our national health care expenditures is expected to grow from its current 40.6% to 42.5% by 2000, with the federal share increasing from 28.7% to 32.6%.[3] Most of these projected increases in both Medicare and Medicaid are due to the increased number of elderly who need care, coupled with the very heavy costs of highly sophisticated technology developed to treat many of the acute-care problems. Because of the projected dramatic increases in outlays to these two programs over the next decade, health care providers must anticipate changes in payment for health care services that embody the concepts of cost constraints to protect the integrity of these programs. For example, Medicare payments nearly doubled between 1981 and 1985 and are projected to increase from $78.9 billion in 1987 to $320.8 billion by 2000.[3] Medicaid too will increase more than 50% every 5 years from its fiscal year 1990 base of $61.1 billion to $138 billion by 2000.

Medicaid is a jointly sponsored state federal program that provides both acute and long-term services for about 20 million poor. Each state may set its own criteria for eligibility based on income standards that have been broadly determined by federal guidelines. Federal guidelines also define a mandatory scope of covered services, such as hospital, physician, and skilled nursing facility care. Although services such as eyeglasses are optional, coverages are determined individually by each state legislature. In 1981, Congress passed legislation that approved Medicaid payment for nurse-midwife services directly. Today, all but two states now offer this coverage service.

Primarily, single-parent mothers and children eligible for Aid to Families with Dependent Children (A.F.D.C.) are the ones who benefit mostly by acute care and preventive services. Although the elderly are less than 20% of the enrollees, the outlays for long-term care for them averages about 45% of all payments. Since 1981, there has been continued emphasis on cost containment within the Medicaid program. This has given rise to intergenerational debates about the appropriateness of services available between acute and long-term care.

Looking only at health care, statistics show that the poor and elderly accounted for 44% of all admissions to hospitals in 1986, up from 40% in 1981. As the trend continues, the government's influence on health care delivery systems will continue to escalate, and shortfalls in payments to hospitals by Medicare and Medicaid will compound the current payment problems. The government's search for further efficiencies will cause even further restructuring in the delivery of services. More attempts to rationalize the delivery of adequate care will lead more providers to negotiate with preferred provider organizations (PPOs) as well as with health maintenance organizations (HMOs). One of the major attractions of managed care is the reduction in utilization of selective services without an appreciable denial of access to quality service.

According to the National Center for Health Care Statistics, inpatient hospital days per 1000 population have already declined since 1980 by 27%, from 1.134 days per 1000 to 833 in 1986.[6] Many HMOs report usage rates of around 400 inpatient days per 1000 population. As we move into an era of even more managed care, one can anticipate a continued movement to less care in our high-cost hospitals and more services provided in other patient care settings. Expansion of services in home care is reflected in the enormous growth in the number of home care agencies between 1981 (3169) and 1987 (5887), an 85% increase; skilled nursing facilities expanded 39%, and ambulatory surgical centers, virtually unknown before 1981, grew at a 516% rate.[4] These increases have had an enormous impact on nursing, because each agency needs registered nurses to supervise and give care. The rapid increase in these alternatives to health care have helped to increase the demand for nurses and have also helped create today's national nursing shortage.

In the acute-care hospital sector, payments have been controlled since 1983 by the initiation of an incentive-based prospective payment system utilizing diagnosis-related groups (DRGs). This sytem has enabled the government to reduce its payment outlays to hospitals by many billions of dollars. For example, the hospital market-basket inflation increased 18% between 1984 and 1987, yet Medicare, whose beneficiaries account for 39% of hospital revenues, raised prices paid to hospitals only 9%. This has caused hospital net profit margins to decline precipitously since 1984, with small rural hospitals experiencing the most problems. The American Hospital Association (AHA) recently reported that more than half of all community hospitals actually lost money on Medicare inpatient care in 1986, a fact that the AHA cites as a reason some hospitals have closed or merged.

Meanwhile, employers have grown increasingly concerned about payments for health insurance to cover their employees and retirees. Within 7 years, employer payment for health insurance doubled,[2] spurring interest by businesses in cost-containment measures such as those initiated by the federal sector. Utilization review has emerged as a major enterprise among businesses, along with coverage options that encourage the use of PPOs and HMOs.

The blending of both private-sector and public-sector concern for financing escalating health care services has led to a new emphasis on productivity and the need for more information to better manage the delivery system. Although hospitals have initiated major marketing strategies and developed contractual relationships with multiple PPOs and HMOs to assure an adequate group of patients, they are only now beginning to measure productivity and quality of care through the use of new hospital information systems. The Health Care Financing Administration's new initiative to determine medical effectiveness of specific procedures should, over the next decade, produce some startling savings—as much as $20 billion to $50 billion—and change the way health care is delivered in our country.

The strategy to study the medical effectiveness of physician practice decision grew out of the work of Wennberg, a physician who found major variations in practice patterns between different communities, even those within the same state. Robert Brooks, M.D., of the Rand Corporation, has also investigated selected procedures, such as coronary artery bypass graphs, cataract surgery and carotid, and endarterectomy and concluded that as much as 20 to 30 percent of these procedures may not be necessary and may not improve the quality of a person's life.

The Department of Health and Human Services is now planning to invest between $75 and $200 million over the next several years in research to analyze the outcomes of selected procedures in order to determine the best practice patterns by comparing large volumes of claims data with actual outcomes for patients. Although the focus thus far has been on medical decision making related to patient outcome, new interdisciplinary research studies are beginning to indicate a significant relationship with nursing. Nursing practice should initiate further interdisciplinary studies related to outcome of care.

IMPACT ON NURSING

From the beginning of the Medicare prospective payment system, immediate changes were noted. Length of hospital stay dropped precipitously, and review for appropriateness of admission caused a concomitant decrease in admissions, thus causing occupancy to plummet in many hospitals. As hospital budgets became tighter, new responsibilities were defined for the nursing staff. Registered nurses were utilized to deliver total patient care, and nurses' aides and licensed practical nurses (L.P.N.s) were laid off because of declining occupancies.

Cost of nursing services began to be examined more closely, because these services represented a large share of the hospital budget. Discharge planning assumed a major new role in importance as patients were discharged to after-care facilities, such as home care and skilled nursing facilities. Within several years, the hospitals diversified into major new ambulatory services, and all these settings demanded registered nurses, causing an increase in demand for R.N.s just as enrollments into schools of nursing were experiencing sharp declines. As the impact of these increased demands were being felt, hospitals began to request that nursing leadership take a new look at the appropriate utilization of nursing personnel. Nursing has recognized the enormous impact of "substitutions" for other care givers and is beginning to restructure the nursing environment to better utilize the skills of both clinical and nonclinical care givers, while retaining the primary role of case manager for the registered nurse.

As quality of care issues became a central concern to hospital trustees and management, the role of nursing was highlighted. The enormous role that nurses play in assisting patients to recuperate is finally being recognized. Concern has escalated over patient complications that cause increased lengths of stay that affect a hospital's fiscal stability, especially when the extended stay results in an "outlier" (an extended stay costing the hospital more than the amount Medicare pays); registered nurses are a valuable asset that can prevent these occurrences. Nurses are using their clinical skills at the bedside to monitor and spot complications and intervene appropriately to prevent complications serious enough to alter a patient's treatment pattern or length of stay. Ever so slowly the contemporary image of nursing is changing to recognize this vital role that nurses have in the provision of care.

The central value in the health care system seems to be the maintenance of a proper balance between quality of care, access to care, and cost. Ideally, quality of care should be increased, access should be increased, and cost should be decreased. Some people do not believe this is possible, and others believe that by restructuring the system and demanding more productivity, along with more appropriateness of therapeutic interventions, quality can be increased while reducing cost and enhancing access.

Hornbrook recently wrote that the value of nursing and hence its economic rewards ought to be derived from its contributions to access, quality, efficiency, equity, and health status.[5] Recently during hearings on the nursing shortage, the Commission on Nursing heard many nurses testifying to the need to pay more for experienced clinical nurses. One of the 16 recommendations of the commission suggests that attention be given to fixing the "wage compression" problem to retain nurses at the bedside. Indeed, some hospitals have recognized the problem and are designing clinical career ladder programs with salaries approaching $50,000 to $60,000 for selected nurses with significant clinical experience. This is an important breakthrough for nursing because it recognizes the enormous contribution nurses are making to the patients' care regimes. However, hospital administrators are becoming uneasy thinking about the fiscal problems they already have even without these salary increases. Thus it is up to the nursing leadership to demonstrate that the nursing department is willing to restructure itself to become as efficient and productive as possible and that not all nurses will be paid the $50,000 figure.

Some hospitals will continue to use all registered nurses because of the type of patients and care that is needed, but many other hospitals will redistribute the care-giving functions among many levels of nursing personnel. Demonstration projects are already being designed to encourage hospitals to evaluate these restructured delivery systems focusing on the quality of care being delivered by these nursing units.

To assist nursing in its management of patient care services, hospitals may need to introduce computerized patient care management information systems. Nurses must recognize the need to utilize modern management tools such as information systems in order to better track patient care and account for errors of omission in care. By enhancing productivity through restructuring the patient care environment and using new technology, nurses may have more time to focus on case management of their patients. Unless nursing is willing to embrace these recommendations, the shortage of nurses will probably continue, causing some hospitals to reduce services, close beds, or incur higher operating costs in overtime and agency fees. Concern for bottom-line budgets could cause some organizations to lower their standards of care, unknowlingly and thus jeopardize their fiscal situation even further, because the government can deny payments to hospitals for substandard care.

As hospitals track patient care, it will become more apparent that nurses have a major role in preventing poor care. Nurses may be able to win a larger role in decision making about therapeutic care plans once they quantify the cost benefits of their activities.

Managed care has long recognized the talents of nurse-practitioners as cost-effective care givers, especially for maintenance of chronic care, and will continue to seek qualified individuals to deliver these services. Because business and industry are now encouraging the use of managed care, it follows that nurses will be increasingly recognized as cost-effective providers of services. The decade of the 1990s will be an important era for nurses, as we will see continued awareness of the importance of nursing in the delivery of health care services.

A rational allocation of resources means changing expectations. Expectations need to be changed about the length of stay in an inpatient care setting as well as whether inpatient care is the most appropriate choice. Consumers, providers, and payers must adjust their expectations. Technological change has forced physicians and nurses to examine their practice patterns and adjust to sweeping psychological changes demanded by the new delivery system. Nurses must be willing to change their expectations about how and where health care services are to be provided, insisting only on cost-effective quality services that promote optimum outcomes in the quality of life for patients.

REFERENCES

1. Dychtwald K: Age wave, Los Angeles, 1989, Jeremy Tarcher, Inc.
2. Employee Benefit Research Institute: The changing health care market, 1987.
3. Health Care Financing Administration: national health care expenditures 1986-2000, Health Care Financing Review 8(4), 1987.

4. Health Care Financing Administration: Health Care Financial Review 9(2), 1987.

5. Hornback M: Economic Models of Nursing Practice. In Alternate conceptions of work and society: implications for professional nursing, Washington, DC, 1988, American Association of College of Nursing.

6. US Department of Health and Human Services: Health in the United States, Pub No 88-1232, Rockville, Md, 1987, National Center for Health Statistics.

CHAPTER 49

National Center for Nursing Research

A commitment to excellence in science

ADA SUE HINSHAW

Excellence in nursing science has been a continual goal and commitment of the nursing profession. This commitment is linked to the efforts of the discipline's scholars to develop a knowledge base that can accurately guide nursing practice. The decisions made in daily practice are numerous and complicated, regardless of their nature or target: enhancement or promotion of health, prevention of disease, or care of individuals and families with acute and chronic illnesses. The generation and testing of data using systematic research methods are critical to the provision of responsible health care. Nursing care must be based on solid, accurate information if therapeutic interventions are to be effective. Research-based practice "reflects the characteristics of the research from which it is derived. It is precise and replicable and produces predictable patient outcomes."[12] Thus the quality of the research by which nursing science is generated and information is provided to guide practice becomes one of the major keys to improving patient care for our discipline.

One of the major goals of the National Center for Nursing Research (NCNR) is the promotion of excellence in developing a knowledge base for the profession. The initiatives and programs of the NCNR are structured to enhance excellence in science and to promote high standards in the scientific community's research. Several areas need to be considered in terms of facilitating excellence in nursing science:

- Definitions and characteristics of "good" science
- Strategies for promoting excellence in science
- National facilitation of nursing research

CHARACTERISTICS OF "GOOD" SCIENCE

In general, the sciences are defined as bodies of knowledge based on general principles about a delim-

ited range of phenomena derived from empirical observations, that is, experiences of the senses, that can be or have been tested. The interrelated generalizations that constitute such a body of knowledge do not reflect idiosyncratic individual experiences but rather the consensus of the scientific community and its collected research.[8] This conceptualization of science emphasizes that it is the "consensual, informed opinion" that provides an understanding and explanation of the natural world.

The traditional definitions of nursing science as a body of knowledge suggest that it consists of defined concepts or constructs describing various human responses to health and illness as well as therapeutic nursing actions in systematically specified relationships.[14] Nursing science is defined by Feldman[6] as a discrete body of knowledge. The purpose of nursing science is "to explore, identify, explain and predict phenomena relating to man, his environment, health and nursing, in order to guide practice."[9] Gortner[7,8] suggests that nursing science encompasses an understanding of human biology and behavior and health and illness, including the processes by which changes in health status are brought about, the patterns of behavior associated with normal and critical life events, and the principles and laws governing life states and processes.

Although science is not the same as the process of systematic inquiry by which it has evolved, science is characterized by certain characteristics of the inquiry process. Thus the characteristics of "good" science reflect both the body of knowledge and the process by which it was generated and tested.

Several criteria for judging excellence in science have been suggested: significance, theory-observation congruency, generalizability, reproducibility, precision, and intersubjectivity.[8] Significance is considered both in terms of the contribution of the research findings to practice as well as the contribution of the findings to the broader body of knowledge. By definition, science involves the empirical testing of theory at some level of development, for example, factor isolating to the predictability of substantive relationships.[5] For knowledge to be used in practice, the concepts and relationships as theorized must have been substantiated with data or empirical observations. The data or empirical observations could be collected under a variety of methodological approaches. Gortner and Schultz[8] label this characteristic of science theory-observation compatibility. Reproducibility simply refers to the ability to reproduce the results under similar conceptual, clinical, or methodological circumstances.[4] Conversely, generalizability refers to the applicability of the findings across multiple clinical conditions, diverse health care settings, and other changing conditions. Precision is defined as the degree of sensitivity and accuracy with which the results can be expected to be repeated in additional research or when transferred into practice. The final characteristic—intersubjectivity—combines attributes of several of the others because it is defined as "evidence and knowledge claims which can be corroborated by others." This last criterion underlies the consensus characteristic that is a major defining attribute of science. These criteria are familiar to nurse investigators but need to be summarized to provide a common base of understanding for defining excellence in science.

These criteria are in themselves generalizable; that is, they are applicable for examining knowledge regardless of the methodological or philosophical approaches used to develop the knowledge. Norbeck,[16] in her "Defense of Empiricism," refers to several of these criteria, and Benner,[3] in discussing the phenomenological perspective on explanation, prediction, and understanding in nursing science, also speaks of criteria that include theory-observation compatibility, significance, reproducibility, and generalizability. Thus the criteria are meant to be broad and applicable under diverse methodological conditions. The criteria need further delineation and comparison across various philosophical approaches and research designs.

STRATEGIES FOR PROMOTING EXCELLENCE IN SCIENCE

As suggested earlier, excellence in science has been a hallmark of nursing's research programs, with an emphasis on scientific rigor merged with societal relevance. The dilemma for nursing is to promote excellence in terms of the characteristics of science while the demands for scientific inquiry escalate rapidly. Promoting such excellence will require enhancing several aspects of the discipline's approach to science:

* Developing depth in the knowledge base
* Adopting scientific career patterns
* Enhancing the scientific community
* Systematically pursuing the dissemination and utilization of research findings

Developing depth in nursing science

There are a number of strategies that can be used to systematically develop depth in nursing science. Depth in nursing science is defined as a substantive area in which there are a number of investigations with replicated, consistent findings. These strategies include the development of individual investigator programs and facilitation of critical masses of scientists working in the same or similar substantive areas of study.

Individual investigator programs. Research needs to be seen as a program of study by nurse-scientists. A research program is a continuing line of study consisting of interlocking investigations that build on one another. Examples of individuals with known research programs are Barnard's work with premature infants,[2] Anderson's work with nonnutritive sucking for premature infants,[1] and Johnson's work on sensory information and its effect on distress responses under different types of clinical situations.[13] Nurse investigators must think of research programs in phases or stages, with each research program consisting of a number of investigations. The strength of this particular view of research in terms of developing nursing science is the opportunity for the individual to build on prior work, substantiate and replicate that work, and add other aspects to the work that are related to the central phenomenon and the evolving base of findings. In such a way depth of knowledge is developed in a substantive area of study.

Critical masses of scientists. Another strategy for developing depth in nursing science is to begin to build a critical mass of investigators functioning in the same area of research and pursuing a line of research in tandem, either within one site or across several sites. In this way scientists are able to build on one another's work and to understand findings from various perspectives in a substantive field of study. Many of the universities have built solid scientific research communities. What is now being recommended is that subgroups in common areas of research be formed within these communities. This kind of arrangement would have implications for resource allocation and funding strategies, as well as for the way in which faculty, predoctoral, and postdoctoral students could be recruited into positions and programs, that is, on the basis of their research and identified areas of scientific expertise or interest.

Adopting scientific career patterns

Training for scientific research is a career commitment that should include periodic retraining or further education. No one understands better than finishing doctoral students that the earned doctorate is only the beginning of a research career, both in terms of the conduct of research and the continual fine tuning necessary for advanced research. Nurse-scientists will have to be able to recognize points in their careers when they need additional training because of the kind of study they are conducting or the proliferation of information in a field they are investigating. Programs and awards need to be developed to facilitate the acquisition of the necessary training not only for postdoctoral study but also for career development study for midcareer and senior-level scientists.

Enhancing the scientific community

Three of the characteristics of a scientific community are crucial to the ability to promote excellence in nursing science: communality, colleagueship, and competition. Communality involves the sharing of scientific endeavors among colleagues within the discipline. As Gortner and Schultz[8] noted in their recent *Image* article, only through open professional scrutiny can knowledge claims be examined in terms of their contribution to the understanding of a phenomenon. Sharing involves not only the communication of activities but also the active involvement of all participants in systematically and rigorously examining the ideas from the perspective of scientific merit, that is, both the rigor of the investigation and the relevance of the phenomenon to the discipline. Colleagueship refers to the support scientists offer one another for trying creative or new theoretical approaches and for being willing to scrutinize their own research endeavors. Thus colleagueship includes creating an environment of support and reinforcement for risk taking, creative thinking, and scientific action. Constructive

competition promotes communality and provides a stimulus and motivation for involvement that permits open discussion of the issues surrounding the phenomenon under study. This type of examination and scrutiny of the discipline's scientific endeavors can lead to consensus on areas that are well researched, highlight important new areas for study, and promote collaborative endeavors among colleagues as different areas of research are understood.

NATIONAL FACILITATION OF NURSING RESEARCH

The National Center for Nursing Research was established in April 1986 to facilitate national programs in nursing research and promote excellence in the knowledge base developed for the profession. It serves as a focal point for federal funding of nursing research. The general purpose of the NCNR is "the conduct and support of, and dissemination of information respecting, basic and clinical nursing research, training, and other programs in patient care research."[17] Nursing research focuses on investigations related to the "diagnosis or treatment of human responses to actual or potential health problems."[15] Such research involves scientific inquiry into basic and clinical biomedical and behavioral processes as well as examinations of nursing therapeutics or interventions that are effective in patient care. The conceptual and methodological approaches are interdisciplinary in nature, reaching across a number of fields. The ultimate goal of nursing science and research is the improvement of nursing practice for the purpose of preventing disease, promoting recovery, and maintaining health.

The broad mission of the National Institutes of Health (NIH) is to improve the health of the people of the United States by increasing our understanding of the processes underlying human health and by acquiring new knowledge to help prevent, detect, diagnose, and treat disease. This broad mission is consistent with the purpose and defining characteristics of nursing research as cited earlier.

The placement of the NCNR within the broader base of other health care research at NIH was believed to have several benefits. First, nursing research, with its orientation to health promotion and disease prevention as well as its emphasis on basic and clinical care processes, provided a natural complement to the biomedical research orientation that is traditionally supported by NIH. Second, nursing science needed to be developed within the context of other basic and clinical health care disciplines. Nursing research is often interdisciplinary and benefits from the knowledge of experts representing other sciences. In addition, as science was developed from a nursing perspective, such knowledge could be incorporated more easily into health care knowledge in general and thus be more accessible to other disciplines as well as our own profession. Third, moving nursing research into a well-recognized structure for biomedical and behavioral research was expected to provide a stability in resource allocation for nursing research as it had for the research programs of other health care disciplines. Thus a number of benefits were expected from the move of nursing research to NIH.[11]

Extramural programs for research

The extramural program at NCNR provides support for the conduct of research and research training. Such support, in the form of grants and awards, is offered to researchers in the university and clinical practice communities who are judged to have scientifically meritorious projects. The extramural program is organized in three broad substantive areas or branches. The branches are defined by the NCNR as follows.

Health promotion–disease prevention. Research in this area is designed to decrease the vulnerability of individuals and families to illness or disability across the life span. Health promotion research addresses the general health of the population and is not directed at any particular illness or disability. Examples include, but are not limited to, studies of the nutritional requirements of the various developmental phases of life and studies of the relationship between the biomedical and behavioral dimensions of human health. Disease prevention research, on the other hand, focuses on a particular illness or disability and how to prevent the onset of the illness or disability. Examples include, but are not limited to, the identification of biomedical, behavioral, and environmental risk factors, and the development or refinement of methods that enhance the abilities of at-risk individuals and their families to respond to potential health problems.

Acute and chronic illness. Research in this area deals with human responses to acute and chronic illness and disability. It is concerned with the biological, biomedical, behavioral, and environmental factors that contribute to the causes, prevalence, amelioration, and

remediation of illness and disability. Examples include, but are not limited to, studies on adaptation and functioning in chronic illnesses, such as arthritis, diabetes, hypertension, and renal disease; technological developments in rehabilitation therapies; adherence to therapeutic regimens; nursing interventions, including physical, behavioral, and educational interventions; biochemical factors and changes associated with acute and chronic illness and disability; and biomedical, behavioral, cognitive, and perceptual responses to illness or disability.

Nursing systems. Research in this area examines the environment in which nursing care is delivered and includes projects that investigate promising approaches to nursing management and nursing care delivery. Some examples are investigations of the outcome of home care, long-term care, and hospital care; identification of the mechanisms responsible for different outcomes in various care settings; development and refinement of methods to improve the delivery of nursing care in underserved areas; development of innovative approaches to the delivery of nursing care in nursing homes, including investigation of alternatives to nursing home care; factors underlying the quality of nursing care; assessment of the cost of providing nursing care; development of models to illustrate effective collaboration among nurses, physicians, and other members of the health team; application of prospective payment systems as it relates to the provision of nursing care; and the use of automation to improve the effectiveness of nursing care. One special program emphasis deals with ethical issues relating to patient care and patient care research. Examples include issues of death and dying; transplantation; prolongation of life; and ethical decision making on the part of nurses, other members of the health team, patients, and relatives.

A number of grant mechanisms are used to support different types of research projects. A series of fellowships, traineeships, and awards are available to assist at different stages of a nurse's research career. The NCNR must provide resources for a cadre of well-trained nurse-scientists to meet the nursing investigative needs of the future.

NCNR initiatives

Several initiatives have been taken to enhance excellence in science and facilitate a national environment for nursing research.[10] The initiatives include identifying a set of nursing research priorities, developing a trajectory for research training and career development, and increasing collaborative interdisciplinary research endeavors.

The first initiative involved the construction of a National Nursing Research Agenda (NNRA) to set priorities for nursing research. The NNRA has three purposes: (1) to provide structure for selecting scientific opportunities and initiatives, (2) to promote depth in developing a knowledge base for nursing practice, and (3) to provide direction for nursing research within the discipline. The driving force behind the development of the NNRA was the need to identify specific areas of research to pursue in depth and to target resources for this research. Nursing research is quite broad in scope. Numerous clinical phenomena and problems could be chosen for study. All these possibilities need to be pursued eventually, but it is important to begin to build depth in areas defined as most critical to provide a body of knowledge that is usable for nursing practice.

The NNRA will consist of defined priorities set by the scientific community, each of which has been refined and will guide use of federal resources for the national center in terms of allocating funds for research and training. However, the majority of the resources available for nursing research will continue to go to individual investigator-initiated proposals, with a smaller amount of those resources being targeted for the defined priorities.

The second major initiative of the NCNR is the development of a career trajectory for research training and development. The career trajectory consists of two components. One is a philosophical statement concerning the lifetime commitment that must be made to research training and staying on the cutting edge of science. The second is the development of a series of awards to enable individuals to obtain additional training at various stages in a research career.

Three other objectives are included in this second initiative. First, increasing the total cadre of nurse-scientists to develop the science base for nursing is critical. Second, it is also important to increase the number of individuals in postdoctoral study to insure that nurse-scientists have ample opportunity to begin and stabilize their research careers before accepting busy academic and clinical positions. Third, it is important to increase the number of institutional research training awards provided to research-intensive schools

of nursing so that individuals in such environments will be trained with seasoned and active nurse researchers as role models.

The third initiative for the national center is the facilitation of collaborative endeavors with other scientific disciplines. The research problems that are pursued by nurse-scientists are complex and diverse and often require perspectives from other disciplines as well as nursing. It is important to foster such a multidisciplinary perspective to develop depth and to provide the most recent and relevant base from which to build nursing science.

CONCLUSION

Nursing is at a very exciting, stimulating point in its development of knowledge for the discipline. The major challenge posed by a number of scholars in our profession is to turn from dealing with the processes—philosophical, theoretical, and methodological—for acquiring knowledge and begin to delve seriously into the actual phenomena that represent the core of nursing practice. To make this turn risks identifying and taking a position on what the business of nursing actually is and what it can offer society. The major goals of the National Center for Nursing Research are promoting excellence in the science of the discipline and facilitating a national environment for the profession's research programs. The initiatives taken in the early formative years of the national center are focused on strengthening nursing's ability to fulfill these two goals.

REFERENCES

1. Anderson G: Pacifiers: the positive side, MCN 11(2):122, 1986.
2. Barnard K: Nursing research related to infants and young children. In Werley HH and Fitzpatrick JJ, editors: Annual Review of Nursing Research, volume 1, New York, 1983, Springer.
3. Brenner P: Quality of life: a phenomenological perspective on explanation, prediction, and understanding in nursing science, Advances in Nursing Science 8(1):1, 1985.
4. Connelly CE: Replication research in nursing, International Journal of Nursing Studies 23(1):71, 1986.
5. Dickoff J, James P, and Wiedenbach E: Theory in a practice discipline. I. Practice oriented discipline, Nurs Res 17(5):415, 1968.
6. Feldman HR: A science of nursing—to be or not to be? Image 13:63, 1981.
7. Gortner SR: Nursing science in transition, Nurs Res 29:180, 1980.
8. Gortner SR and Schultz PR: Approaches to nursing science methods, Image 20(1):22, 1988.

9. Hinshaw AS: The tao of nursing research: the creative principle ordering nursing science and research. Keynote address, Sixth Annual Research Conference of the Southern Council on Collegiate Education for Nursing, Shreveport, La, December 1986.

10. Hinshaw AS: The National Center for Nursing Research: challenges and initiatives, Nurs Outlook 36(2):54, 1988.

11. Hinshaw AS and Merritt DH: Moving nursing research to NIH, Perspectives in nursing 1987-1989, New York, 1987, National League for Nursing.

12. Horsley JA and others: Using research to improve nursing practice: a guide, Orlando, 1983, Grune & Stratton.

13. Johnson JE: Effects of accurate expectations about sensations on the sensory and distress components of pain, J Pers Soc Psychol 27:261, 1973.

14. Kerlinger FN: Foundations of behavioral research, ed 3, New York, 1983, Holt, Rinehart & Winston.

15. Merritt DH: The National Center for Nursing Research, Image 18(3):84, 1986.

16. Norbeck JS: In defense of empiricism, Image 19(1):28, 1987.

17. US Public Law 99-158 (Health Research Extension Act), November 4, 1986.

CHAPTER 50

Third-party reimbursement

MAUREEN BEIRNE STREFF
ROSEANN NETZER

INTRODUCTION

This chapter has evolved from 5 years of extensive, on-the-job experience of designing, lobbying, and implementing third-party reimbursement for certified psychiatric clinical specialists; lobbying and collaborating with nurse-midwives on the implementation of third-party reimbursement; and lobbying with and for nurse-practitioners and nurse-anesthetists to move their legislation around the obstacles encountered in the journey through the legislative process. Behind these struggles is the conviction that because nurses are fully licensed and have been granted credentials by their professional organizations to provide the services within the scope of their nursing practice act, these services should be third-party reimbursable. Nurses should not explain away their role by identifying themselves as "physicians' extenders" or substitutes; they should stand strong in their unique role to effect positive change in the delivery of health care services, which stresses concepts of disease prevention and health promotion through education.

The research and design of any legislative strategy should be based on the history of third-party reimbursement that has been gathered by the American Nurses' Association (ANA) and the experiences of our colleagues across the nation. This chapter will illustrate the evolution of this process for nurses in Massachusetts. The movement for third-party reimbursement for nursing service is growing throughout the United States; to keep it moving we must understand it.

THE HISTORY OF THIRD-PARTY REIMBURSEMENT
Impact on the nursing profession

In 1948 the ANA identified third-party reimbursement for nursing services as a priority and included it in the association platform. However, the issue of reimbursement did not fully bloom until the nurse-practitioner movement toward role autonomy pointed to the identification of potentially reimbursable services. The ANA House of Delegates (in 1972, 1974, and 1976) adopted resolutions urging vigorous support of direct reimbursement for the services of nurses by both public and private third-party payers. The state nurses' associations also began to explore possible avenues to accomplish that goal. The process on the national level of the ANA and the state nurses' associations evolved through the formation of groups to research currently operative reimbursement policies and the potential effects of third-party reimbursement of nurses on the health care system. The ANA in a report in June 1983, "Third Party Reimbursement Legislation for Services of Nurses . . . A Report of Changes in State Health Insurance Laws," addressed the reimbursement status of nursing services in particular states. In 1984 the ANA published the work of the Council of Primary Health Care Practitioners Joint Task Force on Third-Party Reimbursement for the Services of Nurses. This publication has been a useful tool for designing a route to reimbursement. At the time of that publication, the states of Alaska, California, Maryland, Minnesota, Mississippi, Montana, New Jersey, New Mexico, New York, Oregon, South Dakota, Utah, Washington, and West Virginia had legislation affecting specific or all-inclusive nurse groups. By 1986 a review of the national precedents set by the federal and state governments and private commercial insurance carriers added to the above list the states of Alabama, Arizona, Connecticut, Florida, Iowa, Maine, Massachusetts, Michigan, Mississippi, Montana, Nevada, New Hampshire, North Dakota, Ohio, Pennsylvania, Rhode Island, Vermont, and West Virginia. The nursing specialty affected by the legislation is spelled out specifically by each state. Even in 1988 the concept of reimbursement for nursing services is revolutionary in a number of states. Some states have chosen the incremental approach as opposed to the comprehensive approach to reimbursement.

For example, in 1981 in Massachusetts the state nurses' association filed a reimbursement bill to include nurse-practitioners, nurse-anesthetists, nurse-midwives, and psychiatric specialists. The legislators seemed to be overwhelmed by the projected cost of such services and were not familiar with the scope of practice of each group. After 3 years of seeing that bill die in committee, the nurse-midwives and psychiatric clinical specialists, with the blessing of the state nurses' association, filed separate bills, which were passed in 1985 and 1986. The Nurse-Practitioner Reimbursement Bill filed by the state nurses' association and Nurse-Anesthetist Bill filed by their particular group are pending as of this writing. With each of these skills, another important variable was the view that legislators had regarding credentials: advanced level of practice, manifested by a graduate degree or specific certification, was a given. The concept of reimbursing all nurses was not acceptable because the education required of nurses was being compared to the education required of other health care providers (e.g., medical doctors, psychologists) who were currently reimbursable. Nurses involved in the legislative process were asked frequently, "How can *you* provide psychotherapy services? What is your training to perform this role?" According to Richard McKibbon of the Center for Research at ANA, data from states currently offering reimbursement for services of nurses (specifically or inclusively) has been collected by a survey tool designed by the ANA, which explored the status of developments relevant to nursing practice within the United States. According to Nancy Barr of ANA, the results of this survey include the states previously mentioned and Arkansas, Delaware, Hawaii, Nebraska, Oklahoma, and Tennessee. These states now are reimbursing services of all nurses or particular specialties, either because state legislatures have mandated the payments or because insurance companies have recognized nursing services as reimbursable. There is also legislation pending in other states for 1989.

The public and private components of third-party reimbursement

The public component of the third-party reimbursement system includes Medicaid, Medicare, and CHAMPUS (Civilian Health and Medical Program of the Uniformed Services). Medicaid and Medicare are administrated at the federal level by the U.S. Department of Health and Human Services, Health Care Financing Administration. CHAMPUS is administered by the Department of Defense.

Medicaid is a federally assisted and state-administered program providing medical assistance to family members with dependents who are aged, blind, disabled, or under the age of consent (minors). Each state designs and administers its own program and can designate health care providers as long as the state design complies with federal guidelines; by state legislation the general law can be amended, as it was in Massachusetts in 1987 to include podiatrists' services. In 1988 a bill was filed to include the private practice services of certified clinical specialists in psychiatric and mental health nursing. This latter legislation is currently in a committee.

Nurse-midwifery services to Medicaid subscribers have been reimbursable since 1982 when the Medicaid law changed and required all states to meet the needs of pregnant women. In 1977 the Rural Health Clinic Services Act was passed, which provides Medicaid and Medicare reimbursement for services provided by nurse-practitioners and physicians' assistants in health centers located in medically underserved rural areas with or without a supervisory physician on site.

Medicare is a nationwide health insurance program authorized under Title 18 of the Social Security Act, which provides benefits to persons 65 years of age or older. Medicare Part A is the Hospital Insurance program; Part B is the Supplementary Medical Insurance program. The current Medicare law requires that a physician supervise the nurse or nurse-practitioner, that nurse-practitioner services supplement physician services, and that services by nurse-practitioners be incidental to physician services. Payments are made directly to the physician or clinic. These Medicare regulations severely hamper the role of nurse-practitioners and clinical nurse specialists in psychiatric and gerontological nursing who practice privately and who could render effective quality home care as well as care in nursing home facilities. The ANA lobbied federal legislation bill S101, which would have authorized nurse-practitioners and clinical nurse specialists working in collaboration with a physician to certify and recertify the needs for patient care in nursing homes, as well as to perform the mandatory patient visits under both Medicare and Medicaid. The bill would also have provided direct payment to the nurse for patient visits. The bill evoked strong opposition from organized medicine. It was amended to allow nurse-practitioners and certified nurse specialists to certify and recertify patients in nursing homes without physician supervision until 1990; it is limited to Medicaid patients; and direct payments for patient visits were not included.

CHAMPUS recognizes and provides payments to certified nurse-midwives, nurse-practitioners, and psychiatric nurse specialists for services rendered to spouses and children of active-duty or retired uniformed-services personnel, and to family members of deceased active-duty or retired personnel.

The private component of the third-party reimbursement system includes Blue Cross and Blue Shield, which is a nonprofit corporation with plans located across the United States. The national organization of Blue Cross and Blue Shield provides coordination of standards and contract provisions for nationwide programs.

Commercial insurance carriers are usually organized on a for-profit basis and sell other types of insurance in addition to health insurance. They are free to design their policies to suit their own companies.

Health maintenance organizations (HMOs) were created in the 1970s as an alternative to traditional health care plans. They have effectively utilized nurse-practitioners. However, current patterns of health care delivery in HMOs are showing an increasing number of physicians, thereby decreasing the opportunities for nurse-practitioners, who in some states are limited or denied prescription-writing and hospital-admission privileges.

Another trend is toward preferred provider organizations (PPOs), wherein services are provided by established practitioners under a capitation arrangement rather than at an established HMO site. Nurses in independent practice are being invited to join some of these groups.

Another model is the independent physician association (IPA), a group of physicians who have come together to provide managed health care. One particular health care group has invited psychiatric clinical specialists to be providers; however, if that specialist is in private practice in an area in which the health care group has already contracted with an IPA, the nurse may not be able to treat the consumer unless the IPA is willing to have the consumer be seen out of its association. A 1988 publication of ANA suggests that nurses in private practice take the IPA model

(which traditionally has been made up of physicians) and design an independent professional nurses' association and contract with organizations to provide services to a specific population. This trend should be vigorously encouraged by the nursing profession.

DESIGN OF STRATEGY FOR A REIMBURSEMENT POLICY

The enactment of a reimbursement policy required a design that would address the credentials and the scope of practice of the nurse, the responsibility and accountability of the nurse to the patient and the third-party payer, the relationship of the nurse to other providers with whom she might need to collaborate, and a projected cost analysis of the policy. There is general agreement among health care providers that graduate-level (i.e., master's degree) preparation is mandatory for nursing specialists as it is for other health care specialists. In addition, it is presumed that each profession establishes its standards and policies for practice and methods for licensure and granting credentials within the states. The legislators are concerned about the needs of the consumer as well as the wishes of their constituents. Consumers have the right to select from many providers, individuals, or groups who best meet their health care needs and from whom they can be assured of receiving competent services. The consumer's right to choose health care services is enhanced by a reimbursement policy that includes services within the scope of practice of professional nursing.

In establishing eligibility to be a provider and receive reimbursement, the nurse has created an atmosphere in which certain services can be rendered to patients that will be documented and evaluated as designed by the standards for practice, and for which the nurse is responsible and accountable to the patient and third-party payer, as agreed by a contract. Nurses practicing independently do establish collaborative relationships with other health care providers as may be required to maximize treatment benefits. Institutions readily provide that opportunity for nurses as members of interdisciplinary teams as well as occasions for networking within the institution.

Nurses interested in reimbursement are attempting to make available to the consumer nursing services that are unique and different from those of physicians, psychologists, social workers, or any other health care provider. The nursing specialist, regardless of particular practice, has training and experience in physical health and medical sciences. The practical skills in all of the nursing specialties and knowledge of psychopharmacology assure the consumer as well as the third-party payer that the nurse is prepared to assess, diagnose, treat, teach disease prevention, and promote self-help. The latter two services will require more documentation to convince insurers that those services should be reimbursable. The assignment of fees for nursing services should be based on the kind of service offered, the level of expertise of the provider, and the responsibility incorporated in the delivery of the services; the assignment of fees should also take into account a just and equitable income for the provider as a professional who wishes to continue to offer such services.

Nonlegislative strategies for third-party reimbursement

The nonlegislative strategies for third-party reimbursement require a major commitment on the part of the leadership and membership of the ANA and the state nursing associations to interact effectively with elected officials in government, as well as with administrators of major corporations who have or should have an investment in advocating cost-effective health care for all.

In addition, networking with the national insurance organizations such as the National Association of Insurance Commissioners (NAIC) and the Health Insurance Association of America (HIAA) is of major importance. A state insurance commissioner promulgates regulations that are meant to protect the consumer as well as the provider. Members of the nursing profession should attend meetings of these associations, serve on task forces and boards, and present written or oral testimony at hearings. These particular approaches will educate the public about the scope of practice of a credentialed professional nurse and illustrate the services that warrant reimbursement.

Many community action groups want the support of nurses and want to join with nurses to lobby for consumer services. Such groups are very important to the nursing profession because they represent the consumer's viewpoint of nursing services to the legislators. In Massachusetts, for example, this community support was especially effective in gaining passage of the reimbursement bill for psychiatric clinical specialists, because patients did not give testimony for ethical reasons. Another group that helped was the "Friends of the Nurse-Practitioners" who wrote letters to legislators in support of the prescription writing bill. A uniformed police officer who had received health care services from this group came to the statehouse to testify at a health care hearing, and his testimony carried weight with the committee.

Legislative strategies for third-party reimbursement

Developing a legislative strategy for third-party reimbursement is a major task. We believe this is the most effective path to reimbursement because it is a more permanent solution. Receiving reimbursement based on a waiver or petition could be subject to change when the leadership of a particular agency or organization changes.

The ANA has recommended guidelines for the development of legislative strategies. One of these guidelines deals with seeking reimbursement for services of all registered nurses, not merely a specific group. Nurses in each state must assess the political climate when preparing to submit a reimbursement bill and must know who the proponents and opponents of such legislation will be. In Massachusetts an all-inclusive bill proved to be a mistake and was defeated at the first hearing because of concern about the broad financial implications, educational preparation of nurses, and quality care issues. The greatest opposition came from the medical associations and the insurance associations. In mental health and other specialties, turf issues have surfaced, and rivalry among specialties has been acute in relation to fees assigned for nursing services. Any nurse practice act has to be interpreted clearly to the legislators so that the role of nursing can be properly defended. The federal and state insurance laws and codes need to be reviewed so that decisions can be made about amending existing laws. It is advisable to have legal counsel from within the association or hired by the group filing the legislation to review the current statutes.

Decisions about which insurers will be affected and whether the reimbursement will be mandatory or optional are crucial in getting the legislation passed and must be kept in mind when filing. We believe the more insurance companies that are included, the more options the consumer has to choose specific plans and still be assured of access to the provider of choice. However, the group filing the legislation should be willing to omit a specific payer if it appears that the bill would be defeated with that inclusion. For example, in Massachusetts we chose to delete Medicaid because the reimbursement law in the state did not address Medicaid's exclusion of nonmedical mental health providers. We chose to file separate legislation to address this issue at a later date.

In considering mandatory versus optional reimbursement, we chose mandatory because it assured us of payment for services, and, just as important, assured us of recognition by colleagues and consumers as qualified to provide such services. For the most part, insurance companies and business organizations were opposed to the mandatory concept, claiming that an increase in the number of providers increases the demand for the services. We found it necessary and helpful to meet with representatives of these groups to present our positions, to educate them regarding our role and scope of practice, and to better understand their position. These meetings set the tone for potential negotiation.

Selecting bill sponsors from among the senators and representatives was a key element in designing effective strategy. Sponsors were selected on the basis of their support of the role of the professional nurse who is qualified to practice at an advanced level. The particular political affiliation of the legislators and their positions on relevant committees through which the bill would have to pass were of prime consideration.

THE LEGISLATIVE PROCESS

Vigilance best describes the position the bill's sponsors and supporters must assume throughout the legislative process. Passage of a reimbursement bill requires a clearly stated fact sheet, a definition of the scope of practice, a cost analysis, and a projection of the impact of the bill. Each legislator must have this information because the bill's opponents will be developing their own fact sheets and information to present.

A grass-roots organization made up primarily of psychiatric clinical specialists called Nurses United for Reimbursement of Services (NURS) was begun in Massachusetts in 1975; this group took the initial steps toward proposing reimbursement legislation for mental health services by nurses. The leaders and members were a major force in lobbying for this piece of legislation, offering support to one another and networking extensively with the state nurses' association, legislators, other health care providers, and community groups. They did not give up even after the bill had been left in committee for several years in a row, despite valiant efforts to move it along. Victory came when Blue Shield of Massachusetts, one of the strongest opponents, finally acknowledged that nurses could provide cost-effective, quality health care.

IMPLEMENTATION OF THE REIMBURSEMENT BILL

Implementation of the reimbursement bill has been an ongoing and time-consuming process. A necessary part of the work has been the education of insurance companies concerning the role of the professional nurse. We have had to send a copy of the statute to some companies and, in a few cases, invoke the assistance of the insurance commissioner to convince companies to accept nurses as eligible providers. The nurse-midwives have experienced greater difficulty in designing provider contracts with insurance companies that require specific documentation of procedures that are more cumbersome to define than psychiatric services. Some insurance companies offered orientation programs for new providers. NURS and the state nurses' association offered educational programs designed to facilitate the implementation of the bill.

Data on the impact of third-party reimbursement on the health care system continues to be gathered. Despite the initial difficulties in implementation, the independent practice of psychiatric nursing is flourishing in Massachusetts.

CONCLUSION

Third-party reimbursement for nursing service will benefit consumers in their search for cost-effective, quality health care. Nurses are licensed and have the credentials to practice. They must be able to document ways in which their services can be reasonably reimbursed, and they must work for the success of third-party reimbursement in all 50 states. NURS in Massachusetts continues to be actively involved in health care issues. In 1987 its name was changed to Nurses United for Responsible Services and includes nurse-midwives, nurse-practitioners, and nurse-anesthetists. The organization is dedicated to designing, lobbying, and implementing legislative efforts, to clarifying health care issues for consumers and legislators, and to collaborating closely with the state nurses' association in efforts to facilitate access to cost-effective, quality health care.

BIBLIOGRAPHY

American Nurses' Association. Report in the 1988 state nurses association survey on nursing practice. May, 1989.

American Nurses' Association Council of Primary Health Care Nurse Practitioners and Joint Task Force on Third-Party Reimbursement for Services of Nurses: Obtaining third-party reimbursement: a nurses' guide to methods and strategies, Kansas City, Mo, 1984, The Association.

American Nurses' Association Division of Governmental Affairs: 1988 legislative and regulatory fact sheets, Kansas City, Mo, 1988, The Association.

Aydelotte MK and others: Nurses in private practice: characteristics, organizational arrangements and reimbursement policy, Kansas City, Mo, 1988, American Nurses' Foundation, Inc.

Briggs N and Cummings BS: Insurance reimbursement of pediatric home care, Pediatric Nursing 12(6):449, 1986.

Brown BS: Practice management, Pediatric Nursing 10(6):429, 1984.

Burda D: Nursing lobby exerting new found power in Washington, Modern Healthcare 5(17):28, 1987.

Ferber S: Non-MDs move in, Medical Economics 5(62):99, 1985.

Gibson KW: Third-party billing, Nursing Management 18(5):37, 1987.

LaBar C: Third-party reimbursement legislation for services of nurses: a report of changes in state health insurance laws, Kansas City, Mo, 1983, The Association.

CHAPTER 51

Government intervention in a developing country

The Botswana experience

VUYELWA NDIKI NGCONGCO
GEETA LAWOT PFAU

INTRODUCTION

The form of government intervention in health care development is greatly influenced by a government's political philosophy and principles. Botswana's commitment to rural development and social justice seems to have served as a framework for its major intervention in health policy: the development of a primary health care system.

This chapter examines the evolution and progress of government intervention in setting both the stage and the pace for health care development in Botswana since independence was won in 1966. To this end, the goals, objectives, priorities, and strategies adopted through multiphased 5-year national development plans (NDPs) are briefly discussed to bring out the thrust of the government's move to provide primary health care services. The impact of that intervention and the major issues impinging on the quality of health services in Botswana are discussed. An attempt is also made to draw attention to those factors that are likely to either enhance or inhibit the effective provision of primary health care services in Botswana.

Finally, there is a discussion of ways government interventions can be modified to take into account the future needs of Botswana's rapidly changing society.

BOTSWANA

Botswana is a landlocked country that is spread across the center of the Southern Africa Plateau. The total area is about the size of Texas or France. It shares borders with the Republic of South Africa, Namibia, Zambia, and Zimbabwe. About 84% of the land surface is covered with Kgalagadi sand. It is estimated that less than 5% of Botswana's land area is arable.

Most Batswana belong to Setswana-speaking tribes or clans. About 90% live in rural areas. The annual population growth rate was estimated at 3.7% in 1984. The infant mortality rate was 102 per 1000 live births in 1971, but the 1981 census reflected a decline to 68 per 1000.

The people of Botswana are plagued by communicable diseases, intestinal infections, diseases related to maternal and child health, nutritional diseases, diseases of the respiratory tract, cardiovascular diseases, skin infections, ear and eye diseases, metabolic disease, injuries, and a host of parasitic diseases such as malaria and schistosomiasis.

EVOLUTION OF HEALTH SERVICES
A historical perspective

At independence in 1966, the government of Botswana inherited a highly curative, predominantly hospital-based, underdeveloped health care system. The only preventive services provided in the hospitals were antenatal, intrapartal, postnatal, and child welfare care. Most Motswana depended on traditional doctors, midwives and herbalists for health care. Modern health services were mostly crisis oriented, characterized by sporadic campaigns to combat diseases such as diptheria, polio, tuberculosis, typhoid fever, and smallpox. Health care was not geared to meet the needs of the masses, and emphasis was on medical intervention rather than on purposefully planned health intervention.

Major thrust of government intervention

In its third national development plan (1970 to 1975), Botswana decided to pursue an integrated development policy for rural areas, its major goal being rural development. The government actively promoted interventionist economic and social policies. In 1973 the government articulated its accelerated rural development plan, which was to be achieved through the application of the following principles: income policy, employment creation, and equitable allocation of resources. The major thrust of the government's intervention focused on district development—specifically on education, health, economic growth, agriculture, and the establishment of a rural land policy. Allocation of financial resources to education increased from P2,445,000 to P16,505,000; allocations to social and community development services increased from P170,000 to P1,620,000; and government subventions to health increased from P1 million to P3,250,000 by 1973. The government set specific targets for the provision of basic health services. The emphasis was on the provision of integrated basic health services to the rural community, which constituted 90% of the population. By the end of 1974, 85% of Batswana were within a 15-kilometer radius of a health facility. These facilities provided integrated curative, preventive, and health-promotive services with emphasis on maternal and child health, nutrition, communicable disease control, and health education. Health posts and clinics catered to the general population, whereas health centers and district hospitals served as referral facilities.

The government's integrated development orientation was founded on four national principles: democracy, development, self-reliance, and unity. These gave rise to four planning objectives: rapid economic growth, social justice, economic independence, and sustained development.

Although each national development plan had specific objectives, strategies, and targets, the government stressed the following approaches:

- mobilization and management of local and international resources for health development
- provision of balanced health service to rural and urban communities through primary health care
- pursuance of a collaborative relationship for health provision between government, traditional, mission, and private sectors to ensure that all provide a comprehensive community-focused service

- development of specific health programs in support of primary health care
- encouragement of community participation in the provision of health care through decentralized district health services
- implementation and evaluation of national health development plans

The capacity of the Botswana government to create and sustain a stable political environment has facilitated a systematic planning process for health development since 1966. As a result of this stability, the series of 5-year plans for national health development reflect continuity and consistency in theme and purpose.

How the intervention occurred

The third, fourth, fifth, and sixth 5-year national development plans covering the period 1973 to 1991 mark the emergence and development of Botswana's primary health care approach. During the third national development plan, in 1973, the government proposed and implemented a district-based health care system. Local authorities under the Ministry of Local Government and Lands were responsible for the provision of health to communities, but the Ministry of Health retained the portfolio responsibility for providing professional supervision and guidance. This decentralization was accompanied by the construction of many new health posts and clinics, which pointed to the need for an increase in the number of health personnel. Botswana's National Health Institute was asked to hire and train large numbers of nurses and environmental health assistants.

To meet these needs, the government of Botswana cooperated with the Norwegian Agency for International Development (NORAD) in constructing health posts, clinics, staff houses, and village roads. Cognizant of the need to provide effective integrated services, the government negotiated with NORAD for the recruitment and placement of district medical officers, who directed the design, development, implementation, and evaluation of these services. An important element in a health care service is the availability of essential drugs. The government, in collaboration with NORAD, the United Nations Children's Education Fund, and the World Health Organization, provided the health posts and clinics with drugs, basic equipment, and supplies. Of significance is the fact that none of the above-mentioned international organizations initiated the collaborative relationship; instead, they reacted to the government's goals, objectives, and priorities by agreeing to cooperate.

The government emphasized that existing district administrative structures established by local authorities for facilitating rural development should serve as the machinery for the planning and implementation of district health services at the home, village, and district levels so that health development would be seen as an integral part of district development. Community participation in health development was enhanced by the formation of a village health committee in each village that would act in concert with the village development committee. Through the village health committee, families and community groups identified their health problems and health needs as well as their strengths and weaknesses as far as health actions were concerned. The committees decided on the best ways to meet health needs and identified areas for which they required government intervention or assistance. Toward the end of this period the government of Botswana recognized the importance of strengthening existing support programs for primary health care. Thus the fourth plan, in addition to emphasizing the growth of integrated rural health services, also stressed the purposeful development of special support programs.

Whereas the development of a district-based health care system during the third plan was more a consequence of the policy of integrated rural development, the fourth health development plan (1976 to 1981) focused on deliberate strategies to consolidate the effectiveness of the rural basic health services through the implementation of a 5-year health-personnel development plan—a plan to establish special health program units and to set up a planning section within the Ministry of Health that would organize a health information system and formulate a health policy, as well as work out a rational budgetary strategy to ensure the rational allocation of recurrent and developmental health-sector expenditures. The priorities for government intervention were spelled out as follows: (1) personnel development, (2) support programs for health, (3) improvement of planning and statistics, and (4) improvement of physical infrastructure.

Personnel development

The government embarked on a plan for health-personnel development that defined the types, numbers, and roles of individual health groups. The plan also emphasized an integrated approach to curriculum design. In this context, the curricula for training health

personnel were to emphasize disease cure and prevention and health promotion and also to include public health, health education, maternal and child health, and family planning. The plan further stressed the need for a series of in-service education programs for health workers in order to reorient their practice to primary health care. To enhance the team approach to the provision of district health services, health personnel were to be trained in the multidisciplinary training institution, the National Health Institute. During this period the government increased capital as well as recurrent expenditures. Out of a capital health expenditure of P181,133 from 1973 to 1974, P105,785 (58.4%) was spent on basic rural health units, and P22,284 (12.3%) was committed for training. By 1976, out of a total capital expenditure of P1,782,700, 53% was spent to train health personnel and 39.1% to maintain basic rural health units. Between 1977 and 1982, capital expenditure on health had risen to P10,218,400. It is significant to note that out of this amount, P3,400,000 (33.3%) was spent on training facilities, and P1,430,000 (14.0%) was committed to the improvement of basic rural health units. Similarly, recurrent expenditures on training of health personnel increased from P62,320 (3%) in 1973 to P379,450 (7.1%) by 1976.

The government, cognizant of the role of nursing in primary health care, emphasized the training of registered nurse-midwives, enrolled nurses, enrolled nurse-midwives, public health nurses, family nurse-practitioners, nurse-anesthetists, and nurse-educators. In addition to nurses, the following groups were to be trained: dental therapists, health administrators, health assistants, health education officers, health inspectors, family welfare educators, pharmacy technicians, laboratory assistants, medical social workers, and nutrition officers. Medical doctors, dentists, and pharmacists were to be trained outside Botswana. The focus of the training was on nursing and family welfare educators. Nurses formed the backbone of the health service; family welfare educators (i.e., community workers) played a key role in enhancing community participation as well as in serving as the link between the health care system and the community.

Special programs in support of primary health care

The following units were established in order to handle the special support programs considered crucial in the provision of an effective, integrated primary health care service: epidemiology unit for communicable disease surveillance, control and health information development, environmental unit, health education, dental health, occupational health, maternal and child health, nutrition, and a special services unit for the handicapped. These units were designed to operate as integrated support units for district health services, and together with these services were coordinated by a senior medical officer based in the Ministry of Health.

Improvement of the national health planning capacity

A planning unit was established in the Ministry of Health consisting of economists, health planners, and statistical officers. Policy proposals and projects were refined within the Ministry of Health before submission to the Ministry of Finance and Development Planning. Review of progress in the implementation of plans took place within the Ministry of Health. Similar developments occurred in the Ministry of Local Government and Lands, so that district-level health planning and evaluation became ongoing activities. The merging of the medical statistics unit with the planning unit enhanced both the development and effective use of statistical information for health planning and program implementation review. Major efforts were made to incorporate missions in the process of health planning to ensure that the role of the nongovernment health network was both predictable, measurable, and well focused. Researchers studied the role of traditional medicine, eliciting information on the number and activities of traditional healers and laying the foundation for cooperation between modern and traditional medicine. Traditional healers and birth attendants ceased to operate in secrecy, and consultation between traditional and modern practitioners was initiated.

Budget strategy

The government decided to promote more egalitarian and cost-effective distribution of recurrent expenditures. For most of this planned period the government worked toward increasing the proportion of the recurrent budget going to preventive and public health services as well as to the development of human resources.

Improvements to the physical infrastructure

The government, mindful of the need to strengthen the effectiveness of the referral facilities for the health posts and clinics, improved the physical structures of some clinics, health centers, and the outpatient departments of some district hospitals. Laboratory and pharmaceutical services were improved.

Priorities in the fifth national development plan in 1980 to 1985

A review of the ministry's performance in NDP III (1973 to 1978) and NDP IV (1976 to 1981) formed a strong foundation for the setting of targets, objectives, and priorities for NDP V (1980 to 1985).

The major emphases in the fifth national development plan were on consolidating primary health care, achieving maximum community participation, and providing support for all frontline health workers. The following five priorities were set within these three major areas:

1. Primary health care
2. Training and personnel development
3. Strengthening of special health programs and special units
4. Statistics and planning
5. Physical infrastructure

A study conducted by the government in 1982 using global indicators for assessing progress toward the achievement of health for all citizens revealed among other things that the infant mortality rate had dropped from 97 per 1000 in 1971 to 68 per 1000 in 1981, that life expectancy had increased from 55 years in 1975 to 56 years in 1981, and that the gross domestic product (GDP) per capita rose from P550 in 1975 to P900 in 1982.

These changes demonstrate the impact of government health and social intervention on the quality of life of the average Motswana.

In 1984 the Ministry of Health, in collaboration with the World Health Organization, conducted a country resource utilization study. The findings set the pace for the development of the health chapter for NDP VI (1986 to 1991). During the sixth national health development plan, the government set the following priorities:

1. Primary health care development
2. Training and health personnel development
3. Planning and statistics
4. Hospital services development
5. Technical support services development
6. Management services development

A midterm review during 1988 is planned to enable

Table 51-1   Maternal and child health targets and achievements

Service	Actual 1980 (%)	Actual 1983 (%)	NDP5 Target (%)
Pregnant women attending antenatal clinics	87	96	85
Supervised deliveries	52	62	70
Women of reproductive age using family planning	11.7	15	15
Vaccinations	**Children immunized (%)**		
DPT	71	82	80
Polio	71	77	80
BCG	92	94	85
Measles	64	75	60

Source: Ministry of Health (1985)

Ministry of Health departments to review their targets and strategies and make any necessary adjustments.

During the period of NDP VI, the government continued to increase its financial provision for health. As a result, the projected health recurrent expenditure for 1990 to 1991 is set at P35,432,000, a growth rate of 6.3% over the last plans' health expenditures.

The impact of government intervention can be seen from the use of available services in maternal and child health, as illustrated in Table 51-1.

Evidence of government intervention over the past 22 years shows that significant progress has been made toward improving the quality of life of Batswana through the implementation of comprehensive and integrated national health plans. Through a systematic collaboration and integration of existing health systems (namely, government, missions, private, and traditional), a partnership in the provision of primary health care services has been achieved in Botswana. The government has also taken full responsibility for financing the bulk of national health services as well as for the training of health care personnel. For example, by the end of the fifth plan (1980 to 1985) 2017 more multidisciplinary healthworkers were trained in Botswana, and projections are for another 2312 to be trained during the current sixth plan (1986 to 1991).

ISSUES EMERGING FROM GOVERNMENT INTERVENTION AND POLITICAL ORIENTATION

1. The average Motswana has become aware of the benefits of using available health services. Batswana have also learned to regard health as an important element of social development. They have thus become more aware of the need to invest in disease-prevention and health-promotion services (rather than in sophisticated curative services). The demand for the services has increased drastically, and the supply will soon be unable to meet the demand. How will government respond to the demand? What alternatives are open to the government?

2. Along with the government's decision to recognize the existence of traditional medicine and its role in the provision of primary health care services is a need to provide information on the safety and effectiveness of traditional health care. The government has to consider the ethical and professional implications of its decision to support traditional medicine.

3. The government has resolved to invest more resources in the provision of primary health care services to ensure that health care is equitably distributed throughout Botswana. This is in keeping with the development principle of social justice.

On the other hand, Botswana has an emerging group of affluent citizens, some of whom hold key positions in the public and private sector, who are pressing the government to invest in highly sophisticated curative, care-centered hospitals that would be located mainly in urban areas. Invariably these services would cater to only a few, and only the wealthy would be in a position to afford them. It is argued that these sophisticated services will reduce the country's dependence for such services on South Africa. How will government respond to such pressures? Will the government be guided by the effective health-planning process, or will it yield to the political pressure? Will the government strive to sustain the momentum achieved in primary health care development, or will it change direction? What would be the consequences of changing direction?

4. The government has embarked on an aggressive policy of decentralizing the provision of health services at the district level. The local authorities and communities are destined to play a leading role in planning, implementing, and evaluating health services. Will the Ministry of Health hand over the control and management of health services to the local authorities, or will it continue to orchestrate and direct primary health care services from its headquarters? Where will primary health care decisions be made? Are local authorities truly in control of district health care?

5. Whereas the government of Botswana encourages strong community participation in the provision of primary health care services, health personnel in Botswana see themselves as leaders in the provision of health care. As such, they regard themselves as the main source of information on health issues. How can the government achieve full community participation in the development of primary health care services as well as reduce professional dominance?

6. The government has continued to finance all forms of health service. Patients pay a nominal fee of 40 thebe (approximately 25 cents in U.S. currency) for inpatient and outpatient services. This includes hospitalization, food, medication, investigation, and treatment.

Will the government be able to continue financing services at the existing level? The population of Botswana is projected to reach 2 million by the year 2001. This raises the issue of cost containment in providing health care. So far the government has discouraged the privatization of health services. Will rising medical costs and an increase in population influence government decisions in favor of privatization? What would be the impact of such a decision on the provision of primary health care services?

PRIORITIES AND PLANS FOR GOVERNMENT INTERVENTION IN THE FUTURE
Strengthening personnel/management

Although Botswana has invested a lot in the training and development of health-workers, especially in nurs-ing, large shortfalls exist in skilled health personnel. Nurses form the backbone of the health care system and provide strong leadership in the provision of integrated health care. The challenge for the government lies in the development of a more effective health personnel management system to ensure that the existing limited national health personnel resources are effectively utilized, motivated, and retained within the health system. An improved system of incentives, provision of continuing education, training in leadership development, and improvement of working conditions should be initiated to enhance staff morale and increase productivity levels. Currently very little attention is being paid to such important issues, and as a result a number of competent nurses have left the health services. The government must realize that individual job satisfaction is a crucial element in the retention of effective and committed health care providers.

New approaches to health-sector planning

To date the goals and targets of national health plans have focused entirely on community health needs to the exclusion of the health providers who are the main instruments for translating the plans into concrete action. No deliberate strategies as such have been developed to accommodate the personal growth and social needs of health providers. Soon Botswana will have a revolt within the health services. The government will have to adopt recipient- as well as provider-oriented health development plans.

Although the government has commendable health plans, care should be taken to ensure that these plans not only focus on identified existing problems but also anticipate problems likely to emerge in the future, and anticipate possible solutions as well. For example, if our primary health care service focuses on reducing infant mortality, malnutrition, and infectious diseases as well as on increasing life expectancy, then government should plan for an older population and the consequences for health needs of such a population. To take another example, if the government promotes rapid economic growth and development, the health sector should prepare to cope with health problems related to modernization, such as stress, accidents, disabilities, alcoholism, and substance abuse.

Although government interventions have been in the right direction and achievements have been registered in several areas, complacency with the current levels of planning and intervention may slow down the momentum. On the other hand, government may wish to reconsider its priorities in line with the rapidly changing health scene.

BIBLIOGRAPHY

Ministry of Finance and Development Planning: National development plan 1986–1991. Gaborone, 1986, Government Printer, p.307.

Ministry of Finance and Development Planning: National development plan 1979–1985. Gaborone, 1980, Government Printer, p.259.

Ministry of Health: Manual of health services. Gaborone, 1979, Government Printer, p.37-41.

Ministry of Finance and Development Planning: National development plan 1976–1971. Gaborone, 1977, Government Printer, p.237-238.

Ministry of Health: Medical Statistics Gaborone Central Statistics Office, 1978/79.

Ministry of Health. 1977 Medical statistics. Gaborone, 1977, Government Printer, p.20-25.

Ngcongco, VN: Family-centered approaches to the provision of comprehensive healthcare for primary healthcare services. Implications for the development and design of training programmes for health workers in Botswana. (Doctoral Dissertation University of South Africa, 1988).

World Health Organisation: Alma-Ata Declaration. Geneva, 1978, World Health Organisation.

PART EIGHT

COST-EFFECTIVENESS

Nursing economics

JOANNE COMI McCLOSKEY
HELEN KENNEDY GRACE

Economics is a concern for all health care providers in these times. More than ever, nursing is concerned about the cost and price of its services. In the debate chapter Grace addresses the pressing problem of rising health care costs. The implementation of prospective payment was supposed to halt the risk in costs, but has not. While health care costs consume 12.7% of the gross national product, one in four Americans is uninsured or underinsured and many people are in poor health. Grace argues that medical costs, in fact, cannot be controlled and that alternatives to medical care are needed to contain health care costs. She reviews four factors contributing to the escalation of medical costs: an excess of hospital beds, physician influence over costs, insurance plans that benefit hospitals and physicians rather than patients, and lack of consumer involvement in health care decisions. Grace proposes four ways to contain health care costs: restructuring health care services, breaking the monopoly of hospitals and physicians, emphasizing health promotion and disease prevention instead of disease treatment, and increasing the mix of health care providers with expander opportunities for nurses and paraprofessionals. Nursing is capable of providing high quality, cost-effective care both inside and outside hospitals, particularly to those populations most in need—the elderly and the poor. If nurses are to become part of the solution, they need to take an active role in reshaping the health care system and in collectively addressing barriers such as reimbursement and practice constraints.

Continuing this theme of change and restructuring, Maraldo addresses the question, How can nurses prepare for the new order in this era of health care deregulation? As the title of her chapter indicates, the aftermath of DRGs brings a time of transformation. First, she outlines the positive forces working in favor of nursing. These include the fact that nursing has a new opportunity to work closely with consumer groups to gain a position of greater influence. Maraldo discusses three problems that continue to fuel health care expenditures: overutilization of hospital care and costly technology, the cost of treating AIDS patients, and the cost of caring for an aging population. The most pressing health care problems are chronic and require primarily nursing, not medical, care. She cites many examples of the inadequacies of the medical model. She challenges nursing to develop a strategy that gives attention to "pressure points": concern for costs, shifting of care to the community, changing demographics, concern for quality, and the gender gap. Maraldo outlines a three-track strategy: positioning, reimbursement, and politics. Her vision positions nurses in the public's mind as case managers and has nurses contracting with hospitals for services. Her analysis of the situation seems correct, but her solutions require skilled and risk-taking nursing leaders and individual practitioners. Are we ready?

The importance of identifying nursing costs is evident in efforts since DRG implementation to "cost out nursing service." Scherubel briefly reviews the history of nursing in this area and then reviews several methods used to identify the costs of direct (hands-on) nursing care. These include relative intensity measures (RIMs), nursing care categories, the GRASP classification system, patient management categories, nursing diagnoses, and the Nursing Intensity Index. Scherubel also points out that there are many methods for measuring indirect costs such as nursing support services and institutional overhead costs. She discusses the value of knowing nursing costs and spells out dilemmas and future needs. Her chapter includes an impressive reference list that those interested in studying or determining nursing costs will find helpful.

In the succeeding chapter, Fralic and Brett link efforts to identify costs to recent concerns about quality. Readers may want to read this chapter in conjunction with those in Part Five on quality assurance. According to Fralic and Brett, "The basic premise underlying contemporary health care services is that desired levels of quality must be achieved at acceptable levels of cost." First, they examine six quality and six cost elements of a nursing management system. Readers will find their choices helpful and may want to discuss the implications of choosing these rather than others. Next, they describe a theoretical model of these elements and report the results of a study testing the model. The study was conducted on one unit at their hospital and the chapter includes the actual measures used for each element. Several of the relationships were not in the predicted direction and some demonstrate the problems of measuring these variables. However, this illustrates the great need for similar research to identify the important variables to measure for accurate information about cost and quality. All nurse administrators and researchers should read this chapter. The model could and should be tested in many other places. Are we ready?

Efforts to determine costs have moved beyond the inpatient acute-care setting. In the following chapter, Alfano discusses payment of health services in long-term care. Chronic illness poses a particular challenge to the health care system because patient needs are not constant and the type of assistance that is necessary varies. She says that long-term care is not high tech but high skill. By and large, however, the best-prepared nurses and physicians have not seen long-term care as an exciting specialty. Alfano outlines several cost issues in long-term and home health care. She challenges readers to examine whether several existing methods—for example, the multidisciplinary approach to care—are really necessary and cost effective. Like Gamroth and Smith in Part Five, she wants to refocus the purposes of the long-term care facility to be more residential than clinicial. Alfano points out that people do not have the same needs for care and asks why it is necessary to have one plan for everyone. She would like to see the government and its regulations exit from the health care field. At the end of her chapter she proposes that nurses grapple with the difficult questions related to rationing of care. Students in issues courses may want to address the increasingly important notion of rationed care in a class debate.

The issue of government involvement in paying for health care costs is addressed by Biscoe in the concluding chapter. She says that the degree to which an individual agrees with the national approach to health care depends on that individual's perspectives. No country can please all its citizens. There may be an infinite demand for health care, but what direction should governments take in fulfilling this demand? Biscoe takes a world view, reviewing the health care and financing patterns of several countries: Singapore, Poland, Denmark, Belgium, West Germany, Japan, Canada, France, and Switzerland. Readers will find it interesting to compare the health care practices of these countries with their own. Few nations, says Biscoe, know what they are trying to buy for their health care money, and strategic plans for health care are noticeably lacking. She points out that politics is a major variable in any plan and no one model is right for all countries.

Taken together, the chapters in this part raise many interesting health care issues and related challenges for nursing. A partial list might include rationed care, government involvement in health care, focus of long-term care facilities and types of practitioners for the chronically ill aged, reliable measures of quality and cost, nurses as case managers, and relationships with physicians. Nursing's ability to identify and deal with economic issues has come a long way in the past few years. There is still much to do. Are we ready?

CHAPTER 52

Debate

Can health care costs be contained?

HELEN KENNEDY GRACE

Currently the costs of health care in the United States continue to rise at a rate of 10% per year—a rate far exceeding the inflation rate of the rest of the country. Health care costs consume 12.7% of the gross national product (GNP) and are expected to rise to 15% by the end of the century. In contrast, costs of health care in Canada consume about 7% of the GNP. The increasing consumption of the GNP for health care services means that resources are being shifted from other areas of need, such as housing, social services, or defense, to cover the increase in costs of health care. Despite the alarming rise in health care costs, the general public seems remarkably unconcerned. As Reinhardt[10] notes:

The notion continues to spread that health care is one of those commodities to which every citizen in a civilized society is entitled regardless of ability to pay. This sentiment now threatens to engulf *all* technically available health care regardless of its costs.

Despite the continued rise in costs of health care, it is estimated that 65 million Americans, or 1 in 4, are either uninsured or underinsured. Thirty-five million Americans have neither private nor public insurance and another 30 million have minimal or only seasonal coverage.

With the high rate of expenditure for health care in the United States, the health of the population as measured by a number of standards is not good. For example, a 1987 report by the Children's Defense Fund[4] summarizes 10 key findings about the health of America's children:

1. U.S. progress in reducing overall infant mortality is at a virtual standstill.
2. The U.S. infant mortality ranking among 20 industrialized nations declined from sixth in the 1950 to 1955 period to a tie for last place in 1980 to 1985.
3. Black infants continue to die at nearly twice the rate of white infants.
4. Between 1983 and 1984 infant mortality rates increased in 20 of America's 22 largest cities.
5. After a nationwide increase in 1983, 1984 postneonatal mortality rates declined only back to the unacceptable 1982 levels.
6. There were enormous geographic variations in 1984 in the survival rates of infants.
7. In 1984, for the fifth consecutive year, there was no progress in reducing the percentage of infants born to women who received late or no prenatal care.
8. At the current rate of progress, the nation and the states will fail to meet nearly all of the Surgeon General's 1990 objectives for reducing infant mortality, the number of low-birthweight births, and the number of women who receive late or no prenatal care.
9. Teenage childbearing was a nationwide problem in 1984 that contributed disproportionately to the prevalence of low-birthweight births and stagnating infant rates.
10. Vital maternal and child health and nutrition programs are decreasing while maternal and child health needs are increasing.

Although this is but one area, assessment of progress in meeting health goals for the nation for 1990 points to similar problems in the areas of adolescent health, health of minorities of all age groups, and in health of the elderly.

Given this situation, this chapter will first argue that health care costs (largely for medical care) cannot be controlled. Restructuring health care services, breaking the monopoly of hospitals and physicians on the medical care marketplace, an emphasis on health promotion and disease prevention, and expanded opportunities for nurses and paraprofessionals in the delivery of health care as opposed to medical care, offer the only viable long-term solutions

THE HIGH COST OF MEDICAL CARE

There are four major contributors to the escalating costs of medical care: (1) the overcapacity of hospitals, (2) the surplus of highly specialized providers, (3) the financing of health care services, and (4) the role of the health care consumer.

Hospitals

Early hospitals were designed to care for those without family members to assume the responsibilities of medical and nursing care. These institutions were directed toward patient *care* rather than *cure*. Particularly after World War II, with accompaning advances in technology and anesthesia, the focus of hospitals was on cure, and the care function was deemphasized. As Renn[11] notes:

The Hill-Burton program, begun in 1946, provided a massive infusion of federal and state governmental monies, and helped construct over 400,000 hospital beds between then and the early 1970s. The most current data indicate that there are now just under 5800 community hospitals containing nearly 1 million beds. Community hospitals admitted slightly less than 36 million patients in 1985 . . . with an average length of stay of 7.4 days. The average hospital's occupancy rate, a measure of the industry's capacity being utilized, was 64%. Hospitals now employ 3.6 million people, or about one out of every thirty U.S. workers.

Until 1977 there was a continuing increase in demand for hospital beds. The demand then plateaued until 1982, and since that time there has been a steady decline in both number of admissions and length of stay in hospitals. Renn[11] attributes this decline to four factors:

1. The change in incentives that has resulted from moving from a retrospective reimbursement system that paid for actual costs of treatment that were incurred to a prospective payment system that provides payment based upon average costs of treatment for patients within a particular diagnostic category;
2. Growth in capitated financing arrangements that provide disincentives for admitting patients to hospitals;
3. A proliferation of treatment settings that can serve as substitutes for hospitalization; and
4. The increased burden of cost sharing which shifts part of the cost of care directly to the patient.

Despite the decrease in utilization of hospitals, profit of the overall hospital industry has increased. Schramm[12] reports; "Although hospital occupancy declined by 12% in the first year of prospective payment, profits doubled and reached record levels. In 1984,

hospital profits were 6.2% of total revenues—3 times higher than a decade earlier."

How can the increase in hospital profitability be explained? First, the estimated costs of treatment for diagnostic-related groups (DRGs) exceeded the actual costs and certain hospitals profited from the treatment of particular categories of patients. Fast patient turnover increases the profitability of hospitals. Three patients hospitalized for ten days generate more income than one person hospitalized for thirty days. And even though fewer hospital beds are being occupied, most hospitals remain open. Costs of patient care cover the overhead involved in keeping these facilities open and are included in the rate-setting formulas. Renn[11] estimates that in 1984 there was an excess of 140,000 beds, or roughly 800 average-sized community hospitals. Despite a decline in patient numbers, the costs of care remain fairly constant because of the costs of keeping hospitals open.

The decline in numbers of hospitalized patients has been achieved in some instances by keeping out those patients likely to be most costly, by shifting costs for the care of patients from private nonprofit hospitals to public hospitals, and by early discharge of patients, thus shifting costs from the hospital onto the family and community.

Physician influence on health care costs

Although the fees charged by physicians for services account for only 20% of medical costs, decisions made by physicians represent 80% of expenditures. As Eisenberg[1] notes:

Physicians serve a dual role in the provision of health services. Like the player-manager of an athletic team, the physician is responsible for calling the plays in medical care as well as working with others to carry them out. In the parlance of economics, this dual role means that the physician influences the cost and quality of medical care in two ways: first, by organizing and directing the production process; and second, by providing some of the productive output.

Physicians make decisions as to when patients are to be hospitalized, for how long, and the treatments to be employed. Decisions about diagnostic tests and therapeutic regimes are all part of physician decision-making. Hospitals, in many ways, have become the physician's workshop, and the tools for doing physician work are provided by the hospital.

Factors contributing to the escalating costs of health

care are the increase in physician numbers and the high incomes of physicians. In noting that health care costs in the United states are three times that of Britain and five times that of Japan, Menzel[7] raises the questions of whether that money is well spent and whether doctors should be "more than equal." Noting that physician salaries are twice and sometimes up to five times those of other professionals with equal training, he quotes George Bernard Shaw[13]: "That any sane nation, having observed that one could provide for the supply of bread by giving bakers pecuniary interest in baking for you, should go on to give a surgeon a pecuniary interest in cutting off your leg, is enough to make one despair of political humanity." Menzel[7] concludes; "It is utterly hypocritical for doctors, health care administrators, academic analysts, and policymakers to close their eyes to the level of doctors' income amidst an otherwise vigorous concern for making health care worth the increasing money we pay for it."

Under normal marketplace conditions an increase in the supply of physicians would drive their income downward and would also address another problem, that of physician maldistribution. For example, Massachusetts has 308 physicians per 100,000 residents, whereas Mississippi has less than half that number, 122 physicians per 100,000 residents. A Michigan study of the health professions indicates that increases in the total number of physicians results in a concentration of physicians in urban areas. The costs of medical care rise in proportion to the number of physicians practicing in an area. While in Michigan the number of physicians has increased dramatically since 1960, there are more Michigan counties without physicians in 1985 than there were in 1960.[8]

One of the reasons for the escalation of costs is greater physician specialization. The more highly specialized the physician, the higher the consumption rate of health care services to support specialty practice. Renn[11] cautions:

If physicians continue to make most of the allocative decisions in the delivery system, if the emphasis on treatment in acute-care inpatient settings persists, and if payment mechanisms continue to insulate physicians from the financial risks associated with their decisions—then growth in the supply of physicians will probably translate into corresponding growth in health care spending.

One of the problems related to physician decision making and health care costs is that the physician holds

that the physician-client relationship is "sacred" and that no one should interfere with the physician's right to care for each individual patient, including ordering the tests and treatments defined as necessary for good patient care without regard to their costs. However, the physician is looking at care only in terms of the individual patients and does not have to weigh the treatment of those individual patients against the broader issue of the needs of all patients. The individual child in need of a kidney transplant to survive can garner considerable support for expensive treatment, while the large number of homeless are often held responsible for their plight and therefore are considered not worthy of treatment. Because the homeless do not make their way through the doctor's office door, the doctor does not need to consider them in making his or her treatment choices.

Financing medical care services

A further complication in controlling health care costs concerns the way medical care services are financed. Payment for health services usually comes from some third party rather than from the individual's direct payments to hospitals or physicians. Public payers—federal, state, or local governments—paid for slightly more than 40% of health care expenditures in 1985, while private insurance supplied an additional 31%. Direct out-of-pocket payments by patients accounted for 27%.

One of the unique features of U.S. health care financing is the role of private insurance. Started in 1929, the Blue Cross plans became a major force in the financing of medical care. These plans were originally provider-based and involved service agreements with all the providers in an area. Fein[3] clarifies: "Blue Cross and similar plans were brought into being by the hospital representatives with active support of the AHA . . . acting in response to serious problems they and their patients faced: how should hospital bills be paid and how should stable hospital revenues be assured?" The insurance plans were largely for the benefit of hospitals and physicians rather than for the welfare of patients.

The interlocking relationships between physicians, hospitals, and insurers have dominated decision making regarding the financing of health care. Rather than the interests of the patient constituting a primary consideration, the economic well-being of hospitals and physicians has been a priority. Renn[11] notes, "Physicians and hospital representatives often dominate the plans' boards of directors and saw the plans, like most participants, as a means of ensuring the financial solvency of the community's providers." Blue Cross established the approach of reimbursing hospitals on a retrospective, cost-plus basis, thus building in disincentives for economy. Payment of bills related to hospitalization also provided incentives for physicians to hospitalize patients and thus contributed to the overbuilding of hospital facilities.

Another complicating aspect has been the ability of insurance companies to link with businesses so that the provision of health insurance became a major part of the benefits paid to workers. Thus the provision of health care insurance began to be expected by employees as part of their benefits thereby assuring the eocnomic viability of hospitals and physicians. Until recent years the employer has accepted this obligation, but now costs have escalated to a point beyond the ability of many employers to pay. Currently 10% of the cost of an American automobile goes to pay the health care costs of workers. Employers are saying that they can no longer pay these costs and are requiring employees pay a portion of their own health care expenses. This factor is considered partially responsible for reduced use of health care services. Initiated in 1966, the Medicare program provides a number of health care benefits to the elderly covered by the Social Security system. Twenty-eight percent of the income of hospitals currently comes from Medicare. Medicare extended the concepts established by Blue Cross-Blue Shield for working people and the elderly and gave the responsibility of financing these services to the federal government. Thus public funding was used to support the private services offered by physicians and hospitals:

Medicare paid hospitals retrospectively on the basis of the costs incurred by covered beneficiaries at participating providers and paid physicians their reasonable, customary, and prevailing fees. While originally resisted by organized medicine as an instance of the federal government becoming an intervening force between the physician and his or her patient, Medicare payments have become a major source of income for both physicians and hospitals. In addition to paying physicians and hospitals, Medicare became a major stimulant for capital growth without reference to community needs and priorities or regional planning efforts.[3]

Although insurers of public sources pay for over 70% of health care costs, as Renn[11] points out, "Ul-

timately individuals pay for all health care expenditures: While health care is financed by a mix of public and private payers, the original sources of funds are the consumers, workers, and taxpayers, with the dollars taking merely different routes to the providers." Although the process is not directly visible, health care is paid for out of reduced wages for workers or increased taxes for the taxpayers. If this is so, why are consumers not more involved in the debates about reducing health care costs?

Consumer participation

Because much of the cost of care for those without adequate insurance coverage was paid for by overcharging for the actual costs of care, much of this cost was subsidized by insurers and directly by other consumers. This was a hidden problem up until the change to a prospective payment system. Now the costs of care for the uninsured and underinsured cannot be paid for in this way. As a result, some worry that a two-, three-, or four-tiered system of medical care is emerging. Thurow[14] has labeled 3 levels as follows: one for people on government assistance, one for people with health care insurance, and another for the wealthy who can afford the private health care market. To this Reinhardt has added a 4th tier at the bottom for indigent patients who have no insurance.[10] The results of this separation into tiers are that

each tier is increasingly forced to care for its own patients using only the resources available to that tier. And as each lower tier is less well funded than that above, a serious question arises: should physicians still be expected to deliver the (roughly) same standard of care to all patients regardless of their resources?[6]

As this debate regarding differential treatment dependent on ability to pay emerges, it is important to bear in mind that despite perceived lack of resources, the health care costs continue to escalate far beyond other costs in our economy.

Because physicians and hospitals primarily control medical care, the consumer has little or no choice over the types of treatment received. Although options exist in every situation, the consumer often is purposely kept ignorant of these options and therefore the decision-making control is in the hands of the provider. As a result, the most costly form of treatment is usually that provided. The consumer assumes that "the doctor knows best" and rarely challenges the prescriptions that are made. Reinhardt[9] observes that although physicians resist the intrusion of government into their relationships with patients, they are not averse to using regulations to restrict the practice of other, less expensive health care professionals.

He recommneds a litmus test for marketers that ask questions such as whether one favors dental practitioners who practice prophylaxis or pediatric nurse practitioners delivering well-child care, concluding:

As is well known, the organized medical and dental professions have so far answered all questions on the test in the negative, and they have never failed to engage the coercive powers of the government—in the forms of licensure laws—in imposing their view on this matter on the rest of society. These providers, then, do not oppose government intervention in principle. Rather their opposition to such intervention has always been judiciously selective, and has certainly not extended to interventions, such as mandatory licensures that serve to enhance the market power of these professions.

Reinhardt further points out that physicians' argument is always that they are protecting the public from low-quality care. Even if it could be demonstrated that other practitioners provide inferior care (and indeed the evidence shows quite the contrary), should not the consumer have the option of choosing such care as a trade-off against high cost? Information is systematically withheld from the consumer, who is unaware of less costly forms of care. Restriction of licensure and the control of payment to other service providers further constrains less costly care.

The public is becoming increasingly more knowledgeable about the issues related to costs of health care. Health care professionals are confronted by hard choices: Do we continue to address problems of health care costs by withholding services from those who cannot pay? What are the long-range consequences of this approach? What is the legacy to future generations if we opt to deny services that could prevent illness and instead pay the costs associated with chronic illness and disability? Fein[3] summarizes the challenges:

Health care and the way we pay for it is a matter of efficiency, and today's sytem is inefficient. Health care and the way we pay for it is a matter of equity, and today's system is inequitable. We can do better; and, since we can, we should. Will we? It depends upon whether enough of us are concerned about costs, recognize that a less costly system will free resources for other private and public purposes, and support the notion of health care budgets. It also depends upon whether enough of us care enough to work at

translating concepts of decentness, humaneness, cooperation, universality, and justice into actions that would protect all members of the American family. At stake is not only our health care system, but the very nature of our society. While it may appear that in this scenario the consumer is a passive participant, the health care dilemma has indeed been consumer driven and is a reflection of (1) the American inclination to prefer being "fixed" as opposed to "avoiding getting broken," and (2) the American inclination to deify doctors and to assume that the most expensive advice/care is the best. This fascination with high technology continues to fuel the system and technology creates its own demand.

FROM MEDICAL CARE TO HEALTH CARE

Entohoven and Kronick[2] have characterized the situation of rising health care costs and decreased access as a "paradox of excess and deprivation." Although it is possible to describe the current situation in great detail, what are the avenues for addressing the problem? Two recent proposals have been set forth and have received widespread attention, particularly in the medical community.

Enthoven and Kronick[2] have proposed universal health insurance coupled with managed competition in which the insurers (private and public) contract with competing health plans to "manage a process of informed cost-conscious consumer choice that rewards providers who deliver high-quality care economically." The costs of implementing their plan would be a one-time increase of $15 billion in additional costs in the first year (3% of GNP). In the long term this approach is projected to decrease the rate of escalation of health care costs, but does not hold forth the promise of decreased cost.

An alternative approach, "a national health program for the United States," has been proposed by Himmelstein and White[5] on behalf of a working group of physicians. The central elements of this proposal are summarized as follows:

We propose a national health program that would (1) fully cover everyone under a single, comprehensive public insurance program; (2) pay hospitals and nursing homes a total (global) annual amount to cover all operating expenses: (3) fund capital costs through separate appropriations; (4) pay for physicians' services and ambulatory services in any of three ways: through fee-for-service payments with a simplified fee schedule and mandatory acceptance of the national health program as the total payment for a service or procedure (assigment), through global budgets for hospitals or clinics, or on a per capita basis (capitation); (5) be funded, at least initially, from the same sources as at present with all payments disbursed from a single pool; and (6) contain costs through saving on billing and bureaucracy, improved health planning, and the ability of the national program, as the single payer for services, to establish overall funding limits.

It is important to note that this proposal does not address any changes in either hospital or physician practice, but merely proposes a way of paying for them. Nor does this proposal address payments other than those for physicians, hospitals, and nursing homes.

Although both proposals contain very important strategies for paying for the high cost of medical care, it is important to bear in mind that both continue to emphasize the interests of the *providers*, the hospitals and physicians, in how bills will be paid for business as usual; the interests of the consumer for more appropriate care are secondary. In addition, these proposals continue to focus on *medical* care. Although the terminology *health care* is used, these proposals do not address broader issues of health care. Some might argue that truly expanding the definition from medical to health care would further escalate the problem, but an alternative argument is that if health care were provided, the medical care system would be used more appropriately, thereby reducing costs.

Medical care focuses on the diagnosis and treatment of disease, whereas health care has as its aim the well-being of the individual and family at an optimal level of health. Within this broader framework, individuals and their families have primary responsibility for maintaining health with support from health care specialists. Although individuals still will experience illnesses that require expert care and treatment, a broader orientation to health care would result in earlier identification of problems at less acute stages, and therefore treatments would be less costly. Furthermore, a reduction in the incidence of chronic diseases, most of which are preventable, and maintenance of mobility as people age would do much to reduce costs of care in the long run. For example, in the area of maternal-child care there is growing evidence that early, comprehensive prenatal care, including provision for adequate nutrition, social services support, and health education, results in reduced infant mortality rates, increased infant birthweight, and fewer mentally or physically damaged infants. Rough data drawn from one mid-size community indicate that the provision of such comprehensive services to about 500

uninsured and underinsured mothers by a nurse-managed clinic using nurse-midwives will cost about $250,000 over the available compensation for such care from both public and private sources. However, the local community hospital has experienced a total decline in demand for a neonatal intensive care unit, a "savings" to the hospital of $650,000. Although simple mathematical calculations would lead to the conclusion that $400,000 had been saved, from a provider perspective (hospitals and physicians) the conclusion is somewhat different. The hospital looks at this situation as a loss of revenue, in that the $650,000 previously spent on neonatal intensive care was collectible revenue. From the physician's point of view, these "savings" were largely a result of services provided by nutritionists, social workers, nurses, and midwives. Physician revenues, for both obstetrical and pediatric care were reduced.

Similar examples can be drawn from the areas of well-child care, women's health, and care of the elderly. Returning responsibility for health care to the individual and family, engaging a wide range of specialists in supportive roles to the individual and family, demystifying health and illness through education of the public, and appropriate use of the capacity of the medical care system to treat only acute diseases are the only long-range solutions to the problem of escalating medical care costs.

What are the steps toward change in this direction? There need to be some carefully controlled demonstration projects, such as the one described above, that illustrate the benefits to be achieved by comprehensive *health* care. Examples of such studies are beginning to appear in the literature. Generating data, however, is merely the first step. These data must then be made known to those who pay the bills,—ultimately, everyone in the United States. In the scenario related to prenatal care, nothing will change for the community if the financing for expanded prenatal care to create this degree of long-range improvement is left to the discretion of the providers. These data need to be translated and publicized so that community members know the choices that are open to them and ultimately can make informed decisions as to how health care is to be provided. In this community the $400,000 (not to mention the savings in terms of long-range human suffering resulting from brain-damaged infants) saved through adequate prenatal care could result in fewer dollars going for insurance, either directly or indirectly, and could be redirected toward other pressing societal issues such as adequate housing for the homeless.

Nurses have a crucial role to play in creating change. First, movement from a medical care system to health care requires nursing intervention and leadership. Nurses can set up the demonstrations that lead to necessary data, and can publicize these findings for individuals and policymakers. Ultimately citizen action is the only force to create change in a democracy. Nursing has the capacity to educate the consumer to create such changes.

A second essential component is to articulate the components of health care, enlist individual responsibility for maintenance of health, and clearly describe the supportive roles of health specialists, including nurses, in promoting individual health. The myth that anything less than care provided by physicians is second best must be dispelled. In fact, there is mounting evidence that the physician is perhaps the least qualified to provide *health* care.

To take this role in educating consumers, nurses must first have confidence in the ability of the individual to participate in health care, and nurses must have confidence in themselves to provide support to the individual in promoting health. At the heart of change is the need for consumer education, and nurses have the expertise to provide this education.

What hinders this type of change? Nurses have been socialized to be co-conspirators with hospitals and doctors in maintaining the current medical care system. They have been reticent to let the public know of the unnecessary and invasive high-technology procedures that are being done every day in the interests of the medical care system. Nurses are intimidated and fear the loss of their jobs when the hospital is their main employer and all avenues for practice independent of physicians or hospitals are constricted. With nurses comprising the largest number of health care workers in the United States (an estimated 1.8 million), the profession has the collective capacity to speak with one loud voice. However, one of the largest constraints lies within the profession itself and its inability to mobilize this potential for change on behalf of the consumer. Energies have become focused on the profession itself rather than on the broader issues of health care. Fragmentation of the profession results in a feeling of abandonment on the part of nurses engaged in practice, who perceive the leadership as preoccupied with the self-interests of the profession. If nurses unite on the ground of a common concern for health care for all people at an affordable cost, they can join with consumers to create such change and thereby "heal" themselves.

In summary, change is possible but unlikely. Such change depends on (1) a fundamental change in focus from a medical care delivery system to participatory health care for people, (2) breaking the monopoly of hospitals, physicians, and insurers in the decision-making process that preserves the current system, (3) engaging the consumer in assuming greater responsibility for personal health and decision making regarding broader health policy issues, and (4) greater involvement of nurses and other health-related specialists in joining with the consumer in supportive roles and relationships emphasizing health promotion and disease prevention. Nurses are central in making the difference. The ability to become one strong voice on behalf of the American public is essential if nursing is to be a force for positive change.

REFERENCES

1. Eisenberg JW: Doctors' decisions and the cost of medical care, "Health Administration Press Perspectives", Ann Arbor, MI, 1986.
2. Enthoven A and Kronick R: A consumer-choice health plan for the 1990s, N Engl J Med 320(1):30, 1989.
3. Fein R: Medical care, medical costs: search for a health insurance policy, Cambridge, Mass, 1986, Harvard University Press.
4. Hughes D et al: The health of america's children, Washington, DC, 1987, Children's Defense Fund.
5. Himmelstein DU and Woolhandler S: N Engl J Med 320(2):102.
6. Maureim EH: Cost containment: challenging fidelity and justice; Hastings Center Report 18(6):22, 1988.
7. Menzel PT: Medical costs, moral choices, New Haven, Conn, 1983, Yale University Press.
8. Michigan State Health Plan 1983-1987, vol III, Health personnel.
9. Reinhardt UW: Health insurance and cost-containment policies: the experience abroad. In Olson M, editor: A new approach to the economics of health care, Washington, DC and London, 1981, American Enterprise Institute for Public Policy Research.
10. Reinhardt UW: Health insurance for the nation's poor, Health Aff 6(1): 101, 1987.
11. Renn S: Health care delivery in the 1980s. In Schramm C, editor: Health care and its costs: can the United States afford adequate health care? New York, 1987, WW Norton & Co.
12. Schramm CJ and Gabel J: Prospective payment: some retrospective observations, N Engl J Med 318(25):1682, 1988.
13. Shaw GB: The doctor's dilemma (preface). New York, 1981, Garland.
14. Thurow LC: Medicine vs. economics, N Engl J Med 313(10):611, 1985.

CHAPTER 53

Viewpoints

The aftermath of DRGs

The politics of transformation

PAMELA J. MARALDO

Over the past several years health care in the United States has entered a period of fundamental change. After decades of soaring health costs, major change in health care began when The Reagan administration tried to fix the problem and rectify the ills of a system built on the assumption of unlimited resources. So a prospective system of payment to hospitals was enacted and hospitals are now given a certain amount for diseases they treat. After much ado about diagnosis-related groups DRGs, economists such as Eli Ginsberg and Jeffrey Merrill assert that little more has been done than shuffling the deck chairs. That is, in real terms health care inflation has barely abated. In fact, health care inflation is currently increasing at a rate three to four times that of general inflation. Yet the era of DRGs has precipitated revolutionary change in health care and greater changes are yet to come. All the major players in health care have been fundamentally affected, including consumers and of course nurses.

This new method of payment has thrust the U.S. system of health care into deregulation, just like the airlines or the banking or communications industries. The United States is on the verge of developing a true health care marketplace where anything goes. But the crux of what has happened can be summed up in one major change: the centers of power have shifted from the providers of health care to consumers and others who pay the bills—the primary purchasers of care being business, industry, and third-party payers.

There have already been political winners and losers under the new payment system. Physicians, who have always been the captains of the health care ship, are threatened because they are now in the position of having their costly practice patterns monitored and altered because of spending excesses. There has been tremendous turnover among hospital administrators in recent years because administrators are under increasing pressure to maintain a healthy revenue stream in the face of federal policy directed at reducing costly acute care. They also are facing increasing competition from new provider arrangements such as preferred provider organizations (PPOs), health maintenance organizations (HMOs), and community nursing organizations (CNOs). Physicians and hospital administrators are fighting because hospital administrators are forced to control medicine's costly behavior. To make matters worse, the entire industry is caught in the middle of the worst nursing supply crisis it has witnessed since World War II, and there is no end in sight. Clearly things are not business as usual in health care. The question remains, how can nurses prepare for the new order of things? How can nurses influence the politics of transformation to work to their advantage?

It is helpful to keep in mind the positive effects of the changes in health care in assessing the health care climate and nursing's position in it.

- These political battles and the crisis in health care are positive forces for the nursing community. In any system, whenever those holding power are challenged, others have a chance to make strides and gain influence. The major power holders in health care—physicians and hospitals—are being challenged to relinquish decision-making power to consumer agents or to those who pay the bills. Now that consumers have more to say about health care decisions, nursing has a new opportunity to work closely with consumer groups and to gain a position of greater influence in health policy decision making.

- Nurses are in high demand. The reason for the present severe nursing shortage is that better-prepared nurses are in increasingly greater demand.
- Diversification of the health care marketplace into new forms of health care is good for nursing—because nursing's options have increased. Prior to DRGs nurses worked almost exclusively in hospitals. Since DRGs, nursing's employment options have increased substantially to include new opportunities in home care, HMOs, PPOs, or independent practice. These opportunities existed before DRGs, but not to the same degree.

In addition, nursing as a discipline is older and wiser now. Since the enactment of DRGs, nursing has learned many difficult lessons. Diminishing resources have created a heated political climate in health care. As a consequence, national nursing organizations have had to learn that it is essential to cooperate and to take unified policy positions. There has indeed been much greater accord among nursing organizations on important policy issues in recent years.

Through the Kellogg-sponsored National Commission on Nursing Implementation project, representatives from the nursing community have also had the unprecedented opportunity in recent years to work with key leaders from other sectors in health care to discuss and debate important policy issues such as the concerns of the business community over costs, cost and quality concerns of insurers, and third-party payment for nursing services in hospitals. This consistent involvement in broader health policy discussions has been an invaluable exercise for the nursing community, consistently challenging nursing organizations to reach agreement, to present defensible solutions to the need to meet the nation's nursing requirements, and to understand and deal with the political realities of health care.

Thus trends in health care have definitely shifted since the enactment of DRGs to provide new opportunities for the nursing profession. In addition, the nursing shortage has worked very much to nursing's advantage. Very importantly, the shortage has precipitated a generous infusion of funds from several key foundations, for example, the Pew, Robert Wood Johnson, and Macy foundations. The shortage has also captured the attention of the American public. There are many reasons to consider that the nursing policy glass is half full, and the shortage is major among them. Arguably, the reason for the dire nursing shortage stems from the move to prospective payment according to DRGs.

SHORTCOMINGS OF U.S. POST-DRGs HEALTH CARE SYSTEM

Because nursing's future is closely tied to larger national health care trends, a closer look at these trends is called for prior to considering possible strategic steps the nursing community might take to improve its position in the health care delivery system. To be sure, national pressures to cut health care costs will persist indefinitely. Health care is a constant budget target. The Department of Commerce predicted that the nation's health care tab would rise to $550 billion in 1988, or about $2,135 per person. To many Americans and policymakers that is an unacceptable increase. Many people believe that some formal form of rationing of health care is inevitable if the three factors that continue to fuel growth in health care expenditures are not adequately addressed. These factors are (1) overuse of hospital care and costly technology, (2) the costs of treating acquired immunodeficiency syndrome (AIDS) patients and (3) the costs associated with an aging population. Any one of these problems has the potential to bust the public financial bank.

The most difficult health care problems faced by society are not just cost related. The entire system of American health care is in jeopardy. A huge medical-industrial complex exists that is no longer suited to respond to people's health needs or to socioeconomic imperatives. The United States is witnessing the limits of medical science. There is unmistakable evidence that emotions, lifestyle, and psychosocial factors have an infinitely more far-reaching effect on health than the medical community is willing to acknowledge in its activities. In fact, policymakers are increasingly grappling with the reality that the old ways are not working, and evidence of the inadequacies of the medical model of cure, the basis for our current biomedical enterprise, is everywhere:

- Despite immense strides in American medicine and technology, the United States has one of the highest infant mortality rates in the world.

- More than half of Americans living in poverty without any access to health care are children.
- Notwithstanding the huge amounts spent on Medicare, almost half of what the elderly spend for their health care is out of pocket.
- The majority of Medicare dollars are spent on life-sustaining technology to maintain individuals over 80 in the last year of life.
- The leading causes of death in the nation—heart disease, cancer, stroke, chronic obstructive pulmonary disease, cirrhosis of the liver—are in large part preventable, yet less than 0.3% of the health care dollar is spent on prevention.
- It has been estimated that over 81% of the decrease in the incidence of heart disease is attributable to dietary and lifestyle changes; that is, many people have stopped smoking and have cut down on fats. The other nine percent of the decrease is due to cardiovascular drugs and surgery, not a very substantial return on a considerable monetary investment.
- Autoimmune diseases such as systemic lupus, rheumatoid arthritis, and possibly ulcerative colitis defy cause-and-effect approaches, but have been found to be associated with typical personality profiles. Holding back anger, obsessive compulsiveness, conscientiousness, and conformity constitute a fairly consistent picture.
- Health care is far from victory in limiting the causes of certain infectious diseases. Obvious examples are legionellosis, or Legionnaire's disease, related to open air-conditioning vents; genital herpes, related to sexual behavior; and the most frustrating and frightening of all to date AIDS, which is related to sexual behavior, intravenous drug use, and blood transfusions.
- The quality of U.S. health care is increasingly unsatisfactory and at times borders on the hazardous. Recently *American Health* magazine, with a readership of 1 million, warned its readers that "hospitals are dangerous places" and should only be used as a last resort. Peters and Waterman, in the widely read best-seller *A Passion for Excellence,* also exhibit a typically critical public perspective on the matter of care in hospitals in a section entitled "Poor Dumb Patients," which elaborates on the disdain health care workers seem to have for patients.

Nurses, to be sure, are not exempt from blame when it comes to the poor quality of care patients receive. In a recently published exposé on the poor care provided in a major prestigious New York medical center, a patient's letter to the institution was cited:

> Between the indignant confrontative attitude, the incompetence, the forgetfulness, and the lack of follow-through of the nursing staff and their helpers, how could I believe I was getting the proper care or that, in an emergency, they'd be there.

Quality has been declared a number one public policy problem by the Health Care Financing Administration and the situation is destined to worsen. Just as concerns over cost have prevailed during the past two decades, concerns over quality will be predominant in the late 1980s and 1990s. At the root of these problems in the health care delivery system is the inordinate emphasis on the medical model and its inability to meet the changing needs of society for different kinds of care.

The medical model of disease, on which the entire health delivery system is built, grew out of and was most appropriate to the infectious disease era. In this simpler world diseases had causes (germs) and the task of the bioscientific enterprise was to identify the cause and to devise an appropriate and specific cure. The success of this approach is dramatic: there has been a 99% reduction in the frequency and severity of infectious diseases such as smallpox, typhoid fever, syphilis, polio, tetanus, and diptheria.

Today's most pressing and serious national health problems are mostly chronic in nature, and they simply will not succumb to direct application of the medical model. They primarily require nursing care, just as acute disease states primarily require medical intervention. The social and behavioral roots of the current problems run deep, and our system and patterns of care must shift to address these new imperatives. In short, although the United States spends 12% of its gross national product (GNP) on health care—more than any other industrialized nation—American health, judging by death, illness, and infant mortality rates, is no better and is in many cases worse than in European nations that spend a far smaller share of their GNPs on health care.

Thus the United States is at a juncture in health care where the limits of the present system are becoming apparent. At one time it was believed that eventually medical science would know all that there is to know about health: now it is apparent that such is not the case. The question becomes, what are the implications for the nursing profession? In an era witnessing the limits of medical science, of resources, and of consumer willingness to tolerate expensive substandard care, what should nurses do?

THE NURSING SOLUTION

Nurses have the power to direct and refocus a badly needed transformation; nurses have the power to change the face of things in health care. A recent study found that nursing is the third most important reason consumers choose particular hospitals. Nurses have a great deal to offer a health care system that is badly in need of low-cost options and the compassion, continuity of care, and comprehensiveness of care nursing can provide. But for nurses to fully function as professionals in a system badly in need of what they have to offer, a sound, viable strategy giving attention to the following five pressure points in the post-DRGs health care delivery system is essential.

Concern with costs

What government is most focused on, what most concerns the business community, and the major problem in health care—costs—is nursing's greatest advantage. Research in hospitals has demonstrated that nurses can decrease length of stay, sometimes by three to four days, and can prevent readmissions. Poor nursing care can lead to atelectasis, nosocomial infections, phlebitis, and other postoperative complications that increase length of stay.

In ambulatory settings, outpatient departments, and home care, numerous studies have demonstrated nursing's cost-effectiveness. A recent report by the Office of Technology Assessment cites instance after instance of quality care given by nurses at lower costs. The American Association of Nurse Anesthetists (AANE) is on the verge of bringing suit against the Joint Commission on Accreditation of Health Care Organizations for omitting the AANE from the development of newly proposed standards governing the administration of anesthetics. Chances are the nurse anesthetists will emerge victorious—because of their ability to lower costs to the consumer. Thus as columnist George Will put it at a recent National Association for Home Care convention, these days and in the foreseeable future, anyone who comes to Washington, D.C., with the promise of lowering health costs will be heard. Clearly the cost-containment climate is to the advantage of the nursing community and, more important, to the consumer.

Shifting demand from hospital to community

The general push to decrease length of hospital stays, to keep patients out of hospitals altogether, and to use community-based services in lieu of costly inpatient services, means increased demand for services where nurses are the predominant care givers. The inpatient volume of hospitals continues to shrink while home care admissions soar.

There are 25% fewer hospital beds in the United States since the enactment of DRGs. A study conducted by Arthur Anderson and a recent report by Lewin and associates predict the closing of 700 hospitals by 1995; in fact, the Department of Health and Human Services predicts that the number of registered nurses working in hospitals will decrease to 47% by 1995 and 40% by the year 2000—down from the present figure of nearly 70%. But this too can be good news for the nursing community. Because of financial pressures facing health care, policymakers and insurers are far more receptive to diversifying and developing alternative modes of health care delivery. Very often the nursing department can be the key to identifying and developing new markets for the hospital.

In this post-DRGs era, hospital administrators also are seeking creative ways to increase the hospital's market share to offset the decrease in inpatient numbers. One solution is to decentralize the nursing organization and move it into the community. A variety of arrangements can be envisioned, including clinical specialists in group practice, wellness centers, and adult day care.

The wave of the future for hospitals is contract management. Even physicians will be forming contractual arrangements with hospitals in the future. Nursing can be in the vanguard of this movement by offering nursing services on contract to the institution. Entrepreneurial strategies such as seeking hospital funding for a nursing subsidiary for the chronically ill, a mental health counseling center, or a community nursing center—all of which can be sources of referrals for the hospital—will be increasingly well received in the future. If occupancy rates are low, chances are that hospital administrators will be more than receptive to such proposals.

Nursing should think of itself in terms of potentially separate corporate entities that have the flexibility to enter into new markets and new lines of business. In fact, these new arrangements have the potential to become nursing's 1990 version of collective bargaining. That is, these corporate formations will be capable of providing nursing control over costs and the quality of nursing care.

Changing demographics

The number of elderly persons in the United States is expected to double within 10 years. The greatest health care problems of the elderly lie in the area of chronic illness, and the treatment for chronic illness is of course nursing care. In this context, the role of the nurse as case manager is an idea whose time has come. Policymakers know well that chronic illness will never succumb to the medical model for treatment—by definition it has no cure. As the aging population grows and the need for community-based services to manage the chronically ill increases, nursing case management can be implemented to maintain quality, access, and continuity by managing patient care along a continuum that extends through all types of clinical settings. Collaborating with nursing education to prepare nurses for this role in the near future is an essential step and a key opportunity for nursing.

Greater concern with quality

Since DRGs the preoccupation of consumer groups and the federal government with the quality of health care has been a gift for the nursing community. Providers and consumers alike will increasingly look to the nursing community for the quality component, whether quality is defined in terms of patient outcomes, customer service, or compassion. It is the nurse who is looked to to provide quality care because it is primarily the nurse who delivers around-the-clock patient care.

Quality has become a number one public policy concern to nursing's advantage. Now that hospital mortality data have been released to the public as a measure of quality, nursing will likely have a much more receptive ear from administration for changes that should be made to improve quality. Mortality data are just the beginning of a major trend that will consider the quality of care from the consumer perspective. The American Association of Retired Persons is about to release data disclosing rates of infection, readmission, costly duplicative procedures, and unnecessary surgery in major U.S. hospitals. Such actions will sound a clarion call for fundamental change in the current biomedical enterprise.

Gender gap

Because of the simple fact that women vote in greater numbers than men, nursing as a female-dominated profession was able to challenge the medical establishment at the National Institutes of Health (NIH) and to overcome a presidential veto, and achieve a National Center for Nursing Research at NIH. This strategy could and should be used to achieve greater influence in many other spheres of the health policy arena.

These five pressure points in the system should form the basis of a strategy to professionalize nursing and, most important, to gain power during the current period of transformation in health care. The next step will then be, taking these pressure points as a framework, to muster nursing's resources in areas that will have the greatest impact on the most people. Questions to be asked are, Where will nursing gain the greatest amount of strategic leverage? Where will an investment of resources yield the greatest power for nursing? A three-track strategy is suggested:

1. *A positioning strategy that in the minds of the public will position nurses as professionals and as case managers in group practice arrangements, in subsidiaries, and in contractual relationships.* The nursing shortage provides an appropriate public relations angle for such a positioning strategy.

   The key is not numbers but utilization. It is through utilization that nursing's role will be professionalized. With nurses positioned as case managers, nursing will become more prestigious in the public eye. Using a "value-added" approach nursing can develop, through the case-management model or clinical specialist model. The authority and responsibility to make decisions about—and be accountable for—patient care. For instance, if the nurse is strategically positioned to control the case, she or he should be able to direct and monitor the work of the laboratory, EKG, pharmacy, and so forth to eliminate duplication, inefficiencies, and lack of coordination.

   The nurse should be empowered to manage a case as case manager or as the clinical specialist in charge. If nursing fosters this model effectively, patients will win because the providers in closest proximity—nurses—will be able to address those things most important to and most frustrating for patients. Vital decision making in the current health care delivery system is too removed from the patient to be effective. With central responsbility for managing and coordinating the case in nursing's hands, there will be a continuity and coordination of care. The nurse's proximity to the patient will allow them to see through the same lens.

2. *A reimbursement strategy that will reimburse nurses, in and out of hospitals and across settings, for nursing services.* Nursing should work to acquire financial independence, to acquire admitting privileges, and to eliminate the need for doctors' orders to practice nursing. Nursing's dependence is an outmoded and antiquated arrangement that by its very nature mitigates against collaboration with physicians.

   Fortunately for nursing the current Medicare program will soon be restructured to accommodate the increasing numbers of the elderly and the increasing numbers of chronically ill patients. With the growing elderly population, financing adequate long-term care will continue to be a major item on the national agenda, and nurses have solutions to offer that will provide cost-effective, affordable care. It should not only be made very clear that nursing is essential to long-term care, but nurses should strongly emphasize to state and national government officials that Medicare as presently structured is no longer adequate or appropriate for such care.

   Nursing should move now to present a strong case that nurses are willing and available to undertake care of the nation's elderly, and at a reasonable cost. Track two thus focuses nursing's energies on the inclusion of nurses as providers under Medicare and on the restructuring of Medicare's benefits.

3. *Political strategy: it is frequently true that a poor plan well executed is better than a good plan poorly executed.* While the health care delivery system is in a state of massive trasformation, it is essential to identify strategic goals shared by the entire nursing community and to create a common agenda around which we can unite and from which to move forward. This will require cohesion, communication, and open, honest exchange, as well as compromise to maintain the unity that is essential.

In this post-DRGs era nursing, older and wiser, has a golden opportunity to make great strides to advance the nursing profession and, most important, to improve the quality of health care for consumers.

CHAPTER 54

Costing out nursing services

JANET C. SCHERUBEL

The shift to prospective payment for health care with the advent of diagnosis-related groups (DRGs) has placed new emphasis on the necessity of identifying the costs associated with nursing care. Historically the patient day was the unit of measure used by hospitals to quantify services, and costs were reimbursed according to a retrospective formula. Under this system it was difficult to allocate expenses to specific departments, particularly those associated with nursing services. New methods were needed to identify and budget hospital expenses in an equitable and efficient manner.[48]

Today, with improved cost accounting practices, providers have a much better understanding of resource consumption in health care delivery. Methods have been developed to determine the profitability of differing patient services, highlight wasteful practices, and introduce needed practice changes to streamline service delivery.

Nursing departments now have access to more accurate information and have been able to identify and isolate nursing costs from other hospital services.* As a result, long-range planning and timely monitoring and management of nursing productivity have benefited. Moreover, the cost-effectiveness of nursing practice has been repeatedly demonstrated.†

Historical development

Interest in the cost of nursing services is not new. Nurses, primarily independent nursing practitioners, have sought reimbursement from third-party payers for services since the late 1940s.[57,59] In addition, nurses have successfully used a fee-for-service approach in the allocation of costs for hospital-based nurse specialists.[59,61] This effort continues in many settings and has been partially effective.[27,47] In the late 1970's, researchers studied the costs of nursing education in service settings.[1,8,11,21,45] At the same time, a number of hospitals identified the costs of nursing services provided and in some cases billed patients for these services.‡ These nursing administrators recognized the need to differentiate costs related to nursing care from other hospital services. This requirement is even more important today.[36]

METHODS OF COSTING OUT NURSING SERVICES
Direct nursing care costs

Efforts to quantify nursing costs have been addressed by a variety of means. One well-known system is the New Jersey Relative Intensity Measure (RIM).[10,31,40,41] Designed to work within the DRG structure of patient classification, RIMS assign relative values based on minutes of time devoted to particular nursing care activities. RIMs are allocated to homogeneous nursing resource clusters in primary diagnosis, admission and discharge status, presence of surgery, and length of stay. An allocation statistic within the nursing resource cluster is then used to determine the appropriate cost allocations for nursing care delivered to patients. The statistic is derived from patient data categorized according to the DRG classification system rather than a conceptual model or separate free-standing classification system.

Nonetheless, there are critics of the RIM system. One criticism of the method is its linkage to patient length of stay rather than the acuity of the patient's condition.[13,84] Grimaldi and Micheletti[32] cited other deficiencies in the RIM studies, particularly methodological limitations.[32] They noted that small numbers of patients from limited geographical areas were used in generating cost equations. In addition, one quarter of the equations generated were estimates derived from

---

*References 4,25,37,64,70,74,82.
†References 14,16,27,58,71,81.

‡References 7,18,26,75,79,86.

others due to small sample sizes. Thompson[80] and Trofino[84] concurred, adding that little was done to test the reliability and validity of the RIM methodology. These methodological problems created difficulties in data analysis. In initial reports, none of the hypothesized relationships between nursing intensity and length of stay were supported by the actual data.

A somewhat different method has been proposed by Curtin.[12] This method is also useful with the current DRG classification system. Curtin suggests development of 23 major nursing care categories (NCCs) divided into 356 general nursing care strategies (NCSs) to parallel the major diagnostic categories and DRGs currently in use. NCSs would in effect be the detailed nursing care plans incorporating the direct and indirect care needed by patients. The NCSs would be graduated in terms of increasing nursing time required by patients. The system is attractive, in that NCCs and NCSs would complement the DRG model currently in use across the country. There are, however, limitations to such a program. As Curtin notes, the integrity of DRG coding and nursing classification systems is essential.

Several systems have been developed that do not rely on either the DRG classification system or the traditional patient classification systems.[53] One well-known system is the GRASP classification system, which has several advantages. First, patients are classified on an individual basis rather than aggregated into composite levels. Second, the system allows for recording substantially more nursing activities per patient. Although such methods are advantageous, recordkeeping may become complex and cumbersome. In contrast, many classification systems use selected key indicators to represent many nursing activities.

Yet another system involves Patient Management Categories.[91] Developed by physician panels to represent clinically discrete patient types, the system incorporates different levels of illness severity. Patient management paths identify a variety of medical treatment modalities. Nursing services are allocated to the categories either by use of a patient classification system or through identification of nursing "intensity" as determined by the medical management strategies.[91]

Two systems have been developed based totally on nursing frameworks. Halloran[33] advocates documentation of nursing care based on nursing diagnoses. He demonstrates that nursing diagnoses are twice as effective as DRGs in explaining nursing workloads. Reitz[65] bases her Nursing Intensity Index on a pro-

totype nursing classification system. The Index includes 11 functional categories encompassing both biophysical and behavioral health parameters. In addition, the Index is based on the nursing process.

There is wide agreement that to accurately cost out nursing services it is necessary to use a reliable and valid system to identify nursing services provided to patients.[14,23,38] Perhaps the most frequently used system is the patient classification system. Originally developed for the allocation of nursing staff to patient care units, these systems are now being employed to identify the costs of these services.[39,75,77,84]

Use of an acuity based system to allocate costs has many proponents.[28,64,84,87] Such a system allows the nurse to retrospectively tally nursing care needs for each patient each day of hospitalization. Costs are determined from the nursing time associated with particular tasks through work sampling studies. Thus nursing costs are generated for the services delivered to patients and may be assigned on an individual basis.

Another method of apportioning costs is initiated using aggregate patient data. Ratings obtained from patient classification systems are compiled to determine the total direct nursing care costs for all patients in an institution during a given period of time. Costs may then be allocated to future patients based on their classification scores for total length of stay.

Indirect care costs

A variety of classification systems have been developed to identify the costs of direct care needs of patients. However, there is a second component of nursing care costs to be identified: the indirect costs of patient care, including nursing support services and institutional overhead costs allocated to the nursing department. Several methods have been developed to measure these costs.[23,26] Indirect costs may be determined for the total patient population or the total patient days in a given time period, and then are equally divided among all patients on a per capita basis. Indirect costs may then be distributed based on individual patients' lengths of stay. In other systems indirect costs are allocated based on the level of the patient's need for nursing care as determined through a patient classification system. In some instances, combinations of these approaches may prove more useful to an institution depending on the sources of indirect costs and the characteristics of its cost accounting system.

Regardless of the method selected for cost allocation, it should accurately measure the costs incurred in the delivery of care. Further, the method chosen must be employed consistently across all departments within an institution to ensure equitable allocation of expenses. Each institution must carefully examine the alternatives available and select the most appropriate method for its needs.

USES OF COSTING OUT NURSING SERVICES

A major outcome of costing nursing services has been the quantification of the services nursing provides.[54,76] Nursing care costs may be determined for specific patient groups, such as DRGs, within institutions. Lagona and Stritzel[43] used a patient classification system to determine the differences in the cost of nursing care for patients in two DRGs.[44] Data derived from the classification system were used to calculate the hours of nursing care required for each DRG. The cost of delivering this care was then determined by assigning costs to each DRG based on staffing formulas associated with the classification system. Lagona and Stritzel demonstrated that nursing costs were in fact different for the two DRGs. Direct nursing costs averaged over $1000 for patients with complicated myocardial infarctions (DRG 121), whereas the average cost of caring for patients with uncomplicated infarctions (DRG 122) was less than $800. This information proved valuable to nursing management for planning and decision making.

Using a slightly different methodology, McClain and Selhat[51] determined average direct nursing costs for three different DRGs (DRG 88, DRG 195, and DRG 197). In their study nursing costs were calculated not only for registered nurses, but for each level of personnel: registered nurses, licensed practical nurses, and an aggregate cost determined by staff mix. Although the authors acknowledged the limitations inherent in small sample sizes, they noted the advantages of the data collection methods for future costing studies. Other nurse researchers have successfully extended this methodology to compare nursing resource consumption of different health care institutions.[3,83]

Variability in patient needs

A second outcome of quantifying nursing services is that the quantity and quality of these services may be distinguished among and between patients.[5,50,62,83] Identification of the costs of nursing care has led to a better understanding of the variability of nursing needs of patients with similar problems. Nurse researchers have demonstrated significant differences in nursing care needs and costs for patients within DRGs as well as differences over time for individual patients.*

Giovannetti[29] found wide variability in nursing hours of patients within DRGs. She noted patients with chronic obstructive pulmonary disease (COPD) required fewer hours of care when hospitalized for two weeks, while those hospitalized for only one week required more nursing care. This pattern was reversed in patients hospitalized for hysterectomies. For these patients, nursing care hours increased with length of stay. Similar findings have been reported by others. Many nurse researchers have described changes in patient care needs over time.[3,43,51,52]

The results of fiscal studies undertaken to determine the costs of nursing care have provided new information on the variability of nursing care needs of patients with similar illnesses as well as those with different problems. Such variations in patient care needs are important for management decisions ranging from daily staffing patterns to long-range program planning and budgeting activities. For example, the development of product line or service line management has been enhanced by the identification of needed resources and the appropriate allocation of these resources.[2,9,18]

Cost-effectiveness of nursing services

A third benefit of identifying nursing costs is the ability to recognize nursing as a source of revenue to the hospital rather than as a cost center within the hospital.[3,33,67,68,76] Some nurses have extended this position and proposed the organization of independent nursing staff corporations to make nursing a for-profit entity.[78,84] Others feel a need to define the nursing product and to demonstrate that it may be offered at a competitive price.[78]

Through the identification of nursing costs it has also been possible to evaluate current practices in nursing care delivery. Nurses have compared the costs of team and primary nursing in an effort to determine the most efficient and cost-effective means of nursing care delivery. Results of these studies have shown repeatedly the cost savings of a primary nursing delivery system as opposed to team nursing practices.[5,15,58,90]

---

*References 3,32,52,55,56,60,72,73.

A further advantage of costing out nursing services has been the development of more cost-effective techniques in nursing care delivery. Nursing practices have become more efficient and streamlined.* More productive methods of care delivery have been instituted. The development of nursing case management has improved the continuity of patient care without undue expense.[22] The patient's family members may serve as cooperative care partners to meet patient needs not requiring professional nursing services.[89] The institution of unit assistant programs has led to better use of professional nursing staffs and a decrease in nursing performance of nonnursing duties.[24,68] Through these and other innovations, nursing has made valuable contributions to improved health care delivery and has participated in controlling the rising costs of health care.[30,72]

Costing activities have been extended beyond the acute inpatient environment. Ambulatory nursing services, emergency departments, nursing centers, and home health agencies all have recognized the need to quantify the costs of their services to maintain sound financial bases.† Cost identification is essential in nursing homes to respond to regulatory definitions of skilled and intermediate nursing care classifications. Systems that classify nursing work load based on patient problems have been developed and tested to provide more efficient and cost-effective services.[43] Harris and her associates[35] have developed outcome criteria for nursing care to examine not only the costs of services, but also their quality.

Efforts to quantify the costs of nursing services are not limited to direct patient care delivery costs. In a period of increasing fiscal constraints, nurse executives are reexamining the costs of all nursing activities, especially those not involved in direct patient care. Staff reductions have occurred in continuing education departments.[85] There is a pressing need to identify the costs of continuing education within organizations. As a result of these pressures, methods have been developed to quantify the costs of these departments.[6,20,46,85] Studies report the cost-effectiveness of continuing education programs, particularly when these programs contribute to improvements in nursing practice.[20,46] These activities may be expected to continue and to expand to include other nursing support services.

*References 19,34,35,37,56,58,66,69.
†References 35,42,49,62,88.

Dilemmas of costing out nursing care

Costing out nursing care services is not without problems. Identifying the actual costs of care may create difficulties for the nurse executive. Costing out services carries the potential of decreased allocation of resources to nursing departments.[66] If nurses are able to provide services at decreased costs, nursing budget requests may be reduced.

There are limitations to the use of patient classification systems for deriving costing formulas.[23,60] Many systems classify based on nursing care delivered, not nursing care required. Thus, if nurses are unable to provide necessary care for any reason, including staffing, available support services, or time, this care—or lack thereof—is not documented. If budgeting decisions are based on care delivered rather than on nursing care normally required by patients, these decisions may not accurately reflect the true costs of appropriate nursing care.[23]

Nurse executives must acquire new skills to successfully manage the nursing department budget. A sound working knowledge of cost accounting and budget management is essential in today's health care environment. Managers need to develop effective working relationships with their colleagues in finance and hospital administration to effectively articulate the goals and resources necessary to provide cost-effective quality nursing care.

The process of costing out nursing services may be resisted by others, due to the potential power inherent in establishing nursing as a revenue-producing health care service.[48] Other disciplines may view the establishment of nursing independence as an encroachment on their territory.

Despite the potential problems inherent in costing out nursing services, the benefits are considerable. In the current health care environment cost effective and efficient care has become essential. Identifying the costs generated in providing nursing care is the first step in this process.

FUTURE NEEDS

The process of identifying nursing costs began as a response to cost-containment efforts. Activity accelerated as reimbursement programs shifted from a retrospective to prospective basis. Great strides have been made in quantifying nursing services and the costs of these services. At the same time, nurses have gained new knowledge of the patterns and variations in care required by patients. Methods of care delivery have been streamlined and the cost-effectiveness of nursing demonstrated repeatedly. Nurses may well be proud of these accomplishments.

However the work is not done. As health care funding programs evolve, continued efforts are necessary. Changes in funding and the increased focus on alternative health care delivery systems will dictate additional studies of the cost of nursing care.[57] Further research is needed to demonstrate the cost-effectiveness of nursing practice in settings other than the acute care institution, especially in long term care environments.[18]

The costing studies of nursing care completed thus far have been impressive. These efforts have provided a sound basis for the continued efforts of nurse administrators, practitioners, and researchers to expand and develop new understandings of the fiscal impact of nursing on the health care system.

REFERENCES

1. Analyzing the cost of baccalaureate nursing education, New York, 1982, National League for Nursing.
2. Anderson R: Products and product-line management in nursing, Nursing Administration Quarterly 10(1):65, 1985.
3. Arndt M and Skydell B: Inpatient nursing services: productivity and cost. In Shaffer FA, editor: Costing out nursing: pricing our product, New York, 1985, National League for Nursing.
4. Bargagliotti L and Smith H: Patterns of nursing costs with capital reimbursement, Nursing Economics 3(5):270, 1985.
5. Betz M, Dickerson T, and Wyatt D: Cost and quality: primary and team nursing compared, Nursing and Health Care 1(3):150, 1980.
6. Boston CM: Justifying costs for continuing nursing education departments, Nursing Economics 4(2):83, 1986.
7. Brewer C: Variable billing: is it viable? Nurs Outlook 32(1):38, 1984.
8. Bruekner SJ and Blair E: Cost of education in a department of nursing service at a university medical center, J Nurs Adm 8(3):21, 1977.
9. Bruhn P and Howes D: Service line management: new opportunities for nursing executives, J Nurs Adm 16(6):13, 1986.
10. Caterinicchio RP and Davies RH: Developing a client-focused allocation statistic of inpatient nursing resource use: an alternative to the patient day, Soc Sci Med 17(5):259, 1982.
11. Cost-effective management in schools of nursing, New York, 1982, National League for Nursing.
12. Curtin L: Determining costs of nursing service per DRG, Nursing Management 14(4):16, 1983.
13. Curtin L: DRG creep, DRG weights and patient acuity: determining costs of nursing services, Nursing Management 15(10):7, 1984.
14. Curtin L: Who says "lean" must be "mean"? Nursing Management 17(1):7, 1986.
15. Dahlin A and Gregor J: Nursing costs by DRG with an all-RN staff. In Shaffer FA, editor: Costing out nursing: pricing our product, New York, 1985, National League for Nursing.
16. Davis C: The federal role in changing health care financing, Nursing Economics 1(2):98, 1983.
17. Davis C: Health care reform: what can we expect? Nursing Economics 4(1):10, 1986.
18. de Mars MP and Boyer F: Developing a consistent method for costing hospital services, Healthcare Financial Management 39(2):30, 1985.
19. del Bueno D and Bridges P: Providing incentives while reducing costs: an employee suggestion plan, Nursing Economics 3(4):212, 1985.
20. del Bueno D and Kelly K: How cost effective is your staff development program? Nursing Educator 5(5):12, 1980.
21. Derby VL: Financing nursing education, Nurse Educator 5(2):21, 1980.
22. DeZell AD, Comeau E, and Zander K: Managed care via the nursing case management model. In Scherubel J, editor: Patients and purse strings II, New York, National League for Nursing.
23. Dijkers M and Paradise T: PCS: one system for both staffing and costing, Nursing Management 17(1):25, 1986.
24. Donovan MI and others: The unit assistant: a nurse extender, Nursing Management 19(10): pp. 70-71, 74-76, 1988.
25. Edwardson S: Measuring nursing productivity, Nursing Economics 3(1):9, 1985.
26. Ethridge P: The case for billing by patient acuity, Nursing Management 16(8):38, 1985.
27. Fagin C: Opening the door on nursing's cost advantage, Nursing and Health Care 7(7):353, 1986.
28. Giovanetti P: Understanding patient classification systems, J Nurs Adm 9(2):6, 1979.
29. Giovannetti P: DRGs and nursing workload measures, Comput Nurs 3:2, 1985.
30. Grace HK: Can health care costs be contained? In McCloskey JC and Grace HK, editors: Current issues in nursing, ed 2, Boston, 1985, Blackwell Scientific Publications, Inc.
31. Grimaldi P and Micheletti J: DRG reimbursement: RIMs and the cost of nursing care, Nursing Management 13(2):12, 1982.
32. Grohar M, Meyers J, and McSweeney M: A comparison of patient acuity and nursing resource use, J Nurs Adm 16(6):19, 1986.
33. Halloran EJ: Nursing workload, medical diagnosis-related groups, and nursing diagnoses, Res Nurs Health 8:421, 1985.
34. Harrell J and Frauman A: Prospective payment calls for boosting productivity, Nursing and Health Care 6(10):535, 1985.
35. Harris M, Santoferraro C, and Silva S: A patient classification system in home health care, Nursing Economics 3(5):276, 1985.
36. Hartley S: Effects of prospective pricing on nursing, Nursing Economics 4(1):16, 1986.
37. Hayes SH and Carroll SR: Early intervention care in the acute stroke patient, Arch Phys Med Rehabil 67(5):319, 1986.
38. Herzog T: Productivity: fighting the battle of the budget, Nursing Management 16(1):30, 1985.
39. Higgerson NJ and VanSlyck A: Variable billing for services: new fiscal direction for nursing, J Nurs Adm 12(6):20, 1982.
40. Joel L: DRGs: the state of the art of reimbursement for nursing services, Nursing and Health Care 4(10):560, 1983.
41. Joel L: DRGs and RIMs: implications for nursing, Nurs Outlook 32(1):42, 1984.
42. Joel L: Costing out nursing in nursing homes. In Shaffer FA,

editor: Costing out nursing: pricing our product, New York, 1985, National League for Nursing.

43. Lagona T and Stritzel M: Nursing care requirements as measured by DRGs, J Nurs Adm 14(5):15, 1984.

44. Lauver E: Where will the money go? Nursing and Health Care 6(3):132, 1985.

45. Lazinski H: The effects of clinical teaching on the budgets of schools of nursing, J Nurs Educ 18(1):21, 1979.

46. Lesser JE: Cost-effectiveness of continuing education. In McCloskey JC and Grace HK, editors: Current issues in nursing, ed 2, Boston, 1985, Blackwell Scientific Publications, Inc.

47. Lubic R: Reimbursement for nursing practice: lessons learned, experiences shared, Nursing and Health Care 6(1):23, 1985.

48. Maraldo PJ: DRGs: implications for nursing practice. In McCloskey JC and Grace HK, editors: Current issues in nursing, ed 2, Boston, 1985, Blackwell Scientific Publications, Inc.

49. Martin K and Schut N: The Omaha system: implications for costing community health nursing. In Shaffer FA, editor: Costing out nursing: pricing our product, New York, 1985, National League for Nursing.

50. Mason E and Daugherty J: Nursing standards should determine nursing's price, Nursing Management 15(9):34, 1984.

51. McClain JR and Selhat MS: Twenty cases: what nursing costs per DRG, Nursing Management 15(10):27, 1984.

52. McKibbin RC and others: DRGs and nursing care. ANA Publication Sept 1985 (D-86) p 1-65.

53. Meyer D: Costing nursing care with the GRASP system. In Shaffer FA, editor: Costing out nursing: pricing our product, New York, 1985, National League for Nursing.

54. Mezey M: Securing a financial base, Am J Nurs 83(10):1297, 1983.

55. Mitchell M and others: Determining cost of direct nursing care by DRG, Nursing Management 15(4):29, 1977.

56. Mowry M and Korpman R: Do DRG reimbursement rates reflect nursing costs? J Nurs Adm 15(7,8):29, 1985.

57. Mundinger M: DRGs: a glass half full for nursing, Nurs Outlook 33:265, 1985.

58. Olsen S: The challenge of prospective pricing: work smarter, J Nurs Adm 14(4):22, 1984.

59. Palcini J: Perspectives on level of reimbursement for nursing services, Nursing Economics 2(2):118, 1984.

60. Piper L: Accounting for nursing functions in DRGs, Nursing Management 14(11):26, 1983.

61. Powell P: Fee for service, Nursing Management 14(3):13, 1983.

62. Ransien T: Recognizing emergency department price components, Healthcare Financial Management 38(12):12, 1982.

63. Redford JB and Harris JD: Rehabilitation of elderly stroke patients, Am Fam Physician 22(9):153, 1980.

64. Reitz J: The development of a cost-allocation statistic for nursing. In Shaffer FA, editor: Costing out nursing: pricing our product, New York, 1985, National League for Nursing.

65. Reitz J: Toward a comprehensive nursing intensity index. I. Development, Nursing Management 16(8):21, 1985.

66. Reschak G and others: Accounting for nursing costs by DRG, J Nurs Adm 15(9):15, 1985.

67. Riley W and Schaefers V: Costing nursing services, Nursing Management 14(12):40, 1983.

68. Selby TL: Nurses find ways to ease shortage; recruit, retain, American Nurse, p 1, Oct 1988.

69. Servellen GM and Mowry MM: DRGs and primary nursing: are they compatible? J Nurs Adm 15(4):32, 1985.

70. Shaefers V: A cost-allocation method for nursing. In Shaffer FA, editor: Costing out nursing: pricing our product, New York, 1985, National League for Nursing.

71. Shaffer F: Nursing power in the DRG world, Nursing Management 15(6):28, 1983.

72. Shaffer F: Nursing: gearing up for DRGs. II. Management strategies, Nursing and Health Care 5(2):93, 1984.

73. Shaffer F: A nursing perspective of the DRG world, part I, Nursing and Health Care 5(1):48, 1984.

74. Sovie M: Managing nursing resources in a constrained economic environment, Nursing Economics 3(2):85, 1985.

75. Sovie M and Smith T: Pricing the nursing product: changing for nursing care, Nursing Economics 4(5):216, 1986.

76. Stanley M and Luciano K: Eight steps to costing nursing services, Nursing Management 15(10):27, 1984.

77. Stevens B: What is the executive's role in budgeting for her department? J Nurs Adm 11(7):22, 1981.

78. Strong B: Nursing products: primary components of health care, Nursing Economics 3(1):60, 1985.

79. Thomas S and Vaughan RG: Costing nursing services using RVUs, J Nurs Adm 16(12):10, 1986.

80. Thompson JD: The measurement of nursing intensity, Healthcare Financial Management 11:47, 1984.

81. Thompson JD and Diers D: DRGs and nursing intensity, Nursing and Health Care 6(8):435, 1985.

82. Toth R: DRGs: imperative strategies for nursing service administration, Nursing and Health Care 5(4):196, 1984.

83. Trofino J: A reality-based system for pricing nursing service, Nursing Management 17(1):19, 1986.

84. Trofino J: RIMs: skirting the edge of disaster, Nursing Management 16(7):48, 1985.

85. Urquhart AL and others: Perspectives on nursing issues and health care trends, J Nurs Adm 16(1):17, 1986.

86. Vanderzee H and Glusko G: DRGs variable pricing and budgeting for nursing service, J Nurs Adm 14(5):11, 1984.

87. Vanputte A and others: Accounting for patient acuity: the nursing time dimension, Nursing Management 16(10):27, 1985.

88. Verran J: Patient classification in ambulatory care, Nursing Economics 4(5):247, 1986.

89. Weis A: Cooperative care: innovative care in a time of change. In Scherubel J, editor: Patients and purse strings II, New York, 1988, National League for Nursing.

90. Wolf GA, Lesic LK, and Leak AG: Primary nursing: the impact on nursing costs within DRGs, J Nurs Adm 16(3):9, 1986.

91. Young W, Patterson M, and Groetzinger S: Patient management categories and the costs of nursing services. In Shaffer, FA, editor: Costing out nursing: pricing our product, New York, 1985, National League for Nursing.

CHAPTER 55

Nursing's newest mandate

The cost-quality imperative

MARYANN F. FRALIC
JUDITH L. BRETT

Cost has become a preeminent concern in the U.S. health care system, and the quality of the services provided will be central in the future. In an increasingly managed health care system, outcomes and costs are continually linked. The trend has been clear and inexorable. The Joint Commission for Accreditation of Health Care Organizations (JCAHO) has announced a program that tests outcome indicators rather than simply defining quality in terms of structure or process. The objective is to provide data so that each hospital can compare its performance against other hospitals and against standards that are being developed. It is expected that by the early 1990s hospital accreditation will be determined by the degree of conformity to clinical performance standards.[15]

The basic premise underlying the delivery of contemporary health care services is that desired levels of quality must be achieved at acceptable levels of cost. Nursing traditionally has focused on quality achievement, but more recently it has broached the actual measurement of the level of quality produced. The essential and logical progression is to the quantification of the cost of nursing care, and its linkage to the quality of the nursing product.

Historically, nursing administration has scrupulously accounted for the "input" side of the nursing equation. Records stretching back for many years document exactly how many nurses provided care on a particular shift. Within the last decade nurses have developed sophistication in determining the level of patient care needs by using patient classification systems. Thus data exist regarding the requirements of patient care and the number of people involved in providing that care. However, as nursing research moves from tallying inputs to measuring outcomes, the equation lacks two crucial elements. First, what is the quality of the product delivered? Second, at what cost is this specific level of quality delivered?

Any future nursing management system that is appropriate and sustainable must include all of the components of the cost-quality equation. The present and future environment demands this, and nursing must provide it to identify the actual contribution margin of nursing practice to today's health care organizations. The strength and support of nursing practice lies in this identification.

Donabedian[4] notes that the true management of quality in health care requires definition and measurement, a balance of quality against cost. He calls for addressing quality, measuring it, protecting and enhancing it, evaluating how it relates to cost, and then examining the consequences that flow from that relationship. Results must be precisely quantified. Nursing needs to proceed quickly to develop systems that measure effect rather than simply effort.

A MODEL

In this chapter we examine the characteristics of such a system, called QualDex.© First, it should consist of key data elements and indicators that separately measure both cost and quality (see box on p. 400). Informed judgments can then be made as the two are compared.

Quality elements

Patients are unique and complex individuals. Explanations of the cause-and-effect relationship between nursing activities and patient outcomes are thus extremely difficult to articulate, let alone measure. In addition, identifying a basis for evaluation of quality is even more complicated because definitions of quality

---

**QUALITY AND COST ELEMENTS
ESSENTIAL TO A COMPREHENSIVE
NURSING MANAGEMENT SYSTEM
QUALDEX©**

Quality elements

Compliance with standards of nursing practice
(nursing process)
Compliance with standards of nursing care (patient
outcomes)
Occurrence of untoward patient incidents★
Occurrence of hospital acquired infections★
Patient length of stay★
Patient satisfaction

Cost elements

Labor costs
Nonlabor costs
Census
Nursing acuity/intensity
Hours worked by permanent nursing staff
Hours worked by nonpermanent nursing staff

---

*Attributable to nursing action or inaction.

are inherently value laden (what is quality to one nurse may not be shared by a second nurse or the patient).[10,13] The existence of a wide variety of instruments to monitor quality of care also confounds comparison of the results of care across institutions.[7,8,17] However, standards that are "nationally accepted, legally defensible, and ethical" and define "competent, accountable professional nursing practice"[2] provide an alternative basis for evaluating quality of nursing care that is applicable to all nursing institutions.[1] Standards can be patient-specific as necessary and have been suggested as a basis for pricing nursing services that would "facilitate rational and effective decisions regarding cutback or expansion."[12] Standards for practice (nursing process) guide the provision of care, and standards of care (patient outcomes) predict expected outcomes. Thus compliance with these standards is a fundamental determinant of the quality of care provided by a nursing division.

The number of incidents that occur on a nursing unit reflect untoward events, errors, accidents, or other happenings that nurses try to avoid or prevent during the course of the delivery of care. The very nature of these events makes them negative indicators of the quality of the care delivery system; thus they are essential to any model of the cost-quality relationship.

The number of hospital acquired infections is also a negative indicator of the quality of service provided. A patient should not develop an infection as a direct result of the hospital stay or the professional staff members' various interventions. Given the normal circumstances of hospitalization (i.e., increased potential exposure to infection sources) it is likely that a certain proportion of patients may contract an infection despite appropriate care. The level of tolerance for infections should be identified for each nursing unit and used as an indicator of the quality of care.

Nurses play an important role in facilitating the timely discharge of patients. The longer a patient remains hospitalized, the longer he or she is exposed to such negative risks of hospitalization as incidents or infections. Therefore, in addition to the need to discharge patients promptly to minimize their hospitalization costs, it is important to discharge patients as soon as the risks from potential complications of discharge are less than the risks associated with continued hospital stay. Initial assessments should identify potential problems that may delay a timely discharge, and nursing care plans should document the required early interventions to assure that all possible delays are avoided. Thus variations in length of stay (i.e., greater or less than an acceptable standard length of stay for the respective diagnosis-related group, or DRG) represent an additional element of the quality of care.

Finally, despite reports that the definitions of quality of care as defined by health care personnel and patients may be inversely related,[5,11] many authors have suggested that patient perceptions of care are important to a complete understanding of quality.[9,16] Some measurement of patient satisfaction with nursing care must be included in any model of the cost-quality relationship.

Donabedian[3] makes another key point that provides direction in the attempt to define and measure quality. He notes that a reduction in the level of quality is not in and of itself intolerable. Certain levels of quality may actually be associated with very high costs that far outweigh their benefits. Under these circumstances, somewhat lower levels of quality are not only acceptable but even preferable. One will readily agree that luxurious levels of care achieved at exorbitant levels of cost will not be tolerated in any health care system, present or future. Therefore the clear objective is to identify a level of quality that is important for desirable patient outcomes, that is achievable, and that will be supported and sustained.

Cost elements

The cost elements that are important to understanding the effectiveness of a nursing management system must also be valid and reliable. These elements include measures of the work load (the number of patients to be cared for and the associated level of nursing intensity), and the quantity and price of labor and nonlabor resources used to meet the work load.

A valid and reliable patient classification system, preferably a factor-evaluative type, is essential to identification of work load. A classification system can be used to prospectively or retrospectively identify the amount of care, usually expressed as the hours of nursing care that patients require. Some systems are sophisticated enough to identify the specific number and "mix" of care providers required (for example, how many registered nurses, licensed practical nurses, or nurse assistants).

Census is an additional component of work load assessment. Even though the patient classification system's total "points" (the required hours of care) may be equal on two different days, if the number of patients those points refer to is vastly different the work load is affected. Thus both census and nursing intensity totals should be measured.

The number of hours of care provided by all members of the staff, differentiated by type of provider, also should be carefully measured. Since the care provided by a largely temporary work force (consisting of significant proportions of agency or pool personnel) is theoretically different from that provided by a stable staff, the proportion of temporary as compared to permanent staff also needs to be monitored.

Expense data, including total salary and nonsalary dollars paid, must be measured to ensure that the cost of delivering care is within the institution's range of affordability. Nonlabor expense is an essential component of the cost of providing care. Adequate patient care supplies of appropriate quality and quantity are needed to deliver effective care. However, waste and unnecessary expense are not tolerable in today's cost-controlled climate. Thus managers need to track and control supply costs carefully through an appropriate management control system.

Management models, no matter how logically planned or well executed, are of value only if they are proven to work. In order to test the interrelationships of the elements previously described, a two-year research project was designed and conducted within the nursing division at Robert Wood Johnson University Hospital (RWJUH). A theoretical model (Fig. 55-1) was developed using all the elements and predicting their relationships. Measures of each of the elements were identified and the model was tested using structural equation analysis (LISREL).

For purposes of the study, elements in the model were operationalized as follows:

1. Permanent hours worked: total hours worked during a day of the study by nursing staff permanently assigned to the unit.
2. Extra hours worked: total hours worked during a day of the study by nursing staff temporarily assigned to the unit. This variable included hours worked by personnel from an outside agency or in-house pool, or nurses reassigned from other units.
3. Salary expense: all salary dollars paid for a day of the study, including sick, vacation, and premium pay, conference days, and agency costs.
4. Nonsalary expense: included costs of nonchargeable items for a day of the study.
5. Census: the number of patients in the unit as of midnight on a day of the study.
6. Acuity: the total number of patient classification points for all patients on the unit for a day of the study.
7. Compliance with standards of practice (PROCESS): the number of RWJUH nursing process criteria achieved, divided by the number applicable.
8. Compliance with standards of care (OUTCOMES): the number of RWJUH nursing outcome criteria divided by the number applicable.
9. Incidents: the number of incidents attributable to nursing action that occurred during a day of the study.
10. Infections: the number of infections attributable to nursing action that originated during a day of the study.
11. Length of stay: the ratio of the actual number of days of hospitalization to the standard days of hospitalization for the patient's specific DRG. A ratio greater than 1 indicated the patient had been hospitalized longer than the standard.
12. Patient satisfaction: patients' scores on the patient satisfaction instrument (PSI) developed originally by Risser[14] and modified by Hinshaw and Atwood.[6] Higher scores represented higher levels of patient satisfaction.

Most models undergo several tests of validity and frequent modifications before general acceptance is

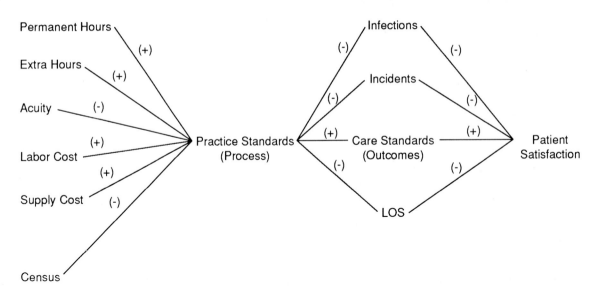

Fig. 55-1 Conceptual model of the relationship of cost and quality of nursing care. Model developed by J. Brett and M. Fralic, 1986.

warranted. The initial test at RWJUH involved one nursing unit, and the results must be interpreted with caution. Extension and refinement of the model is planned as additional time, energy, and resources are made available. However, the model and the initial results are useful for illustrating cost-quality measurement concepts.

Results

Figure 55-2 is a diagrammatic depiction of the results of the initial test of the model comprising the quality-cost relationship. Overall, statistics used to test the fit of the depicted model to the data were favorable.

Five relationships were statistically significant as predicted by the model. The variable "compliance with nursing practice (process) standards" was significantly related to three others: permanent hours worked, census, and compliance with nursing (outcome) standards. In addition, patient satisfaction was significantly related both to the number of infections and to compliance with standards of care. Several relationships, although not significant, occurred in the direction predicted by the model. These were found between "compliance with nursing practice standards" and the variables of labor costs, and number of incidents, and length of stay.

The remaining six relationships were opposite in direction to those predicted by the model. For example, the relationship between patient acuity and compliance with nursing practice standards was sta-

tistically significant, but was positive rather than negative. The data suggest that the higher the patient acuity and the more complex the care requirements, the better nurses are at complying with nursing practice standards.

Both extra hours worked and supply expense had weak inverse relationships with compliance with nursing standards. Measurement of the supply cost for a day on a nursing unit was difficult, so this relationship may be a product of measurement error. The inverse relationship between extra hours worked by nonpermanent agency or pool nurses and compliance with nursing practice standards is perhaps not surprising. Although an extra pair of hands may be useful, a temporary employee is likely not to know the patients or routines of a unit as well as a permanent employee. Thus the quality of care as measured by compliance with nursing practice standards may be compromised.

The observed relationship between compliance with nursing practice standards and the number of infections was significant and positive. Pinpointing the start of an infection to a day on the nursing unit (the unit of analysis) was the result of expert opinion and yet may have been imprecise. The amount of error in the measurement of the day of origin of an infection may have resulted in the unexpected nature of this relationship. Additional study using a month as the unit of analysis should minimize this measurement error.

The final two relationships not taking the expected direction were both nonsignificant and involved pa-

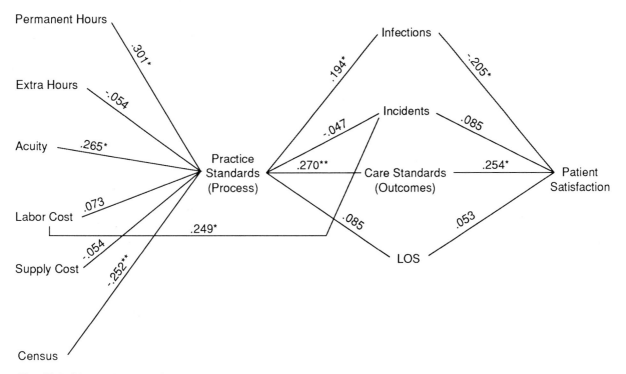

Fig. 55-2 Observed model of the relationship of cost and quality of nursing care. Model developed by J. Brett and M. Fralic, 1986.

tient satisfaction. The observed positive relationship with length of stay suggests that as hospital stay increases, patient satisfaction also increases. Hospital and patient objectives concerning length of stay appeared to be at odds. Are "too short" hospital stays too hectic and therefore dissatisfying to patients? The unexpected positive relationship between incidents and patient satisfaction needs additional study. One explanation for this finding might be that the occurrence of incidents may generate increased attention for patients as staff attempt to protect the patient from additional accidents. This increased attention then can result in patient satisfaction with care.

An additional relationship not in the original model was identified in the data analysis. A significant direct relationship between salary and incidents suggests that the higher the salary expense, the greater the number of incidents. It is important to note that the salary variable included expenses due to vacations, conference days, orientation, overtime, and the extra costs of any agency nurses used. These costs represent the most expensive yet potentially least productive nursing hours. This finding has important implications for nursing management.

Future analysis of the model will need to separate

some of the components of the broad variables and to clarify measurement in variables where the relationships were weak or unexpected.

SIGNIFICANCE AND IMPLICATIONS FOR PRACTICE

What is the importance of illustrating such a study? First, it is extremely useful to visually depict the strong associations between certain variables that in effect represent professional nursing activity. This is how theory builds, and it is how nurses develop a scientific base for practice, decisions, and actions. For example, with such a model it will quickly become clear that there is a strong positive relationship between the quality of care and the number of professional nurses involved in direct care. Also, it can be seen that nurses react negatively to increased work load but do not react negatively to increased patient acuity. That is, nurses are equipped and trained to provide care in highly complex cases, but they become overwhelmed if the number of patients is unmanageable.

Of major importance is tracking of nursing's contribution to reducing patient infections, untoward patient incidents (falls, medication errors), and lengths of stay. These are potent indicators that have tangible financial import for every health care organization. Once nurses acquire the sophistication to model, predict, and illustrate the fiscal impact and contributions of high-quality clinical nursing practice, these will be clearly evident in meaningful measures that every organization can understand and support.

We believe that with a system such as that described here, nursing divisions can produce defensible, precise, and substantiated annual budgets, using specific quantitative data on the actual cost and quality performance of each nursing unit each month. Nurse managers and nursing staff members will be able to see how their own units have performed against each individual measure during the month, with respect to previous months, and as compared to other nursing units. Each individual element (for example, infections) can be evaluated, promptly discussed with the staff, and remedial action targeted. This system is designed to control for a predetermined level of quality of patient care while keeping costs appropriate and within accepted institutional levels. Such systems will meet the new imperative, meld the elements of cost and quality, and, most important, move nursing beyond the simple measurements of inputs and process. This model accomplishes the meaningful and previously elusive measurement of professional nursing practice—its outcomes, its values, its contributions, and its innate worth.

REFERENCES

1. Bloch D: Criteria, standards, norms—crucial terms in quality assurance, J Nurs Adm 7(7):20, 1977.

2. Dirschel K: A mandate for standards of care, Nursing and Health Care 7:27, 1986.

3. Donabedian A: Quality, cost, and cost containment, Nurs Outlook 32(3):142, 1984.

4. Donabedian A: Five essential questions frame the management of quality in health care, Health Management Quarterly 9(1):6, 1987.

5. Eriksen L: Patient satisfaction: an indicator of nursing care quality? Nursing Management 18(7):31, 1987.

6. Hinshaw A and Atwood J: A patient satisfaction instrument: precision by replication, Nurs Res 31(3):170, 1982.

7. Horn B and Swain M: Criterion measures of nursing quality care. US Public Health Service Pub No 78-3817, Washington, DC, 1978, US Department of Health, Education and Welfare.

8. Jelinek R and others: A methodology for monitoring quality of nursing care, US Department of Health, Education, and Welfare Pub No HRA 76-25, Washington, DC, 1974, US Government Printing Office.

9. La Monica E and others: Development of a patient satisfaction scale, Res Nurs Health 9:43, 1986.

10. Lang N: Issues in quality assurance in nursing, ANA Publication G-124, p 45, 1976.

11. Larson P: Cancer nurses' perception of caring, International Journal for Cancer Care 9(2):86, 1986.

12. Mason E and Daugherty J: Nursing standards should determine nursing's price, Nursing Management 15(9):34, 1984.

13. Nicholls M and Wessells V, editors: Nursing standards and nursing process, Wakefield, Mass, 1977, Contemporary Publishing.

14. Risser N: Development of an instrument to measure patient satisfaction with nurses and nursing care in the primary care setting, Nurs Res 24:45, 1975.

15. Sneak preview: JCAHO's quality indicators, Hospitals 62(13):38, 1988.

16. Taylor P and others: Development and use of a method of assessing patient perception of care, Hospital and Health Services Administration, 26:89, 1981.

17. Wandelt M and Ager J: Quality patient care scale, New York, 1974, Appleton-Century-Crofts.

CHAPTER 56

Payment for health services in long-term care

GENROSE J. ALFANO

If the predictions are correct about the number of aged persons in our society increasing, it seems only logical that if chronic illness and its resultant disabilities continue to afflict them at the same rate, the number of older persons requiring some form of health care over an extended period of time will increase. I believe that despite the increasing age of the population, the proportion of the aged using health care services in long-term care, specifically nursing home care, will not increase appreciably. However, as others have pointed out, the dependency of persons admitted to long-term care facilities will be greater, and the age of individuals entering nursing homes will be concentrated in the eighth, ninth, and tenth decades of life. If this is true, the questions that must be answered are what services will be necessary, who will need them, where will they be given or delivered, who will provide them, what will they cost, and who should pay?

SERVICES TO THE CHRONICALLY ILL AND AGED

Chronic illness has posed an interesting challenge to the health care system because the care required by individuals is not constant and often runs a cycle of acute medical and intensive nursing care to maintenance medical and intensive, rehabilitative, and supportive nursing care. An individual's competency to carry out activities of daily living may fluctuate. Thus the need for services and assistance may also vary. Eligibility requirements for care and services that are subject to acts of the legislature may impede timely intervention at a lesser cost and result in a need for more extensive care and services at a later date.

Considerable confusion and debate has centered around what services are necessary; because of this confusion, no criteria have been established for sites where services could most appropriately be delivered and for personnel would be most able to deliver them. By and large the best prepared nurses and physicians have not seen long-term care as a rewarding or exciting specialty, so for the most part the chronically ill and aged have had to rely on well-intended, minimally prepared healthworkers.

COST ISSUES
Home care

A number of surveys, one of which was done by the U.S. General Accounting Office, have already determined that the greatest need of the chronically ill and the infirm, frail elderly is assistance with activities of daily living.[1] Most of these services do not require a full-time homemaker or personal attendant. Nor do they require a nurse, a social worker, or a physical therapist and certainly not all three. And they rarely require the services of a physician. The functional capabilities of individuals who need long-term care may be assessed initially by a physician, a nurse, a physical therapist, or an occupational therapist. They can evaluate the patient's potential for improvement or change and can do periodic reassessments at intervals determined by the patient's clinical history, the existing pathology, or any new crisis or exacerbation of the original pathology.

Institutional reimbursement

The inability of hospitals and nursing homes (which represent the bulk of long-term care facilities) to identify their specific costs has led to the predetermined payment system based on diagnosis-related groups (DRGs) and, in nursing homes, resource utilization groups.

The prospective payment system presumably discourages abuse, but it also encourages overpayment and waste when only minimal services are required.

For instance, for years patients were hospitalized for diagnostic tests that could have been done conveniently on an outpatient basis because Blue Cross would only cover inpatient care. It was the shortages of hospital beds and rising inpatient bed and board costs that finally motivated Blue Cross to cover the cost of tests on an outpatient basis.

Reimbursement for inpatient nursing services

To reimburse for nursing services on the basis of a mathematical ratio of hours per patient is unrealistic. Admission to a nursing home is an acknowledgment that someone needs the care of others to maintain a human quality of life or that someone's clinical status indicates a need for daily supervision and treatment to prevent an acute illness or death through neglect. Nursing care thus becomes the primary nursing home service, so it must command the largest portion of the institution's budget, and the director of nursing services must be a key policymaker within that setting.

There are many who believe that nursing care can be itemized so that the cost can be determined, and staffing, salary, and appropriate reimbursement can be apportioned more accurately. If we are looking at care, comfort, education, and rehabilitation, I do not believe that nursing services can be broken down into cost units. These are qualitative, not quantitative, components of care. Only tasks can be itemized.

Cost out a bed bath for a person with severe osteoarthritis and exertional dyspnea, cost out feeding a patient who has dysphagia. How does one cost out care? I would like to see us develop a concept of nursing needs related groups similar to that of the DRGs or RUGs. It might then be feasible to establish an average cost for these procedures with the possibility of adding outliers, as in DRGs? This will require some very sophisticated approaches to nursing diagnoses and many more nurses in practice will have to develop this sophistication.

Proliferation of healthworkers

Another important reason for the increased cost of long-term care has been the insistence on multidisciplinary teams and approaches for all patients and the mandate that all care must be directed by a physician. Those who have worked in the area of chronic illness and care of the aged know that many physicians consider it primarily a social rather than a medical problem. Because they are less sophisticated in the use of social agencies, functional aids, and emotional support systems than are nurses or social workers they fail to make appropriate referrals.

The growth of specialists in the field of long-term care for the aged has been phenomenal. Fractionalizing care and increasing the number of people to carry out similar and closely related tasks have always resulted in the duplication of effort, poor communication, and increased costs. In the face of this history, some groups such as the AMA still want to solve the present-day shortage of all health personnel by adding yet another worker, the registered care technician. We are facing these shortages because of the ever-increasing role specificity for health professionals. What we need are larger numbers of broadly prepared generalists in nursing and in medicine—people who know how to care for people instead of parts.

A nurse clinician carrying out a thorough initial assessment with input from the patient and family can identify and prioritize health and social needs and determine what specific help may be required. The majority of patients in the community will not need more than good nursing care and periodic medical evaluation and treatment.

Changing focus in community and public health nursing

Public health and visiting nurses have long provided the bulwark of care for the chronically ill in the community in terms of health teaching, family counseling and morbidity care. However, because patients are now being discharged to their homes still requiring hi-tech procedures and treatment, home health agencies have proliferated, many of them hospital based. They employ nurses with hospital experience to carry out these procedures. Unlike their public health colleagues, these nurses visit to carry out specific care techniques or treatments and do not concentrate on overall health or family care issues. Consequently, a whole spectrum of health care and disease prevention is going unattended because of a concentration on services that are quantitatively assessable and deemed reimbursable.

Personnel

Understanding of motivation for living, individual differences among people even in the same age group, value systems of others, knowledge of the interrelational effect of psyche and soma, and the complexities of physiological response and reaction to external and internal stimuli, real or perceived, become important competencies in the care of the long-term chronically ill person.

There is a prevailing myth that hiring registered nurses (R.N.s) would be more costly than hiring licensed practical nurses (L.P.N.s). It is certainly true that the base salary of the R.N. would have to be higher, particularly if this nurse were expected to function with a scope and span of responsibility commensurate with a professional level of practice rather than that of a technical apprentice and gatekeeper. And if the R.N. were to function in this way, then most of the care delivered would be rehabilitative in nature rather than caretaking or custodial. Although such care might not result in a larger number of discharges from institutions, it might result in patients who were more functional and who needed less nursing care time. Thus fewer nursing personnel would be needed on the unit at any given time. If R.N.s were the care coordinators, there might be less need for as many health professionals.

If L.P.N.s became the preferred workers by virtue of availability and then experience, it is foolish to assume that they would be content to receive less money. L.P.N.s would expect to be paid a salary worthy of their hire.

And what about nurses' aides? As of September 1988, The Secretary of Health and Human Services is expected to present a plan to the states outlining the regulations for the employment and retention of aides in the care of patients in long-term care facilities. They will be required to have at least 70 hours of training before employment and to be certified as aides for nursing home care. Although not a federal stipulation, some states will require licensure, either under boards of education or nursing.

Considering that the essential reason for hiring aides for long-term care was that they were inexpensive, unskilled labor, it will be interesting to see what happens to salaries when nurses' aides become certified. And will hospitals facing a shortage of qualified, suitably prepared nurses rationalize that aides certified in long-term care will be good substitutes for professional licensed nurses after a little extra inservice training and supervision? The nursing home and home health industry may find itself under added pressure to pay competitive salaries.

There is a common saying that the more things change, the more they stay the same. The issue is still whether adequate nursing care can be given by people prepared at the level of nurses' aides. My conviction is that it cannot and that the care and cost for long-term care will never be different until we are able to recruit and retain persons broadly prepared in nursing. What they are called is not so important as whether they have the knowledge, skills, and competencies to do the job.

The one certainty about cost for the long-term care of patients in institutions is that it will go up. But will it go up without any appreciable improvement in care, or will it go up accompanied by qualitative improvements in care delivery and the competencies and characteristics of the personnel most immediately involved?

Generally, the daily cost of long-term care has been less than that of acute care, but with longevity increasing among the chronically ill, the overall expenditure for long-term care is beginning to equal if not exceed that of acute care.

Megacenters

The trend toward multiservice centers must be examined very closely, whether medical center, nursing home outreach programs, or those managed by corporate chains of health care providers with many differing types of facilities. Costs of affiliated outreach programs often run higher than those of free-standing or unipurpose facilities. Often the programs that cost less to operate have costs allocated from the more expensive services or must pay a proportion of the cost of services for the entire corporation, many of which the smaller unit does not use.

The rationale is always that the affiliation or relationship gives the patient access to total services, and the care given is of higher quality. In some instances this may be true, but there is also the danger that this outreach unit may receive less than it contributes or receive more sophisticated services than it needs. And the third-party and individual payers will be paying for hidden services they rarely receive. Well-run and well-organized free-standing unipurpose units with good working relationships with medical centers may be the most cost-effective and qualitatively good situations.

FLEXIBILITY NEEDED TO REDUCE COSTS
Refocusing purpose for the long-term care facility

As the long-term care facility is seen more as a residence that provides necessary clinical and personal care, unit structures and allocation of staff can vary, and patients or residents will be assigned to units based on their most immediate clinical or physical need. Some residents might be able to go out to work after receiving the needed assistance to get ready. When they required treatment, they could attend the nursing clinic within the facility or, if necessary, be transferred to the infirmary for a course of treatment and care.

Such an arrangement would make possible a base rate relevant to room and board charges, with specific charges for nursing or medical care and treatment on a per visit basis. Under this system, daily rates for room and board would be constant, and other charges would vary. Individuals would not have to be transferred to skilled nursing units when temporarily in need of more intensive nursing services; the flexibility would allow a more efficient use of beds; and a more explicit and accurate cost-accounting approach to care would be possible.

Whether the ambience is clinical or residential, the process of ensuring safety, comfort, and growth, including hope and enjoyment of daily living, is more complex than soap and water, monthly birthday parties, television rooms, and a well-meaning, caring staff.

Respite care

Day-care hospitals, which can supply daily assistance and facilities with beds allocated for respite services to provide relief to the primary care giver, are other alternatives and can either defer or avoid nursing home or hospital admission.

Vacation camps for the cognitively or physically impaired who have no active pathology serve not only to enhance their quality of life but also to maintain them in their homes and provide needed relief for the family or care givers.

Case management

Competent, knowledgeable case management can avoid duplication of function, introduce care appropriately, and discontinue services in a timely fashion. Patients needing a constellation of services will have them coordinated effectively by a knowledgeable advocate. Family members who might otherwise have considered a nursing home because of the obstacles and red tape they faced in trying to obtain health care services will be able to cope with the problems of home care of a dependent parent a little longer. Patients at home will not feel as isolated from an organized system of help. And nursing home admission will occur in a planned and appropriate manner.

OPTIONS FOR PAYMENT

When Secretary of Health and Human Services Otis R. Bowen proposed a MedIRA as a way of giving people an incentive to save for potential long-term or nursing home care, the proposal was dropped from the package on coverage for catastrophic illness under Medicare. The explanation for dropping it was, first, that most people did not want to think about needing long-term or nursing home care, and, second, that people would have to begin very early in life to save enough to cover the costs of such care. Although these objections may be valid to some extent, a MedIRA is still an option that ought not to be dismissed even if only a few persons opt to take advantage of it.

Private health insurers such as Aetna, Prudential, and Travelers have already begun to cover long-term care. Perhaps insurers might consider a plan to allocate a percentage of unused acute-care days each year into a long-term care bank for those individuals who do not use their health insurance. Another possibility is that contributions to a long-term care insurance fund could become a payroll deduction like Social Security, with employers contributing an equal amount. Still another option is to cover individuals for health care without specifying the type of care: acute or chronic, inpatient or outpatient, high-tech medical or low-tech clinical and personal. The only stipulation would be that the care is necessary to promote the health and welfare of the client.

People do not have the same needs for medical coverage or health care. Why should there be only one plan for everyone?

SUMMARY
Rationing care

There are some unpleasant questions to be faced. Can we afford to offer care indiscriminately to all who seek it? Is it time to begin to ration health services? Should we pay for extraordinary care for those whose life is limited to bed or chair or to pain and confusion? Should we pay for extraordinary measures, or any care at all, for those whose illnesses are a direct result of unhealthful behaviors and who refuse to alter those behaviors even after they have been warned or advised to change? If such a health promotion course were adopted, then the government or other health insurers would have to make provision for payments for health teaching and health maintenance or behavior modification counseling.

A decision to ration care might mean that those who can afford to pay for their own health care could receive services despite the rationing. Would the wealthy then drain the existing services to the extent that those who are eligible for services could not receive them?

Let us assume that the choice is for the lowest level of care possible within the realm of common humanity. In this environment, high-tech bionic engineering and complex surgical and chemical therapies would be reserved for those below the seventh decade, whose pathology is arrested, and who have potential for full recovery. Care for people with chronic illnesses and increasing pathology or residual functional impairments would be confined to conservative medical and nursing care at home or in pleasant, safe environments. Even with this structure, the cost of long-term care for the aged infirm or permanently impaired will still represent a major chunk of health care expenditures for this society. And as long as we continue to hire minimally competent personnel, it will cost more than it should.

The fact is that long-term care may not be considered high tech, but it is high skill. Perhaps the only way to prove this is to try to program a patient care plan in response to patient behaviors of the cognitively impaired, or a plan for the patient with osteoarthritis or the patient with both disabilities and perhaps a little congestive failure due to cardio-renal insufficiency. We could conjure up some interesting nursing diagnoses to respond to the behavior of an individual with these physiologic and pathological problems. The care would require any number of adaptations depending on which problem was predominant at any given time. Patient comfort and mobility would certainly vary according to the treatment given, and the treatment given would certainly be dependent on the assessment made by the care giver.

CONCLUSION

One thing is certain: we must find a way to get the government out of the health care field. Legislation and regulations protect, but they also constrain. We must seek ways to safeguard the quality of care by strengthening moral and ethical codes within the professions, and we must police and maintain the integrity of the individuals who practice within each discipline. Peer pressure must be the watchdog for good quality care, not regulations.

Ultimately it all comes down to where we want to spend our money and concentrate our resources. For me, the issue is clear. Our only claim to humanity is a respect for life.

REFERENCE

1. US General Accounting Office: Medicaid and nursing home care: cost increases and the need for services are creating problems for the states and the elderly. Report to the chairman of the Subcommittee on Health and the Environment, Committee on Energy and Commerce, House of Representatives, October 21, 1983.

CHAPTER 57

Who pays for the costs of care in other countries?

GILLIAN BISCOE

At one end of the continuum of health care financing is the marketplace approach; at the other end, government monopoly. Each country's position on this continuum arises from a complex interaction of culture, politics, economics, and management ability. No model in the world is agreed upon as the best for health care delivery and financing. The models used by various countries have their own particular advantages and disadvantages and are developed for a particular socioeconomic, cultural, and political environment.

There are also marked differences between developed and developing countries in terms of financing health care systems. Mortality is much higher in developing countries, as is morbidity. However, both developed and developing countries face an increasing gap between the costs of health care and the money available to meet those costs. There is increasing critical analysis of how health care might best be financed to reduce this gap. In some countries this resulted in the rationing of services. Around the world there is concern for problems that may arise in the future because of the increasing elderly population and a declining number of taxpayers contributing to health care costs.

The World Bank[4] has defined three main problems in the health care sector: allocation issues, such as insufficient spending on cost-effective health programs; internal inefficiency issues, such as wasteful public programs of poor quality; and inequity issues, such as inequitable distribution of the benefits of health services. The World Bank's view is that the fundamental cause of these problems is inappropriate approaches to health care financing.

In low-income developing countries (for example, Ethiopia, Uganda, Pakistan) the average spending on health is about $9 per capita per year. In middle-income countries (Poland, Thailand, Greece) the fig-

ure is $31. In developed countries (Singapore, France, Japan) the average figure is $670.[4]

The percentage of gross national product (GNP) spent on health in 1984 ranges from 2% by Ethiopia to 9.3% by the United States. In terms of total government spending, this figure becomes 3.4% for Ethiopia (the most recent figures available are from 1980) and 11% for the United States. In addition to government financing sources, more than half of the health care costs in developing countries are born directly by individuals. In developed countries this fraction is less than one fourth.

Definitions of what constitutes spending on health vary from country to country. In developing countries, for example, clean air and clean water may be included. In developed countries, these and other aspects of health may not be included in the health care accounting equation. However, these figures do serve a useful purpose for macro-level comparisons between countries.

Health care can therefore be said to cover an indefinable range of needs and services. The general view is that there is also an infinite range of demands made by consumers on any health care system. This issue can be put in a philosophical perspective: Is equity and access to health care a right, or should it be contingent on the ability of the consumer to pay?

An analogy might be the demand for luxury automobiles. A survey in the United States might result in 100% of the respondents replying "yes" to the question, "If you could afford a Mercedes-Benz, would you want one?" Not everyone drives a Mercedes-Benz because not everyone can afford one. The desire for a Mercedes-Benz does not entail satisfaction of that desire. Similarly, there may be an infinite demand for health care, but does that mean that countries have to fill that demand? The issue of need versus demand,

and the associated ethical debates, is receiving increased attention from both health care providers and consumers.

This argument cannot be fully developed in this chapter, but such issues are already influencing decisions on how health care is financed. Philosophical and ethical issues of needs versus rights, together with economic factors, will shape the future of health care financing.

The World Health Organization's 1981 goal of health for all by the year 2000 has resulted in increased attention to raising health status as distinct from providing curative services. Curative services is in many cases necessary precisely because both society and the individual do little to maintain health. At the crux of achieving health for all is the question of how to finance primary health programs while maintaining curative services in the transition period from an illness-oriented health system to a health-oriented system. In its simplest form the issue can be viewed as how to redirect the financing of expensive, hospital-based curative care to health-promotion and health-prevention strategies, in order to reduce the need for curative care.

INTERNATIONAL OVERVIEW
Singapore

Singapore's system of health care financing is based on aspects of its cultural philosophy. In Singapore the family is the basic social and economic unit. Although there is a collective responsibility on the part of society to care for the family, Singaporeans believe that personal responsibility also exists. Singapore is particularly concerned with the imbalance between an aging population and its younger members, and hopes to promote financial independence among the future elderly so that they may shoulder their own health costs.

Since 1984 employees and employers in Singapore have been required to make equal payments to employees' personal saving accounts. Interest is paid on the money deposited, the balance is the property of the account holder, and it can only be used to pay for the medical expenses of employees or their families. At retirement age (55 years) the account can be accessed but a minimum balance must be maintained. On the death of the account holder, any balance remaining in the account is paid to the estate's beneficiaries, free of estate or death taxes.

In 1983 health expenditures in Singapore were 6.4% of total government expenditures. The ratios of phy-

sicians and nurses to the general population were 1:1100 and 1:340, respectively, and the corresponding ratio for hospital beds was 1:340.

Poland

Prior to World War II Poland was regarded as an underdeveloped capitalist country. Since the war the organization and funding of its health care sector reflect the country's socialist political and economic structures. The Ministry of Health and Social Welfare not only directs 95% of Poland's health facilities, but also all of its medical education, medical research, and other research institutions.

Because of Poland's socialist political structure—and in contrast to Singapore—the salaries of health workers vary only slightly across all categories and are among the lowest in Poland in comparison to other occupational groups. This is based on the premise that health workers do not "produce," they "cost," which has resulted in an interesting social phenomenon. After 1945 the majority of men chose to enter careers that "produced," such as engineering, rather than the health professions. The end result is that medicine, dentistry, pharmacy, and nursing attract a higher percentage of women.

Attempts to bring reform to the health care system have been largely thwarted by the realities of the political infrastructure. Nursing has taken a leadership role, however, in the aftermath of the 1980 industrial difficulties. Following the Gdansk Agreement, a nurse chaired an advisory committee to the government addressing issues such as adequate primary health care; improved training for young physicians not located near hospital centers; improved mechanisms to address alcoholism; increased research, particularly on work-related diseases; more continuing education for health personnel; allocating a greater share of the GNP to health; and increased capital investments for construction and equipment in the health care industry.

The recent political changes in the Soviet Union are beginning to have an impact in Poland. How this will affect its health care system, in terms of process as well as outputs and outcomes is difficult to project. An encouraging sign has been the regular publication of some health statistics over the last few years.

The physician-to-population ratio in 1981 was 1:550. The 1965 figure for nurses was 1:410 (1981 figures were unavailable). In 1984 average life expectancy at birth was 67 years for males and 76 years for females. The infant mortality rate (for children under

1 year) was 46 per 1000 live births in 1965 and 19 in 1984.[4]

Denmark

The health care situation in Denmark reflects its cultural and political perspectives, with the state providing a strong social services infrastructure for the population. All residents of Denmark are entitled to free medical treatment by a medical practitioner or practicing consultant. This right is independent of income, the cost of the services being paid by revenue raised through taxes. Care for the infirm and the aged is closely allied to social services.

In 1981 health expenditures in Denmark were 1.4% of total government spending. The ratios of physicians and nurses to population were, as of 1981, 1:420 and 1:140, respectively. In 1984 life expectancy at birth was 72 years for males and 78 years for females. In 1984 the infant mortality rate had fallen to 8 per 1000 live births from 19 in 1965.[4]

Belgium

Belgium is a hereditary, representative, and constitutional monarchy. Belgian law largely reflects its national philosophy of liberalism and individualism. Paradoxically, its legislation on health financial matters, including physician reimbursement, is highly detailed and regulatory to the extent that it covers issues that in other western European countries might be regarded as infringing on ethical matters.

As in most industrial countries, health care costs in Belgium have been difficult to contain. Health insurance is compulsory, with individuals paying little if anything from their own pockets for treatment or consultation. This has resulted in a situation in which it is the norm to press for second opinions, which tends to overburden diagnostic facilities and increase costs.

West Germany

The Federal Republic of Germany is a democratic and socially federated state with the 11 *Lander* (substates) sharing decision making with the federal government. The federal government is responsible for ensuring that all West Germans have equal access to health care, and the *Lander* take the initiative in encouraging a wide range of health care services.

Health care costs are also rapidly increasing in West Germany. The health care system is funded through a network of programs providing considerable freedom of choice to the consumer. One difference between West Germany's health care funding system and many others is that it provides benefits not only for curative services, but also for the prevention and early detection of illness.

Japan

Japan has a nationwide social health care system, but the delivery of health care services relies heavily on the private sector. The social health care system is based on the West German model.

The Japanese Medical Association is particularly strong and has considerable influence on national medical policy. Physician income is very high compared to that of other professional groups. Japan's health care system is extremely complex, reflecting the complex nature of its society.

As with other nations, Japan faces steep increases in health care costs. Quality and availability of health facilities are assured in Japan. The combination of accessibility, availability, and health insurance programs results in an expensive system.

Canada

Canada's system of health care financing is based on equity and access, with means-testing considered anathema and anything less than 100% participation inequitable.

The Canadian constitution limits the federal parliament to implementing national programs through provincial governments. Private insurance is allowed only for services not covered under the provincial health services plan. Persons may not be excluded on the basis of preexisting conditions.

Canada spends 6.3% of its total government spending on health. This is a 10% increase in real terms over the previous decade. In 1981 ratios of physicians and nurses to the general population were 1:510 and 1:120, respectively. The average life expectancy at birth as of 1984 was 72 years for males and 80 years for females.[4]

France

Since the French socialist party came to power in 1981, there have been many changes to the laws and regulations affecting health. The socialist government has attempted to tackle health expenditures and to permanently modify the health care system through structural reforms such as decentralization and departmentalization. Again, as in most developed countries, health costs have in general risen faster than the nation's ability to pay. The government has sought to halt the rising costs of health care by limiting supply.[3]

France's social insurance system strongly reflects various occupational and class interests. Thus conflict arises along class lines more frequently than in other welfare states where social insurance systems tend to blur class conflict.

Switzerland

Since 1848 Switzerland has been a federation with cantons forming its federal structure. Responsibility for health care falls first on the cantons. Unlike Germany or Canada, Switzerland has no political ideology dictating equal access to health care.[2] Cantons therefore draw up plans to suit their own needs. There is frequent duplication of services, giving rise to additional and unnecessary expense. Some cantons are richer than others, resulting in further inequities. On the other hand, the Swiss view is that decentralization of decision making means that health care services can be adapted with considerable flexibility to the differing cultures and philosophies of the various cantons.

In 1983, 13.4% of Switzerland's total government spending went for health care, an increase of some 3% over the previous decade. 1981 ratios of physicians and nurses to the general population were 1:390 and 1:130, respectively.[4]

SUMMARY

The structure and financing of national health care systems is the result of complex interactions of culture, politics, and economics. For all countries the growth in national resources allocated to health care outweighs the growth in available resources.

The World Health Organization's philosophy of health for all strongly emphasizes equity.[1] There is, however, a basic economic principle having to do with choice. Choice means that not everything is available, that resources are limited, and that trade-offs must be made. Few countries have a strategic plan for health care. Few countries know what it is they are trying to buy with the large amounts of money expended on health care. Few countries measure what it is they have bought for those large amounts of money.

There are many who say that health care is first and foremost about care, that its social benefits outweigh any costs. There are others who respond that that may be so but decisions have already been made that entail that some people have access to treatment and others do not (for example, age restrictions for admission to coronary care units, or labor restrictions in delivering community-based health care).

There is no one model of health care that is right for all countries. Each different culture requires that health care delivery be tailored to those cultural needs. Each country's economy will determine to a large extent how much money is available to purchase health care. Politics is a key variable. The purchase of health care is expensive and the effective management of that purchasing process is critical.

Notwithstanding these complexities, the key to health cost containment is the national definition of milestones to be achieved and health goals to be attained. Strategic plans can then be developed that address allocation, efficiency, and equity issues in achieving those goals. A clear road map will then emerge, enabling each country to restructure health care to best suit its own unique situation.

REFERENCES

1. Andreano R: The challenges to health for all and primary health care: an economist's perspective. Unpublished background paper to joint WHO/ICN consultation on Nursing for primary health care: 10 years after Alma-Ata and perspectives for the future, 1988.
2. Veska: Health services in Switzerland, AARAU and the Swiss Hospital Association.
3. Walliman I: Social insurance and the delivery of social services in France, Soc Sci Med 23(12):1305, 1986.
4. World Bank Policy Study: Financing health services in developing countries, Washington, DC, 1987, World Bank.

PART NINE

PERSONAL AND PROFESSIONAL ASSERTIVENESS

Nurses must be personally and professionally assertive

JOANNE COMI McCLOSKEY
HELEN KENNEDY GRACE

Many of the previous chapters have raised problems; some have offered solutions. One ingredient of any solution is to "get involved"; frequently it is the only solution. Concepts related to career, image, women's work, and power are central. Part 9 is a discussion, then, of that solution recommended most often as the answer to many of nursing's professional problems—the act of getting involved.

Getting involved requires commitment. In the debate chapter for Part 9, Swanson explores the career development of nurses. If nurses do not view nursing as a career, how will they be able to find the energy, time, and commitment that getting involved requires? Swanson first reviews three career development theories including the 10 postulates of Super. Although these theories are mostly based on the career development of men, they are applicable in many ways to women. Using the theoretical framework as a base, Swanson asks whether there is career development in nursing. Most nurses are women and do not seem to look beyond the expectations of employment when they choose their occupations. Nursing is continually challenged by the lack of planning, which is critical to career development. Recent evidence does support more career development in nursing, but many nurses are still job rather than career oriented. Swanson's chapter indicates that career commitment in nursing needs to be fostered most during the middle stages of a nurse's career. Education and service must provide opportunities for nurses to do career planning. Anyone interested in the retention of nurses will find a number of provocative ideas in this very comprehensive, theory-based chapter.

To be retained, nurses must first be recruited. Interest in nursing among freshmen in junior and senior colleges has fallen from 8.4% in 1983 to 4.0% in 1987. The image of nursing has been identified as a factor in the nursing shortage. In their rich chapter on nursing's image, Donley and Flaherty examine the impact of nursing's image on the recruitment, employment, and retention of nurses. Nurses and others who are attempting to meet the crisis of the nursing shortage will want to pay particular attention to this chapter. In times of shortage, the image of the nursing profession becomes everyone's concern. Nurses who read this chapter in conjunction with Swanson's will want to debate the relative responsibilities that the individual nurse, the profession, and society have for the current situation in nursing.

In the next chapter, Curran focuses on strategies for changing nursing's image in the media. She argues that it is not necessary for nursing to project a single image, just a positive one. She examines two types of media: internal and external. Internal media include such products as catalogs, brochures, and newsletters produced for an institution. These are relatively easy to influence because they are developed and controlled by the institution. Nurses in the institution should examine the image of nursing being portrayed and whether nursing receives proportional representation. External media, or the popular press, include television, films, and books, among others. The press is very interested in information about health care but journalists do not understand nurse expertise. Curran urges us to avoid the tendency to be humble, apologetic, and timid when interacting with the press. She proposes that we make more use of media groups to work with the media. To influence the internal media, she proposes organized media committees in each institution. To monitor and react to the external media,

Self-concept is a significant element and is defined generally as the individual's perception of the circumstances or conditions of existence. Super[38] states that it is imperative to define self-concept in this way because the situation surrounding an individual always affects the individual's behavior and understanding.

"The process (item 4 of career development) may be summed up in a series of life stages characterized as those of growth, exploration, establishment, maintenance, and decline. These stages in turn may be subdivided into (a) the fantasy, tentative, and realistic phases of the exploratory stage, and (b) the trial and stable phases of the establishment stage."[38] The growth stage refers to the physical and psychological dimensions of development. Opinions and behaviors that are significant elements of the self-concept evolve during this stage. As these components of the self-concept are forming, individuals are involved in numerous experiences that will be of assistance to them in making their tentative and final occupational determinations.

In the exploratory stage, individuals understand that work is part of life. But their verbalized choices may be unrealistic and have no long-term significance for the individual, especially if they are expressed during the fantasy phase. After the fantasy phase, individuals advance into the tentative phase, in which occupational choices are limited to a few alternatives. It is also possible that all of the choices made will be eliminated due to the uncertainty about ability, educational offerings, or employment opportunities. During the final phase or the realistic phase, the list of occupational choices consists of those that individuals perceive are realistic for them to attain.

The establishment stage, as the name suggests, involves early efforts of actual work situations.[38] Using these work experiences as a testing ground, individuals evaluate whether the choices made in the previous exploratory stage have any merit. They may change jobs if the situation is not satisfactory. But if the work situation is appropriate, gains are made in confidence, experience, and proficiency, and the individuals become stabilized.

On advancing through the stabilizing phase of the exploratory stage, individuals enter the maintenance stage. As a part of this stage, individuals try to continue in or improve their occupational situation.[38] Because the work situation is always changing, individuals are always trying to alter those components of their work that are less than satisfying. It is interesting to note that individuals do not continually try to change their work situation. This becomes evident during the final stage of the career development process.

The decline stage is when individuals work to keep their jobs and are not concerned about enhancing their positions. This period ends at retirement. This stage is the last one of career development proposed by Super, but other authors have suggested another stage.

Murphy and Burck[20] propose a revision of Super's developmental theory that would include an additional stage occurring at midlife. They suggest that the stage of renewal be added between the stages of establishment and maintenance. Murphy and Burck[20] contend that a stage of this nature currently exists. It is when individuals reevaluate earlier goals and plans and either recommit to those goals or decide to refocus and make a midlife career change.

"The nature of the career pattern is determined by the individual's parental socioeconomic level, mental activity, and personality characteristics, and by the opportunities to which he or she is exposed."[38] All of an individual's experiences are relevant in forming attitudes and behavior. Some factors may be more significant than others, and parental socioeconomic level may be one of the most significant. This particular factor exposes individuals in the earliest stages of development to their parents' work, associates, and family, all of which can greatly influence later work patterns.[38] Additional factors that may be important are an individual's mental abilities and subsequent academic successes, the ability to work with others, and the gift of being in the right place at the right time.

"Development through the life stages can be guided, partly by facilitating the process of maturation of abilities and interests and partly by aiding in reality testing and in the development of the self-concept."[38] This postulate emphasizes the role of the secondary education system and its guidance program. The role of these programs is to assist individuals to develop abilities and interests and to help them obtain a perspective of their own strengths and weaknesses so they can make appropriate occupational choices.

"The process of vocational development is essentially that of developing and implementing a self-concept: it is a compromise process in which the self-concept is a product of the interaction of inherited aptitudes, neural and endocrine makeup, opportunity to play various roles, and evaluations of the extent to which the results of role-playing meet with approval of superiors and fellows."[38] Individuals develop and create mental images of themselves. One way in which the development of self-concepts is influenced is through the educational process. Before entering the workforce, individuals seek out experiences to maintain or improve their self-concepts. During these educational experiences, individuals encounter forces that may have a negative impact on their self-concepts, and they may have to compromise or accept less than what they want.[38] The work world provides similar experiences that affect one's self-concept.

Another component of this postulate is described in "A Life-Span, Life-Space Approach to Career Development."[37] Super emphasizes the variety of roles played by individuals during their lifetimes and the significance these roles have on lifestyle and career. Common roles that most people engage in are child, student, sibling, citizen, worker, spouse, and parent. These roles affect individuals' mental images of themselves and reinforce the lifelong aspect of career development.

"The process of compromise between individual and social factors, between self-concept and reality, is one of role-playing, whether the role is played in fantasy; in the counseling interview; or in real-life activities such as school classes, clubs, part-time work and entry jobs."[38] Individuals experiment with different activities to evaluate whether the vocational aspects of a job align with their images, but they cannot always experiment in real work situations or activities. Consequently, they may have to try to match self-images and vocational demands in situations that relate abstractly to the occupational choice.[38] Individuals may seek out related experiences to evaluate the fit between the occupations of choice and their self-images. Perhaps individuals interested in a health care occupation would volunteer at day-care centers, senior citizens' centers, or hospitals.

"Work satisfactions and life satisfactions depend on the extent to which the individual finds adequate outlets for his or her abilities, interests, personality traits, and values; they depend on his or her establishment in a type of work, a work situation, and a way of life in which he or she can play the kind of role that growth and exploratory experiences have led him or her to consider congenial and appropriate."[38] Super states that when experiences encountered at work correspond to the individuals' images, there is ample opportunity for individuals to be as they wish to be. In contrast, if work does not afford opportunities for individuals to act in accordance with their mental images of themselves, they are discontented. This dissatisfac-

tion could easily provoke them to look for work situations in which their mental images corresponded more to their work experiences.

Many studies have been conducted to evaluate Super's developmental theory and supporting concepts. In general, the research findings confirm the idea that occupational choice represents the implementation of a self-concept. The results also provide an impressive volume of empirical support for the general aspects of Super's theory.

Although these three theories are of primary importance in understanding the process of career development, some researchers contend that they do not adequately explain the vocational behavior of women.[22,24] For instance, these stages may be delayed or interrupted due to marriage and childrearing responsibilities. Fitzgerald and Crites[5] contend that the development of a vocational self-concept for women may be very complex because of the divided role expectations of a wife, mother, and worker.

Women career theories

With the paucity of theories directly applicable to women, other efforts have generated constructs relevant to a woman's career development. Psathas[28] delineated some of the factors affecting women's entry into occupational roles and stated that gender is the most noticeable of all factors.

A second attempt at constructing a career development framework for females can be attributed to Zytowski.[42] His nine postulates attempt to take into account the distinctive differences for men and women in work life, development, and patterns of vocational participation. For example, the woman's main role is that of a homemaker, which is dynamic yet orderly and developmental. Zytowski[42] also perceives that vocational participation of women will cause a departure from her main role in life. He concludes his postulates by stating that selected factors are responsible for a pattern of vocational participation for men and women. Interestingly, both Psathas[28] and Zytowski[42] focus on the homemaker's role as the primary one in the occupational life of a woman.

It appears that the difficulty with developing a theory uniquely for women relates to the everchanging role of women.[22,42] Fitzgerald and Crites[5] support this contention and continue by stating that women are a much more heterogeneous group than men with regard to life-career patterns. These factors do make the formulating of a relevant theory difficult, but the lack of theory for women does not mean that established theories of career development are of no value. "It seems reasonable to assume that all individuals, regardless of sex, share the basic human need for self-fulfillment through meaningful work."[5] In other words, theories can provide a practical means of viewing career development for women. Fitzgerald and Crites[5] believe that these theories can apply in some degree to everyone. Super[38] suggests that the general concepts of career development are applicable to women if modifications are made to provide for the childbearing role. Therefore, it seems appropriate at this time to apply selected aspects of the career development theories to women.

CAREER DEVELOPMENT: NOT IN NURSING

Career development in nursing can be evaluated using Super's theory with the incorporation of Murphy and Burck's renewal stage.[20] For example, the stage of utmost importance to the new graduate nurse is the establishment stage. The establishment stage includes employment with a commitment to that particular choice. The final occupational choice is accepted as the one that provides the best opportunities to meet the individual's goals and expectations. Another stage of career development that is applicable to this discussion is the renewal stage. To reiterate, the renewal stage, as defined by Murphy and Burck,[20] relates to the midlife career changes persons may experience between the ages of 35 and 45. Individuals reconsider occupational goals and plans and decide either to rededicate themselves to the original goals or to move in other directions with a midlife change. During the maintenance stage, as identified by Super,[38] individuals attempt to continue or improve their occupational situation.

Keough,[16] in her editorial "The Need for Nursing Career Development," defines a nursing career development program for nurses. It "is an organized system in which goals are set, needs are identified, counseling and guidance are available, plans are implemented, activities are evaluated in order to revise plans as needed." This approach resembles the components of Super's last three stages because of the focus on behavior and its action-orientation. In both processes, the person must become actively involved in career development and not just verbally communicate the intent of behavior. Otherwise no advancement can be made toward the achievement of the individual's desired career. Theoretically, I have adapted Super's vocational stages to nursing via Keough's[16] defined system of organization. But does career development exist within nursing? It is my contention that career development does not appear within nursing because nurses cannot move through the vocational developmental stages of establishment into a satisfactory position within the maintenance stage. Nurses can secure entry-level employment, but they do not develop stable positions, so retention becomes a problem. Evidence from across the United States shows that hospitals are having trouble retaining registered nurses.[4,6,7,27] Parker and Drew[23] and Colavecchio,[2] using similar terms, tie this inability to retain nurses to inadequate staffing, poor hours, low status, limited recognition, and changing assignments.

Surveys conducted by Donovan,[4] Gulack,[10] and Wandelt, Pierce, and Widdowson[41] support certain factors identified by Colavecchio. These factors of discontent can be grouped into three categories: content of the job itself, working conditions, and organizational factors. The major source of dissatisfaction in relation to job content is that of a quantitative overload.[41] Nurses identify the high patient-staff ratios, the volume of paperwork, and the intense time pressure to complete work as components of this overload phenomenon. Pines and Maslach[26] contend that it is the overload that leads to burnout rather than the intense interpersonal nature of the work.

The second major issue contributing to the nurses' dissatisfaction stems from concerns about their working conditions. Nurses are concerned about (1) the variable schedules, long hours, and floating from unit to unit; (2) the sufficiency of fringe benefits; (3) the problems of interacting with a support staff of questionable competence; and (4) compensation.[4,10,41]

The third source of discontent among nurses concerns organizational factors.[4,10,41] The specific factors were the lack of support and recognition from both hospital administration and medical staff. Nurses were also dissatisfied with the lack of recognition they received for their professional competence, the lack of input into the job, and the need for improved nurse-physician relations.[41] Another factor was the inability to advance within the system due to the flat organizational structure. The organizational structure, as it exists, offers the professional very few positions for promotion and upward mobility.

Thus when disenchantment occurs, the nurse

moves on to another job, another occupational choice, or withdraws from the work world entirely. National League for Nursing statistics reported in the *Journal of Advanced Nursing* support this changing of jobs or withdrawing from the system. Data showed an increase in the proportion of nursing graduates employed in nonnurse positions as the years increased since graduation. After 5 years, 1% of the graduates were in nonnurse occupations, whereas 6% were in those types of positions after 10 years. There was also a sizable shift in full-time work to part-time employment. For example, 1 year after graduation 85% of the graduates worked full-time and 5% worked part-time; 10 years after graduation the percentages were 37% full-time and 22% part-time.[21]

Data collected by Donovan conveys a similar picture. "Two out of every five nurses drop out of the job market at some point. . . ."[4] Other statistics from Donovan's article support a declining job stability within the profession. Nurses in the 45 and older age bracket have stayed in each of their jobs for at least 7 years, whereas, nurses in the 25 to 34 age bracket have held each of their jobs for approximately 2½ years.[4]

Although burnout has been given as a reason for increased mobility and temporary or permanent withdrawal, Kleinknecht and Hefferin[17] indicate that indecision about professional goals is also an important factor. Limited opportunities for professional development and the inability to determine and direct their own future produce turnover and a low sense of achievement. Now the problem of nurses not focusing on career development goals is complicated by the nursing shortage. Administrators have to float or relocate nurses from specialty area to specialty area to provide patient care or to maintain financial solvency. These moves are made without considering the interests, goals, or experiences of the nursing staff involved. Price and Randolph[27] contend that this scenario makes career development unrealistic.

Two other factors are relevant in considering the lack of career development for individuals within nursing. Nursing is still a predominately female occupation, although the number of males is increasing.[31] But with nursing being female oriented, certain behaviors associated with women are bound to exist. Mahoney[18] contends that women do not plan. Consequently, they do not think about employment-related possibilities. Smith[31] perceives that nurses do not think in terms of a planned series of steps of development or advancement. Friss[6] also examines this idea in relation to the

individual nurse. Nurses are not geographically mobile; they tend to fashion "their careers around local labor markets."[6] Carr[1] relates this lack of planning to the system. He believes that nothing exists within the system to allow talent and ability to be used at higher levels.

Mahoney[18] comments on another behavior common to women that, if true, would suggest that it would be extremely difficult to operate in nursing with a career-development orientation. She contends that women do not look beyond the expectations of employment when they choose their occupations. Women pick up an occupation that is easy to enter and leave without being demoted. Several nurse authors unknowingly have applied these attitudes about employment to nursing. Masson's statement regarding career appeal could be related to the implications of Mahoney's statement: "Experienced professional nurses believe today that early appeal as a career eludes them. . . ."[19] Friss[6] again comments on the relationship of nursing or nurses to a career. Nurses have minimal career aspirations, and those who want to develop a paying work career do not choose nursing.

In summary, a nursing career could provide greater satisfaction as a profession. Nursing is continually challenged by the lack of planning, which is critical to career development. As Keough[16] points out, staffing crises occur frequently because vacancies exist. However, the major deterrent to career development in nursing is nurses' inability to enhance or improve their vocational positions, a factor that contributes to the high rate of staff turnover and professional dropout.[7] Thus because nurses cannot change those unpleasant aspects of their work situation, they are driven out of their positions and the profession. They do not advance through the maintenance stage of Super's career development theory *or* remain within the profession.

CAREER DEVELOPMENT IS POSSIBLE IN NURSING

There are opportunities within nursing to assist new graduates in securing appropriate positions. Reres[29] and Smith[31] present the idea of an appraisal tool that helps nurses recognize their goals, skills, and personal needs. Furthermore, this entire process is usable in attaining a position compatible with one's lifestyle, talents, and goals. Reres[29] supports this contention but approaches it from a benefit perspective. It allows the nurse to maximize and realize the rewards of the system. This knowledge of one's own skills allows the nurse to view opportunities for advancement more positively. Similarly, Hefferin and Kleinknecht[11] suggest an assessment of work-related preferences for certain kinds of nursing activity. Using a research approach, they developed the Nursing Career Preference Inventory (NCPI) to "assist individual nurses in identifying their personal patterns of nursing work interests or preferences and determine the primary nursing practice areas and the hospital-based nursing role positions that most often reflect the identified work interest patterns."[11] Although the researchers state that the instrument is based on an inpatient health care setting, the results of the instrument may be useful to nurses in other traditional and nontraditional settings in assessing their career goals.

Super[38] stated that persons within a stabilization phase are secure and comfortable. Nurses are becoming more comfortable psychologically within the profession. Smoyak[32] reports that nurses value one another more than they did 10 years ago. For example, nurses are seeking each other out for consultation, acknowledging one another, and are more positive with regard to what they have to offer.

Another aspect of either the establishment stage or the maintenance stage related to financial gains. Granted, nurses have not made sizable gains financially, but because most nurses are females, one point needs to be reinforced. The economic motivations of women and men are not different, as people once believed. Smoyak[32] and Osipow[22] argue that although their motivations are not different, discrimination with respect to pay still exists. Smoyak[32] believes that this discrimination is being countered by intelligent women with an activity-oriented approach.

Once an individual has secured a position, decision making and goal setting can be used to formulate a career path that points to future opportunities and advancements. Of importance within Super's maintenance stage and Murphy and Burck's renewal stage are not only goal setting and decision making but the availability of informational resources as well. Smith[31] comments on the variety of resources accessible to nurses: counselors, career planning literature, university courses, continuing education offerings, and personnel and staff development offices, for example. Specifically to address the issue of professional career development, the nursing department of Mount Sinai Hospital in New York City established the Nurse Career Counseling Services in 1982. According to Vezina,[40] the nurse career counselors assist the nursing staff by providing counseling and guidance on pertinent career development issues.

Other aspects of career development are evident within nursing. Smoyak perceives that nurses' interests in one another's development has created an "upsurge of mentorships."[32] Smith[31] believes that the entire profession is active in career development, not just individual nurses. An example is the presence of nursing programs assisting students to formulate their career plans. Faculty members act as role models when they maintain their clinical skills. Smith[31] perceives that this clinical orientation reinforces for students the reality of a hospital career commitment. Other faculty members promote the career planning of their students from a different perspective. Jarczewski,[14] in "The Career Plan: A Luxury Item?", presents the format for a career planning unit of a trends course offered the final semester of a nursing program. Content for the career planning unit includes the selected concepts of "professionalism, career planning, and management of various roles of career nurses."[14] Students also become knowledgeable of the process of career planning.

Sossong and associates[33] describe how managers who recognized the significance of staff nurses to patient care were able to create a stimulating environment for career development. The program provided nurses with the opportunities to advance professionally and financially within their area of choice. With the staff nurse as the center of the "RN Career Opportunities Program," the career options branch into the areas of nursing management, education, practice, or research.[33] Each of the three work options is influenced by the nurse's interests, goals, and desires. "Since most career advancement options required national certification or advanced degrees, the administration worked to bring opportunities to attain them. . . ."[33] Subsequently, advancement to the next higher level position is based on position availability, performance, educational degrees, and recommendations by superiors. Thus career opportunity programs do exist within medical centers to assist in the professional development of nurses.

Other examples of the profession's commitment to career development exist. Kleinknecht and Hefferin explain the open and closed models for career development.[17] The open system includes all appropriate persons in the assessing and planning of the individual nurse's career, with knowledge that all are benefited.

But the focus of the closed system is to prepare the individual for one particular position within an organization. Kleinknecht and Hefferin[17] mention the similarities and differences of the systems. The similarities focus on the nurse currently being employed by the primary organization, all persons are interested in the career chosen, and the models are relevant for any identified occupational group. But the major difference is the breadth and depth of career paths available. The closed system looks primarily at opportunities within the employing organization, and the open system allows for opportunities outside of the organization as well. But regardless of whether the system is open or closed, the models are operating to provide opportunities to learn new skills and meet the requirements for newly established positions—positions that offer the nurse a choice for professional development and advancement. Shaffer and Moody[30] view models such as these as a means of keeping nurses out of the traps that can occur at certain job levels.

In her article on staff development, Sovie[34] identifies a systematic approach to hospital career development. This career pattern incorporated the aspects of professional identification, professional maturation, and professional mastery. Within each of the components, Sovie[34] identified activities or behaviors to be accomplished. Specifically, for nurses to move toward professional maturation, they must master their job functions, display meritorious performance with clinical competence, and formulate a psychological contract with the employing organization. On completion of these tasks and others, one would be eligible for staff development for eventual career advancement and, subsequently, professional mastery. A number of tasks must be completed at each level before movement within the process, however.

Another option for nurses within the Sovie model[34] assists those who may not choose to progress through the three phases. A nurse may consciously decide to stay in the first or second component. Sovie believes that the individual should be given every opportunity possible to make this career decision and be viewed as a valuable professional. Sovie in the second article[35] of the two-part series perceives that the career model she has identified is applicable to other hospital nursing careers, not just nurses practicing patient care.

Shaffer and Moody[30] and Kleinknecht and Heffjferin[17] write in separate articles of the career-development approach operating within selected units of the Veterans Administration Nursing Service in the United States. Kleinknecht and Hefferin present its major elements as orientation to career development, self-assessment techniques, and program implementation sessions. During the orientation, the nursing career facilitator gives material on the focus of the program, the career opportunities available within the system, and the experiences offered through the program to help nurses advance. Then selected tools are completed to gain pertinent information about the nurse's past experiences, interests, strengths, and professional goals. In the third component the nurse is involved with a facilitator in individualized counseling sessions. During these sessions, the nurses gain insight into their qualifications, potentials, interests, and career opportunities.[17]

Evidence of career development does exist within nursing. Programs exist to help nurses evaluate their own interests, goals, and values. These approaches also allow for the formulating of activities to ensure the advancement and career fulfillment. Programs of this nature not only exist but serve vital functions to nursing. They can provide a means to meet the particular needs of each agency or individual while expanding the talent and achievement aims of the present nursing work force.[17]

CAREER DEVELOPMENT: PROMOTE MORE IN NURSING

Whether career development exists within nursing is still an issue, but the promoting of career development is not. Sovie[34] reports that 35 of 41 studies identified professional recognition, career mobility, and advancement opportunities as professional needs of nurses. Nurses in health care settings do want more career opportunities. But most important, the individual nurse will not be the only one to profit from career development; the profession will as well. Smith[31] contends that through careful career planning, the profession can meet the demands of the nursing shortage. Furthermore, nurses desiring leadership positions or displaying leadership potential can outline career plans and obtain the appropriate training. Sovie[35] views the benefits from a different perspective. She believes that career-oriented nurses cannot exist within an organizational system in which they are the bottom rung of the ladder. Thus to secure and retain these persons in the positions for which they chose nursing—*nursing practice*—career development must be a realistic possibility within the profession.

I believe the individual nurse as well as the profession should have a commitment to career development. Nurses need to be knowledgeable of their own interests, values, and aspirations. The development of key attributes has a direct effect on a career. They must be cognizant of tasks or opportunities that will increase their chances for advancement, not hinder them. Nurses must learn to capitalize on their professional opportunities through planned career development.

Professionally, career-development models like Sovie's[34,35] and Kleinknecht and Hefferin's[17] need to be applied to a variety of nursing settings. Other career models need to be generated. More staff educators should be involved in career development experiences with nurses of differing educational and work backgrounds. Assessment tools and strategies need to be devised and tested, with the results being communicated in the professional publications. Nurses need to review these materials and use them in personal and health care settings. It is only through applications of these tools, strategies, and models that ones relevant and pertinent to nursing can emerge.

In closing, nursing service and nursing education must work together on career development. They can work to change the individual nurse's view of nursing as a haphazard series of jobs. Both can help a nurse to see nursing as a challenging, interesting, and rewarding profession with satisfaction deriving from direct patient care. Both can be vehicles through which to discuss ethical issues, personal values, and trends that can assist nurses to evaluate their own career development. But of utmost importance, education and service can provide opportunities for career planning. Nursing has much to offer its practitioners, but career development with the involvement of nursing education and service must be part of nursing's future.

REFERENCES

1. Carr A: Promotion: family vis-à-vis career, Nursing Mirror 150(11):14, 1980.
2. Colavecchio R: Direct patient care: a viable career choice? J Nurs Adm 12(7):17, 1982.
3. Davis DA, Hagen N, and Strouf J: Occupational choice of twelve-year-olds, Personnel and Guidance Journal 40(7):628, 1962.
4. Donavan L: What nurses want (and what they're getting), RN 43(4):22, 1980.
5. Fitzgerald LF and Crites JO: Toward a career psychology of women: what do we know? What do we need to know? Journal of Counseling Psychology 27(1):44, 1980.
6. Friss L: An expanded conceptualization of job satisfaction and career style, Nursing Leadership 4(4):13, 1981.
7. Gibson LW and Dewhirst HD: Using career paths to maximize nursing resources, Health Care Management 11(2):73, 1986.
8. Ginzberg E: Toward a theory of occupational choice: a restatement, Vocational Guidance Quarterly 20(3):169, 1972.
9. Ginzberg E and others: Occupational choice: an approach to a general theory, New York, 1951, Columbia Univ. Press.
10. Gulack R: Why not fit the job to the nurse? RN 45(5):27, 1982.
11. Hefferin EA and Kleinknecht MK: Development of the nursing career preference inventory, Nursing Research 35(1):44, 1986.
12. Henning M and Jardin A: The Managerial Woman, New York, 1978, Pocket Books.
13. Hollender J: Development of a realistic vocational choice, Journal of Counseling Psychology 14(4):314, 1967.
14. Jarczewski PH: The career plan: a luxury item? Nursing Success Today 3(10):6, 1986.
15. Kelso GI: The influence of stage of leaving school on vocational maturity and realism of vocational choice, Journal of Vocational Behavior 7(2):29, 1975.
16. Keough G: The need for nursing career development, Journal of Continuing Education in Nursing 8(3):5, 1977.
17. Kleinknecht MK and Hefferin EA: Assisting nurses toward professional growth: a career development model, J Nurs Adm 12(7-8):30, 1982.
18. Mahoney ME: Part-time for a life-time: the limits facing most working women. Presentation, Wellesley College, October 24, 1981.
19. Masson V: Nursing: healing in a feminine mode, J Nurs Adm 11(10):20, 1982.
20. Murphy PP and Burck HD: Career development of men at mid-life, Journal of Vocational Behavior 9(3):337, 1976.
21. National League for Nursing: Summary report on American nurse career pattern study: baccalaureate degree nurses ten years after graduation, Journal of Advanced Nursing 4(6):687, 1979.
22. Osipow S: Theories of career development, ed 3, Englewood Cliffs, NJ, 1983, Prentice-Hall, Inc.
23. Parker JE and Drew KF: Women, work and health, Occupational Health Nursing 30(7):27, 1982.
24. Patterson LE: Girls' careers-expression of identity, Vocational Guidance Quarterly 21(4):268, 1973.
25. Pietrofesa JJ and Splete H: Career development: theory and research, New York, 1975, Grune & Stratton.
26. Pines AM and Maslach C: Characteristics of staff burnout in mental health settings, Hospital and Community Psychiatry 29(4):233, 1978.
27. Price JL and Randolph G: Career trajectory in nursing: the Randice approach, Nursing Success Today 1(2):21, 1984.
28. Psathas G: Toward a theory of occupational choice for women, Sociology and Social Research 52(2):253, 1968.
29. Reres M: Self-assessment and career choice, Imprint 26(3):13, 1979.
30. Shaffer MK and Moody YK: A model for career development, J Nurs Educ 19(8):42, 1980.
31. Smith MM: Career development in nursing: an individual and professional responsibility, Nurs Outlook 30(2):128, 1982.
32. Smoyak SA: Women/nurses in 1982: how are we doing? Occupational Health Nursing 30(7):9, 1982.
33. Sossong A and others: An expanding universe: professional career opportunities, Nursing Management 18(2):46, 1987.
34. Sovie MD: Fostering professional nursing careers in hospitals:

the role of staff development (Part 1), J Nurs Adm 12(12):5, 1982.

35. Sovie MD: Fostering professional nursing careers in hospitals: the role of staff development (Part 2), J Nurs Adm 13(1):30, 1983.

36. Super DE: Vocational development in adolescence and early adulthood: tasks and behaviors. In Super DE and others: Career development: self concept theory, New York, 1963, CEEB Research Monograph No. 4.

37. Super DE: A life-span, life spacer approach to career development, Journal of Vocational Behavior 16(3):282, 1980.

38. Super DE: Career and life development. In Brown D and others, editors: Career choice and development, San Francisco, 1984, Jossey-Bass.

39. Tiedeman DV: Decision and vocational development: a paradigm and its implications. In Zytowski DG, editor: Vocational behavior, New York, 1968, Holt, Rinehart & Winston, Inc.

40. Vezina ML: A new approach to professional development nurse career counseling, Journal of Nursing Staff Development 2(1):38, 1986.

41. Wandelt MA, Pierce PM, and Widdowson RR: Why nurses leave nursing and what can be done about it, Am J Nurs 81(1):72, 1981.

42. Zytowski DG: Toward a theory of career development for women, Personnel and Guidance Journal 47(7):660, 1969.

CHAPTER 59

Viewpoints

Strategies for changing nursing's image

ROSEMARY DONLEY
MARY JEAN FLAHERTY

The nursing shortage of the 1980s has focused public and professional attention on the profession of nursing. In analyzing the parameters of the crisis, public image emerges as a factor in the shortage. The enhancement of nursing's public and professional image also has been proposed as one strategy for remedying the crisis. Borrowing from the outline provided by the Commission on Nursing of the U.S. Secretary of Health and Human Services (HHS),[65] in this chapter we will examine the impact of image on the recruitment, employment, and retention of nurses. Nursing's image will be studied from the viewpoint of significant publics: prospective students, practicing nurses, and their administrative and medical colleagues. Strategies for image enhancement will be suggested.

THE PUBLIC IMAGE OF NURSING

Some analysts report that nursing is no longer attractive to career-oriented young women, socialized by the women's movement to seek new challenges. These women have been taught to shun fields that are predominantly female. For example, interest in nursing among freshmen in junior and senior colleges fell from 8.4% in 1983 to 4% in 1987.[11] In 1968 freshmen women aspiring to nursing outnumbered future physicians 3:1. In the fall of 1986 more college women wanted careers in medicine.[25] A longitudinal study of college freshmen supports these findings.[11] Its 20-year tracking of college freshmen suggests that gender differences no longer explain career aspirations or college majors. Austin, Champion, and Tzeng[12] explain that nursing is associated culturally with weakness. Feminist writers outline the concerns commonly expressed by nurses and identify them as concerns of women. The problems on the job, in the economic marketplace, and in professional and social situations that have filled nursing journals are common themes in the evolving women's literature.[27] Cleland[17] says quite clearly that the source of nursing's problems, as with the historical problems of women, is alienation from sources of power.

Literary perspectives on nursing

There is a tendency in much modern writing to disregard and devalue not only the handmaiden role but also other traditionally feminine responses associated with nursing. Newton[50] presents a provocative minority view when she argues that the "gentle sister" image of the nurse may be important to ill and dependent patients and, in fact, aid in their recovery. Curran[18] acknowledges that when nurses gave up uniforms and caps, on the assumption that clothing has no effect on competency, they ignored the symbolic power of uniforms. Webster[66] notes that it is not wearing white that is important, but public beliefs about the meaning of the white nurse's uniform. Little[43] identifies the movement away from nursing uniforms as a "strip-tease" that began with psychiatric nurses in the 1950s, spread to pediatric nurses, and became normative with the women's movement. She pleads for nurses to return to the uniform, embrace the values of tradition, and dress for success as professional nurses. However, Little's position is not in vogue. Today people anxious to make a difference in health and human welfare are free to select "power" careers in medicine or health care financing.

If the selection of nursing is not seen as avant-garde

or challenging by young women or by the public, what is it seen as by more traditional high school students and their parents? How are ideas about nursing shaped? In study after study, the social class of the respondents has influenced their perceptions of the field. Upper-class respondents in one study ranked nurses with waitresses; those from lower classes considered nursing to be a noble profession.[59] In a very insightful study of registered nurses in Kansas City, Deutscher[20] not only reported that nursing image was inversely correlated with social class but also presented a nursing typology or set of stereotypes: the Sairey Gamp, the alcoholic nurse described by Charles Dickens; the ministering angel; and the trained professional. If nursing images relfect the views of beholders, it is not surprising that these images have changed over time. Kalisch and Kalisch[29] traced those changes in image: the nurse as angel of mercy (1854 to 1919), girl Friday (1920 to 1929), heroin (1930 to 1945), mother (1945 to 1965), and sex object (1966 to the present).

Bishop[14] believes that the public, unaware of nurses' expertise, thinks that nurses do what they are told by physicians. Physicians and hospital administrators seem inordinately concerned about the image of nursing. In fact, the handmaiden-of-the-physician image or its modern expression, the physician substitute or the registered care technician, vies with the angel of mercy as the most recognized image of nursing. The work of Kelly[34] suggests that hospital administrators and physicians project an image of nursing more congruent with their respective roles than with the statements of nurses. Health care consumers, particularly patients, tend to act out their images of nursing. Sometimes their positions are passive and reflect the expectations that nurses will perform personal health services or carry out the wishes of physicians. At other times, support from consumers has enabled nurses to obtain practice privileges in hospitals or to develop alternative health care delivery systems that support client independence and decision making.

When Clark[16] examined behavioral expectations in the area of professionalism she found that nurses, the largest and most adaptable group of health professionals, have little influence on health policy and decision making. Nurses, who see themselves as undervalued, having no status, and receiving few economic rewards, respond with apathy, boredom, and a lack of professional commitment.

On the other hand, Maher[44] thinks consumers are beginning to recognize the value of nursing and its contribution to health care. She cites as evidence the APACHE 11 study conducted at the George Washington University Hospital, which demonstrated that nursing care makes a difference in patient survival rates in intensive care. Simmons[59] noted 25 years ago that the significance of an image is related not to its validity but rather to the vigor with which it is held and to the influence it exerts over behavior. Later research showed that different groups hold different images. Beletz[13] found patients in her study described nursing behaviors that varied considerably from accepted definitions of professional nursing activities. In 1988 a report of the American Hospital Association (AHA) Special Committee on Nursing[5] questioned whether the word *nurse* reflected professional responsibilities and duties.

Media Perspectives on Nursing

A natural question arises about the kinds of information prospective students receive through the media, a dominant influence in the late twentieth century. What do young people see on television and in the movies? What do they read in newspapers and books that contributes to their impressions of nurses?

Stereotyping remains the greatest obstacle to the accurate protrayal of nurses on television.[8,15,52,57,61] Bohn,[15] a free-lance writer, examined televised images of nurses and concluded that nurses were generally shown as dumb and silly sexpots or as battle-axes. These portrayals carry the message that nurses are inferior, subservient, or decorative in the world of medicine. Speculating as to how writers acquire their notions about nurses, Bohn suggested that nurses create their own images in their interactions with patients and visitors.

These reflections support beliefs that inaccurate public images of nurses will change when nurses take the initiative in self-portrayal.[46,52,61] Miaskowsky and Zwerlein[46] pleaded with the Oncology Nursing Society to assume leadership in the promotion of positive images of oncology nursing as a strategy to generate public interest in the work and image of nursing. In 1988 the National Commission on Nursing Implementation Project (NCNIP) received a favorable response from the Advertising Council in support of a major national media campaign to clarify and improve the image of nursing.[48]

The lack of consensus about the image of nursing evident in the literature occurs among and within nursing's reference groups. Aroskar[9] calls this phenomenon the fractured image, and suggests that the different perceptions existing between and within groups are harmful to the nursing profession and to its contributions to health care. In defense of her thesis that cracks and conflict exist in the image of nursing, she presents the traditional contemporary view of nursing proposed by Olesen and Whittaker.[53] Ashley[10] describes a system in which nurses are taught to care for the "hospital family" and to meet the needs of patients and staff. In her classic study of new graduates, Kramer[36] describes conflicts played out in the hospital culture between new nurses with baccalaureate degrees and diploma nurses.

Long before the present shortage, the "image problem" was identified as bad for nursing's health. In 1975 the House of Delegates of Sigma Theta Tau, the international nursing honor society, concluded that improvement in the public's image of nursing is a major professional challenge.[58] A Delphi survey of the members of the American Academy of Nursing[42] ranked as the three top priorities (1) developing public awareness of the unique contribution nursing makes to health care, (2) improving the public image of nursing, and (3) creating public acceptance of nursing as an independent profession.

Kalisch and Kalisch are among several researchers who have documented what needs to be changed about images of nursing. One of their nurse-physician comparative studies found media nurses to be less intelligent, rational, and individualistic in their behavior.[33] They were also less important to story plots. The fictional nurses of 1920 to 1980 were less likely to value scholarship or achievement, made fewer clinical judgments, valued service and helpfulness to patients less, and showed fewer nurturing and empathic behaviors than physicians. The researchers concluded that the image of nursing declined over the span of 60 years, while medical images stayed the same or improved.

A parallel study examined 2561 articles in the lay press between 1978 and 1981 for references to nurses. Operating room nurses ranked above community and psychiatric nurses in capturing media attention.[32] It appeared that the professional Association of Operating Room Nurses (AORN) was instrumental in highlighting the clinical activities of its members. The Kalisches noted that community health nurses, successful in generating news, managed news coverage poorly.[30] The work of psychiatric nurses was rarely noted in the lay press during the period of study.[31]

In another comparison, Krantzler[39] studied how nurses and physicians were represented in advertisements in the *Journal of the American Medical Association* and the *American Journal of Nursing*. He noted that although both professions were highly ritualized and represented by traditional symbols, physicians gradually exchanged their classic symbols (white coats and stethoscopes) for business suits and emerged as senior consultants and entrepreneurs. In the meantime, nurses gave up their caps and put on white coats and stethoscopes. The author observed that doctors and nurses were depicted in their respective journals as idealized and independent of each other. Krantzler found little congruence between the advertisements and the social reality of nursing and medicine.

The absence of nurses in television programs is instructive. In 1984 NBC aired a series of 20 10-minute health sequences during National Health Month. Psychologists, registered dieticians, pharmacists, doctors, and safety control experts made presentations. Nurses were not pictured in the series and the word *nurse* was used to describe the potential for school nurses to identify vision problems. The information booklet sent to 250,000 people made no reference to the nursing profession. Later, when a survey was sent to a sample of nurses and nursing students, all 300 respondents perceived a need to include accurate, detailed information about the value of nurses in health promotion. However, only one respondent of those who saw the series (n = 94) noted the absence of nurses. No one suggested that nurses should have been included in the series.[63]

Nurses are being urged to protest every unflattering representation in the media, such as the portrayal of a nurse accepting a cash tip from a patient in an episode of "Murder, She Wrote," or the appearance of nurses in magazines such as *Playboy*.[51] The nurses featured in the November 1983 centerfold of *Playboy* precipitated angry reactions in the professional literature. Critics expressed feelings of betrayal and discouragement that nurses would contribute to the sexual exploitation of women[19] and the perpetuation of the stereotype of nurses as sex symbols.[35]

Proposals for Changing Nursing's Image

It is generally accepted that nursing's image needs to be changed. Smith[60] proposed a tripartite approach that includes (1) the transformation of self-image into a professional image; (2) the development of a favorable public image in which presentation behaviors, personal appearance, and public relations reflect the transformed self-image; and (3) the expression of a corporate self-image. Smith argues that in today's highly competitive health industry cleanliness and neatness are no longer hallmarks of a positive nursing image.

The Kalisches[31] recommend several approaches to changing the public's images of nursing: developing skills in responding to questions about important issues, writing letters to the editor for local newspapers, submitting articles about nursing to small papers and newsletters, and regularly using newspapers' calendars of events. There is no formula to alter inaccurate or inadequate presentations. However, several nuggets about newsmaking can be drawn from lay interest in clinical events. High-tech nursing, like high-tech medicine, captures public attention. Dunn[23] believes that nurses can change their public image by working within nursing agencies and professional organizations. She suggests that nurses capitalize on the drama of their work and report their observations reliably. Diers[2] puts it another way when she asserts that positive professional image lies in the development of professional practice. The instructive message is that nurses should present themselves and their work to fit the public interest agenda.

There is ample evidence that nurses are of interest to the media. Most nurses, however, believe that the negative portrayal most recently exemplified by the televised series "The Nightingales" diminishes public respect and discourages talented people from seeking careers in nursing. The literature offers three suggestions—communication[62], public education[56] and campaigning[54]—for combatting negative media images of nurses.

Image as a Factor in Employment

Images of nursing in the workplace are complex and contradictory. People who look to the workplace for an explanation of the nursing shortage are intrigued by the seemingly insatiable demand of hospitals, nursing homes, and home care settings. The nursing shortage has dominated the agendas of national and regional meetings of provider groups. The U.S. Congress, poised to increase significantly the federal budget for nursing has placed special emphasis on the workplace in its 1988 revision of the Nurse Education Act.[6] Schools of nursing and health care institutions are stimulated by the promise of grants to plan innovative

schedules, benefits, and proposals to change the scope and division of work. Private foundations are sponsoring demonstration projects to entice hospitals to reform their nursing services.[55] As noted earlier, the Secretary of Health and Human Services has launched a blue-ribbon Commission to make recommendations about the nursing shortage. Major newspapers, including the *New York Times*, the *Wall Street Journal*, and the *Washington Post*, and television talk show hosts Phil Donahue and Oprah Winfrey, all have discussed the work of nursing as a factor in the shortage.

It can be argued that high visibility and high demand for nurses in all sectors of the health environment support the image of a desirable and sought-after profession. However, the demand for nursing services has a dark side. Identification with visible, coveted fields usually brings high salaries, highly selected colleagues, and the ability to exert influence and control. A recent American Nurses' Association (ANA) survey of 3500 nurses listed sources of dissatisfaction in the workplace.[28] More than one half the sample reported lack of support from nurse administrators (76%); inadequate salaries (70%); lack of available help when a patient needs extra care (70%); inadeqaute registered-nurse-to-patient ratio (67%); a sense of not being an important member of the health team (60%); and undesirable work schedules (50%). When nurses in this study were asked to identify what was bad about nursing, they cited child-care facilities (78%), support from hospital administrators (66%), support from nurse administrators (65%), salary (52%), and benefits (42%). The AHA Special Committee on Nursing[5] identified 24-hour industrial positions, task-oriented functions, lack of support staff, complex technology, severity of patient illness, and required documentation as environmental hazards in the hospital workplace.

Autonomy

The NCNIP[47] describes the work of nursing as undifferentiated practice. Put another way, anecdotal information and some literature indicate that nurses are seen as interchangeable by administrators, who ignore differences in age, experience, education, or specialty preparation in assigning responsibilities to their registered nurse force.

In the U.S. the dazzling array of educational choices in nursing (the 2-, 3-, 4-, 5-, and 6-year curricula) and the generalist meaning of the term *registered nurse* contribute to confusion about identity, appropriate scope of nursing practice, and disparity between clinical authority and responsibility. The blurred image of the registered nurse makes indiscriminate substitution of one nurse for another a convenient but inadequate response to the shortage. Substituting nurses for other health professionals (dieticians and pharmacists) and ancillary personnel (housekeepers, ward clerks, and messengers) as a strategy of cost containment is an equally ineffective response, and adds to the shortage of nurses. The Magnet Hospital Study[3] and Kramer and Schmalenberg's revisiting of selected magnet hospitals during the nursing shortage[37,38] suggest that autonomy in clinical nursing judgment, control of nursing practice, and participation in governance and in determining conditions of work are critical to professional self-image. Autonomous professions set boundaries around their scopes of practice. These borders create a mystique that discourages others from assuming the profession's work or assigning its responsibilities. The level of autonomy in nursing as illustrated by substitution in the workplace reflects the feminist perspective that the work of nursing is undervalued and unrecognized.

Status

The literature on status looks at the nurse in the health care hierarchy, examining the nurse's position relative to health care administrators and physicians. The parochial tendency to look to hospitals or physicians for validation distracts nursing from seeking influence in the worlds of policy, finance, and business. It is possible to name the few nurses who sit at buisiness and policy tables. Sheila Burke and Carolyne Davis, members of a small group of influential nurses, are described in the press as ex-nurses. Nurses' limited participation in board rooms,[40] and the tendency to bring early closure to nursing careers,[22] conspire against personal and professional actualization by denying nurses access to some traditional paths to career advancement. Although the women's movement has raised the sights of many women, too many nurses see head nursing, a deanship, or a nursing vice presidency as the end of the rainbow. The so-called shortage studies, although colored by the number of hospital-based nurses who struggle with organizational and professional authority, indicate that support from administration is essential to self-esteem and professional actualization.[28] Hafer and Joiner[26] addressed the problems of image and role conflict among health partners in their research on hospital environments. Nurses perceive organizational environments as insensitive

and uninterested in employee satisfaction. Nurse-physician relationships, perhaps the most studied yet least understood factor in clinical care, have deteriorated during the nursing shortage.

The 1988 American Medical Association (AMA) proposal to introduce "registered care technicians" into fragmented hospital environments has been seen as yet one more indication that physicians do not respect nurses as colleagues. The proposal was presented for action to the AMA's House of Delegates over the objections of the ANA and without review by other major nursing associations.[7] That physicians think they can solve the problems of nursing gives insight into the fragility of collegial relationships between organized nursing and medicine's rank and file.

Nurses' search for professional status has not been understood or accepted within organized medicine or the hospital industry. Physician "captains of the ship" are made uncomfortable by the independent practices of nurse-midwives, nurse-anesthetists, and nurse-practitioners. These nurse providers are perceived to be competitive with the financial and professional interests of practicing doctors. Most doctors argue for interdependent or dependent roles for nonphysician providers and for medical leadership of the health care team. Nurses have been systematically denied status under Medicare, Medicaid, Blue Shield, and most private insurance plans. Many nurse-midwives and nurse-practitioners are refused admitting privileges in hospitals. Nurses are not members of the Joint Commission on the Accreditation of Health Care Organizations (JCAHO). The bid by the National League for Nursing (NLN) to have its home care program, CHAP, given deemed status under Medicare is stalled in a bureaucratic maze in the Health Care Financing Administration. The status of nurses as underlings, dependent workers subject to organizational and medical whims, creates morale and image problems in the workplace and dampens enthusiasm for professional nursing practice among practicing nurses.

Compensation

The members of the HHS Secretary's Commission on Nursing pondered the question, Why, in the face of an ever-increasing number of graduates from schools of nursing, is there an insufficient number of nurses to meet the demands of the workplace? After public hearings, sensitive reviews of the literature, and frank discussions, the attention of the commission members was drawn to salaries and compensation. Admittedly nurses are a bargain in the workplace.[41] Their starting salaries, estimated in 1987 to average around $21,000,[41] increase slowly. Salary compression produces situations in which nurses with 10 years of continuous experience earn only about $9000 more than neophytes.[4] Nurses are not adequately compensated for hardship duties such as working alone; working on weekends, nights, or holidays; or working rotating or double shifts. Graduates with baccalaureate degrees ordinarily earn no more than two-year graduates. Licensed practical nurses earn 75¢ for every $1 paid to registered nurses.

Image, especially the feminine image, may be a factor in wage depression. Gardner's study[24] of hospital benefits led him to an examination of the hospital worker. Hospital employees are likely to be female and slightly younger than other workers. They frequently have working spouses (70.5% of hospital nurses are married) and young children (21% have children under 6 years old). They have skills that allow them to change employers easily. The difference in economic outcomes for male and female workers is apparent when the link between salary, gender, and education is explored. The U.S. Department of Education's Center for Educational Statistics[64] reports that male workers with 4 years of college have a median income of $32,000, while women with comparable backgrounds earn $21,000. Hospital workers tend to be underpaid when compared to other workers.[24]

A portion of the nursing work force is employed part-time. Although they earn about the same as their full-time colleagues ($11.90 per hour as compared to $12.10 per hour), part-time workers receive few benefits.[5] The employer's ability to build a full-time work force with part-time employees contributes to the depression of salaries and to the image of nurses as "seasonal" workers. In highly technical societies workers are paid for what they know. For example, engineers and lawyers almost double and quadruple their salaries, respectively, at the end of six years.[1] Teachers, on the average, earn 19% more than nurses.[2] An average nurse's income is 17% of the average physician's income.[5] Nurses are not perceived as scholars or as posessing highly valued specialized knowledge. They can be called on to carry out a wide range of custodial and clerical tasks. Their work can be delegated to less-prepared technical workers. Nurses have failed to establish themselves as "knowledge workers". This failure has diminished nurses' abilities to demand professional wages and benefits.

IMAGE AS A FACTOR IN RETENTION

The report of the HHS Secretary's Commission on Nursing[65] blends issues related to nurse employment with the retention of a competent, experienced work force. This mix represents an interesting development, because retention has not been given much attention in the health care workplace. Throughout its history the hospital industry has relied on the educational pipeline. Student nurses staffed hospitals into the 1950s. Later, hospitals counted on the yearly crop of new graduates to fill vacancies and to carry out the "hardship work". Adjusting to the turnover of nurses has been a necessity in health care. Hospitals institutionalized the management of turnover in their budget planning, setting money aside for recruitment and dedicating staff development personnel to the care and training of newly hired nurses. There were no incentives to develop retention programs.

There is some evidence that hospitals will reexamine their salaries and personnel policies when the need arises. This represents a market orientation, not an altruistic response to the requests of organized nursing. The negative image of nursing, the women's movement, and the economy all have had a profound effect on enrollment in preservice programs. NLN data show that enrollments have decreased by 26% since 1983.[49] Adherence to the traditional formula—increasing starting salaries and offering extra incentives to attract nurses during periods of shortage—ignores enrollment trends. Enlightened administrators are showing concern for their experienced work forces. The work of the AHA committee indicates an awareness that hospital fringe benefits do not compare favorably with industry models.[5] However, successful retention strategies require more than the unfreezing of salary ranges and the elimination of salary compression. The development of professional personnel policies cannot hinge on "frequent flight" bonuses for nurses who accumulate months of employment. Structural reform of health care financing must occur if lasting changes are to be made in nurses' compensation.

Nursing's perennial concerns about compensation, scope of work, and status offer a reasonable framework in which to examine strategies for improving retention and changing nursing's image. Fixed reimbursement and prospective budgets are indicators of the no-growth philosophy of health care costs. With the majority of nurses employed by institutions, unique opportunities are afforded by the new pattern of hospital and long-term-care reimbursement. It may be in the best interest of hospitals to break out the costs of nursing care from routine operating costs. The grouping of nursing services with room and board produces two undesirable effects. Nursing service appears as an expense rather than a revenue-generating center on the hospital budget. It is a strange phenomenon that accounting protocols produce the perception that nursing services cost money but do not produce income. Under prospective payment formulas, nursing care is the reason for admission, yet budgeting frameworks do not recognize that the need for nursing care brings people to hospitals. The second negative factor associated with the current financing arrangement undermines the value of professional practice. The grouping of nursing service with room and board charges contributes to the vision of the nurse as homemaker-caretaker.

The current system of health care financing does not enable the public to choose nurse providers. The same financial policies that ignore nursing services as health care benefits deny qualified, nurse-midwives, nurse-practitioners, and nurse-clinicians the status of providers. Until a major reorganization of the third-party-payer system is achieved, adjustments to salary and compensation for hospital and nursing home nurses will be merely cosmetic.

There is a bright side. The present crisis has brought public attention to the career patterns of nurses who expect recognition from their years of experience and professional development. The health care industry and professional nursing organizations have appeased these practitioners by calling for clinical career ladders and better salaries. Other industries that employ professionals provide experienced workers with opportunities for increased responsibility and influence. University presidents usually come from the ranks of the faculty. Physicians become presidents of foundations and phamaceutical houses. Businesspeople become board members and presidents. However, there is little career advancement in nursing. For example, head nurses become coordinators. Experienced staff nurses become nurse IIIs, the most advanced level of nursing practice.

It is essential to ask why people are attracted to or remain in particular fields. What can be said of a profession where the work is frustrating, hours are uncertain, rewards are few, recognition is limited, and salaries are poor? Who remains in a field that can be described in such negative terms—the entrapped, the ignorant, or the holy?

Nursing has not been taken seriously as a career because society traditionally has considered the work of nursing—or other female endeavors—to be preparation for the more important work of women: marriage and motherhood. However, Labor Department statistics and professional data provide a picture that does not fit the stereotypical careers of nurses of the 1940s or 1950s. Today, the percentage of employed nurses is the highest among traditionally female work forces. Diversification of health delivery patterns, the growth of nurse pools, and new jobs in quality assurance, ambulatory care, and case management have made it possible for nurses to control their own working schedules.

Perhaps attention to retention issues, taking the form of long-range strategies to change the scope and conditions of work and to redefine compensation, is the key to resolving the present crisis and the more significant problem of image. These problems will abate if a revolution occurs in health care that recasts the work of nursing as an autonomous, proud professional practice whose members provide nursing service, who work collegially with other health providers and with the public, who plan more sensible and cost-effective systems of delivery, and who develop public policy in support of these initiatives.

REFERENCES

1. Aiken LH: Nurses for the future: breaking the shortage cycles, Am J Nurs 12(Suppl):1616, 1987.
2. Aiken LH and Mullinix C: The nurse shortage: myth or reality, N Engl J Med 117(10):641, 1987.
3. American Academy of Nursing: Magnet hospitals: attraction and retention of professional nurses. Kansas City, Mo, 1983, American Nurses' Association.
4. American Hospital Association: Surviving the nursing shortage: strategies for recruitment and retention of hospital nurses, Chicago, 1987, The Association.
5. American Hospital Association: Report to the Special Committee on Nursing, Chicago, 1988, The Association.
6. American Nurses' Association: Capital update, Washington, DC, 1988, The Association.
7. American Nurses' Association House of Delegates: Reference Hearing, E Nashville, Tenn, June 1988, ANA.
8. Angelone R: Nursing's media image: overcoming the stereotypes, Journal of Practical Nursing 34:28, 1984.
9. Aroskar M: The fractured image: the public stereotype of nursing and the nurse. In Spicker S and Gadow S, editors: Nursing images and ideas: opening dialogue with the humanities, New York, 1980, Springer Publishing Co.
10. Ashley J: Hospitals, paternalism and the role of the nurse, New York, 1976, Columbia University Press.

11. Astin A, Korn W, and Green K: Retaining and satisfying students, Educational Record, Winter, 1987, p 36.

12. Austin JK, Champion VL and Tzeng OCS: Crosscultural comparison on nursing image, Int J Nurs Stud 22(3):231, 1985.

13. Beletz E: Is nursing's public image up to date? Nurs Outlook 22:434, 1974.

14. Bishop B: Don't wait to be asked (editorial), Maternal Child Nursing 12:85, 1987.

15. Bohn VL: The image of nurses in television, Nursing Success Today 3(2):20, 1986.

16. Clark MD: The historical basis for nursing's troubled self-image, AAOHN Journal 34(4):169, 1986.

17. Cleland V: Sex discrimination: nursing's most pervasive problem, Am J Nurs 71:1542, 1971.

18. Curran C: Seeing ourselves as others see us. Today's OR Nurse 6(18):23, 1984.

19. Dains JE: Nurses' image: an act of betrayal, Journal of Education in Nursing 10:20A, 1984.

20. Deutscher I and others: Social and occupational characteristics of an urban nursing complement: a study of the registered nurse in a metropolitan community, Kansas City, Mo, 1956, Community Studies.

21. Diers D: To profess to be a professional, J Nurs Adm 16(3):25,1986.

22. Donley R: Don't say no to success, Nursing Success Today 3(12):29, 1986.

23. Dunn A: Tricks of the trade, Nursing Times 80(9):48, 1984.

24. Gardner E: Flexible benefits plans help boost employee morale, reduce costs, Modern Health Care 17(7):51, 1987.

25. Green KC: The educational "pipeline" in nursing, J Prof Nurs 3(4):247, 1987.

26. Hafer JC and Joiner C: Nurses as image emissaries: are role conflicts impinging on a potential asset for an internal marketing strategy? Journal of Health Care Marketing 4(1):25, 1984.

27. Heide W: Nursing and women's liberation, a parallel, Am J Nurs 73:824, 1973.

28. Huey FL and Harley S: What keeps nurses in nursing: 3,500 nurses tell their stories, Am J Nurs 88(2):181, 1988.

29. Kalisch PA and Kalisch BJ: Anatomy of the image of the nurse: dissonant and ideal models. In Williams C, editor: Image-making in nursing, Kansas City, Mo, 1983, American Academy of Nursing.

30. Kalisch PA and Kalisch BJ: The press image of community health nurses, Public Health Nurs 1(1):3, 1984.

31. Kalisch PA and Kalisch BJ: Psychiatric nurses and the press: a troubled relationship, Perspect Psychiatr Care 22(1):5, 1984.

32. Kalisch PA and Kalisch BJ: Newspapers and nursing, AORN J 42(1):30, 1985.

33. Kalisch PA and Kalisch BJ: A comparative analysis of nurse and physician characters in the entertainment media, J Adv Nurs 1(1):179, 1986.

34. Kelly L: A frame of reference for nursing education, doctoral dissertation, School of Education, 1965, University of Pittsburgh.

35. Kinney M: Nurses are people too, Focus on Critical Care 11(1):7, 1984.

36. Kramer M: Reality shock: why nurses leave nursing, St Louis, 1974, The CV Mosby Co.

37. Kramer M and Schmalenberg C: Magnet hospitals: part I, J Nurs Adm 18(1):13, 1988.

38. Kramer M and Schmalenberg C: Magnet hospitals: part II, J Nurs Adm 18(2):11, 1988.

39. Krantzler NJ: Media images of physicians and nurses in the United States, Soc Sci Med 22(9):933, 1986.

40. Kusserow RP; Management advisory report: Nurse participation in hospital decision making—potential impact on the nursing shortage. OAI-03-88-01120, 1988.

41. Landers RK: What is causing the nursing shortage? Editorial Research Reports, Washington, DC, March 25, 1988, Congressional Quarterly, Inc.

42. Lindeman C: Priorities within the health care system: a Delphi survey, Kansas City, Mo, 1981, American Academy of Nursing.

43. Little D: The "strip tease" of nurse symbols or nurse dress codes: no code, Imprint 31:49, 1984.

44. Maher AB: Now that we've finally arrived (editorial), Orthopaedic Nursing 6(3):10, 1987.

45. Meade CD; Control the media with power, Nursing Success Today 3(12):24, 1986.

46. Miaskowski C and Zwerlein L: Reflections and reactions to nursing's image in the media, Oncology Nursing 13(5):95, 1986.

47. National Commission on Nursing Implementation Project: Timeline for transition into the future nursing education system for two categories of nurse and characteristics of professional and technical nurses of the future and their educational programs, Milwaukee, 1987, NCNIP.

48. National Commission on Nursing Implementation Project: Personal communication, August 1, 1988.

49. National League for Nursing: Nursing student census with policy implications 1986 Pub No 19-2202, New York, 1987 NLN.

50. Newton L: A vindication of the gentle sister: comment on "the fractured image." In Spicker S and Gadow S editors: Nursing images and ideals: opening dialogue with the humanities, New York, 1980, Springer Publishing Co.

51. Nursing can do without... St. Elsewhere, Nursing '86 16:1, July-Dec. 1986.

52. O'Heath KA: The challenge: nursing's accurate portrayal, Imprint 31:53, 1984.

53. Olesen V and Whittaker E: The silent dialogue: a study in the social psychology of professional socialization, San Francisco, 1968, Jossey Bass.

54. Raleigh ED: Promoting a professional image through campaigning, Nursing Success Today 3(2):4, 1986.

55. Robert Wood Johnson Foundation: Personal communication, 1988.

56. Seidenberg A: Controversies in school health, school nurses: improve the reception and sharpen the image, J Sch Health 54(9):363, 1984.

57. Siegel FA; Lights, camera, action! the nurse's image in theater and film, Nursing Success Today 2(8):20, 1985.

58. Sigma Theta Tau: Avenues of action: proceedings of the 1975 biennial meeting, Indianapolis, 1975, Sigma Theta Tau.

59. Simmons L: Past and potential images of the nurse, Nursing Forum 1:16, 1962.

60. Smith BA: Toward a more profitable nursing image (interview), Nursing Success Today 1(4):18, 1984.

61. Smith SJ: Nursing's public image: what they see versus what you know, California Nurse 81(4):8, 1985.

62. Tellem SM: Building a positive public image, Dimensions of Critical Care 3(1):30, 1984.

63. Turnbull E: Nurses respond to NBC over "accurate portrayals," Nursing Success Today 3(6):4, 1986.

64. US Department of Education, Office of Educational Research and Improvement: Digest of education statistics, Washington, DC, 1987, Center for Education Statistics.

65. US Department of Health and Human Services, Secretary's Commission on Nursing: Interim report, July 1988.

66. Webster ML: Professional style: an update, Nursing Life 5(2):63, 1985.

CHAPTER 60

Effective use of the media

CONNIE R. CURRAN

Not since Nurse Ratchett in the film and novel *One Flew over the Cuckoo's Nest* have nurses been portrayed as negatively as those in the 1988 to 1989 weekly television series *Nightingales*. In these popular media pieces, nurses are nonprofessionals who contribute to patients' suffering. Research by B. and P. Kalisch reveals that the general public views nurses as angels, mothers, physician's handmaidens, sexually promiscuous, and coldhearted. Yet nurses perceive themselves as patient advocates, patient educators, care givers, coordinators, technicians, and researchers. Why does this vast difference exist between public perception and self-perception?

In 98% of all U.S. homes there is at least 1 television set that is operating approximately 6½ hours a day. Most American homes subscribe to at least one newspaper and one or more magazines. Over 90% of all automobiles have radios and approximately the same percentage of homes have radios. Annual movie attendance is in the billions. The media bombards Americans in their homes and cars and during work and leisure hours.

The media educate, inform, evaluate, and entertain Americans. According to Lenore Hershey, a noted journalist, "The press has the responsibility to report the news, to inform the general public and to evaluate the society they reflect." The Kalisches' research indicates that the media perpetuate negative stereotypes of nursing. The media do not intentionally malign nursing but present what their representatives perceive as accurate. Nursing must present information that accurately describes nursing to the public and the media. There are several approaches that nurses and the nursing profession must take to use the media to promote a positive image of nursing.

Because nursing is many things and nurses work in a variety of settings with a variety of individuals and families, there are many opportunities for confusion and communication. The great heterogeneity within the profession can be very positive in portraying nursing to the public as versatile, specialized, and a broad-based profession. It is not necessary to project any single image; it is, however, imperative to project a positive image.

The public is often unaware of the many roles nurses play. Nurses are care givers, coordinators of other health team members, patient advocates, and health educators. They are the largest group of employees in most health care institutions. Nurses spend more time caring for the ill than any other professional group. Their educational and experiential backgrounds are a rich resource to the general public, yet nurses are often anonymous. Rarely do nurses introduce themselves as "*Ms* ____, your registered nurse." First names tend to be commonplace. What type of professional accountability and authority is communicated by using first names only? Physicians do not introduce themselves using their first names: they refer to themselves as "*Doctor* ____." Teachers, attorneys, social workers, and even airline attendants use the titles *Mr.* or *Ms*. These groups recognize that authority and accountability are essential to accomplishing their jobs. Nursing must examine the use of titles, credentials, and last names, and the messages they send.

Individual and group efforts can promote a more positive image of nursing. In the early 1950s the American Medical Association (AMA) formed a group to work with the media. This group has been very effective in preventing the media from projecting negative images of physicians. Nursing can have this same effect by working through groups. Media committees should be organized in hospitals, schools of nursing, and in local, state, and national nursing organizations. When working with the media, the position of the individual is strengthened by the impact of the group.

INTERNAL MEDIA

Internal media are catalogs, brochures, newsletters, annual reports, advertisements and other forms of publicity developed by an institution. It is important to collect and analyze the material distributed by an institution. What kind of visual message do these materials communicate about nursing? Are nurses shown caring for patients, or are they following the physicians? Are the nurses in "high-tech, high-touch" situations, or in handmaiden roles? Is the nurse shown as the primary patient care giver or as a victim?

Nurses are the largest group of hospital employees. Do they receive proportional representation in the institution's media? Is nursing included in the annual report and other significant documents? The type and amount of coverage given to nursing sends an important message about how much an institution values nursing. Advertisements should be analyzed for both their verbal and visual content. Do ads use professional language? Are there references to "professional nursing practice?" The words may communicate one image and the photographs a conflicting one.

Recruitment materials send a message to the general public as well as to potential employees. The recruitment and retention of nurses can be greatly influenced by the message communicated through the internal media. Realistic photographs of nurses (including older nurses, minority nurses, and male nurses) shown caring for patients, studying, or in leadership roles visually communicate the career opportunities available and the commitment the institution requires. If the message conveyed is "come here to meet a husband," an institution may well lose nurses who are career centered and attract nurses who are husband hunting. When the institution's message is "we want caring, committed professionals," it will attract nurses who perceive themselves in those ways. If the message conveyed is "we value our nurses," the public's perception is that nurses are very important to health care.

Internal media are relatively easy to influence because they are developed and controlled by the institution. The institution's public relations department usually coordinates internal media production. Public relations staffs are usually composed of journalists with little or no experience in the health care field. They also may have inaccurate stereotypical images of nursing. Therefore it is important to educate the public relations staff about nursing. Invite staff members to spend time on nursing units. Direct experience will create an accurate nursing image and allow the journalist to observe the nurse in various roles. For example, how many journalists know exactly what the nurse does on the night shift in critical care? Or the

diversified and sometimes conflicting roles of the nurse administrator? Nursing is a field rich in human interest and patient success stories. These are the types of stories that public relations personnel will use to tell the institution's story.

Nurses also can work directly with the public relations department to affect the staff's orientation to nursing and to ensure the better representation of nursing in the institution's internal media. Some institutions have developed nursing media committees that work with the public relations department. Media committees are active in developing public relations materials. The media committee submits nursing news items to the institution's internal media, creates "draft copies" for publications, and provides photographs that communicate accurate visual messages about nursing. In large institutions media committees are often effective because of the number and variety of nurses they include. Committee members can assist the public relations staff in gaining access to expert staff nurses for needed information, or may serve on internal editorial boards to exert influence on the institution's publications.

Media committees are intriguing to nurses who may have had their fill of quality assurance or nursing diagnosis committees. Even in a very small hospital with a very limited (or nonexistent) public relations department, the nurse executive can use a small nursing media committee to write a nursing newsletter for distribution throughout the house. The nurse executive in a small or large institution can be a public relations committee of one simply by writing intradepartmental and interdepartmental memos to share the accomplishments of the nursing staff.

Successful media committees, in time, can expand beyond their influence on internal media to more fully affect the institutional image. The news media often fail to accurately report nurses' contributions to health care. Media committee members can encourage participation by staff nurses in community health-related activities and can then seek local newspaper coverage for the events. This may lead to coverage of more innovative nursing accomplishments, such as effecting shorter hospital stays. Nurses have been leaders in innovative health care practices such as home care, hospices, and birthing centers, but the news media rarely give credit where credit is due. (However, nursing strikes always get a lot of publicity.) The media committee can ensure that the public relations release credits nursing appropriately—or committee members can write it themselves. In addition, the committee can solicit from staff nurse experts—perhaps even from the nurse executive—letters, editorials, or articles for the local newspaper on health care issues pertinent to the community. Surveys of the general public consistently indicate the public's desire for more information related to health. Nurses can be excellent resources for health-related information. Well-written, informative articles that identify the writer as a nurse from a particular institution reflect well both on the institution and on nursing as a profession.

Media watch groups are an effective way to sensitize consumers, advertisers, and producers to media that are positive or negative in their portrayals of nursing. The function of such groups is to react to the media and reward or reprimand journalists for their health-related material. This positive or negative feedback can be in the form of letters, phone calls, or personal visits to editors, producers, writers, and commentators. The public relations department can acquaint the media watch group with appropriate media contact persons; frequently this information is only a phone call away.

Image is important to all that nurses do. There is increased concern for nursing's personal image in light of the current focus on nursing as a product and as a result of well-documented projections of even more severe problems in nurse recruitment and retention. There is also increased concern for the institutional image in light of the current competitive health care market. The general public and nursing value competent, professional care. The great majority of nurses deliver such competent, professional care. It is time for nurse executives to define and communicate that message in a clear and consistent manner, to successfully market nursing.

Nursing must assume a role in creating public relations materials that portray nursing in an accurate and positive manner. In-house media tell the institution's story. It is vital that nursing receive acknowledgement for its contribution to that story.

EXTERNAL MEDIA

External media, or the popular press, include television, radio, films, newspapers, magazines, and books. Nursing is often portrayed inaccurately in the popular press. The media have projected nurses' images as angels, handmaidens, mothers, naughty, and sexually promiscuous. Soap operas, films, and magazines constantly reinforce these inaccurate stereotypes. Because of the control the popular press exerts over public opinion, it is very important to influence and shape these vehicles.

The popular press makes money and gains power through the numbers game. The greater the circulation and the higher the ratings, the more money advertisers are willing to pay. Therefore, the media are interested in stories that will capture viewers or listeners or sell copies. Public appeal is their common goal. Surveys of the general public consistently indicate the public's desire for more information related to health. Nurses are an excellent resource for health-related information. They can be very valuable resources to the popular press.

Nurses can access the media directly; they can communicate through television, radio, newspapers, and magazines. Nurses are experienced health educators and their communication skills and educational abilities are great assets in communicating with the popular press. Before making contact with the press, nurses must prepare to sell themselves and their ideas. It is essential that nurses establish themselves as experts. Journalists usually do not know about nursing expertise. They often share the same stereotypes of nurses held by the general public. Therefore, it is advisable to prepare a résumé and a written statement that assures the journalist that the nurse is representing a constituency and speaking as an expert. A résumé should stress the number of patients cared for and the number of hours worked with a particular illness, as well as a nursing background that includes health communication and education. Nurses should avoid the tendency to be humble, apologetic, and timid. The nursing media committee can review the material and ensure that it is suitable for the popular press. The media committee can assist individual nurses in presenting their materials in a nontechnical fashion with a human interest focus.

A brief written statement must be developed to sell the ideas for the story, emphasizing through statistics and facts the number of people who might have an interest in the topic. Because the media are concerned with the extent of public interest, emphasize the numbers involved. Communicate in a clear, concise, visual, and positive manner. Avoid the use of technical language and medical jargon. Include visual material such as graphs and pictures of equipment. These props are especially significant for the visual media.

Conceptualize the task as selling ideas to the general

public. Timeliness is important to the popular press. When something is in the headlines, the media attempt to capitalize on the public's interest in that topic. When Nancy Reagan had breast cancer, there were innumerable stories on cancer, breast surgery, and medical technology. Journalists were searching for health professionals who could discuss these topics. Nurse media committees should take advantage of this type of interest by matching interested journalists with nurse experts. Journalists often are responsive to nursing's offerings that are related to topics of national and local interest.

Specific access routes for contacting the media vary. Newspapers and magazines include names and addresses for submission of manuscript ideas. A telephone call to a radio or television station will yield the name and address of the producer of a particular show. It is important to determine the correct fit between the show or column and the information to be offered. Attempt to match the material to the particular audience of the show or column.

The employer's public relations department is another access route to the media. Public relations employees usually have relationships established with members of the community's press. The media committee should meet with the public relations staff members and discuss ideas with them. Presenting public relations personnel with a brief overview of the material and seeking their advice and assistance in accessing the appropriate media channels can be very beneficial in gaining media access.

REACTING TO THE MEDIA

Because media are driven by numbers there is always great interest in the public's reactions. The press is interested in both the positive and negative reactions of the public. A rule of thumb is that for every letter or telephone call there are a hundred others in agreement. Therefore producers, publishers, and sponsors are very interested in public reaction to their material.

The nursing media committee and media watch groups can offer technical assistance to the press. They can volunteer to review materials for technical accuracy. This type of review creates the opportunity to offer advice regarding material related to nursing, to alter inappropriate images, and to provide an accurate portrayal of nursing and other members of the health care team. This type of technical advice has been pro-

vided to major motion picture studios by the AMA. Its successful results can be duplicated by nursing groups.

Individuals and groups can also write letters to the editors of magazines and newspapers. Television and radio stations provide individuals with the opportunity to respond to their editorial positions. Nurses can also take advantage of public service announcements to inform the public of special health programs. These public service announcements are suitable for such services as blood pressure programs or vision screening programs and inform the public of other services offered by nurses.

SUMMARY

In summary, nursing's public image is often at great odds with the way nurses perceive themselves, and is often inaccurate. The media—both internal, institutional media and external media such as television, radio, and newspapers—are the most effective creators of nursing's image. Therefore, it is important for nurses to work, both individually and collectively, to improve nursing's image. This can be done by forming media watch committees to monitor the outside media and by using internal nursing media committees to influence an organization's publications and advertisements to reflect an accurate, professional image of nursing. It is important to join together to influence the press, television, and other media sources of the public's impressions of nurses. Nurses must work together to ensure that the image of nursing presented to the public is an accurate one and one that reflects professionalism and dignity.

BIBLIOGRAPHY

Curran C: Strategies: marketing nursing, Nurse Executive Management Strategies 9:1, 1988.

Evans D and Fitzpatrick T: A district takes action, Am J Nurs 83:52, 1983.

Kalisch B and Kalisch P: Anatomy of the image of the nurse: dissonant and ideal models. In Williams CA, editor: Image-making in nursing, Kansas City, Mo, 1983 American Academy of Nursing.

Kalisch B and Kalisch P: Improving the image of nursing, Am J Nurs 83:50, 1983.

Kalisch B and Kalisch P: A comparative analysis of nurse and physician characters in the entertainment media, J Adv Nurs 11:179, 1986.

Turck J and Curran C: The hidden deficit behind the hospital nursing shortage, Health Marketing 6:10, 1988.

CHAPTER 61

Nursing and political power
The cutting edge of change

GLORIA R. SMITH

As the health care industry becomes more turbulent, nurses must become more political if they wish to control their future and to influence the direction of the health care system. In the context of a system shrinkage it is important to examine how nurses behave as a group. We must determine whether our implicit model of the political process is likely to yield the results we hope for: professional autonomy and the authority we need to shoulder our responsibilities effectively.[3] Two recent thrusts are particularly instructive: the emergence of nurses in elected and appointed public offices, and a more unified approach of professional organizations to a limited political agenda.

During the first week of May 1988 a number of nurse leaders around the United States were excited about the news that Myra Snyder, Executive Director of the California Nurses' Association, had resigned her job to take a new position—as deputy mayor of the city of San Francisco. The news of Snyder's appointment was broadcast quickly through nursing networks and her new celebrity status is certain to be applauded by nursing colleagues. There is considerable interest among nurses about how to get and use power. There is a heightened awareness of politics and increasingly nurses are sizing up the political scene. More and more in nursing circles the dialog is centered on the relationships among power, leadership, politics, and policy formulation. It is recognized that solutions to world and community problems in health care advanced by nurses to provide optimum cost-effective services will be implemented only if nurses have power as decision makers and access to decision makers. For nurses to have power recognized and acknowledged by communities, they must be more visible and potent in the political arena and they must have agendas that are relevant.

The numbers of women holding public office in the United States have increased over the years. Currently 2 of 100 senators and 23 of 435 congressional representatives are women. During the past decade there has been an increase in the number of women holding state, county, and municipal offices, including a number of nurses (and a smattering of male nurses). One can applaud the increase in public offices held by both women and nurses; however, there is not parity in relation to demographics. Women hold 18,000 of 116,000 public offices in the United States.[2] Although elected office is not the only way to influence the shaping of public policy, it is certainly the most direct way. Many people enter political life through the route of appointment, as did Carolyn Davis, who was appointed Director of the Health Care Financing Agency; Barbara Sabol, Cabinet Secretary of the Kansas Department of Health and Environment; Barbara Nichols, Cabinet Secretary of the Wisconsin Department of Licensing and Regulation; and Gloria R. Smith, Director of the Michigan Department of Public Health.

There are no primers that ensure success in the political game. Thus the tendency on the part of retiring, departing, or exiled politicos to tell their stories may be fueled more by the need for the individual to discover coherence than to do a bit of ego boosting. The apt student of politics understands this and approaches such autobiographical material as if developing gounded theory, that is, in search of emerging themes. How much intelligence has the nursing profession gathered from its first wave of appointees who report directly to heads of state? What has the profession learned from the first nurse to head the Health Care Financing Agency? What is the profession's apparatus for gathering, storing, and analyzing such information? If I were to use my own experience with my colleagues as an example, I would conclude that nursing is not adequately taking advantage of an available opportunity.

The single question most often asked of me by nurses is, how did you get appointed Michigan's Director of Public Health? Too often the unvoiced question is, why you? Just who are you to achieve this honor? Although I hasten to answer the first question, in the hope that what I say will reveal what works best in getting other nurses and women appointed, I don't know how to respond to the latter, unspoken question. Its existence, in any case, shows that the profession needs more from political trailblazers than simple factual descriptions of how they got their jobs.

For more than two decades nursing has grappled with issues pertaining to licensure, certification, and other regulatory concerns. One must conclude that a former American Nurses' Association (ANA) president who has headed a state agency of licensing and regulation for four years (Barbara Nichols) would have gained tremendous insight and a unique perspective on top priorities of the profession. How does the profess access that information? How is it used to redefine policy, legislative agenda and strategy?

For many years the legislative liaisons of various nursing organizations have returned to their various state and national constituents to report that legislators will not take up nursing issues until nurses present a united front. In the last few years nurses seemed to have made progress, agreeing to approach Congress with a single position on issues such as the Nurse Training Act, third-party reimbursement for nurses, and a National Center for Nursing Research. That major organizations in nursing could reach such agreement is progress indeed. However, we must move on to the next phase.

Kingdon[1] has described public policy-making as a set of processes including at least (1) the setting of the agendas; (2) the specification of alternatives from which a choice is to be made; (3) an authoritative choice among those specified alternatives, as in a legislative vote or a presidential decision; and (4) implementation of the decision. In Kingdon's conceptualization, agenda is the list of subjects or problems to which government officials *and* people outside the government *closely associated* with those officials are paying serious attention at any given time.

Given this definition the health agenda would probably include acquired immunodeficiency syndrome (AIDS), cost containment, organ transplants, long-term care, substance abuse, quality of care, and un-

compensated care. These are all issues in which nursing has a major stake. Nursing's own agenda, however, is far more likely to be cast in terms of professional aspirations: the baccalaureate degree as the level of entry into practice, third-party reimbursement for nurses, and control of practice. This agenda may have great relevance for nursing but its relationship to the health agenda must be demonstrated if it is to be advanced. In short, the fact that nursing groups are able to reach a consensus on a limited agenda is progress, but it is not enough.

The following situation illustrates this point. In 1987, Michigan optometrists wanted a bill passed that would permit them to expand their diagnostic capabilities. The optometrists wanted to put eye drops in patient's eyes that would dilate the pupils and enable patients to see the field with more accuracy. The ophthalmologists in Michigan were opposed, asserting that the optometrists were not qualified to do eye examinations and that patients should be referred to ophthalmologists instead. The optometrists felt that they were giving a quality service and providing greater access to larger numbers of patients, particularly the elderly. The optometrists hired a multiclient lobbying firm to represent them. The lobbyist quieried the Michigan Health Department to see if the department had studies or citations indicating that patients would receive inadequate care if eye examinations were carried out by optometrists. The evidence the department had gathered showed there was no difference in outcome. The department also had an interest in facilitating access to care. Clearly, the department of public health could not advocate for one practitioner over another in this case. The optometrists' bill passed, despite opposition from the powerful medical community. I believe they won because the bill was tied to the popular agenda of health care for the aged. The optometrists were presented as a more accessible, quality cost-effective alternative. The fight was waged over consumers' needs rather than professional turf.

I have no idea what set of circumstances might help nursing to move its agenda forward. The nursing shortage crisis certainly seems to offer opportunity. Nurses might have to borrow a page from Michigan optometrists and link the crisis to specific aspects of patient access and quality. If nurses cannot take advantage of this crisis, the potential exists for others to do so to our disadvantage. It is possible to envision the development of proposals for health care technicians, such as the proposal of the American Medical Association for a new type of health worker to augment the diminished supply of hospital-based nurses. As nurses we must ask ourselves, What will be the litmus test? What agency will be asked whether or not there is evidence of diminished quality or safety when registered care technicians are substituted for nurses?

One of the elements included in Kingdon's description for public policy-making was the specification of alternatives from which a choice can be made. What policy alternative have nurses designed and pushed? My experiences with nurses have been consistent with the accounts shared with me by colleagues in public office. During my five years as Michigan's Director of Public Health, nurses approached me on a single issue, third-party reimbursement of nurses.

No matter how many books she reads on politics and how government works, no matter how many powerful mentors she has, and no matter how brilliant or well connected she is, a woman in the political arena is not one of the boys. Women legislators and agency heads must learn to cope with this very difficult reality. I saw four patterns in my work in the state capitol: (1) women who surrounded themselves with other competent women; (2) women who were taken care of and controlled by their male staffs; (3) women who struggled to be in charge of a predominantly male staff, draining energy needed for more vital functions; and (4) women who just drifted.

I believe it is important for organized nursing to deal with the issue of gender in a more direct way. Gender should be one of the variables considered when nurses plan legislative strategies. In their book *Momentum Women in American Politics Now*, Romney and Harrison point out that

> political life is not and never has been an equal opportunity game. Most politicians are men, the power structure of both parties is overwhelmingly masculine, and there is still often a decidedly lower-room atmosphere in the offices and back rooms of elected or appointed officials.

In nursing we like to think that people are impressed with credentials, articulate powerful presentations, and presence. It is difficult to determine how much currency those things actually have in persuading legislators, legislative aides, bureaucrats, and others to accept proposed policy alternatives. It is my observation that when one is a member of the old-boy network, transactions are on a much simpler level. The most useful piece of advice given to me when I arrived

at the state capitol was offered by a woman who sized me up quickly and decided to help. I had been in the waiting room of Michigan's powerful Chairman of the House Appropriations Committee for an hour or more. There was another woman in the waiting room who seemed to know everyone who passed by, but we had not spoken. The door of a nearby conference room opened and people began spilling out. One of the directors of a sister agency walked over, kissed each of us on the cheek, and said that we should get to know each other. After our mutual acquaintance had introduced us and left, this woman said to me "So, you're the new director of public health. Well, my dear, let me give you some advice. No words over three syllables. Do not try to dazzle anyone with your brilliance because no one gives a damn. The name of the game in this town is mediocrity." I did not appreciate this sage advice at that moment, but over the following months I grew to understand that it was the wisest thing anyone could have said to me. I did not know at that moment that only legislators and constituents are allowed to have egos. She was telling me to wear my credentials sparingly, to use plain English, and to play it low key. All excellent advice until one learns the lay of the land and is allowed to be a personality after having earned the respect of the players in the capitol.

Nurses need to select their legislative liaisons wisely. They need to know their own strengths and weaknesses to find ways to complement the nursing team, through staff positions, multiclient lobbyists, or special friends who have special access. For example, after several months in my position I learned that there was a level of access to the locker rooms and other smoke-filled boys-only spots that I would never achieve. I also had identified some ways to increase access, but each contained risks. There were several legislators who would shelter me, but the price—playing the role of a helpless little girl guided by a wiser, stronger man—was too high. I decided to add to my top management team as my deputy a "good ole boy" who had access to the locker rooms. It was the right move but the wrong man. My deputy's ego required that he be seen as taking care of me and doing my thinking for me. He could not adjust to the fact that I was the director and I was capable and in charge. We managed to work together relatively successfully, but managing the relationship was very time-consuming.

Nursing organizations originated for the creation

and maintenance of mutual support systems to advance nursing through the promotion of educational and practice standards and registration of practitioners. Preoccupation with these issues has obscured the need for nursing to be significantly involved in major movements with implications for the larger population, including feminism, the civil rights movement, economic liberation, and antiwar efforts. These larger movements might have provided—and may yet provide—nursing with support for its goals. The drive for professionalism has been an unrelenting and unrequited passion.

It seems reasonable to assume that nurses can effect social change as a result of sheer numbers and the basic need for nursing services. There are 1.9 million registered nurses and another 1.5 million licensed practical nurses, attendants, technicians, aides, and orderlies. This is an enormous force. Nursing can acquire power by using the political system, by creatively collaborating with others within and outside health care in order to influence the direction of the U.S. health care system. If nursing is to resocialize its membership, it should be toward new values that are likely to make a difference in how nurses are perceived by the public and employed by institutions.

Nursing's image will change when some of the realities of nurses' participation in American life change. Nursing will be in a position to help the powerless when nurses are highly visible in public life as elected and appointed leaders. If nurses can be identified and accepted by the public and our colleagues as *nurses* who take on leadership roles in health care, we will have made significant inroads. When nurses are widely dispersed and visible in social institutions (including business, education, recreational organizations, and so on) then and only then can we build new and broader alliances. Only then can we influence the course of the health care system. Nurses must have a power base from which to work. For most of us that will be centered in our profession—our nursing association. Some of us turn to bigger alliances, coalitions, and political parties. To realize our dreams and empower ourselves, we move more in the mainstream.

REFERENCES

1. Kingdon JW: Agendas, alternatives and public policies, Boston, 1984, Little, Brown & Co.
2. Romney R and Harrison B: Momentum women in American politics now, New York, 1988, Crown Publishers, Inc.
3. Smith GR: Nursing power: the political experience, The Oklahoma Nurse 29(5):19, 1984.

CHAPTER 62

Feminism

A failure in nursing?

CAROLE A. SHEA

A century ago a burning issue of the time was women's rights and women's rightful place in the world. Today the issue is no less salient, but it is a smoldering fire, not a tinderbox. Even when changes in the societal wind do cause a burst of flame, as during the 1960s and 1970s, the flare-up is relatively shortlived and damage to the sexist social structure is minor. There are those who try to smother the flames with claims of legislated civil rights and nominal gains of women in the workplace. But the spark to develop human potential to its fullest keeps igniting feminists' efforts to make the world a more humane place. Nowhere is this feminist spark more imminent but less acknowledged than in the modern nursing profession.

Nursing: a women's profession. Feminism: a women's movement. What is their common cause? Where is their common ground? How has ideology shaped behavior? Why have these historic contemporaries—nursing and feminism—evolved toward divergent interests and pathways? After a brief look at the origins of feminism and modern nursing, these questions will be examined in light of practice and education in professional nursing today.

FROM FEMINIST BEGINNINGS

Feminism is an ideology that addresses social, political, and economic inequalities based on gender. It embodies organized activities fostering women's interests, rights, and accomplishment. Its champions, as well as its detractors, include both women and men.

Unity in the woman movement

As Cott[6] noted in her historical account, the origins of modern feminism are grounded in what she calls the *woman* movement of the nineteenth century. In the beginning, the woman movement signaled unity of purpose and membership in the cause for the advancement of women in all sectors of public and private life. In addition to the rights and prerogatives accorded to men, women sought a reexamination and "re-valuing of their own nature and abilities."[6]

The struggle took place in three arenas: (1) social policy and service; (2) political, legal, and economic systems, and (3) intrapersonal and interpersonal relationships. Although the goal of transforming the gender hierachy of power was paramount to each, the ways and means employed in each arena were different, as was the guiding philosophy. Some women sought to reform the existing social order from within, while for others nothing but a full-scale revolution would do.[6]

These differences led to inevitable conflicts among and within the various women's groups. However, the woman movement was able to maintain a "functional ambiguity"[6] by recognizing the need for a Janus-like perspective toward equal opportunity for women *and* special appreciation of women's unique contributions to society. In those early days, the commonality of gender was the bedrock on which all programs for future advancement were built. Women's diversity as individuals was an asset in achieving women's rights in a pluralistic society.

Nursing as an extension of woman's work

Nursing arose as a profession of and for women in the contexts of the social policy and service arenas. Its tradition was heavily influenced by a philosophy of benevolence, altruistic values, Christian morality, and military authoritarianism.[23] Its founders were women with an exceptional gift for social reform. They took as their mission the improvement of public sanitary conditions and home health care for the poor who were flooding the newly industrialized urban centers. Many of their efforts were directed specifically at the welfare of women and children.

Florence Nightingale, a reformer with an upper-class background and a scientific bent, recruited women from the upper and middle classes into nursing. Her intent was to upgrade the provision of health services while establishing a precedent for respectable women to work outside the home. Nightingale viewed nursing as an opportunity to combine the use of scientific principles and women's natural talents in a public service for the social good of others.[22] She was skeptical about the recently discovered germ theory; she had little faith in the physician's power to cure disease.[23] She believed in the recuperative nature of the human body and that nursing has the power to heal by providing a restful environment, clean air, good nutrition, and comforting ministrations. She structured the practice of nursing in hospitals to capitalize on the special abilities and skills learned by middle-class women in the home—to observe, organize, empathize, nurture, and manage housekeeping and health care. She layered knowledge about hygiene and disease prevention on this foundation of feminine attributes and ascribed roles for women.

Contrary to popular myths about her avowed allegiance to the feminist cause, Nightingale[22] advised nurses to remain above the fray created by the movement for women's rights. She wrote:

Keep clear of both jargons about the "rights" of women, which urges women to do all that men do, including the medical and other professions, merely because men do, and without regard to whether this is the best that women can do; . . . and which urges women to do nothing that men do, merely because they are women, and . . . "this is women's work," and "that is men's" . . . Surely woman should bring the best she has, whatever that is, to the work of God's world, without attending to either of these cries.[22]

Her admonitions were only partially heeded.

Many of the early nursing leaders did espouse feminism and were active in the woman movement. As nurses they advanced the progress of all women in several ways. Principally, they expanded their roles as competent managers and care givers from the private domain of the middle-class family to the public domain of the welfare of the sick and poor. In exceptional cases they took the lead in establishing settlement houses, community health services, and birth control clinics that benefited women from all social strata.[6,23] They founded professional organizations to foster the education and practice of women in nursing. However, a dark cloud hung over these accomplishments.

Nightingale and her followers had hoped to increase women's independence from the patriarchal family by moving care of the sick from the home into the institution. In actuality the hospital setting perpetuated patriarchy and male dominance. With the concomitant rise of medicine as a profession, the physician assumed power and control of all health care.[24] Although nursing originally was envisioned as a sphere interlocking with medicine, with both having mutual and distinct goals in health care services, this ideal was never realized. Instead, the nurse became "handmaiden" to the physician. The superior-subordinate physician-nurse relationship in the hospital perfectly mirrored the male-female role set in general society. Indeed, as indicated by Ashley,[1] Nightingale herself advocated standards of conduct for nurses that emphasized deference, obedience, and self-sacrifice. Thus patriarchy was upheld in the health care system.

The entrenchment of patriarchy has overshadowed nursing's contribution to the woman movement ever since. It has also endured as a major preoccupation within the profession of nursing and as a focus of attack by some feminists in the current women's movement.

NOTHING IN COMMON

At the turn of the century the common ground of feminism and nursing dissolved. With victory for women's suffrage imminent, the woman movement became the *women's* movement, signifying the broader scope of its constituents' issues.[6] Feminism emerged as the ideology devoted to women's rights and relations in society. Its adherents became radical, dogmatic, and elitist in their dedication to the cause. As the women's movement shifted into high gear to do battle on all fronts of the male power structure, they left behind those they judged as having failed in the attempt to confront the gender hierarchy—particularly nurses—or as having refused to abandon their traditional roles.

The feminist agenda

Feminists had no interest in pursuing feminine careers such as nursing, social work, or primary education. They sought to invade the male bastions of law, medicine, politics, finance, and the ministry, leaving their mark as equal competitors with their male counterparts. Once seated in positions of power, they hoped to exert influence in the direction of equal opportunity for women and men.

Feminists chose the professions as the battleground in part "because of the close relation of the professions to education and service (where women's contributions were acknowledged, to an extent); and because the professions promised neutral standards of judgment of both sexes, collegial autonomy, and horizons for growth."[6] Initially they achieved some success by entering the professions in significant numbers. However, in the 1920s the door to opportunity slammed shut as it became apparent that women did indeed provide serious competition for the rewards of professional activity. It also became clear that women were intent on transforming the status quo of all social institutions, not merely seeking equal representation. Discriminatory barriers to the hiring and promotion of women were erected throughout industry, and prejudicial quotas were set at institutions of higher learning, the gateways to economic opportunity.

As resistance to the full social participation of women increased, feminists became more militant. They staged conventions, marches, labor strikes, and various acts of civil disobedience and even violence to dramatize the call for equality in all areas of life.[6] They tried to stimulate self-determinism and freedom from male domination among poor and working-class women, those in female occupations, and homemakers. However, the feminist concept of self-determinism did not allow for the choice to retain traditional female roles. Their efforts to end male oppression took little recognition of the fact that some women were not prepared and, in fact, did not want to reorganize their lives to experience the freedom promoted by ardent feminists.

Feminists claimed that those women who resisted the aims of the movement were denying the evidence of their oppression and needed their consciousness raised.[16] However, many women were without the necessary resources to take part in public demonstrations or even in private discussions. Certainly they did not have the means—education, money, and support— to reject the prevailing social norms, mores, and structures in favor of a new life of self-sufficiency and independence. Other women, because of temperament, personality, preference, or situation, were not attracted by the prospect of major upheaval in their lives. They preferred to remain at home and to confine their public forays to volunteer work in their communities.[8]

From the early 1900s the women's movement was faced with fierce resistance from without and discord from within. Unable to generate an identity of compassionate "we-ness" among all women, the leaders of the women's movement set priorities that disenfranchised those who would not or could not embrace the traditional male pursuits of business, politics, and the professions. Woman's place in society was reexamined, but woman's work was not revalued; it was devalued.[11,19] As a consequence, women at home were admonished that the work of homemaking was demeaning, but that money-making in the marketplace was meaningful. In essence, the feminists had turned their backs on the needs and desires of the "traditional" woman.

Nursing predicament
Caught in feminist crossfire

In the 1970s the feminist refrain was "women should be doctors, not nurses." Nurses were chided for only taking orders from physicians, and for their unscientific mind-set and generally subservient demeanor. Muff[21] has suggested that this feminist attack on nursing was essentially rooted in behavior associated with oppressed minorities, that is, identification with the dominant group (men) and aggression against one's own group (women).

Through identification, feminists emulated not only men's work but men's attitudes toward women. When they rejected the work of nurses (98% of them women), the devalued nurses as women by disparaging the feminine attributes and characteristics associated with nursing. Their denigration of the stereotypical nurse was a direct attack on womanhood itself. This anti-woman tactic erected a formidable barrier between the prevailing majorities in both the women's movement and nursing.

For a brief time feminists and nurses did become united in the communal spirit of the early 1970s. The National Organization for Women (NOW) had become a forceful reality. Wilma Scott Heide, an outspoken feminist-nurse, used her dual identity to good advantage.[13] She inspired nurses to form Nurses NOW to exercise their political clout as a critical mass within both the health care system and the larger society. Unfortunately the unity between feminism and nursing was shortlived. The establishment of a separate branch for nurses suggests that the needs and concerns of nurses were not or could not be addressed within the mainstream of NOW. The reasons for the split were embedded in the changing social times and in the fate of the feminist agenda. The sociopolitical climate turned conservative. Traditional values were reasserted and there was a backlash against expanded social roles for women and men. Despite concerted effort, the women's movement failed to capture America's imagination with promises of the benefits of equality for women and men. It achieved incremental gains for women in the workplace but lacked a clear-cut victory. The passage of the Equal Rights Amendment, a high-visibility goal, became stalemated. Debates about the basic tenets of the women's movement flared up within nursing.[7] As the momentum of the women's movement and NOW's influence began to fade, the alliance between feminists and nurses evaporated.

Difficulties on nursing's home front

Nursing itself was not immune to antiwomanism in the form of identification with the oppressor and self-aggression. It has had a complicated history of striving for the knowledge, status, and power of the male physician. The drive to professionalize nursing is replete with examples where nurses eagerly sought to identify with physicians and overtly (or covertly) fought against other nurses. Nursing's identification with medicine is both real and symbolic. Some examples are organizing nursing according to the medical specializations ; using medical jargon to refer to patients ("the MI in room 212"); writing "orders" for the patient; *wearing* stethoscopes; and not giving priority to women's health issues in education or practice. For years nursing has followed the course charted by medicine, accepted the medical model, learned medical language, used medical technology, adopted the content and methods of medical science, and assumed the beliefs and attitudes of the medical profession regarding health, women, and nurses. Nurses may regale one another in private with tales of physicians' foibles, but in public their behavior is often indistinguishable from their medical role models. Many *do* act like junior doctors.

The aggression of nurses against themselves is best exemplified by the conflict over entry into practice. The infighting is centered on *who* should become nurses and *how*. This issue touches all aspects of nursing: admission criteria, curriculum design, academic degrees, licensure, certification, standards of practice, employment policies, organizational structures, patterns of care delivery, reimbursement eligibility, public image, and consumer needs. The socialized desire

to please everyone, coupled with the tradition of bureaucratic hierarchy, strict supervision, nonacademic training, and perfectionism—Nightingale's endowment to nursing—has hampered the resolution of this one issue for decades. In circular discussions and internecine quarrels nurses have dissipated the energy so vital to the creation of a new discipline. The debate has become a form of slow suicide for the profession.

Principally the debate about the future direction for nursing has taken place within professional organizations whose memberships represent a small fraction of the total number of nurses. Nursing leaders have repeated feminist history by setting an agenda that ignores the needs and desires of traditional nurses. The professional agenda does not speak to the grassroots nurse. For example, the philosophical move to reject the medical model (essentially a male model) in favor of a holistic model threatens a large majority of nurses who learned how to nurse according to the medical model and presently practice in a medical setting organized around that model. Theoretically, the holistic model may be good for nursing, but what does it do for practicing nurses? In terms of entry into practice, requiring a baccalaureate degree (a ticket to the American dream for *both* women and men) may be a good strategy to upgrade the profession and clarify roles. But what about the thousands of nurses who do not have college degrees or the resources or motivation to obtain them? In what way does the professional agenda speak to them? What is the base of exchange between the interested parties?

Compounding the problem, nurses have exhibited self-hatred by blaming themselves and each other for failing to solve the complex dilemmas that confront their profession. There is no doubt that the dilemmas in nursing are profound. Consider some of the dilemmas with which nurses are grappling: (1) how to hold to principles that will foster professionalization but limit opportunity for a significant group of individuals interested in nursing; (2) how to recognize the very real contribution of nurses at all levels of the nursing hierarchy yet design a career ladder based on clinical expertise and not academic elitism; (3) how to meet the needs of a practice environment in a shrinking economy while guaranteeing nurses fair compensation and competitive incentives; (4) how to maximize the use of the knowledge and skills of nurses as they and their role partners (administrators, physicians, and other health care providers) adjust to changes within the health care system and their own professions;

(5) how to recruit people into a field that suffers from a distorted public image and a confused professional one; and (6) how to make alliances with stronger professions without losing nursing's fragile identity.

To date no proposal, compromise, or answer has been found acceptable to the various factions in nursing. In part, this is due to the tremendous complexity of the problem itself. However, it is also the result of nurses giving only lip service to the notion of "different but equal." Deep down they believe to be different is bad and that some are more equal than others. The diversities among nurses as women have only served as trigger points for dissension and condemnation. The commonalities inherent in belonging to a women's profession have become submerged in a sea of confusion about what constitutes femaleness and maleness, femininity and masculinity, self-esteem, image, competence, and success. Overriding these issues is concern about the nurse as a product of the sexist society who is trying to survive in an incredibly stressful environment as a nurse, as a woman, and as a person in the process of self-actualization.

MOVING TOWARD NEW COMMON GROUND

As the twentieth century draws to a close, there is mounting evidence that the pathways of feminists and nurses are once again converging. Their coming together is fueled by recent theoretical developments in feminism and nursing. Stressful economic forces in the health care system have catalyzed the move. From their opposite camps, both sides are searching warily for a language of reapproachment, a road to a common higher ground, the establishment of a collaborative community.

The rebirth of feminism

Gradually the expression of feminist sentiments has moved from the vehement protests of the women's movement to the scholarly inquiry of women's studies programs in academia. There, feminist scholars conduct critical micro- and macroanalyses of all aspects of the human condition. They examine the systematic gender biases introduced by androcentric thinkers who have predicated accepted truths, scientific knowledge, and commonsense understandings about personal and social life, all based on the study of men. From their own studies of the female experience, feminists offer alternative explanations contradicting the notion that women are inherently inferior, subordinate, nurturing, masochistic, irrational, or any of a host of other stereotypic feminine qualities.

Perhaps most important to the advancement of feminist thinking is the construction of gender as a *cultural* rather than a *biological* dimension of human beings.[17] The making of this theoretical distinction has led to new insights about women and women's issues. Understanding the female experience in terms of women's thinking, psychology, morality, history, artistry, politics—in short, women's ways of being in the world—has changed perceptions dramatically. For example, Belenky and associates[2] described the development of women's learning about self and reality as occurring in five ways that they characterize as "connected knowing." Miller[18] and others reconstructed the female psyche (after the devastation wreaked by Freud) to show that biology is not destiny. Gilligan[9] challenged the moral supremacy of males by positing that females make moral decisions based on relationships and responsibilities rather than on an abstract notion of justice. These are only a few instances of the feminist revision of the "nature" of woman.

Because of its descriptive richness and explanatory power, the contemporary feminist critique has attracted a wider audience than did the militant rhetoric of either the first or second wave of the women's movement. The sense of integration and wholeness characterizing much of the current writing and discussion of women's issues tends to make the message more accessible to a broader segment of society. The focus on context and relationships heightens the meaningfulness of the theoretical discoveries for women. The explication of differences and similarities as variations rather than discrepancies between women and men short-circuits arguments about one being better or more valid than the other.

Feminism still has its radical component but there is a philosophical mainstream that is inclusive, not exclusive. There is a cooperative spirit in the way that women are sharing feminist knowledge. One sign of this is the attention being paid by feminist academics and the media to the neglected concerns of traditional women, women's work, and class or race discrimination. A particularly clear example of this is the renewed interest in nursing by those outside of nursing. There is Reverby's seminal work[23] on the dilemma between duty and autonomy in nursing and Harding's discussion[12] of the effects of technology on the politics of nursing, to name only two. There is the news media's front-page treatment of the nursing shortage. As a problem that affects everyone [10,14] and the feminist press's promotion of the nurse's work.[15] These initiatives forge a feminist link with nurses who tend to be traditionalists, who do women's work, and who are frequently discriminated against.

The new wave of nursing

In its quest to become a science, nursing has experienced a growth spurt in theory development and research. One source of this growth is the reexamination of nursing's philosophical roots and historical underpinnings by nurses and others.[1,6,20,23] Here, too, some revisionist history is being written. The logical tie to feminism is avidly acknowledged by some,[1,4,10,13] yet remains hidden to others. Nevertheless, its effects are being felt throughout nursing.

Feminism as a conceptual framework is not generally accepted in nursing education. However, the concepts of wholeness, connectedness, relationship, process, and differentiation of self, which are the essence of modern feminism, are an integral part of current curricula in nursing.[4] The nursing content itself is changing. Women's health and women's issues are moving to the forefront of nursing concern.[25] Nursing research using qualitative as well as quantitative methods is illuminating health phenomena by listening attentively to the voices of its subjects, particularly women.

Nurses in practice as well as in academia are becoming conversant with feminist explanations for why people do what they do. There is a greater understanding that the nurse's self-blame and poor self-concept are the result of the dynamics of gender relations as determined by culture and socialization, not inherent personal faults. For instance, the so-called nursing shortage is sometimes explained as the abandonment of nursing by young women for the more lucrative careers esteemed in a materialistic society.[14] However, economic incentives do not tell the whole story. The imperative to function under stress in "high-tech, high-touch" acute care hospitals without professional autonomy and collegial respect has driven more nurses from the patient's bedsides than the lure of Wall Street riches. Nurses who choose to stay in nursing have used the power of collective bargaining to negotiate for better pay and greater autonomy in their workplace. They have lobbied for stronger practice acts and equitable reimbursement procedures. They have advocated patients' rights as well as nurses' rights. The measure of their assertive evolution is their vocal acknowledgement of feminist ideals and political support from the women's movement.[15]

Nursing has learned some important lessons from its feminist heritage:

1. Engender a collective sense of "we-ness" among all nurses that emphasizes commonalities and values diversities.
2. Forge alliances with other women's groups and establish political ties with health care providers to make changes within the health care system.
3. Challenge the male mystique that men are always united in their thinking, incisive in decision making, and effective in achieving goals instead of engaging in self-blame and negative behavior toward self and others.
4. Study feminist ideology as a means to transpose basic philosophical questions and discover new perspectives about human relations and caring as the work of nursing.
5. Acknowledge nursing's traditional roots without shame, while affirming its present-day value as professional work for women.

Above all, there is a resurgence of interest in the importance of caring in nursing.[3] Once conferences were called to discuss the scientific objectivity of nursing; now they are convened to explore the feminist subjectivity embodied in caring as the work of nursing.[5] This deliberate revaluing of the caring component of nursing draws together the historical core of nursing with its feminine qualities, the contemporary struggle for definition of practice, and the feminist commitment to connectedness among people.

Nurses have composed a definition of feminism that suggests the full-circle intertwining of feminism and nursing: "Feminism as an integrative healing process that manifests as a social and political movement as well as a personal therapeutic journey aims to restore women and men to their full stature as joyful, loving, responsible human beings."[4] Does nursing seek to do any less?

REFERENCES

1. Ashley JA: Hospitals, paternalism and the role of the nurse, New York, 1977, Teachers College Press.

2. Belenky MF and others: Women's ways of knowing: the development of self, voice, and mind, New York, 1986, Basic Books, Inc.
3. Benner P and Wrubel J: The primacy of caring: stress and coping in health and illness, Menlo Park, Calif, 1988, Addison-Wesley Publishing Co.
4. Bermosk LS and Porter SE: Women's health and human wholeness, New York, 1979, Appleton-Century-Crofts.
5. Caring and nursing: explorations in the feminist perspectives. Conference sponsored by the Center for Human Caring, University of Colorado School of Nursing, June 17-18, 1988.
6. Cott NF: The grounding of modern feminism, New Haven, Conn, 1987, Yale University Press.
7. Crane M and others: Should nursing support the ERA? In McCloskey JC and Grace HK, editors: Current issues in nursing, Boston, 1981, Blackwell Scientific Publication, Inc.
8. Eisenstein H: On the psychological barriers to professions for women. In Muff J, editor: Socialization, sexism, and stereotyping: women's issues in nursing, St Louis, 1982, The CV Mosby Co.
9. Gilligan C: In a different voice: psychological theory and women's development, Cambridge, Mass, 1982, Harvard University Press.
10. Gordon S: The crisis in caring, Boston Globe Magazine, p22, July 10, 1988.
11. Gornick V and Moran BK: Woman in sexist society: studies in power and powerlessness, New York, 1971, Basic Books, Inc.
12. Harding S, editor: Feminism and methodology: social science issues, Bloomington, 1987, Indiana University Press.
13. Heide, WS: Feminist activism in nursing and health care. In Muff J, editor: Socialization, sexism, and stereotyping: women's issues in nursing, St Louis, 1982, The CV Mosby Co.
14. Hevesi D: Shortage of nurses forces a rise in salaries, New York Times, p1, July 31, 1988.
15. Holcomb B: Nurses fight back, Ms.; 16(12):72, 1988.
16. Hole J and Levine E: Rebirth of feminism, New York, 1971, Quadrangle Books, Inc.
17. Learning about women: gender, politics, and power, Daedalus, Fall 1987 (whole issue).
18. Miller JB: Toward a new psychology of women, Boston, 1976, Beacon Press.
19. Morgan R, editor: Sisterhood is powerful: an anthology of writings from the women's liberation movement, New York, 1970, Vintage Books.
20. Muff J, editor: Socialization, sexism, and stereotyping: women's issues in nursing, St Louis, 1982, The CV Mosby Co.
21. Muff J: Why doesn't a smart girl like you go to medical school? In Muff J, editor: Socialization, sexism, and stereotyping: women's issues in nursing, St Louis, 1982, The CV Mosby Co.
22. Nightingale F: Notes on nursing, New York, 1969, Dover Publications, Inc.
23. Reverby S: Ordered to care: the dilemma of American nursing, 1850 to 1945, New York, 1987, Cambridge University Press.
24. Rosenberg CE: The care of strangers: the rise of America's hospital system, New York, 1987, Basic Books Inc.
25. Woods NF and others: Being healthy: women's images, Advances in Nursing Science, 11(1):36, 1988.

CHAPTER 63

Women and the empowerment of leaders

Lessons from the Geraldine Ferraro case

GLORIA R. SMITH

Both women and men have problems in empowering female leaders, in recognizing and legitimizing them so that they can exercise leadership in public affairs and in private enterprise. All public leaders are vulnerable because everyone has aspects of their personal lives, pasts, family involvements, or family history that can be questioned by people who resist the delegation of authority to leaders as women and as individuals. The Geraldine Ferraro case is very instructive in illustrating the dilemmas of women leaders and the pressures and personal sacrifices that accompany upward mobility in American society.

Geraldine Ferraro ran for Vice-President of the United States on the Democratic ticket in 1984. During the fall of 1984, the trials and tribulations of Ferraro and her husband, John Zaccaro, were a staple of the American media. Many married career women watched the Ferraro-Zaccaro with great interest and sympathy and rooted for a shared national experience to advance the national women's agenda.

Ferraro had been nominated to one of the highest executive offices in the country. She had attempted to separate her career and finances from those of her husband. Her situation provides others with an opportunity to examine the potential for marital and career conflict and male-female role changes that occur as women juggle domestic relations and political advancement.

In brief, the controversy about Ferraro's campaign finances in 1984 grew out of her responses to the Federal Election laws. In 1978, during her first campaign for national office, Ferraro received $110,000 in loans from her husband. The law required that the maximum contribution which could be made by an individual was $1,000. The Ferraro campaign paid $740 in fines for violating the law. When Ferraro agreed to accept the nomination for Vice President, the law required that she file new financial disclosure statements within 30 days of the nomination. Ferraro attempted to interpret the law narrowly so as to exclude disclosure of her husband's financial holdings and transactions. Disclosure of Mr. Zaccaro's finances uncovered illegal financial contributions to Ferraro's campaign as well as highly questionable and unethical conduct in his business practices.

The ambiguities of power itself are amply demonstrated by the unanswered questions raised by Ferraro's finances. No one seems able to define just how much financial disclosure is sufficient, perhaps because the purposes of disclosure are unclear. Did the public want assurance that the Ferraro-Zaccaro family had paid enough taxes? How much is enough? Were the business ethics of the Ferraro-Zaccaro family to be revealed by the care with which they handled their business and tax-related finances? To what extent are spouses responsible for each other's business transactions? Is financial disclosure related to party affiliation?

Why is it that the problems encountered by Ferraro can be considered a microcosm of those of all women aspiring to high national office? Many women achieving national influence today have been financed largely by their husbands, particularly in the political arena, where it has been difficult for women to attract donations. Husbands are frequently the only men willing to invest in their wives' political careers. Historically women rarely have had much money to contribute to political causes, nor have they been likely to see such contributions as a significant political responsibility. Election finance laws have been developed to prevent candidates from accepting large donations from a few backers who might "own" them in office. The political action committees, or PACS, that brought so-called reform merely tapped the male corporate network, further excluding many women from access to political office without juggling family assets to meet changes in electoral law. These changes did not extend greater equity to women, or even recognize their dilemma as outsiders in an increasingly expensive media-dependent political system.

Women must mediate between marital and career roles with tact, particularly if they begin or resume their careers after spending many years as homemakers. The management of family finances is often the cutting edge of power. As a case in point, Zaccaro is much wealthier than Ferraro. He lent his wife money for her congressional campaign, in conflict with government regulations and for which a fine had to be paid. Further, Ferraro played the traditional wife, signing off as a partner in her husband's business, about which she seemed uninformed.

Ferraro is an attorney and should have known that she was legally responsible for having full information about a business in which she was a shareholder and officer (secretary-treasurer) and from which she derived some financial benefit. Yet apparently she merely agreed to her husband's financial statements. The questions raised by her ownership of lots adjacent to their Fire Island home, her sale of a property subsequently purchased by her husband from a mutual associate after a brief interval, and her potential to inherit his assets suggest that the domestic and career issues of the Ferraro-Zaccaro marriage were never sorted out by either party.

The media have given notice that spouses are not being let off the hook if they are involved in each other's careers. When involvement is in one direction (for example, Zaccaro's financial assistance for his wife's congressional bid), then there is speculation about a lack of reciprocal assistance (for example, Ferraro's not informing her husband of the impropriety of borrowing money from an estate for which he is a conservator). These are delicate issues of domestic adaptation and public exposure. There are some lessons to be learned from the Ferraro case for all people, whether in public or private service, who aspire to positions of power and authority in an increasingly conservative political milieu.

1. *Husbands and wives should bear in mind the potential impact of their actions on their spouse's career.* For example, long after the Ferraro-Zac-

caro finances are buried, the fact that a pornographer operated from a building owned by Zaccaro may haunt Ferraro's political career. Likewise, his disregard for legal standards in treatment of an estate as its conservator, along with their income tax underpayment, her financial disclosures to Congress, and the financing of her campaign, raised questions about the family's carelessness with regard to regulation. Men may wish to anticipate the escalation of their wives' careers and behave accordingly, well in advance of the need for justification.

2. *Women in the public arena will be held to the same standards applied to men,* regardless of the potential impact on spouses. Female attorneys especially can anticipate that the public will expect them to understand disclosure regulations, legal sources of donations, and arm's-length transactions. This is not unfair. If women can't take the heat, they should stay out of the kitchen.

3. *The public careers of women are in transition: compartmentalizing domestic and career considerations is impossible.* A woman with power in the public arena inevitably will find her career and home life interwoven. Her marriage may have to be renegotiated, or it may suffer or fail. Independence at work and traditional arrangements at home break down when a woman's career advances or as the result of other requirements—transfer to a different geographic location, business travel, or home entertainment.

Some may believe that women are held to a higher standard than men, but I do not believe this is the case. Recent examples of media attention to the fees received by congressmen's wives from beneficiaries of congressional influence dramatize the increased public concern with ethics in government. The basic issue is the national interest and the public's desire to examine the consistency of candidates' private behavior and political beliefs.

Let me add that I supported the candidacy of Ferraro and I sympathized with her efforts to reconcile her marital pattern with her political visibility in an era of cumbersome electoral law and many Americans' increased suspicion of political candidates. I think it would be an error for women to become defensive about the questioning of Ferraro's finances. Rather, we should explore the unexamined areas of our own behavior to find ways to enhance our abilities as autonomous individuals. This requires sorting out the expectations held by our significant others and by the public as well as those we have of ourselves.

Scrutiny of elected officials will not diminish in the 1990s. Americans have difficulty empowering their leaders, which explains in part the deflection of so much attention to candidates' finances. Ultimately, both men and women will have to deal with the issue of empowerment, the most troubling problem facing all organizational leaders in the late twentieth century.

On a more personal level, I have great empathy for Geraldine Ferraro. I imagine that she has learned what many of us have come to realize, understand, and accommodate, and that is the level of chauvinism hidden beneath the veneer of our supportive, understanding, and encouraging spouses. For years I had described my own husband as an easygoing, generous, secure person who was not threatened by my career achievements. He had been there rooting for me and reminding me that he was there to support me. The first glimpse that I got of a little insecurity was when I received my doctorate, but that was quickly resolved and forgotten. I have imagined that the scene at the Zaccaros' house when Ferraro was being considered by Walter Mondale as a possible running mate was like the scene at the Smiths' house when I was being considered as a potential appointee to the state cabinet by Michigan's Governor Blanchard. My husband said: Right on; I'm behind you; If you want it, go for it; Give 'em hell; and all of the other bon mots that he had verbalized so frequently over the years of our married life.

The metamorphosis began almost immediately after I accepted the position of Director of Michigan's Department of Public Health. No amount of preparation seemed sufficient for my husband to accept the prospect of relocating because of my career needs rather than his. We talked at length about maintaining our home in Oklahoma but decided against it. Although some ambivalence continues, my husband is convinced most of the time that he made the right decision. I must say that having a supportive husband at hand is a tremendous relief.

Our personal lives have changed as a result of this experience in ways I could never have imagined five years ago. We have each become more independent in new areas and we have learned to offer support with less regard for role distinctions. This does not mean that my husband is less chauvinistic; it does mean that he has learned to cook, manage a home, rinse hosiery,

iron blouses, and do work that in the past I would never have asked or expected him to do.

Geraldine Ferraro's marriage may never be the same either. She can no longer merely sign off on her husband's business finances; she will be held responsible for their contents. Their relationship probably has been renegotiated. Zaccaro may never make another business decision without wondering about future scrutiny of his finances because of his wife's prominence. He may always live his business life in a fishbowl now that it has been the focus of a national spotlight. Ferraro's children's lives have also been publicly scrutinized and their career patterns affected.

The Ferraro candidacy polarized women in the United States. After the election, two opposing positions were elicited from women interviewed by reporters. A feminist stated, "Power is a very hard thing for women to deal with. It's not nice. Ferraro gives all women permission to get power." A traditionalist said, "I thought Ferraro would project herself as a lady and let us have her as a symbol. But she's come over as hard and coarse!" Changes in personal relationships and criticism of their professional behavior (especially from other women) plague female political leaders.[1,2,3]

According to Jeane Kirkpatrick, former U.S. ambassador to the United Nations:

There are already more opportunities for women in politics than there are women ready to pay the price. . . . We are making the price of power much too high in this society. I worry that we are making the conditions of public life so tough that nobody except people really obsessed with power will be willing to pay the final price. That would be tragic from the point of view of public well-being.[4]

One can only wonder if Geraldine Ferraro feels the price has been too high. In an interview during the campaign she said of her husband, "I just feel very, very badly for what they've done to him. . . . I know my husband. He's a man of integrity, a man of honor." She added, "We've gone through this much, we're in it to stay. . . . You don't go through a bloodbath like this and then walk away from it." Zaccaro said, "They want us to weaken, we don't weaken. Whatever it is, it is."[5]

To become more influential as leaders, women must arrange their public and private lives without compartmentalization so they can emerge with leadership positions and increased political power. A rational and humane political milieu must involve women as major actors along with men. Women must deal with their work and home roles and attempt to build some consistency between them to avoid a watering down of their public impact and painful, chronic cognitive dissonance.

REFERENCES

1. Mann J: The gender barrier is gone, Washington Post, Wednesday, November 17, 1984, p. B3.
2. Hall C: Charting the women for NOW, determination despite setbacks, Washington Post, Wednesday, November 7, 1984, p. D3.
3. Thornton M: Ferraro loss shadows gains by women, Washington Post, Thursday, November 8, 1984, p. A46.
4. Show and tell: under pressure, Ferraro passes a vital test, Time, p 18, September 17, 1987.
5. More hurt than angry, Time, p 21, September 3, 1984.

BIBLIOGRAPHY

Blackman A: Two-careers dilemma confronts Ferraro, Lansing State Journal, p 3A, August 16, 1984.

Blumenthal R: Ferraro says buy-back by husband was legal, New York Times, p 16, August 22, 1984.

Carrington T and Penn S: Ferraro discloses she, spouse each paid taxes equal to 28% of income since 1979, Wall Street Journal, p 3, August 21, 1984.

Carrington T and McGinley L: Campaign impact uncertain: Ferraro defends tax disclosures in effort to end the controversy, Wall Street Journal, p 2, August 22, 1984.

Ethics act: what it says, New York Times, p 17, August 22, 1984.

Excerpts from Ferraro's news conference about finances, New York Times, p 17, August 22, 1984.

Ferraro seeks to stem political damage by release today of tax, financial data, Wall Street Journal, p 6, August 20, 1984.

Gerth J: Ferraro denies any wrongdoing: second loan by Zaccaro from estate, New York Times, p 1, August 22, 1984.

G.O.P. aides critical of Ferraro role, New York Times, p 18, August 21, 1984.

Greenfield J: Ferraro's friends not helping. Lansing State Journal, p 8A, August 22, 1984.

Herbes J: Full disclosure is now a family affair, New York Times, p 1E, August 19, 1984.

It's no ms-tery, call me mrs.: the times trips on a title, Time, p 105, August 20, 1984.

Joyce FS: Aides to Mondale say Ferraro got limited review as running mate, New York Times, August 21, 1984.

Joyce FS: Mondale elated on Ferraro: twits Bush on disclosures, New York Times, p 18, August 22, 1984.

Joyce FS: Mondale praises Ferraro tax disclosure decision, New York Times, p 16A, August 19, 1984.

Lewis F: A stronger president? New York Times, p 29, August 21, 1984.

McGinley L: Ferraro seeks to bury flap over finances, lambastes Reagan to cheers of teachers, Wall Street Journal, p 9, August 23, 1984.

Orekes M: Ferraro and Zaccaro did not tell agency of fines, New York Times, p 13, August 21, 1984.

Perlez J: Husband plans tax disclosure with Ferraro, New York Times, p 17A, August 19, 1984.

Ferraro Finances Plague Democrats. Wall Street Journal, p 56, Tues. 14, 1984.

Roberts S: Ferraro denies any wrongdoing: second loan by Zaccaro from estate, New York Times, p 1, August 22, 1984.

Schanberg SH: The mondaro credibility gap, New York Times, p 29, August 21, 1984.

Sobran J: Halo is shattered, Lansing State Journal, p 13A, August 23, 1984.

Soda R: Democrats: Ferraro tax disclosure bares errors, Lansing State Journal, p 1, August 21, 1984.

Text of Ferraro statements on loans and Zaccaro properties: campaign loans, New York Times, p 12, August 21, 1984.

The Ferraro file (editorial), New York Times, p 30A, August 22, 1984.

Werner LM: Hatfield's disclosure forms may be weighed in inquiry, New York Times, p 15, August 19, 1984.

Zaccaro's borrowing under fire, Lansing State Journal, p 4A, August 23, 1984.

Zaccaro defends loans he made from an estate, Wall Street Journal, p 40, August 24, 1984.

CHAPTER 64

Traditions, transitions, and transformations of power in nursing

SANDRA S. SWEENEY

Power has held a captivating, almost seductive interest for nurses during the past two decades. Merely mentioning power summons forth diverse reactions. Nurses seem to find themselves liking it, hating it, wanting it, not wanting it, trusting it, distrusting it, wanting more of it, or wanting less of it. Regardless of how nurses react to power, however, they rarely view it as a neutral concept. Some 20 years ago Schutt[20] reported that "nursing is often guilty of extremes in the application of power . . . those who have it . . . fail far too often to use it; while those who wield it . . . tend to abuse it."

This chapter introduces a new perspective on the traditions, transitions, and transformations of power as it relates to nursing. A historical perspective is presented, followed by descriptions of the relationship of power to obedience and traits useful in cultivating and developing power. Distinctions are made with regard to perceptions of the nature, source, and consequences of power, and suggestions are offered as to how resources can be cultivated, mobilized, and used to the profession's best advantage.

Neither nursing nor nurses, collectively or individually, lack power. In 1973 Ashley[2] noted, "It is not that nursing lacks power but that nurses have failed to recognize their power or use it to the profession's advantage." Consider the power inherent in any work force with more than 2 million members![1] Further, in view of the fact that 83% of these individuals are actively employed, few would consider such a group to be powerless. Today nursing represents just such a work force and numerically is capable of being recognized as one of the most powerful groups in American society.

TRADITIONS OF POWER

If nursing and nurses want power, then traditional perceptions of nursing's powerlessness must be aban-

doned and new perceptions regarding its power accepted. The profession must also transform traditional interpretations of sex roles as equivalent to gender roles and distinguish between those roles derived from biological function and those ascribed by society. Nursing must be prepared to wrestle with and alter the philosophical, ethical, and social conventions embodied in existing professional and social systems that prescribe behavior. Such changes can be accomplished if and when the perceptual fields of nurses transform previous interpretations of the past and present into new realities. Thus before nursing and nurses can actualize and exercise power, its traditions—including definitions, sources, and consequences—must be recognized and appreciated.

Throughout history power has had a mystical-magical aura that affects various aspects of personal, professional, and social life and is frequently an integral component of many interactions. One could argue that few, if any, traditions of power have existed in nursing, since the concept did not emerge in the nursing literature until the 1960s. There are other traditional aspects of power, however, that are relevant to nursing.

DeJouvenel,[8] for example, describes how power originated and how it has been used to secure obedience from others. Classically, he suggests, the lineage of power can be traced to early societies and the roles held by individuals within family structures. Whether the power and authority to rule were primarily vested in patriarchal or matriarchal social structures remains open to debate. DeJouvenel[8] infers that paternal authority and power constituted the first form of rule and command, in which the family of families was ruled by the father of fathers. However, he also suggests that many early societies (including those of Greece and some Native American Indian tribes) were actually governed by the matriarch in the family structure. Thus regardless of where one thinks power originally was vested, its original source remains closely entwined with roles ascribed to family and social structures.

Power also has historically enjoyed close connections with spiritual figures or leaders. Some of the earliest forms of "magical power" were vested in tribal priests or priestesses. These individuals presided over rites that governed every act of life celebrated by their society, and fear was frequently used to ensure conformity to family or social rules.[8] Fear continues to play a major role in many of the power equations found in contemporary societies.

The introduction of sovereign rule, the divine right of kings and queens, placed power in individuals whose birth alone bestowed upon them the right to rule. Sovereign power was granted by heredity, was legislated by lineage, and established the rules and policies under which one's subjects lived. The Reformation diminished the influence of sovereign rule and eventually the power no longer vested in sovereign rulers was transferred in many societies to the general populace. This type of power by the populace is, for example, that which the United States places in officials elected to public office.[8]

The industrial age, suggests DeJouvenel,[8] introduced the organic theories of power, in which attention was directed to the ends of power rather than its means, and where the function of command became more important than the right of command. Power as an entity, therefore, became more important than individuals. The industrial age transformed social, political, and economic values from the farm to the city, from human muscle power to machine-driven power, from handcrafted production to mass production, from multigenerational to nuclear families, from family-owned businesses to corporate structures, from education of the few to education for the masses, and from person-to-person communication to worldwide communication.[23] The industrial age created the Vanderbilts, Carnegies, Rockefellers, and other large, family-dominated businesses in which the power to hire, fire, give, take, condemn, or condone was virtually unlimited. Although such families were not sovereign, they commanded substantial resources that enabled them to establish an American aristocracy capable of dividing labor from capital. Thus "power and how it is conceptualized and defined integrally reflects a society, culture, and era in vogue at any one time."[8]

Power presently is entering a new age—the information age—in which the power of specialized knowledge and the ability to communicate and translate knowledge into action is assuming increasing importance and unparalleled prominence in all nations and societies. Once again, power and how it functions in this new age will need to be redefined and reconceptualized.

What can nursing and nurses conclude from this brief overview of some of the traditions of power? Although nurses historically have been involved in healing, they rarely have been considered the healers; they have been female rather than male; and they have been governed, not governors. Nursing therefore has a heritage of few if any opportunities to assume positions of power. However, this lack of opportunity may have resulted as much from socially ascribed gender roles as from a frequently cited dearth of professional and independent functions.

Lipman-Blumen[13] makes a clear distinction between sex roles (roles associated with biological functions) and gender roles (socially created expectations regarding masculine and feminine behavior and occupational patterns). Thus while biological roles are similar across societies, gender roles may differ greatly. Despite the existence of cross-cultural differences, however, it is the "relative roles and positions of men and women in their society, their differing responsibilities and privileges, and their unequal control of resources that combine to form the major power differences between them."[13] However, traditions can be altered and replaced. Nursing and nurses can transcend and transform traditions of powerlessness into new customs and conventions of practice.

Nurses also need to recognize the pervasiveness of social conventions of power and their effects on attempts at change. For example, "Once social arrangements are established, those accustomed to the greater privileges of power will find it only natural and imperative to defend the status quo. . . ."[13] Subsequent generations will then accept these social arrangements as the norm and will guard them vigorously. . . .Thus even when social conditions might change, preexisting systems and institutional arrangements will serve to perpetuate the system.[13]

If Lipman-Blumen is correct, then traditional struggles for power between nurses and physicians may be both a convention and a reflection of our society. If nurses traditionally have accepted these social conventions without challenge, then they must be prepared for the resistance to change characteristic of the present health care delivery system. If it is true that gender roles provide

the premise upon which power relationships have existed for and between generations, social-economic classes, religions, social and ethnic groups, and that every society values men's contributions, resources, activities, privileges, and responsibilities more highly than women's[13]

then if nurses expect to alter the power equation the effort will demand much more than wishful thinking, assertiveness training, and rhetorical challenges.

Change will require new translations of the boundaries and parameters of practice as described by the gender roles customarily assigned to medicine and nursing. Change will require a new interest in and commitment to feminist history and theory, and a renewed pride in belonging to a predominantly female profession. Change in the power equation will require negotiations regarding the appropriate parameters of practice of nurses and other health care professionals, ever mindful that

both the powerful and the powerless tend to take existing social systems for granted and rarely recognize that it is not *talent,* but rather laws, customs, practices, and institutions that, in reality, keep the powerless . . . powerless.[13]

Nurses must recognize the effects of such traditions on the profession and be prepared to transform or at least reinterpret such customs, laws, and practices into new conventions that will be recognized and accepted not only by themselves but by the society being served.

TRANSITIONS OF POWER

Power, recently introduced as a concept into nursing, has undergone several transitions in the literature. Power initially emerged in the nursing literature in the mid to late 1960s, perhaps a reflection of the social unrest of the decade as opposed to any unrest in the profession itself. Although a few articles appeared in state nursing journals in the early 1960s, power actually burst onto the scene as a result of issues and papers presented at the 1968 convention of the National Student Nurses' Association. Dickoff and James[9] addressed the convention on power and excerpts of their speech were later published in the *American Journal of Nursing*. It seems significant that widespread interest in power in nursing came not so much from nurses or their leaders as from the concerns expressed by students and the message delivered by philosophers.

Dickoff and James[9] suggested that power is generally viewed as the use of brute or bodily force designed to create a fear of harm; it involves patronizing permissiveness within rigid constraints. They suggested further that nursing and nurses had confused and confounded the tokens of control with the symbols of power. For example, misconstruing privilege with capacity, permissiveness with independence, and constraint with ill will were, in their judgment, interpretations capable of infecting true conceptualizations of power.[7] But while Dickoff and James[9] may have formally introduced the concept to nursing and illustrated some of the conceptual problems surrounding its definitions and use, they neglected to offer a definition capable of countering the very concerns they so clearly delineated in their presentation.

Today nursing still confuses the privileges of power with the capacities of power, permissiveness with independence, and constraint with malice. The inability to clearly define the parameters of control from those of power, authority, influence, and other closely related but unique entities continues to inhibit individual nurses' and nursing's abilities to use any of these concepts efficiently, effectively, and appropriately. Nurses have relied heavily on the works of Simon,[22] Dahl,[7] Bennis,[3] French and Raven,[12] Mechanic,[12] Parsons,[16] Blau,[4] Etizioni,[11] and Drucker[10] for definitions, interpretations, and applications of power and its related concepts. Although these sources portray the contexts of power from the perspectives of business, sociology, medical sociology, organizational theory, and change; they do not incorporate the nature and contexts of power as defined in the discipline of its birth—political science. Definitional issues have been further confounded by the wide range of topics in which nurses have used the phenomenon of power as a convenient means to explain various relationships, in the absence of a clearly defined context. The focus of published work for and by nurses has moved from early discussions of the differences between power and authority, to using power as a form of advocacy; from concerns about roles to concerns for social change; from health care for women to collective bargaining and, more recently, to the use of power as a means of solving moral and ethical issues confronting the profession. Finally, the vast majority of articles delineate the authors' opinions about power; very few are based on data obtained from research. If power is to be an effective asset of nursing and nurses, a much clearer comprehension of its nature, definitions, sources, and consequences is required to achieve effective, efficient, and appropriate applications.

Sharp[21] suggests two distinctive ways to view the nature of power. One view sees people as dependent on the goodwill, decisions, and support of their government, with power being self-perpetuating, durable, not easily controlled or destroyed, and vested in those holding command. Conversely, the other view suggests that governing bodies are dependent on the goodwill, decisions, and support of the people, with power a fragile commodity drawing on many aspects of society.

It seems obvious, then, that how one views the nature of power greatly influences how one defines and uses power. One view stresses the monolithic nature of the concept and assumes that the power invested in an entity is a relatively fixed property. This position suggests that power is independent, durable, self-reinforcing and self-perpetuating. The second view, however, sees power as pluralistic and fragile, dependent on many people and groups for continued reinforcement.[21]

How one views one's position and role within a profession or organization is also dependent on how one views and interprets the nature of power. However, such philosophical distinctions have been largely ignored or neglected when power is discussed and defined in the nursing literature. For example, although nurse authors have been quick to adapt the work of others, they have failed to make clear distinctions between the *sources* of power and the *definitions* of power. Thus it has been relatively easy for nurses to confuse a source of power with the essence of its real nature or existence.

It is not uncommon for nurses to discuss "position power" within the context of a given entity; however, position is really a source of power, nothing else. In addition to confounding sources and definitions of power, nurses also have interjected the settings in which it is exercised—as, for example, organizational power. This continual confusion of contexts and definitional meanings has only served to cloud the contributions the concept may make to the profession.

Nursing's distortions of the traditional definitions of power have persisted throughout the transitional phase. As the concept has emerged in nursing, definitions of power also have assimilated the separate notions of authority, control, influence, and the ability to achieve goals. For example, Claus and Bailey[5] define power as "ability based on strength, willingness based on energy, and action that yields results." Sanford[19] suggests that "power is the ability to mobilize others in an effort to achieve a goal" and Miller[15] argues that power exists whenever one has authority, control and/or influence over others which can be used for positive or negative effects." The addition of related but separate concepts has limited the usefulness of the concept of power.

As nurses have grappled with this difficult notion, it appears that there has been a tendency to try to portray power as a "nice" concept. Interpreting power as influence, for example, serves only to further weaken both concepts, while ignoring the positive and negative elements of power. Lipman-Blumen[13] has defined power so as to eliminate the vagueness found in most current definitions used by nurses. She describes power as

the process whereby individuals or groups gain or maintain the capacity to impose their will upon others, to have their way recurrently despite implicit or explicit opposition, through invoking or threatening punishment, as well as offering or withholding rewards.

This formulation clearly and succinctly defines the phenomenon of power and its processes.

Sharp[21] asserts, however, that any power equation is dependent on the coexistence of a companion concept: obedience. The interdependence of these two concepts has yet to be acknowledged in the nursing literature on power. Indeed, nursing seems to prefer to ignore power's relationship to obedience rather than to explore its usefulness. Sharp[21] contends that it is obedience as the voluntary willingness to comply that makes power happen, regardless of its sources, and he distinguishes six sources of power from seven reasons to obey. These distinctions provide a rational explanation for power that is presently missing from the nursing literature.

Sharp's[21] six sources of power are (1) authority; (2) human resources; (3) skills and knowledge; (4) intangible factors such as, psychological or ideological influences and habits, attitudes, faiths, and missions frequently associated with power; (5) material resources; and (6) sanctions. Sharp concludes that, . . ."these sources of power depend intimately on obedience and cooperation" to be effective.[21]

The concept of obedience tends to generate negative

reactions among nurses, however, perhaps because of nursing's history of oppression. The early domination of nursing by religious and military orders, coupled with a tradition of subordination to medicine, has resulted in the virtual elimination of the word *obedience* from the profession's vocabulary. The word itself, however, is not the problem. Perhaps the problem is not knowing how and when obedience can and should be used—a problem which, if solved, promises interesting solutions.

Sharp[21] outlines seven reasons why individuals or groups voluntarily "choose" to obey others. Human beings, individually or collectively, will obey as a result of (1) habit; (2) fear of sanctions; (3) moral obligation; (4) self-interest; (5) psychological identification with someone in charge; (6) indifference; and (7) a lack of self-confidence.

Are nurses submissive as a result of their history of oppression and obedience to authority? Or are we victims of our own lack of self-confidence, patterns of habitual response, fears of being penalized, self-interest, or disparate zones of indifference? The historical factors cannot be dismissed lightly, nor should they—but can members of the nursing profession really be expected to effectively use power without appreciating the equally important role of obedience in the power equation? Perhaps nurses have attempted to apply theories of power without systematically analyzing the components and connections necessary to achieve desired results. Power, if it is to be a useful and important concept for nursing and nurses, must not only be clearly understood but must be used in conjunction with obedience in a comprehensive manner.

TRANSFORMATIONS OF POWER

How, then, can nurses begin to transform power into a force to enhance and advance themselves, the profession, and the profession's goals in health care? Robbins[17] suggests seven basic characteristics necessary to develop and cultivate power: passion, belief, strategy, clarity of values, energy, bonding, and mastering communication.

Imagine what it would be like if the nursing literature was replete with discussions of how great it is to be a nurse and how nurses look forward to each day of work, rather than the litany currently recited in which nurses are overworked, underpaid, and burned out. What would happen to the profession if nurses developed a consuming energy and purpose for their

work similar to the enthusiastic spirit of caring often seen in sophomore and junior students of nursing but rarely found in seasoned practitioners? As Robbins[17] states, "Passion gives life power and juice and meaning. There is no greatness without a passion to be great, whether it's the aspiration of an athlete or an artist, a scientist, a parent, or a businessman." And I add, or a nurse! If nursing wants power, it must be ready to pay the price for obtaining and maintaining it—a price that demands more, not less, effort; more, not fewer, hours; increased, not decreased, dedication; and a greater, not a lesser, commitment to caring than currently seems to exist. There must be the desire to constantly improve and the willingness to continue learning throughout one's professional career. Power in this era is earned, not bestowed, and it takes more than rhetoric to possess it.

Nurses must believe in their mission, in their own self-worth, and in their ability to truly make a difference! A former teacher shared the following story from her childhood in an Irish immigrant family. "My mother would have me say every morning before leaving for school: 'Every day in every way I get better and better!'"[6] Imagine the power in those few words! What would happen if nurses adopted a similar attitude, and instead of allowing themselves to feel like failures every time they make a mistake or cannot recall a piece of information, were content to learn from their errors, vowed not to make the same mistake again, and resumed their duties proudly and confidently because their error made them "better and better?"

Nurses continue to assume responsibility for and to provide the major portion of all care administered to patients. This important role and the visibility it has for patients, their families, and society needs to be recognized and valued by nurses regardless of how it is perceived by others in the present health care system. Nurses must develop, nurture, cultivate, and encourage a belief system that allows them to have pride in their work and contributions, to make that important difference.

Whereas passion and belief provide the fuel for achieving power, intelligence and logical strategies provide the road maps by which success is eventually achieved.[17] Strategy is used by military organizations to define and achieve long-range goals or objectives. Nursing and nurses must begin to think in terms of proactive and long-term objectives if they really expect to achieve and hold power. Power is not assuming a posture of continual reaction, but rather developing the foresight to organize the resources needed to produce predetermined objectives and preferred results. This means working together to achieve consensus on nursing leadership, the objectives of the profession, and the role of nursing in health care. Success means working together to resolve internal differences in work environments as well as external problems with other groups and constituencies. It means learning when to take a stand or stage a battle, as well as when to surrender or retreat without losing the war. It means being willing and able to plan, organize, develop, implement, and reevaluate what is important for nursing and how to achieve those results. It means taking action, not just talking, complaining, blaming, disagreeing, and expecting others to act for nurses. It means anticipating and being prepared to meet challenges constructively instead of criticizing new approaches, concepts, ideas and proposals.

Nursing and nurses must have and endorse well-orchestrated strategies if they are to achieve the power they want and need to affect health care.

Robbins's fourth trait, clarity of values, means being able to identify the "fundamental, ethical, moral, and practical judgments" about what the profession and its members truly hold as important and what makes nursing a worthwhile profession.[17] Nursing must come to grips with what it is and what it is about if it is to unify its members and their passions, beliefs, and strategies. The need to articulate nursing's values and purposes is neither new nor novel, but it has not yet been accomplished. We need to reexamine the work of early leaders, such as Robb, Nutting, Wald, Dock, Stewart, and Goodrich, among others, who were able to resolve their differences while determining and clarifying values for a changing profession. Their accomplishments illustrate how nursing and nurses can handle conflicts internally while coalescing efforts for external progress.

If nursing and nurses are successful in developing these four traits, then they will need to marshal the energy required to achieve articulated objectives. "It is impossible to amble toward excellence . . . opportunities must be taken, shaped, and capitalized upon in order to make the most of an opportunity."[17] Nurses have tremendous energy stores that need to be channeled toward achieving positive outcomes rather than wasted in futile, often meaningless efforts that fail to result in productive change. Consider the energy many nurses expend trying to meet the needs of patients assigned to their care!

Nurses work hard and the pressures and demands they face every moment, hour, and shift are rarely recognized, let alone appreciated by others—including some of the patients entrusted to their care. They report leaving work mentally and physically exhausted, often with a sense of despair because they were unable to do more to assist patients in need. Imagine what could happen to the profession if nurses' energies were redirected to satisfaction, if refreshment replaced fatigue, if encouragement replaced frustration, and if cheerfulness replaced depression! But in order to accomplish this, nurses must reconceptualize how best to utilize their energy and be prepared to rechannel it in ways that improve patient care and promote themselves simultaneously. The energies of nurses must be redirected toward what they can accomplish rather than what seems impossible. Energy, given direction, can be mobilized to achieve greatness, and nurses need to capitalize on their energies to bring about the changes that will improve the total health care delivery system.

The sixth trait needed to cultivate and develop power is bonding.[17] Bonding refers to the ability to connect and establish rapport with many diverse groups both within and outside the profession. Nurses must emerge from their protective cocoons and capture center stage, accepting the attendant risks of such a step. First of all, nurses must bond among themselves. Nurses must learn to trust one another despite their differences, and to discuss points of agreement as often as areas of disagreement. Nurses must learn how to handle success as well as failure. Nurses must learn to stand together and support one another before physicians, administrators, and others. If nurses establish bonds within the profession, it will be difficult and perhaps impossible for others to break those ties. Eleanor Roosevelt once said, "No one can intimidate you, unless you allow them."[18] Nurses do not have to be intimidated. Developing the strategies to deal with physicians and others, and with the bonding essential to generating and directing action, nurses can gain control over the delivery of patient care. Only when nurses bond can they expect to achieve their goals and develop the power necessary to ensure nursing's presence and voice in the structures and functions governing health care.

Finally, Robbins[17] suggests, there is a need to master communication if one is to enjoy both the fruits and responsibilities of power. Nursing and nurses need to focus on and appreciate the challenges of the profession, not its limitations. If nurses only continue to identify and define nursing's limitations, then those constraints will become reality. Nurses must communicate with one another, with patients, with physicians, and with hospital administrators. Nurses must articulate who they are and what they can do—from their own perspective, not those of others. Nursing and nurses need to determine what it is that they want, establish the means to achieve it, bond together to work for it, and keep the channels of communication open throughout the process. They can no longer sit by and hope the right thing will happen. If nurses are not part of the solution, they will always remain part of the problem. The opportunities created by the nursing shortage provide an unparalleled occasion in which to individually or collectively, by institution, district, state, and nation, convey our message—if we know what it is we want and how we wish to obtain it.

Power is after all, only a perception; perception is, after all, power.

REFERENCES

1. American Nurse, June, 1989, p. 27.
2. Ashley J: This I believe: about power in nursing, Nursing Outlook 21:637, 1973.
3. Bennis W: Leadership theory and administrative behavior: the problem of authority, Administrative Science Quarterly 4:259, 1959.
4. Blau P: Exchange and power in social life, New York, 1964, John Wiley and Sons.
5. Claus KE and Bailey JT: Power and influence in health care, St. Louis, 1977, The C.V. Mosby Co.
6. Condon Sr MB: Personal communication, Eau Claire, Wisconsin, April 1988.
7. Dahl R: The concept of power, Behavioral Science, 2:201, 1957.
8. DeJouvenel B: On power, New York, 1949, Viking Press.
9. Dickoff J and James P: Power, Am J Nurs 68(10):2128.
10. Drucker P: The practice of management, New York, 1964, Harper and Row.
11. Etizioni A: Modern organizations, Englewood Cliffs, NJ, 1964, Prentice-Hall, Inc.
12. French J and Raven BH: The basis of social power. In Cartwright D, editor: Studies in social power, Ann Arbor, Mich, 1959, Institute for Social Work.
13. Lipman-Blumen J: Gender roles and power, Englewood Cliffs, NJ, 1984, Prentice-Hall, Inc.
14. Mechanic D: Sources of power of lower participants in complex organizations, Administrative Science Quarterly 7:349, 1962.
15. Miller S: Power yesterday, today, and tomorrow, Heart and Lung 10(12):214, 1981.
16. Parsons T: Suggestions for a sociological approach to organizations, Administrative Science Quarterly 1:225, 1956.
17. Robbins A: Unlimited power, New York, 1986, Simon and Schuster Publishing Co.
18. Roosevelt E: In Barwick DD: Great words of our time, Kansas City, Mo, 1970, Hallmark Cards, Inc., p. 19.
19. Sanford NO: Power for the O.R. Nurse, Association of Operating Room Nurses 31(15):787, 1980.
20. Schutt BG: Power, symbols, and substance, Am J Nurs 68(10):2123, 1968.
21. Sharp G: The policies on non-violent action (Part I): power and struggle, Boston, Mass, 1973, Porter, Sargent Publications.
22. Simon H: Administrative behavior, New York, 1945, The Free Press.
23. Toffler A: The third wave, New York, 1980, William Morrow and Co., Inc.

CHAPTER 65

Imagery issues in international nursing

TREVOR CLAY

The desired switch from the medical model of health care to primary health care with the patient as a partner in care is taking place. Most of the effort in this direction is being made by nurses in the southern half of the world, the developing world.

Although the images of nursing throughout the world have been changing radically, are these changes reflected in reality? Have nurses yet addressed the existing doctor-nurse relationship so that their approaches to health care can be seen as sufficiently different from the shackles of the medical model of care? Nurses should be facilitators of care, not simply the providers of care, especially when the "doing" is purely in response to medical prescription based on the medical model.

What images exist among nurses in different parts of the world? Are the world's nurses one big happy family? Even within a single country, nursing has often splintered into disciplines and specialties that override the potential and strength of nurses as a unified profession. Rather than dwell on sectional differences, the profession needs to develop internationally, to build on its potential to be a movement for women in work, as well as to display the necessary assertiveness to work as professional equals with doctors. As the world's largest organization for nurses, the Royal College of Nursing has achieved much in the United Kingdom by uniting disparate branches of nursing toward a professionalism heeded by allied professionals.

NURSES AS A UNITED POWERHOUSE FOR CHANGE

Nurses in the developed world do not realize how lucky they are. They take for granted their freedom to debate publicly and to develop and change the direction, structures, and conditions within health care from both the professionals' and the consumers' points of view. These nurses must not hold back on the rel-

ative progress they are making, especially in acute care, but they must not become so distant from their fellow professionals in developing countries that part of their international unity of purpose—that of achieving health for all by the year 2000*—becomes dispersed or splintered.

What is included in each "half" of the world? The North includes the United States and the United Kingdom, along with Canada, Australia, New Zealand, most Western European countries, and Japan. The South includes the Near East, Middle East, and Far East, Africa, Central America, South America, the Indian subcontinent, and Asia. For brevity I will use the terms North and South.

Although each half of the world can learn from the other—the best of both traditional and modern health care—nurses in the developed world must look beyond their focus on acute care to the concerns of nurses in the South. These nurses have patients whose needs are so great that the nurses have little time to do anything except attempt to meet those needs, including most importantly, aspects of disease prevention and cure. The North can share its great advances in health care technology, from machines to pharmaceuticals and from modern education methods (perhaps not all of them) to modern management systems (most of them). It can also share those aspects of nursing research that seem relevant to the South, much of which has never been applied in the North.

Having set out what the South might gain from the North, what benefits can the North gain from the South, allowing, of course, for the differences in econ-

---

*Nurses throughout the world are increasingly adopting the World Health Organization (WHO) Declaration of Alma-Ata that "a main social target of governments, international organizations and the whole world community in the coming decades should be the attainment by all peoples of the world by the year 2000 of a level of health that will permit them to lead a socially and economically productive life."

omies, cultures, and nursing roles in the North and South. If nurses in the North are sincere about their aim of achieving health for all by the year 2000—largely by shifting the health care emphasis from a repair and maintenance service to a disease-prevention and health-promotion system—they can learn about life in societies unspoiled and unhampered by what Illich[3] calls medical nemesis, the medicalization of life.

More than all clinical iatrogeneses put together, more than the sum of malpractice, negligence, professional callousness, political maldistribution, medically decreed disability and all the consequences of medical trial and error: It is the expropriation of man's coping ability, by a maintenance service which keeps him geared up at the service of the industrial system.

By the year 2000 the North will be coping with a major demographic shift: a huge increase in its elderly population, along with the accompanying increase in demand for health care. In the United Kingdom alone there could be as many as 100,000 more dependent elderly people requiring skilled nursing care.

Illich's alternative to the medicalization of life—an almost anarchic abandonment of professional health care as it now exists—might seem a bit drastic, but he is right in his assertion of the individual's right to self-determination in medical treatment. This is also one of the recommendations of the Royal College of Nursing Commission on the U.K. National Health Service:[8]

We recommend that patients be given more power to choose the treatment they receive, not only in terms of which doctors or hospital treats them, but also the type of treatment used (extending also to alternative or complementary medicine), and, where possible, the time and place of treatment or consultation. Similarly, patients should be entitled to see any health care professional they choose, and not simply a doctor—nurses (particularly nurse practitioners), physiotherapists, homeopaths, and others, should all be directly accessible to individual clients. The value of this radical change in practice is amply borne out by indications that, when given the information and opportunity, patients do correctly self-diagnose and choose appropriate treatment.

The commission also called for the voice of the consumer to be strengthened and accorded more representational power. The professional-dominated health care system does not encourage individuals to believe that they have much or any control over their own health. The prevailing medical model, in fact, has discouraged people from feeling responsible for their own health. "The nursing profession, in particular," the commission stated, "has a key role to play in dispelling this illusion, through adopting models of health promotion and beginning to run a health service rather than a sickness service." The focus needs to shift toward primary health care and disease prevention, with the patient or client as a partner in care. And to succeed in this, the potential of the world's nurses as health care's major untapped resource must be fully realized.

Similar positions have been taken by two U.K. government reports,[6,7] both on change in primary health care. One of them, the Cumberlege report,[7] strongly emphasized the need to make better, broader, and more effective use of nurses and urged reform of the existing boundaries between the different medical professions.

Former WHO director, Dr. Halfdan Mahler, has said of this powerful combination of potential and people in health care, "If millions of nurses in a thousand different places articulate the same ideas and convictions about primary health care and come together as one force, they could act as a powerhouse for change.[4a]

Already great strides have been made, albeit not exclusively by nurses in the South. These nurses, however, need to have access to the same kind of political and governmental power enjoyed by nurses in the North so that their wisdom, motivation, and energy can be put to use for the betterment of humanity.

The high-tech health care half of the world might think that it leads the other half in both quality and quantity of health care. From the perspective of quality, any comparison would be like comparing the nutritional qualities of an apple to those of a fast-food hamburger. In terms of quantity, the majority of the world's health care is performed by untrained personnel, using unsophisticated equipment, often to surprisingly good effect. What of the feldsher, the practitioner of traditional medicine, the barefoot doctor, the witch doctor, the tribal doctor, the relative, and the friend? Folk medicine, grounded in traditional remedies, regardless of whether it is scientific or magical, nature based or based on placebos, still accounts for a significant proportion of health care throughout the world. Nurses in the North have begun to learn from some of these alternative systems of medicine. In cancer nursing, for example, nurses are now stressing the need for the patient to be an active, positive participant in the fight against cancer. They are also advocating touch, stroking, and massage as part of their care. Is this scientific or magical? Who knows?

But nurses are doing it, and these techniques seem to improve the patient's health.

Complementary health care approaches are also increasing in popularity with both professional and consumer alike. Homeopathy, acupuncture and acupressure, chiropractice, herbal medicine, hypnotism— each offers an alternative to orthodox medicine. Such is the poor relationship that still exists between orthodox and unorthodox health care that these alternatives are often tried only as last resorts. Brian Ingles[4] has spoken of the virtues of complementary medicine and the need for orthodox medicine to ally itself more with nature. "Nature has its own healing force," he says, "a force which medical practice should assist, not supplant. For even if based on the soundest scientific principles, orthodox methods can often be sadly and cruelly misguided."

It is difficult to call for change, especially when professional demarcations are endangered, without stepping on a few toes. However, some doctors—particularly an emerging breed of women who are less orthodox—are making changes in the medical model. They must be supported as they join with fellow health care professionals to try to change peoples' understandings, expectations, and activities in regard to their own health care. And especially they must reconsider where nursing fits into this new version of health care.

NURSES, DOCTORS, AND PATIENTS: THE NEED FOR PARTNERSHIP

Among nurses too, there needs to be both a realization of that potential and a major international effort made to harness what must be a power for good. Nurses also need to be aware of who will be learning lessons from whom.

As medical technology and science advance in the North, there needs to be a corresponding move toward the art in medicine and nursing, the human perspective, and what might be termed the laying on of hands. These more human aspects of health care are already a standard part of nursing. The nurse thus is the most appropriate health professional to address the health care needs of the world, to be the agent of change in shifting the emphasis in health care away from the limitations of the medical model. Nurses are a major untapped resource in health care not only because of their numbers but also because of the broad nature of their practice.

Apart from these factors, nurses must also consider the differing images of nursing in the North and South. The assumption used to be that the high-tech professional nurses in the North were forging their way apart from doctors while the less developed professionals in the South were somehow still being held back. But the lines between nurses and doctors are becoming blurred all over the world. Wherever nurses work in hospitals, North or South, it is *they* who are still largely bound by doctors and the medical model of care. It is the nurse in the community, whether in upstate New York, suburban London, or rural Lesotho, who has made the greater strides toward the development of nursing. It may be the community nurse visiting patients' homes with a disease-prevention perspective, nurse practitioners managing their emerging role as part diagnostician and part prescriber of care, or the independent midwife working outside formal health service structures. Nurses are breaking away from their previous reliance on the medical profession and forming new partnerships.

Nurses also need to address their divisions. Are they ready to take on such change? And can they organize that change for their benefit? Dalton McFarland has explored how the types and sources of power apply to American nursing administrators and individual nurses.[5]

Over 90% of today's 1.4 million nurses work for organizations that provide structured job opportunities, resources, planning, goals and clientele—important elements in the nurse's power base. To increase their power, therefore, nurses need a sophisticated experimental knowledge of organizational processes and the behavior of people within them.

. . . Organizations find professionals notably harder to deal with than other types of workers. They band together through kindred interests, thus gaining the power of alliances and coalitions.

Nurses can band together to achieve their aims, forming alliances with fellow health care professionals and others—including consumers—when they take the lead. In spite of their divisions and weaknesses, there is an international family of nurses with the potential to increase its power, and to set the agenda for world health care change. That family of nursing must help those within it who can play no political role in their profession because their professional associations have little or no power. Nurses in some countries may, and often do, receive good training in nursing, but they cannot always put into practice what they have learned. Nor do many of them have nursing departments at the government level to speak and fight for nursing and nurses.

It is nothing short of miraculous that prominent nurses have emerged from such countries in the South. Their achievements are all the more impressive because of the hurdles and obstacles. In one respect they are fortunate, in that they are not saddled with the Nightingale model and the tradition of nursing that it founded. (Modern nursing is said to have been founded in the United Kingdom through the efforts of Florence Nightingale.) They are, therefore, freer to look at primary health care and its new roles for nurses in a way that U.K. nurses and some others find much more difficult.

THREE DISTINCT IMAGES: ONE COMMON AIM

It is invidious to highlight individual nurses, but there are lessons to be learned by looking at the careers of three of the world's most distinguished nurses. If nothing else, the motivation and strength of these women should command our respect and admiration.

Wang Xiuying, Nursing Adviser to the Second Medical College, Beijing, has contributed in important ways to the improved health of the Chinese people. Her enthusiasm for nursing education and public health nursing has led to radical innovations in the delivery of health care services in China. Her high standing as a matron well before China's Cultural Revolution allowed her access to young Chinese nurses, whom she encouraged as she traveled throughout the country. She motivated these young people to devote themselves wholeheartedly to their profession. She has pioneered public health in China for half a century; no wonder other nurses are in awe of her. She has been honored internationally for her contributions, including being made an Honorary Fellow of the Royal College of Nursing of the United Kingdom.

Equally prominent in her own country, Chief Kofoworola Abeni Pratt of Nigeria, also an honorary Fellow of the Royal College of Nursing, has raised the status of nurses and nursing not only in Nigeria but throughout the African continent as well. She has also significantly enhanced the status of women in that country. Her influence has spread well beyond nursing and the struggle for female emancipation and has gained her many honours and awards. Undoubtedly, however, her most significant honour was earned for services to her nation—that of the Chieftancy Title, Iya Agbo of Isheri. This is a crowning glory for an African nurse who started her career at the Nightingale School of Nursing at St Thomas' Hospital in London and who was the first Nigerian nurse to hold the post of ward sister in her own country.

The North has seen its own revolution in nursing care. Fourteen basic principles of nursing care developed by Virginia Henderson, an American nurse, have become the founding principles of late twentieth-century nursing. Her definition of a nurse is a classic:

The unique function of the nurse is to assist the individual, sick or well, in the performance of those activities contributing to health or its recovery (or to peaceful death) that he would perform unaided if he had the necessary strength, will or knowledge, and to do this in such a way as to help him gain independence as rapidly as possible.[2]

Virginia Henderson is a legend in her own lifetime and has received many prestigious honors, including the Honorary Fellowship of the American Academy of Nursing. She has shown how a nurse can effect international change, not only in improving nursing care but also in establishing a power base on which other nurses might build.

These three nurses have been influential well beyond their national boundaries and have shown what nurse power and unity can achieve. In spite of the individual efforts made by these women—and by others, including men—the problems are far from solved. The North cannot yet boast that all of its powerful organizations have truly used their energy, enterprise, and resources to put out a helping hand to poorer countries.

THE POWERHOUSE FOR CHANGE: MAKING THE CONNECTIONS

Not many nurses' associations within the International Council of Nurses have even one staff member allocated to international work. It seems that resources are not the only block to international progress; attitudes and ignorance contribute as well. Do nurses in the North understand what everyday life is really like in the rest of the world? Amnesty International and the International Red Cross know of the torture and imprisonment that nurses have endured in some parts of the world. Progress can be made on issues such as this only through concerted, intelligent, and sensitive campaigns by nurses' associations.

The image of the nurse throughout the world is always one of a person who cares. That image is often accompanied by one that portrays the nurse as worthy and honorable but not necessarily strong academically or politically. There can be no better way for nurses to achieve an image as powerful, competent, and autonomous professionals—and simultaneously to change world health care systems—than to act as a united, international agent of change in health care, a veritable powerhouse for change.

REFERENCES

1. Clay T: Worldwide nursing unity: building a powerhouse for change, Nursing and Health Care 8;7:407, 1987.
2. Henderson V: Basic principles of nursing care, Geneva, 1977, International Council of Nurses.
3. Illich I: Medical nemesis, the expropriation of health, London, 1975, Calder & Boyars, Ltd.
4. Ingles B: Natural medicine, Glasgow, 1979, William Callins Sons & Co, Ltd.
4a. Mahler H: A powerhouse for change, Senior Nurse 8;7:23, 1987.
5. McFarland DE: Power as a change strategy. In Lancaster, Jeanette and Lancaster, Wade, editors: The nurse as a change agent, St Louis, 1982, The CV Mosby Co.
6. Primary health care: an agenda for discussion, London 1986, Her Majesty's Stationery Office.
7. Report of the Community Nursing Review: Neighborhood nursing—a focus for care, London, 1986, Her Majesty's Stationery Office.
8. Royal College of Nursing of the United Kingdom: The health challenge—report of a commission on the national health service and health care in the United Kingdom, 1978, London, Royal College of Nursing of the United Kingdom.

PART TEN

ROLE CONFLICT

Conflicts within nursing

JOANNE COMI McCLOSKEY
HELEN KENNEDY GRACE

Throughout this book, the conflicts within nursing are frequently identified as contributory to diminishing the influence of the profession. Turf battles among organizations, the distance of nursing leadership and education from the concerns of nurses at the practice level, disagreements over educational preparation for nurses, and the vying of specialty groups with one another are all seen as weakening the potential power of the profession. This section examines in greater depth some of these conflict areas.

Addressing the issue of nursing organizations, Partridge in the debate chapter poses the question, "Can There Be One Nursing Organization?" Although the American Nurses' Association (ANA) represents only 10% of the more than 1 million nurses in the United States, it is one of the largest professional organizations in the world. If the ANA merged with other organizations, nursing would be one of the most powerful professional groups.

The issue of consolidation of nursing organizations has been under review at varying times since 1924. Despite a commissioned study recommending the merger of nursing organizations, this proposal was rejected in 1947, primarily over the issue of nonnurse membership. Out of this effort, territorial boundaries were established between the ANA and the National League for Nursing (NLN), making the ANA responsible for practice and professional employment issues and the domain of the NLN nursing service and educational issues. Through the years there has been considerable blurring of these divisions of turf. However, in recent years the proliferation of specialty organizations serves as a threat to both the ANA and the NLN, resulting in increased collaboration between these two major organizations.

The National Federation of Specialty Nursing Organizations (NFSNO) was formed in 1973 and now lists over 80 member groups. To counter the likelihood of the NFSNO becoming an organization separate from the ANA, the National Organization Liaison Forum (NOLF) was created as a part of the ANA in 1983. These organizations have held parallel meetings every year since, each seeking to represent specialty groups in nursing. Noting the obstacles, the author concludes that consolidation is important to change the profession's tendency to be represented by "small, impotent groups primarily concerned with self-interests and self-preservation. Rather than worrying about individual organizational survival, nurses should be concerning themselves with their collective survival."

Moving from the macrolevel of the profession to the microlevel of practice, Mauksch addresses the need for support and recognition of the staff nurse. In a thoughtful chapter, he examines the concept of abandonment as it applies to the bedside nurse. He says that if nurses feel that they have been abandoned, then this is the reality. Focusing on hospital nursing, he points out that anonymity and powerlessness are associated with beaucratically structured positions. The education of beginning nurses, which emphasizes professional status and individual responsibility, does not prepare one for the minimal power and anonymity of the staff nurse position. The result is that nurses feel betrayed and unappreciated when confronting the "reality shock."

Mauksch discusses several changes during the last few years that have intensified the sense of abandonment felt by the staff nurse. These include increased patient care demands with no additional support for the nurse; the increasing differentiation of the nursing intelligentsia and the grass-roots nurses; changes in the organizational structure whereby the director of nursing becomes a vice-president and moves up into institution management but away from staff nurses;

the acceptance of feminism and a sensitivity to the issues of equality that have made the physician's approval less rewarding and less acceptable and, in turn, have decreased the physician's tendency to express appreciation; and, perhaps most important, the fact that the daily routine of hospitals facing the increasing demands of technology and cost containment emphasizes more and more the subordinate and technical dimensions of care at the expense of activities that are unique to nursing. It is no wonder, asserts Mauksch, that bedside nurses feel that "real" nursing has been abandoned. According to Mauksch, neither the bureaucratic model of the hospital nor the individualism model of the educational institution are right for the bedside nurse. Structural changes are needed that promote a system of collective teamwork and group accountability. All nurses, grass-roots and others, will find this a very helpful chapter in explaining the complex and subtle conflicts experienced by the staff nurse.

Continuing with the same issue, Hardin addresses conflict situations arising at the patient care level leading to occupational stress. After an extensive review of research in this area, the author concludes:

> For nurses, occupational distress involves general and specific causes such as task overload, time-and-space-constricted environments, responsibilities, patient crises, and physician demands that are persistent and chronic.

Within this context, the support structure for nurses and perceptions of autonomy and control are important mediating factors. Despite extensive knowledge about occupational distress of nurses, few organizational interventions have been implemented. Most of the emphasis has been placed on individual interventions to assist the nurse in dealing with work-related stress. Noting that psychiatric nurse specialists in private practice do not report being distressed, and reflect high levels of self-esteem, Hardin asserts:

> One essential difference between these two types of practitioners seems to be their autonomy. Nurse-practitioners have power and control to match their responsibility. . . . Moreover, [psychiatric nurses in clinic settings are free] from at least one of the most highly rated stressors in these research reports—physicians.

Just as nurses at the practice level may experience stress because of perceived powerlessness, the difficulty in influencing public policy is reflective of a similar problem at the organizational level of the profession. Beyers asserts that

First nurses, must accept the responsibility to influence and to become involved in public policy decisions. Second, they must develop issues and problems in meaningful positions to offer substance to deliberation and debate by the decision makers. Third, nurses must continue to develop their expertise in processes of influencing public policy.

With these imperatives in mind, the author then addresses some of the difficulties in becoming engaged in the policy-making arena. One of the unfortunate outcomes of many organizations speaking from a variety of perspectives is that the profession as a whole is perceived as lacking in power, and second, that conflicts are resolved in the public arena rather than within the profession. Returning to the original question posed in the chapter title, Beyers concludes that public policy issues will be resolved only if nurses accept responsibility and become expert in this arena.

Moving up the administrative ladder to the position of nurse executive generates a number of role conflicts that need to be resolved. Donaho identifies the following areas of potential conflict: fostering independence on the part of staff while maintaining visibility within the organization; appropriate mentoring of staff members while delegating responsibility; achieving a proper balance of delegation and control; and moving from clinical to organizational management. In addition to achieving an appropriate balance in the internal management of nursing services, the nurse executive also needs to balance requirements for participation in the broader realm of management, in the organization and in the external environment. Given this broader perspective, perhaps the most difficult conflict for nurse executives is offsetting the demands for internal decision making and management against broader futuristic concerns. Donaho, although noting that some nurse executives may opt to focus on the nursing department and today's clinical departmental issues, concludes:

> That decision results in relegating tomorrow's organizational decisions to other professionals. The nurse executive who operates with a vision for the profession will become a strategic player in both the organization and the external environment and will influence decisions.

Although conflict most frequently is portrayed as a negative factor, Johnson argues for using conflict as a positive force. Traditionally nursing has sought to avoid conflict at all costs, which has resulted in acting out conflicts in the public arena rather than reaching resolutions within the field. The positive functions of conflict are identified as (1) unification, through the creation of group cohesion; (2) group preservation, through preventing the accumulation of hostility; (3) integration, through the promotion of group and individual stability; (4) growth, through the promotion of innovation and change; and (5) problem-solving, through the stimulation of the quality of problem solving.

Turning to the international scene, one of the more subtle and confounding issues in nursing is a result of the intertwining of conflicts related to women's roles and those related to nursing. Traditional roles for women in developing countries are more circumscribed than those in the current American cultural environment. Carillo traces the early historical roots of women's roles as food gatherers and bearers and nurturers of children. In early Andean culture women were very active members of the community. The author notes that one's status in society was determined on the basis not of gender but of the leadership role played by the individual. The Spanish conquest changed this situation, making women subordinate to men in Andean cultures. Women's current status is compounded by their poor economic situations in these countries, and the emphasis on the role of woman as wife and mother. Women are employed in low-paying, low-status positions. Nurses in this context are considered "second-class professionals." The challenge for nursing is to transform perceptions and to enable nurses to become complete human beings, to assume responsibilities, to make decisions, and to emerge as confident professionals with the obligation to build a more equitable world for all. This challenge applies not only to developing countries but to nurses in all settings.

CHAPTER 66

Debate

Can there be one nursing organization?

REBECCA PARTRIDGE

Representing about 10% of the 1 million registered nurses in the United States, the American Nurses' Association (ANA) is one of the largest professional organizations in the world. With the consolidation of the ANA and other organizations, nursing could have not only the largest professional organization in the world but also, and more importantly, the most powerful health-oriented professional organization in the world.

The chapter presents a historical review and discussion of the present situation regarding the development of nursing organizations. It is intended to serve as an aid in the current debate on the changing structure and identity of national nursing organizations.

THE EARLY DEVELOPMENT OF NURSING ORGANIZATIONS

Alumnae associations were the first formal organizations established by nurses. The first of these societies was started by graduates of the Bellevue training school for nurses in 1889, and many others were started in the years that followed.[6] Because of the nature of the training school environment and the apprenticeship model, a strong sense of rivalry among schools developed and was maintained.

Hospital-operated training schools successfully inculcated in their students an ardent loyalty to their home institution, a loyalty that persisted throughout a graduate's career.[2] The symbol of this institutional loyalty, the wearing of a cap signifying one's school, persisted in many areas of the country until very recently. School loyalty and the "singular objective of promoting their own schools"[6] kept the focus of the alumnae associations narrow and their impact minimal. Even more important, the rivalry provoked by this myopic loyalty to one's school mitigated against collective action among alumnae societies.[6]

In 1893 nursing leaders began to recognize the need to cooperate on a national level to solve two major problems: the "lack of standardization in nurse training as well as the need for laws to protect the public from poorly trained nurses.[6] Although these problems are inextricably linked, the leaders of nursing formed two separate organizations to seek remedies for them.

The American Society of Superintendents of Training Schools for Nurses was created in 1893 to develop and implement a universal standard for training. This organization was the precursor to the National League of Nursing Education (NLNE) and, finally, the National League for Nursing (NLN), which still exists today as the officially recognized accrediting body for nursing education programs (see Fig. 66-1).

Protecting the public from ill-prepared nurses through the enactment of licensure laws became the task of the second nationally based organization, the Nurses' Associated Alumnae, which was started in 1897. This organization was later to become what we now know as the ANA. Ironically, these first two national organizations were started by many of the same nursing leaders. It was at this point that issues of nursing education and practice were first dichotomized. This initial split was to grow wider and deeper in the years to come. Ashley[2] contends in the following statement that the decision to form two organizations instead of one was a critical error nursing has yet to remedy.

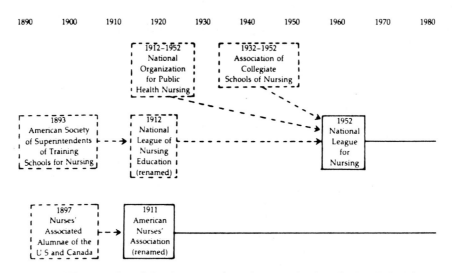

Fig. 66-1 The growth and development of nursing organizations in the United States.

With the control of education in the hands of one organization and the control of practice in the hands of the other, gaps in communication were inevitable. The lack of concerted action by both educators and practitioners created serious problems, as future decades were to prove. With this separation of functions, the foundation was laid for continuing lack of unity accompanied by conflicts and misunderstandings. The two separate organizations still exist today, and so do the conflicts and the misunderstandings.

EARLY PROPOSALS FOR CONSOLIDATION

In 1924 the NLNE and the ANA, along with the National Organization for Public Health Nursing, first discussed the advantages of consolidation, but they decided to remain separate organizations. Again in 1939 consolidation was considered when the ANA formed a special committee to consider the formation of one national nursing organization. But World War II intervened, and the pursuit of one organization was not renewed until 1946, when the ANA contracted with Raymond Rich Associates to conduct a study of the six existing national nursing organizations:

- American Nurses' Association
- National League of Nursing Education (became the NLN)
- National Organization for Public Health Nursing (merged with the NLN)
- Association of Collegiate Schools of Nursing (merged with the NLN)
- National Association of Colored Graduate Nurses (dissolved and joined the ANA)

- American Association of Industrial Nurses (remained independent)

The Rich report identified three issues dividing these organizations: membership of nonnurses, devotion to special interests, and program emphasis.[18] Although special interests and program emphasis were matters of concern, the membership and participation of nonnurses was the pivotal issue, and this fact was reflected in the nature of the two plans Rich proposed. Plan I called for the creation of a single nursing organization, the American Nursing Association, and conferred full membership privileges on nonnurse participants.

Plan II recommended the establishment of two nursing organizations with linkage provided by a national nursing center. One of these organizations would include only nurses, the other would include nurses and nonnurses among the membership.

It is perplexing to note that the ANA provided the impetus for the consolidation study conducted by Rich Associates, and then rejected the recommendation to unite. However, it is clear from the following statements, made at the 1947 convention, that the ANA strongly desired the organizational strength consolidation would provide. "You agree you want a united front organization for nursing. You want a strong, vital organization representing all of the nurses. You want to eliminate duplication, overlapping . . ."[4] But the delegates also wanted the ANA to "remain the national organization representing all graduate professional nurses and [to] retain its status in an expanded form in any unified action which may be undertaken."[17]

In addition to the desire of the ANA to retain its identity, the issue of nonnurse participation was a major obstacle to the consolidation efforts. The plan for one organization proposed by Rich included full membership privileges for nonnurses, and this would have made it impossible for the new organization to be a member of the International Council of Nurses.

To remedy this problem, the ANA suggested the establishment of one nursing organization that would limit the participation of nonnurses, nursing service agencies, and schools of nursing to advisory forums. "ANA's recommendation was not acceptable to the representatives of the other five nursing organizations who argued that such a proposal would hinder the execution of vital nursing-related activities requiring full participation of nonnurse groups."[6] The consolidation effort was not a complete failure, however, as it was successful in combining the six nationally based nursing organizations into three: the NLN, the ANA, and the AAIN.

An attempt at coordinating the endeavors of the ANA and the new NLN was made for the purpose of identifying appropriate domains for the two organizations.

According to Chairman Pearl McIver, the joint coordinating committee attempted to assign "those functions which should be the sole responsibility of the members of a profession" to the American Nurses' Association and "those functions which the members of any profession should share with the consumers of their product and allied professional workers" to the National League for Nursing.[6]

The territorial boundaries were defined by assigning practice and professional employment issues to the ANA, and nursing service and educational matters to the NLN. As pointed out earlier, the division between practice issues and educational issues is nebulous and to an extent artificial. The many areas of overlap fostered competition and rivalry in the years that followed.

For example, the ANA has periodically sought to expand its organizational boundaries by co-opting tasks previously performed by the NLN. The most recent example of this behavior is the ANA credentialing study. The study was conducted in response to a resolution passed by the 1974 House of Delegates that called for the ANA "to move with all deliberate speed to establish a system of accreditation of basic, graduate, and continuing education programs in nursing."[6]

This action was, not surprisingly, perceived by the NLN as a blatant and offensive invasion of its organizational domain. The NLN was invited to cosponsor the study. But this invitation by the ANA was primarily designed to offer the NLN the opportunity to share the financial burden of funding the study rather than to actively participate in it, as the actual study was to be contracted out to an independent research group.

RECENT PROLIFERATION OF SPECIALTY ORGANIZATIONS

During the first half of this century, medicine and nursing relied on general practitioners. In 1934 only 15% of physicians were specialists. By 1960 the trend toward specialization was well established, with 63% of physicians limiting the scope of their practice.[8]

This shift toward specialization occurred in nursing as well, but precise statistics on the volume of specialty nurses are not available. The most dramatic evidence reflecting the trend toward specialization in nursing is the establishment of numerous organizations with a particular clinical focus.

Starting in the 1960s, many specialty nursing organizations have been created to address dozens of emerging specialties. The current roster of national specialty nursing organizations follows.

- Alpha Tau Delta National Fraternity for Professional Nurses
- American Academy of Ambulatory Nursing Administration
- American Academy of Nurse Practitioners
- American Academy of Nursing
- American Assembly for Men in Nursing
- American Association of Colleges of Nursing
- American Association of Critical Care Nurses
- American Association of Neuroscience Nurses
- American Association of Nurse Anesthetists
- American Association of Nurse Attorneys
- American Association of Occupational Health Nurses, Inc.
- American Association of Spinal Cord Injury Nurses
- American Cancer Society
- American College of Nurse-Midwives
- American Heart Association
- American Holistic Nurses' Association
- American Hospital Association
- American Nephrology Nurses' Association

- American Nurses' Foundation
- American Organization of Nurse Executives
- American Psychiatric Nurses' Association
- American Radiological Nurses' Association
- American Society of Ophthalmic Registered Nurses, Inc.
- American Society of Plastic & Reconstructive Surgical Nurses, Inc.
- American Society of Post Anesthesia Nurses
- American Thoracic Society, Section on Nursing
- American Urological Association Allied, Inc.
- Association for the Care of Children's Health
- Association of Nurses Endorsing Transplantation
- Association of Operating Room Nurses
- Association of Pediatric Oncology Nurses
- Association for Practitioners in Infection Control
- Association of Rehabilitation Nurses
- Cassandra: Radical Feminist Nurses Network
- Commission on Graduates of Foreign Nursing Schools
- Dermatology Nurses' Association
- Drug and Alcohol Nursing Association, Inc.
- Emergency Nurses' Association
- Federation for Accessible Nursing Education and Licensure
- Frontier Nursing Service
- Hospice Link
- International Association for Enterostomal Therapy, Inc.
- Intravenous Nurses' Society, Inc.
- Lesbian and Gay Nurses' Alliance
- National Alliance of Nurse Practitioners
- National Association for Health Care Recruitment
- National Association of Hispanic Nurses
- National Association of Neonatal Nurses
- National Association of Orthopaedic Nurses, Inc.
- National Association of Pediatric Nurse Associates and Practitioners
- National Association for Practical Nurse Education and Service
- National Association of Physician Nurses
- National Association of School Nurses, Inc.
- National Black Nurses' Association, Inc.
- National Center for Nursing Ethics
- National Council of State Boards of Nursing, Inc.
- National Federation for Specialty Nursing Organizations
- National Flight Nurses' Association
- National League for Nursing
- National Organization of World War Nurses
- National Nurses' Society on Addictions
- National Student Nurses' Association
- North American Nursing Diagnosis Association
- Nurses Against Misrepresentation
- Nurses' Alliance for the Prevention of Nuclear War

- Nurses' Association of the American College of Obstetricians and Gynecologists
- Nurses' Christian Fellowship
- Nurse Consultants Association, Inc.
- Nurses' Educational Funds, Inc.
- Nurses' Environmental Health Watch
- Nurses' House, Inc.
- Nurses' in Transition
- Nurses' Organization of the Veterans' Administration
- Oncology Nursing Society
- Public Health Nursing/American Public Health Association
- Retired Army Nurse Corps Association
- Sigma Theta Tau International
- Society for Nursing History
- Society of Otorhinolaryngology and Head/Neck Nurses
- Society for Peripheral Vascular Nursing
- Society for Retired Air Force Nurses
- Transcultural Nursing Society
- Visiting Nurse Associations of America

This roster does not include all organizational entities that address specialty practice issues. For example, the following subdivisions within the ANA are devoted to specific domains in nursing.

- Cabinet on Nursing Practice
- Cabinet on Economic and General Welfare
- Cabinet on Human Rights
- Cabinet on Nursing Education
- Cabinet on Nursing Research
- Cabinet on Nursing Services

Although the ANA's Cabinet on Nursing Practice has been active, the organization has clearly devoted most of its energies toward the following two objectives, which transcend the boundaries of clinical specialization:

1. Increasing the minimum education of new professional nurses to the baccalaureate level (commonly referred to as the entry-into-practice issue)
2. Increasing wages and promoting better working conditions for nurses (the union activity known as the economic and general walfare program)

Both these major objectives undertaken by the ANA have resulted in predictable internal conflict and membership losses in the 1960s and 1970s. However, things now seem to be stabilizing. No longer does the mere mention of a baccalaureate education requirement cause heated debate. Most nurses agree that this level of education is both necessary and inevitable for the future of nursing. A similar realization has occurred relative to the ANA's union activities. Although some nurses still view collective bargaining as a vaguely unprofessional and unsavory affair, most readily acknowledge the financial gains that have accrued as a result.

While the ANA was occupied with the universal issues of education and compensation, numerous organizations were created to address clinical issues in the growing number of nursing specialities. In the early 1970s, the rapid proliferation of independent specialty organizations led to the suggestion that they band together to address common issues. Donna Zschoche, executive director of the American Association of Critical Care Nurses, called for a meeting of the first National Nurses' Congress, which later came to be known as the National Federation of Specialty Organizations and ANA.[22]

NATIONAL FEDERATION OF SPECIALTY NURSING ORGANIZATIONS

In 1973 the Federation of Specialty Nursing Organizations was formed. The designation of *specialty nursing organization* refers to a "national organization of which the majority of the voting members are RNs governed by an elected body with by-laws defining its purpose and function for improvement of health care, and a body of knowledge and skill in a defined area of clinical practice."[13] Shortly after its inception, the meetings of this group came to be officially known as the Federation of Nursing Specialty Organizations *and ANA*. The purpose of meeting was "not to take action or make decisions binding on the member organizations, but to discuss matters of common interest and concern."[12]

The fedreation began as and remains a loose affiliation of organizations with divergent interests. It has no formal structure, bylaws, headquarters, staff, or officers. Within the political lexicon, this federation would more accurately be described as a confederation or coalition. This lack of structure precipitated an offer from outside the nursing profession. In 1975 the former staff of the National Commission for the Study of Nursing and Nursing Education made an offer to the federation. The impetus for the offer can be traced to recommendation number 17 in the Commission's 1970 report[11] entitled *An Abstract for Action:*

The national nursing organizations (should) press forward in their current study of functions, structures, methods or respresentation, and interrelationships in order to determine: (a) Areas of overlap or duplication that could be eliminated; (b) Areas of need that are currently unmet, and (c) Areas or functions that could be transferred from one organization to another in the light of changing systems and practice.

The offer extended to the federation by the commission staff consisted of a proposal to

establish an ad hoc committee on planning, purposes, and structure for the organization along with funding from an outside agency interested in the further professionalization of nursing. To the surprise of the grantor, the proposal was rejected on the basis that this, somehow, might lead to a superorganization of nursing that would be more powerful than any of the participating groups including the American Nurses' Association.[10]

Although the federation had rejected an offer of outside assistance that would have expedited the process of collaboration and planning, in 1977 a survey of member organizations revealed only modest progress had been made toward the goal of cooperative activity. Lysaught[10] summarizes their responses:

All felt that the current level of organization was essentially preliminary to more definitive progress on mutual goals. Six organizations felt that the group had already made significant strides toward presenting an effective voice of nursing on issues, whereas nine organizations felt that this had not yet been accomplished.

In the longitudinal 10-year follow-up on the recommendations of the National Commission for the Study of Nursing and Nursing Education, Lysaught[10] reveals in the monograph's title a sense of frustration over the continuing need for unity of action in nursing: *Action in Affirmation: Toward an Unambiguous Profession of Nursing.*

In 1983, after 10 years of meetings, the group, which had by then changed its name to the National Federation of Specialty Nursing Organizations (NFSNO), convened an educational workshop to consider long-range plans and possible incorporation (i.e., a legal action that would require the development of bylaws, structure, and goals). In an address of Margretta Styles,[19] the workshop participants were reminded that they were faced with four alternatives:

1. The Federation could propose to broadly organize all of nursing so loosely and without direction that unity would not likely be achieved.

2. The Federation could propose to broadly organize all nursing to provide unity, leadership, and direction; and therefore promote a competitive stance toward ANA.
3. The Federation could propose to focus specifically upon specialty practice issues and strive toward collaboration with ANA.
4. The Federation could delay action on long-range planning and continue with its current informal structure.

The NFSNO selected the fourth alternative. This delay allowed the NFSNO to consider using the ANA's new Nursing Organization Liaison Forum. The forum was created as part of a major internal restructuring approved at the 1982 ANA convention. The first meeting of the ANA's Nursing Organization Liaison Forum (NOLF) took place in December 1983.[14]

The NFSNO and the NOLF held parallel meetings for the next five years, each seeking to represent specialty interests within nursing. In January 1988 the NFSNO finally made the decision to incorporate, although it has not decided in which state this shall be done. Incorporation may provide the mechanisms needed for this group to take actions and thereby refute the criticism that it is an unneeded powerless conglomerate. This negative image was presented in a 1986 editoral,[15] which began by saying:

It is time for the NFSNO to disband—gracefully. . . . the Federation resembles a ladies' bridge club. All the members play the same game but oppose each other once in awhile, each member takes a turn hosting the party and providing refreshments, and lots of information is exchanged. At the end of the game, plans are made to meet again.

In the meantime, the NOLF continues to meet and function in an advisory role to the ANA's Board of Directors. The NOLF concerns itself with national issues that affect most nurses, such as legislative action, liability insurance, and recruitment into the profession. In contrast, the NFSNO is seen as focusing more on specialty practice issues. However, it seems obvious to even the most casual observer that continuing both the NOLF and the NFSNO is redundant and divisive.

The challenge of achieving collaborative action with such a vast diversity among nursing organizations is great. The difference in size alone presents major obstacles. The ANA has 189,000 members through 53 state and regional associations. The NFSNO has 28 affiliating organizations ranging dramatically in size. There are 59,000 members in the American Association of Critical Care Nurses; 43,000 members in the Association of Operating Room Nurses; many specialty nursing organizations have only a few thousand members; and some have only a few hundred members. One of the smallest affiliating groups is the Nurse Consultants' Association, with 150 members. The combined membership of the NFSNO is about the same size as the ANA membership.[14]

INTERORGANIZATIONAL BEHAVIOR

It may be helpful at this point to examine the behavior of organizations from a theoretical perspective. Interorganizational behavior can be viewed as either *competitive* or *cooperative*. Competition implies that a sense of rivalry exists and that the weaker of the two may be eliminated. The three subtypes of cooperative behavior are bargaining, co-optation, and coalition. Bargaining refers to the negotiation of an agreement through the use of an exchange process. Co-optation is a method of absorbing some elements of one organization into another. And coalition refers to the temporary or partial alliance of two organizations for the purpose of achieving a common goal. To this spectrum of organizational behavior described by Thompson and McEwen,[20] I would like to add consolidation, which is the permanent and complete combination of two organizations, effectively blurring the singular identity previously held by each.

Nursing organizations have much in common and much to gain from consolidation. But there exists a high degree of hostility and distrust that must first be overcome.

Once conflict and hostility exist, we tend to develop supporting stereotypes that maintain the conflict. Thus each side exaggerates the differences that exist—and once the perception is established, only small actual differences are necessary to maintain the stereotype. This is facilitated by a decrease in intergroup communication that accompanies conflict. If forced to interact, each side listens only to its own representatives. Indeed, in the absence of any shared goals, communication tends to reinforce stereotypes, and relations to deteriorate further.

Nursing organizations must continue their dialogue. Members of each should be encouraged to join the other organization, and common goals should be identified. Forming a coalition on important issues facing nursing could be the antecedent to a successful consolidation of organizations.

OBSTACLES TO CONSOLIDATION

There are, of course, areas of disagreement among nursing organizations, and these will continue to be obstacles to consolidation unless each side is willing to compromise. With thoughtful discussions and rational exchanges, an agreement could be reached that would allow organizations to unite for the benefit of all nurses and health care consumers.

A number of issues will require debate, discussion, and, ultimately, compromise before a consolidation can succeed. Some of these issues are the composition of membership, dues structure, union function, educational requirements for practice, and accreditation of educational programs.

Membership

The problem of who should be included among the membership remains. The ANA currently comprises only registered nurses (RNs). NLN members include lay and agency representatives in addition to licensed vocational nurses (LVNs) and registered nurses. Specialty organizations may include RNs, LVNs, and other categories of health care workers. A consolidated organization would best be served by a membership that included all nurses: RNs and LVNs. Nonnurses could participate through advisory councils without full membership privileges. This type of action, the ANA giving up its RN-only stance and the NLN and other organizations relinquishing full membership for nonnurses, is a good example of how compromise might be achieved through the appropriate use of an exchange mechanism. Each participant in a compromise must be willing to give up something to ultimately gain through cooperative action.

Dues structure and union function

The ANA dues structure is relatively elevated and acts to limit membership. Many nurses argue that the tangible benefits derived from ANA membership are too few and, by contrast, the NLN and specialty organization dues appear quite reasonable.

In a consolidation, the memberships of all involved organizations (approximately 180,000 from the ANA and an equal number of nurses from other organiza-

tions) would combine to form a powerful unified body representing nursing. A new dues structure would have to be designed for the new organization and it should be low enough to attract, rather than repel, new members. One method of restructuring dues to achieve this goal is to separate the economic and general welfare program (the union function of the ANA) from the other parts of the new organization and allow members to join the union component of the organization separately. In this way, dues could be reasonably priced and affordable to all nurses. Using this type of fee-for-service dues structure would relieve the nurse who is not working in a contract situation from the responsibility of financially supporting the Economic and General Welfare (E&GW) program, while those who enjoy the benefits of working under a contract would be responsible for paying the costs of negotiation and maintenance of their contracts.

Unionization is still a controversial issue in nursing. Using the fee-for-service mechanism described, the new consolidated organization could meet the needs of nurses who favor, as well as those who oppose, union activities in nursing. Nonnursing unions have repeatedly targeted nurses as a potential source of workers to bolster their declining memberships and if nurses fail to defeat these recruitment attempts by nonnurse unions, nursing will be further weakened and fragmented.

Education and practice

The ANA has long advocated that nursing education take place within institutions of higher learning. This position validates associate degree and baccalaureate education for nursing, but it implicitly calls for the phasing out of non-degree-granting programs (vocational and diploma). The NLN, however, continues to support four educational methods of entering nursing: vocational, diploma, associate degree, and baccalaureate.

In this college-oriented society, it is unjustifiable to continue to prepare nurses outside institutions of higher learning. Not only is it unfair to the nursing student to be denied a degree after years of study, but it is also unfair to the health care consumer to be subject to a system of training that fosters nurse loyalty to an employing institution rather than professional accountability to patients.

The consolidation of the ANA and the NLN would require concessions on the part of the NLN. Undoubtedly, it would be required to abandon support of non-degree-granting nursing programs, but in return its accreditation functions could be preserved in the new organization.

The artificial hiatus between hospital-based acute care and community-based continuing care could be bridged by a merger of the ANA and the NLN. Historically, the ANA has usually represented the interests of nurses involved in acute care, whereas the joining of the NLNE with the National Organization for Public Health Nursing in 1952 incorporated the community nursing focus into the NLN.

With the rapidly escalating costs of acute health care and the increasing attention to prevention, the time is right for nursing to intervene by closing the gap between hospital and community-based care. A consolidation of the ANA and the NLN would bring together nursing leaders from hospital-based and community based nursing services so that more effective nursing care could be provided in a variety of settings.

If nursing organizations fail to unite, it is quite possible for the "conflict to continue indefinitely with neither side able to gain the advantage, to the extent that both sides contribute to the ultimate loss of whatever values each was seeking to uphold."[9] It is for this reason, the potential loss of all that is important to both organizations, that nursing organizations must consolidate.

THE NEED FOR UNITY

Throughout its history, nursing has been represented by small, impotent groups primarily concerned with their own self-interest and self-preservation. Rather than worrying about individual organizational survival, nurses should concern themselves with their collective survival. Continued fragmentation will leave nursing vulnerable to the "circling opportunists . . . who do not recognize the nature of the nursing process . . . and seek to control it."[5]

The conflicts and misunderstandings among nursing organizations have periodically exacerbated into open competition that has had a destructive effect on the profession as a whole. It is time that the organizations join together to work cooperatively. Nursing must put aside its relatively petty "internal struggles [that] have sapped its strength and energy" and defend itself against the "medical profession, health departments, education departments, [and] hospital associ-

ations" and labor unions that "relentlessly pursue their strategy to divide and conquer nursing."[16]

"In the 1890s, it was called esprit de corps; in the 1940s, a united front; in the 1960s, a spirit of oneness; and in the 1970s, collaborative action"[6], and in the 1980s perhaps we shall call it unity, and finally succeed in achieving it through consolidation of the major groups in nursing—the ANA and the NFSNO. Nearly a century ago Edith Draper succinctly stated the prerequisite to our success: "To advance we must unite."[6]

REFERENCES

1. AJN's 1988 directory of nursing organizations, Am J Nurs 88:555, 1988.
2. Ashley J: Hospitals, paternalism and the role of the nurse, New York, 1976, Teachers' College Press.
3. Dolan J: Nursing in society: a historical perspective, Philadelphia, 1978, WB Saunders Co.
4. Densford K: Proceedings of the special sessions of the Advisory Council (1947-1948) and the House of Delegates (1947) of the American Nurses' Association, New York, 1948, ANA.
5. Driscoll V: Beware the circling opportunists, Journal of the New York State Nurses' Association 4:5, 1973.
6. Flanagan L: One strong voice: the story of the American Nurses' Association, Kansas City, Mo, 1976, ANA.
7. Hampton D, Sumner C, and Webber R: Organizational behavior and the practice of management, Glenview, Ill, 1973, Scott, Foresman & Co.
8. Kalisch PA and Kalisch BJ: The advance of American nursing, Boston, 1979, Little, Brown & Co., Inc.
9. Klein D: Some notes on the dynamics of resistance to change: the defender role. In Bennis WB and others, editors: The planning of change, ed 3, New York, 1976, Holt, Rinehart & Winston.
10. Lysaught J: A longitudinal follow-up on the recommendations of the National Commission for the Study of Nursing and Nursing Education. In Action in affirmation: toward an unambiguous profession of nursing, 1981, New York: McGraw-Hill.
11. Lysaught J: National Commission for the Study of Nursing and Nursing Education. In An abstract for action, New York: 1970, McGraw-Hill.
12. Nursing Federation compares notes on certification and continuing education policies and procedures, Am J Nurs 74:416, 1974.
13. Nursing organizations adopt group name, Am J Nurs 73:1306, 1973.
14. McCarty P: Federation for specialty groups studies incorporation proposal, American Nurse 15:3, Sept 1983.
15. Palmer PN: The nursing profession does not need two federations, AORN Journal 43:784, 1986.
16. Powell DJ: Nursing and politics: the struggles outside nursing's body politic, Nurs Forum 15:342, 1976.
17. Proceedings of the special sessions of the Advisory Council (1947-1948) and the House of Delegates (1947) of the American Nurses' Association, New York, 1948, ANA.
18. Rich R: Report on the structure of organized nursing. In Pro-

ceedings of the Thirty-fifth Biennial Convention of the American Nurses' Association, Vol I, House of delegates, New York, 1946, ANA.

19. Styles M: The anatomy of a profession. Paper presented at the Long-range planning committee workshop on future directions for the National Federation of Specialty Nursing Organizations, June 24, 1983, Pittsburgh, PA.

20. Thompson JD and McEwen WJ: Organizational goals and environment, American Sociological Review 23:23, 1958.

21. Two new nursing organizations join nursing federation, Am J Nurs 74:416, 1974.

22. Zschoche D: Letter calling for a national nurses' congress, Heart and Lung 1:589, 1972.

CHAPTER 67

Viewpoints

Has the front-line nurse been abandoned?

HANS O. MAUKSCH

This chapter could have been written from a number of perspectives. After having listened to the despair and rage as well as the dreams and commitment of hundreds of nurses,[3,7] I chose to focus on the nurse's perception of abandonment. What people feel and experience and how they structure their own reality is more significant in influencing their behavior than are external data. Even if rigorously validated, such data may not be meaningful to the population whose experiences they are supposed to reflect. Yet this chapter is not merely a summary of views and expressions but rather an effort to examine the nurse's perceived world as a system governed by a logical, albeit subjective, thought system.

Even the title of this chapter tries to do justice to the legitimate yet apparently conflicting perspectives of subjective and objective truths. Whether the researcher determines that the front-line nurse has been abandoned is less significant than the effort to understand and to respond to the conditions that might explain in what way these nurses feel abandoned. If nurses, collectively and individually, feel this abandonment as a reality, then one must conclude that they have been abandoned, notwithstanding possibly contrary findings produced by collected data. To examine the conditions that are peculiar to the nurse as an employee of hospitals and similar institutions requires an approach in which the observer takes on the perspective of the grass-roots nurse and accepts the relevance of those factors that the nurse claims are meaningful, even though others, such as administrators and researchers, might not give them the same weight.

The aim of this chapter is to synthesize the views of the practicing nurse while screening the nurse's voice through the spectroscope of institutional and professional conditions. We shall start with the implications of corporate employment by contrasting it with the conditions that would prevail for someone who functions as a fully accountable individual practitioner. The nurse in private practice (I prefer not to use the term *private duty*) enjoys more personal recognition, visibility, and individuality than the nurse who functions as a member of the staff of an institutional system or department that is collectively responsible for the rendering of nursing care. Although several dimensions of the abandonment problem will be examined in the following pages, a fundamental and causally significant factor has to be the difference between the attention paid to individually functioning and individually accountable practitioners and the quasi-anonymity of those professionals who are part of organizational systems with collective accountability—a staffing pattern based on assumed substitutability of front-line practitioners.

The difference between the implications of individual and institutional functioning can be observed in other settings. One of the sources of the aura and power of physicians emanates from the deliberate efforts to present the physician as an individually autonomous practitioner rather than to acknowledge the M.D. as part of an institutional system.[8] Some medical departments nevertheless function as bureaucracies. Some of the consequences of institutionalized bureaucratization can be seen in organizations like the public health service or U.S. armed forces, in which one can observe the reduction of the physician's individuality and in which replacement, substitution, and transfers are the norm, with the concomitant reduced consideration of individual capabilities and preferences.

Having made the basic point that feelings of anonymity and powerlessness are associated with being the occupant of a bureaucratically structured position, turn now to the specific case of nursing and to the nurse's preparation before joining the grass-roots level of practice. Unlike the novice in the armed forces and unlike the worker in an industrial bureaucracy, the novice in nursing does not receive an orientation to substitutability, minimal power, and anonymity. On the contrary, most of the educational environment of the nursing student emphasizes professional status, individual responsibility, and the symbolic importance of becoming a nurse. For the sake of nurses' mental health, it would be better to emphasize the reality of the nurse's position, even though the current reality needs to be changed.[10] Notwithstanding the nurse's capability, knowledge, and readiness, the image that seems to describe the real institutional environment within which the nurse functions is that of the industrial worker whose accountability is limited, who can be moved and replaced, and whose expertise is perceived to be the result of situational training rather than of knowledge and inquiry.

The nurse feels betrayed and unappreciated when confronting the reality of the work environment, and several developments during the last few years have actually intensified this sense of abandonment and frustration and have substantiated the grass-roots nurse's belief that "nobody really understands what I am doing." One of these confounding factors is linked to the needs of the patient and the rapidly growing complexity of patient care.[5] As more and more detailed knowledge has been identified, a growing number of specialists have fleeting contacts with the patient. The patient, who may be overwhelmed by so many different people and so much new information, increasingly looks to the nurse as the source of information, reassurance, and as the integrator of diverse and confusing stimuli. To serve as the interpretor of complex events requires, minimally, a sense of security and a sense of being supported. The employment conditions described above are not conducive to providing a feeling of being trusted and being respected. Under these adverse conditions, trying to meet the needs of the patient for knowledge and understanding becomes a fairly risky and stressful activity for the nurse rather than serving as a morale-enhancing reaffirmation of the nurse's worth.

The second, more complex and divisive source of a feeling of abandonment is an unintended result of some of the most desirable historical trends in the development in nursing. The transfer of the major site for nursing education from the hospital to the college campus and the emergence of increasing numbers of nurses with advanced degrees represent changes that the profession appropriately endorses and welcomes. Yet every gain exacts a price. The intelligentsia of the profession, an important and influential group in the 1980s, is characterized by different roots, different concerns, and by a different language than the grass-roots level nurse. This applies even to many staff nurses who have earned the baccalaureate. In the 1930s and 1940s the leaders and administrative chiefs in nursing had social and cultural origins that were similar to those of the front-line nurse. Presumably there was a sense of collective belonging, and the typical leader in nursing was someone with whom the staff nurse could identify.

The differences between the front-line nurse and the academically advanced nursing intelligentsia must be ascribed to attitudes and behaviors on both sides. It may be controversial to assert that among nurses with advanced academic degrees there is little sense of identification with the grass-roots nurse and that even highly motivated programs of research and action appear as if they were done "for them" rather than done "for us." Similarly, grass-roots nurses look with some suspicion at the fancy language, and the emphasis on research and abstraction that leaves them wondering whether they have allies and colleagues in academe or whether they serve primarily as objects of study or, worse yet, sympathy.

As the differentiation between the practicing nurse and the nursing intelligentsia has progressed, we can apply the notion of abandonment even more appropriately. It has been shown that the front-line nurse would like the nurse with advanced academic preparation to show more concern about the contributions of research to daily practice and to demonstrate that all this knowledge can be applied to a unified pattern of action. The word *sympathy* was emphasized above because it points to a pervasive and very significant experiential deficit identified by many grass-roots nurses. A recognition of real worth cannot occur without an acknowledgment of equality. Charity, no matter how well intended and how much motivated by sympathy and caring, implies a difference in social status. Indeed, an act of charity can create inequality, whereas participatory support does not. It does not matter whether such inequality was intended by those who wield the symbolic or structural power. Deprivation gives rise to additional perception of deprivation. Those who have relationships with nurses in front-line roles have to be sensitive to the risk of triggering a perception of inequality regardless of intent.

Another similar yet also profoundly different source of feeling abandoned and frustrated has to be associated with changes in the organizational structure of the hospital.[5] Fifty years ago, nurses working directly with patients became part of a nursing service department headed by a director of nursing. This organizational pattern and its label conveys a message of inequality and of subservience to a departmental authority structure, to management, to the physician, and, above all, to the administrator of nursing. This subservience was intensified because people in deprived situations have greater need for identifiable leadership and of nurturing support symbolisms.[1] The director of nursing was that role model, a visible leader, and someone who spoke for nursing, although there may have been major differences between what was said and what was done. These images of the director of nursing have changed, although nurses' needs remain. In recent years the chief of nursing has become increasingly involved in the complexity of hospital management and issues of organizational efficiency. The director of nursing became redefined as a vice-president within the hospital management structure. Now instead of being the director *of* nursing, the new title was vice-president *for* nursing, if even that specific. It appeared superficially that the status of nursing was elevated by being included in top-level institutional management, but the emotional and role needs of the staff nurse paid a heavy price. The nursing executive became much less visible and, regardless of real intent, appeared to the staff nurse to have abandoned nursing by joining the administrative elite.

That these changes were defined as abandonment has been shown in several studies of nursing morale and of recruitment and turnover.[9,10] The very functions of nursing seem to require more support and recognition for their performance than some tasks in other professions.[4] The reality of a diminished social affirmation of importance has accentuated nurses' needs for support and leadership. This phenomenon is intensified by another historical event that, paradoxically, constitutes a highly desirable development yet exacts a high price from the front-line nurse.

The deference that characterized the behavior of nurses vis-à-vis physicians and that females generally displayed to males was expected and accepted forty years ago. In those days the staff nurse gained satisfaction and symbolic rewards from approval and appreciation given to her by a physician. She thought that her proximity to the physician gave her an advantage over nursing administrators and nursing educators. They had little access to the pat on the head that is the physician's patriarchal gesture of approval. There was a delicate balance between the gratification gained from physician recognition and the benefits derived from the structure of nursing leadership. The slowly spreading acceptance of feminism and of sensitivity to issues of equality has made the physician's traditional form of approval less rewarding and less acceptable and has subtly diminished the physician's tendency to express appreciation in the traditional patronizing way. The rays of sunbeams emanating from the physician's aura may have lost much of their luster, but the parallel warmth derived from the director of nursing also escaped behind the clouds of the management system. The grass-roots-level nurse thus experiences several layers of abandonment. Not only the secondary sources of reward and recognition have been severely diminished, but the very processes that everyone else sees as progress (i.e., modern technology and feminist consciousness) have exacted a heavy price from the staff nurse.[6] No wonder nurses say, "No one understands my situation." Indeed, these powerful subtleties are really not understood by many.

How occupants of social roles and institutional positions are treated by others and how closely they are perceived to be "center stage" depend very much on the perspective and interests of other actors. This is particularly true if these others wield a certain amount of power, and it is even more true if the institution is a composite of widely differing vantage points, interests, and cultures. These conditions prevail in the typical U.S. hospital and have a specifically complicating consequence for nurses. Nursing happens to be placed where the processes of medicine, management, nursing, and patient desires converge. Each of the major participants in the processes of institutional functioning and patient care provision sees the nurse differently in worth, as well as in scope of function. Nursing is caught in a competitive struggle for domain and for control over its own activities. That the perspective of others does not coincide with those of the nurse at the front lines of care should not be surprising. It is better to acknowledge divergent priorities rather than to use patronizing benevolence as a substitute for real understanding.

It is not surprising that physicians prefer to work with nurses who follow orders without questioning them and who acknowledge the physician's power and prerogatives as evidence of wisdom and the natural order.[8] It is equally understandable that the hospital management team finds it advantageous to see the nurse as a substitutable occupant of personnel slots who can be moved according to staffing needs and reassigned without considering specialization, team effectiveness, or the prerequisites of professional control over one's own practice. At the same time the nurse is frequently placed in the position of confidant for the patient, as interpreter, and as advocate in negotiating with those people who come and go hurriedly and leave their decisions on charts and policies. The result of such inconsistency in role expectations cannot but produce stress and disillusionment. This has been particularly true in recent years when the one source of symbolic and real support—the director of nursing—has become more remote and has become suspect of having divided loyalties.

Additional impetus for feeling that one has landed on a blind and forgotten spur away from the main line arises from the images, reputations, and prestige distribution that is conveyed by word of mouth, professional publications, and the media. The researcher, the teacher, and, generally, the academically oriented nurse appear in the limelight. The grass-roots nurse would not mind such attention if it did not occur at the expense of diminishing recognition of direct nursing care and if the direct care nurse could enjoy recognizable benefits derived from the accumulation of impressive knowledge and the delivery of sophisticated practice.

The paradox that seems to exact from the grass-roots nurse the by-products and indirect costs of apparent progress intensifies if one examines the glorified advances in the technology of patient care and what it means for nursing. The record is mixed. Although the technology of the intensive-care nurse has added tactical strength to the nursing side of the nurse/physician interaction, most of the technology of primary patient care has placed limits on nursing judgments and has made the health care practitioner a functionary whose work is controlled by the dictum of technological apparatus. One should not forget that the growth of technology was not accompanied by a reassessment of the labor force and that the management and monitoring of instruments competes powerfully with those activities that are generally seen as the core of direct patient-oriented nursing.

Many nurses feel that notwithstanding changing technology in patient care and resulting changes in the demand on nursing time, nursing skills, and nursing knowledge, the plans for the deployment of nurses essentially have not changed. A comparison of charts of patients with similar diseases in 1945 and in 1985 would show that the number of medical orders and procedures and the complexity of intervention have risen dramatically. Time of hospitalizaton has been reduced dramatically, so the periods of heavy demand on nursing effort occur much more continuously and intensively. There is less per-patient nursing time available, notwithstanding the increased needs of the patient and the range of intervention indicated. Almost always the medical orders, as shown on the chart, will be carried out before those activities that are the most challenging and most central to modern concepts in nursing. The nurse in the 1980s increasingly feels frustrated by being forced to execute tasks initiated by others at the expense of those activities that are properly and exclusively nursing.

It is not surprising that the grass-roots-level nurse concludes that "real" nursing has been abandoned, at least its ability to implement the core of what is unique to nursing. It is not surprising that many nurses rank their identity as conveyors of nursing functions as being less worthy, less significant, and less consequential than their role as agents for medical or management directives. Their daily reality emphasizes the subordinate and the technical dimensions of the nurse's functions, thus conflicting painfully with the lessons learned in the school of nursing. Unfulfilled expectations are much more frustrating and destructive than experiences anticipated without the distortions of rose-colored glasses.

Being forced to accomplish delegated tasks that typically must be recorded and not being able to provide nursing functions per se account for much of the feeling across the country that nurses are understaffed. The objective observer has to concur with the reality of inadequate staffing in most institutions. Furthermore, the observer cannot help but wonder whether one reason for feeling so keenly about inadequate staffing derives from the obstacles to rescuing the actual nursing components from the mix of each day's pressures. Increased staffing may indeed provide some opportunities for doing more and for doing it better. Yet the question remains whether the current structure and organization will ever affirm the importance of the functions that are unique to nursing and also the importance of the nurse's membership in the health care team.

It may be difficult for administrators to appreciate fully the intensity and the focus of the frustration and the sense of undue burdens that characterize the feelings of nurses. On the whole this is not a reaction to "working too hard." The two themes that must be heard clearly and must be distinguished from the mere notion of overwork are: "I can't provide all the care the patient is entitled to," and —even more pervasively— "Everything I have to do as an adjunct to the physician and to others prevents me from really providing nursing as it should be."

If this explanation is understood, it will not be a surprise that the use of the so-called contract nurse is felt to be demeaning and destructive rather than a welcome help, as many administrators believe it should be interpreted. For most front-line nurses, knowledge about the patient and commitment to the patient's nursing needs supersede concern with work per se. The contract nurse shares neither familiarity with nor commitment to the patient of regular staff nurses. Most nurses feel that the contract nurse creates additional work and additional stress; they need interpretation, assistance, and a tolerant link, which is normally what strangers require to function in a new environment.

Earlier the conflict between two models of the nursing presence was mentioned. One, emanating from educational socialization, stresses the "professional" client-oriented perception of the nurse as an autonomous, fully accountable, decision-making functionary. The other pattern, a by-product of actual employment, presents the quasi-industrial model of a labor force with personnel slots to be filled and with the occupants of these positions being replaceable and movable. Many morale and performance problems derive from this dualism. Worse yet, neither model seems to satisfy the nurse's experience and the grass-roots-level nurse's felt needs for satisfying and secure working conditions. Interpreting comments, reactions, and themes of interviews leads one to conclude that the actual experience of the grass-roots-level nurse resembles neither model but, rather, approximates an organizational reality resembling the social structure of a symphony orchestra or a football team. These social models combine a group of individually skilled and specialized performers who demonstrate a deliberate interdependence. The orchestra and the football team alike do not succeed solely because of the individual artistry of team members but because of the cooperation characterized by mutual respect and skilled anticipation of collectively supported behaviors.

The application of this model to nursing becomes more persuasive after examining other approaches. Neither the authoritarian, bureaucratic system nor unbridled individualism satisfied the sophisticated understanding of most bedside nurses. Structural changes are desperately needed that combine more effective individual involvement by nurses with a system of collective, group-based accountability.

Exemplifying the general thrust of this need are the pervasive comments about head nurses.[2] In group interviews, professional nurses as much as nurses' aides voiced their concern about needed support for the head nurse. They ranked the strengthening of the head nurse position and the concomitant need for the head nurse to be educated and supported as the single most important area of change. The support and the recognition accorded to the head nurse appear to be viewed as an indicator of the value and dignity given to the work of the grass-roots-level nurse.

Among the most pervasive indicators of respect involve acknowledgment of the head nurse's position as one that requires effort, time, and concern. In institutions in which the head nurse is expected to carry a full patient load and squeeze her managing responsibilities into the remaining time or into off-duty hours, the staff nurses and the nursing assistants uniformly conclude that nursing is not competetive in the hierarchy of respected jobs. Sensitivity to the symbols of recognition is intensified by some of the characteristics of the occupants of nursing positions and by their organizational positioning. A study by Mauksch[4] revealed a high level of the need for succorance combined with an even more pronounced need to avoid blame-producing situations. Recognizing that the need to receive nurturing support is among the most important for nurses, one can easily see that organizational practices that feature rewards, recognition, and active support are directly related to the nurturant and caring themes characteristic of nursing functions.

This constellation of needs makes the current institutional placement of the front-line nurse a dramatic paradox. Any effort to deliberately minimize a supportive structure could not do better than to place the nurse at the interface of medical authority, administrative authority, nursing authority, and patient demands. Nurses feel that they are exposed to the risk of being blamed and held responsible without having the institutional authority or support to back them up. Being exposed also gives rise to the phenomenon called "dumping," which is usually associated with the expectation that some functionaries, because of their image of commitment, will be willing to absorb extraneous tasks that have been neglected by others.[2]

The perception that "nobody understands" easily changes during low morale–high stress situations from "nobody cares" to "nobody thinks it is worthwhile to understand." Almost all of the researchers who have tried to elicit the worldview of the grass-roots-level nurse agree about the dominant thrust of their results. Nurses in the front ranks feel deprived if they are not recognized as individuals, if they are not involved in the development and modification of policies, and if they cannot find a willing ear to listen seriously. They demand to be accorded dignity. To be devalued, discounted, and trivialized is tantamount to feeling abandoned. These issues are linked to matters of dignity and courtesy, such as being known by name, being treated as a competent practitioner, and receiving credit for sharing through action and concern in the drama of care. On a different level, the practicing nurse wants to receive the recognition that the total range of nursing competence far exceeds the mere implementation of medical orders; she wants to invest in the well-being of her patients but also in the stability and effectiveness of her team. Being frequently pulled to another patient care unit is experienced as an amputation from a delicately balanced team. Pulling diminishes the opportunity to gain satisfaction in rendering comprehensive, high-quality nursing care. Being moved arbitrarily is felt to be a denial of the crucial importance of the nursing team and of the special competence of the nurse. Pulling does not nurture the team by maintaining mutual support and reciprocity of function. It is a recurring experience of nursing researchers to observe that although other issues may be mentioned more frequently, none is protested with as much feeling and fervor as pulling.

In these pages the questions of existence and worth as they affect the front-line nurse have been explored. It was emphasized that a distinction should be made between abandonment as a list of objectively demonstrable and measurable conditions and abandonment as a pervasively felt perception of working realities. It was further suggested that abandonment is frequently conveyed through organizational restraint or neglect of uniquely nursing functions. Lack of dignity and respect characterizing professional interactions are destructive, devaluing experiences. Most of the proposed changes to improve the situation are administratively very feasible and require only modest financial outlays. Fostering customs of courtesy, face-to-face respect, and recognition of the importance of participation are not difficult to implement if the current power wielders, be it the medical staff or the administrative hierarchy or even nursing management, are willing to acknowledge that giving respect and dignity does not diminish their own status. A system based on mutual respect will benefit all participants and, according to some suggestive data, may actually improve the quality of the product.

Every working person needs a degree of control commensurate with responsibility and accountability. Hardly any position in the repertory of human work demonstrates as wide a gap between expectations and responsibility on one hand and institutionalized control over conditions of work on the other hand. To feel included, the nurse must be a participant in policies, regulations, and the formulation of objectives. To be in control of the conditions of work, the nurse should be free from the notion that nurses must absorb whatever others dish out. Assertiveness should stem from the right to ensure quality and should not be labeled a quasi-militant display of insubordination.

REFERENCES

1. Ashley J: Hospitals, paternalism and the role of the nurse, New York, 1976, Columbia Univ Press.
2. Corley MC and Mauksch HO: Registered nurses, gender and commitment. In Statham A, Miller EM, and Mauksch HO, editors: The worth of women's work: a qualitative synthesis, Albany, 1988, State Univ of New York Press.
3. Kalisch BJ and Kalisch PA: An analysis of the sources of physician-nurse conflict, J Nurs Adm 1:51, 1977.
4. Mauksch HO: Becoming a nurse: a selective view. In Skipper JK Jr, and Leonard R, editors: Social interaction and patient care, Philadelphia, 1963, JB Lippincott.
5. Mauksch HO: Ideology, interaction and patient care, Soc Sci Med 7:817, 1973.
6. Morgan A and McCann JM: Problems in nurse-physician relationships, Nursing Administration Quarterly 7:1, 1983.
7. Nursing shortage poll report, Nurs 88 18(2):33, 1988.
8. Prescott P and Bowen SA: Physician-nurse relationships, Ann Intern Med 103:127, 1985.
9. Wandelt MA: Work conditions causes nurses to leave, American Nurse 12(10):5, 1980.
10. Wandelt MA, Pierce PM and Widdowson RR: Why nurses leave nursing and what can be done about it, Am J Nurs 1:72, 1981.

CHAPTER 68

Nursing occupational distress

SALLY BROSZ HARDIN

STRESS: THEORETICAL CONSIDERATIONS

"Complete freedom from stress is death," pronounced Hans Selye, the founder of stress theory.[39] Selye defined stress as the body's nonspecific response to any demand. He distinguished "eustress," a positive phenomenon by which persons cope with daily living, from "distress," a negative experience with destructive physical and psychological effects. The Institute of Medicine, following its 5-year review of stress research, recommended the inclusive systems model of Elliot and Eisdorfer, which defined stress as a dynamic, interactional phenomenon that involves stressors, effects, the person, and the environment.[10] Selye noted that the average person incorrectly relates stress exclusively to nervous exhaustion. In fact, the literature frequently uses the constructs stress and distress interchangeably. Although Fuller[13] discussed the beneficial effects of stress in enhancing immunological and analgesic physiologic responses, most authors and researchers discuss stress as though it were a negative experience.

A second feature of the stress literature is that it defines stress in numerous ways. Stress, distress, tension, anxiety, burnout, and crisis are treated as though they were synonymous. Stehle,[41] in her excellent review of research on intensive-care nursing stress, points out that this theoretical confusion presents major problems in stress research. Timing and duration of stress are other elements that the literature treats in a confusing manner. Few authors differentiate acute from chronic stress; others imply that crises and chronic stress are similar. Selye, however, argued that the stress process occurs in three phases: (1) alarm reaction, (2) adaptation, and (3) stage of exhaustion.[38] He noted that it is chronic, persistent, high-level stress that produces deleterious effects. Exhaustion occurs, he explained, because adaptation energy is finite; if stressed individuals have prolonged or chronic exposure to stressors, they become exhausted.

NURSING OCCUPATIONAL DISTRESS

Nurses are subject to crises and instances of anxiety at work; yet, these two phenomena do not seem to be the elements critical to nursing occupational distress. A crisis, episodic anxiety, or acute stress and its alarm reaction should mobilize the nurse. In most instances, nurses respond and adapt without becoming exhausted. It seems that nursing occupational distress occurs because of persistent, chronic stressors that cause exhaustion. In a burnout-prevention group session for head nurses, one member spoke for many others when she described her routine scenario of work distress.[16] "I can see I have all my 9 o'clocks sitting waiting for me to pass and lots of call lights are on. I still haven't made out the hours for my next schedule. Day after day, it's the same thing. I can actually feel my stomach tighten up and I'd cry if I could." Another nurse concurred: "I seem to handle emergencies o.k. It's the day-in-day-out stuff that gets me!" Nurses feel not only that this nursing stress is chronic and persistent, but also that they are unable to escape the field or to believe that conditions will improve.

Literature on nursing occupational distress

The explosion of articles on nursing occupational distress would seem to be evidence, in and of itself, that such distress does indeed exist. Lyon and Werner found that since 1956, 976 articles on nursing stress appeared in the nursing literature and that between 1974 and 1984, 82 studies related to nursing stress.[29] Major stress series were offered by the *American Journal of Nursing* in 1979 and 1980.[36,37,40,43] Other articles offered nurses helpful, if somewhat folksy, strategies for dealing with stress.[24,26] Most of these strategies, such as good nutrition, exercise, meditation, or relaxation techniques, concentrated on individualized coping mechanisms.

Another whole series of articles appeared about

the environment in which nursing distress occurred. There were studies of intensive-care (ICU) nurses,[1,2,31,41] operating room (OR) nurses,[33,35] and oncology nurses.[42] For the most part, these studies offered conflicting results. Some found ICU, OR, or oncology nursing stress was high; others did not.* It seems counterintuitive that ICU, OR, or oncology nurses would not be stressed, especially because ICU and oncology units have persistent staff shortages even when other intensive nursing units do not.[22] However, occupational distress is more complex than merely the conditions in the work environment.

Research began to take on broader dimensions. Researchers started to ask questions other than, "Are nurses stressed?" Moreover, nurses themselves, rather than physicians, psychologists, and sociologists, began to do this research. (Stehle[41] showed that only 37% of the original ICU stress studies were done by nurses; in half of these studies nurses took second, third, or fourth authorships.)

Variables in an occupational distress model

Causes. A simple way to study occupational distress is to examine its causes and effects and the role of support factors, coping, and interventions as intervening variables. Nurses have examined potential causes of work distress and have found that general and specific factors in the work environment were stressors. General environmental stressors include the need to perform numerous physical and psychosocial tasks quickly and in time-constricted settings. Hospital nurses also practice in space-constricted environments, because they are not free to leave the unit as are other members of the health team. Also nurses have major responsibilities for the lives of patients who are often in life crises, and the amount of responsibility in one's work is strongly related to work distress. For example, air-traffic controllers' jobs are labeled as highly stressful primarily because the controllers are called on to make many instantaneous life-and-death decisions. Similarly, Hay and Oken[18] reported high responsibility as a major stressor for ICU nurses, whereas Olsen[33] showed that in the operating room, nurses who were not working directly with patients had the least stress. Another general stress factor that few authors note is that most nurses are women and mothers[32] and, as such, are vulnerable to stress as dual-career nurses.[12]

Workloads, patient crises, and physicians have been shown to be specific stressors for nurses. Anderson and Basteyns[1] and Huckabay and Jagla[20] reported that of the sixteen most frequent specific sources of work stress for nurses, six concerned physicians, three understaffing and overwork loads, three dying patients or their families, and two the nurses themselves (i.e., making a medication error or being aware of one's responsibility for patients' lives). When Olsen[33] ranked OR nurses' specific stressors, she found abusive physicians ranked number one. Hyman and Woog[21] concluded that the magnitude, intensity, and duration of general and specific stressors must be taken into account when examining work stress. Moreover, they believe all stressors must be considered, because the impact of stressors is most likely additive.

Effects. It seems that every possible symptom that the human body and mind can experience has been related to work distress. Anxiety; aggression; frustration; low self-esteem; fatigue; emotional outbursts; excessive drinking, smoking, or eating; loss of appetite; inability to make decisions; hypersensitivity to criticism; mental blocks; psychosomatic complaints; family problems; job dissatisfaction; disorientation; disorganization; depression; burnout; fear; helplessness; withdrawal; bizarre behavior; and psychoses have all been blamed on work distress. Obviously, if work distress is everything, it is nothing. A more reasonable approach was taken by Stewart and others,[42] whose formal study reported nurses' major stress symptoms were physical and emotional exhaustion and daily mood swings. Nurses working with cancer patients also reported negative effects on their long-term relationships and withdrawal from patients or burnout.

Support Factors. Support factors are important intervening variables in mitigating the negative effects of work distress. Hyman and Woog[21] showed that higher income and prestige residence and strong, lasting interpersonal relationships were effective in mediating occupational distress. Stewart and others[42] found that nurses identified supportive family and friends, religious beliefs, and vacation days as most effective in keeping their stress levels manageable as they worked with cancer patients.

Coping. Hyman and Woog,[21] in a solid review of the stressful life events and illness literature, noted that the effects of stressors are also mediated by individual personality characteristics. They categorized these characteristics as psychological, which included the perceptions and expectations of an individual; and

---

*References 1, 14, 18, 20, 31, 33, 35, 42.

cognitive, which involved problem solving, abstract thought, and intelligence.

Similarly, Olsen said that the "stress response is a function of the perception, expectations, and cognitive appraisal the individual makes of the situation."[33] Dohrenwend and Dohrenwend and others found that persons who experienced objectively stressful lives did not necessarily feel distress.[8,21] Selye agreed: "Stress has various shades of meaning to different people."[38] He continued, "It is not so much what happens to you, but how you take it that matters in producing stress."[38] Kobasa[28] found that high-stress–low-illness executives, in comparison to high-stress–high-illness executives, had a great sense of commitment to and feeling of meaningfulness about their work and saw change as a challenge.

In this respect, shopping-list life stress event scales may be relatively useless because they address neither the context within which an event occurs[21] nor the meaning that subjects give to events. As an illustration, a colleague who is a therapist knowingly remarked: "Ask a man how stressful Christmas is, then ask a woman. Do you suppose there would be any differences?"

The perception and definition of a situation, commitment, motivation, intelligence, and problem solving ability all have to do with an individual's internal resources to deal with stress. Experience is another factor to be considered. Olsen found that the greater the experience of operating room nurses, the less stress they perceived.[33] Hyman and Woog, on the other hand, felt that the evidence about whether experience increased or decreased perceived distress was inconclusive.[21]

In the 1980 Harvard study on stress, women who perceived that they had little control over events felt highly stressed.[17] Hay and Oken[18] found that distressed nurses also reported feeling helpless in their work situation. Huckabay and Jagla[20] conjectured that certain events, such as dealing with physicians or patients' deaths, were viewed as distressful because they were beyond nurses' control. Anderson and Basteyns agreed.[1] Hospital nurses' control and autonomy are often deeply curtailed[4,23]; nurses' roles may be reduced to troubleshooters (team leaders) and traffic managers (head nurse), with hospitals, government, and physicians exerting more influence on nursing than nurses themselves.[27]

Defenses can be quite functional in helping nurses deal with occupational distress. Oncology nurses described how they "block out the unpleasant features of their work" or "throw themselves into their work" to defend against distress.[42] Hay and Oken[18] reported that ICU nurses also used the defense of submergence into the ICU system to deal with their distress. Olsen[33] believed that the perception of distress depends on the demands of one's job situation in relation to beliefs about the self and level of self-esteem.

One can conclude, then, that stress or distress are multidimensional concepts that include causes, effects, support factors, and coping skills. For nurses, occupational distress involves general and specific causes such as task overload, time-and-space-constricted environments, responsibilities, patient crises, and physician demands that are persistent and chronic. Primary effects of occupational distress are physical and emotional exhaustion, mood swings, withdrawal from patients, burnout, and negative effects on interpersonal relationships. These effects are mediated by the perception, cognition, and problem-solving ability of the affected persons, as well as by support factors, especially significant others, religion, higher income and prestige, and vacation time. Finally, the meaning and definition given to stressors and the perception of autonomy and control versus helplessness are important in the distress paradigm. Hyman and Woog[21] and Smith and Selye[40] offered models for the stress-distress process that included many of these facets: causes of distress, support factors, and coping skills. Preston, Ivancevich, and Matteson[35] operationalized this model at the University of Houston, where they compared causes (work stressors such as work overload, responsibility for people, relationship with physicians, colleagues, and supervisors) with coping skills (mental health, self-esteem, mood, type A or B personality) and physical health and inclination to leave nursing. Few studies, however, are based on multidimensional models such as this.

INTERVENTIONS FOR NURSING OCCUPATIONAL DISTRESS
Administrative and organizational interventions

Several authors have offered practical administrative or organizational solutions to decrease nursing occupational distress. These, however, have not been based on research results.[41] Anderson and Basteyns[1] recommended 4-day, 40-hour schedules with long weekends, rotations out of presumably high stress nursing units, and a 1:2 nurse-patient ratio in critical care areas. Maloney[31] suggested humanistic support training for head nurses and supervisors, staff group meetings to provide opportunities for emotional catharsis, and increased use of auxiliary personnel for nonnursing functions. Several writers have suggested that psychiatric nursing consultation be available to nursing staff on a regular basis. Tierney and Strom[43] urged nurses to take control of the nurses' station and the clock and not allow themselves to be summoned by anyone. To my knowledge, none of these interventions has been systematically or longitudinally tested.

Individual interventions

On an individual level, nurses have been advised to accept their inability to meet some patients' needs and their irritation at certain patients, decrease unrealistic self-expectations, use their work group as a support group, and recognize that they do have control over stress's negative aspects.[37] Tierney and Strom[43] also urged nurses to see that nursing, like life, is always unfinished. They believed that graceful acceptance of this would decrease nurses' tendencies to be Type A personalities who do many technical tasks in short time periods. Keelan[26] suggested humor was beneficial as an antidote for nurses who take themselves too seriously or see potential crises in mundane daily nursing events. He continued, "Anything that controls you will cause stress . . . put yourself above your careers. It's easy to confuse your role with your identity."[26]

None of these suggestions seems extraordinary; most would probably be beneficial in decreasing nursing occupational distress. There are also certain counterbalancing mechanisms that may prevent or reduce negative work stress. Surprisingly, none of the stress models or nursing literature addressed the issue of rewards. Money, prestige, autonomy, the ability to effect change, power, or adventure may all be considered external rewards that can counterbalance the negative effects of stress.

If one considers the stressors inherent in nursing in relation to its counterbalancing rewards, the scale is tipped in the direction of stress. Nurses are responsible for life-and-death decisions, and they often deal with patient life crises. Society and the profession demand that nurses be nurturant and caring, yet assertive and decisive. The rewards that counterbalance nurses' occupational distress are few and probably insufficient to dilute the corrosive effect of negative stress.

High motivation levels of nurses might account for their reported ability to deal with high job stress. In earlier times, when nursing was a "noble calling," this may have been especially true. In more recent times, however, self-sacrifice may be yielding to other social pressures of a less altruistic nature. As a former classmate complained in a recent survey, "Nursing is plain, old hard work and humanitarian zeal goes only so far!"

Increased rewards may decrease nursing distress. Increasing nurses' salaries could not worsen the situation certainly. But, even more important, the actual monetary costs for categorized nursing care, called for by Fagin[11] and others, would allow nurses to see their dollar-and-cents value in a dollar-and-cents society.

Psychiatric nurse specialists in private practice who were surveyed in recent research[9,15] did not report being distressed; further, they reflected high levels of self-esteem even though they made approximately the same salaries (with more education) as the average hospital nurse. One essential difference between these two types of practitioners seems to be their autonomy. Nurse-practitioners have power and control to match their responsibility. Hoeffer's suggestion for nursing clinics modeled after health maintenance organizations could provide nursing with an alternative to inpatient practice in which autonomy is often squelched by rigid bureaucratic structures.[19] Moreover, these clinics would offer nursing freedom from at least one of the most highly rated stressors in these research reports— physicians. Nursing education should continue to determine and evaluate effective ways to prepare nurses who have the coping skills to deal with job stress. Kahn[25] showed that nursing students' self-esteem steadily decreased from the beginning to the end of their nursing programs. Finally, the nursing profession, especially in these times of a catastrophic nursing shortage, should continue to exercise organized, political pressure to enhance nursing's occupational rewards.

CONCLUSION

As nursing research indicates, nurses are subject to frequent job-related stress. Several organizational and individual interventions to decrease nursing distress have been offered. There are, of course, other important avenues for investigation. Although some might assume that nursing distress is decreased in outpatient settings, this has not been proved in fact. Second, it would be helpful to study nursing's "success stories";

that is, to determine how nurses who do not report subjective distress cope in presumably high-stress units. It may also be useful to determine the extent to which nurses increase their own stressors by obsessively adhering to unnecessary routinizations and procedures in clinical practice. On a personal level, studies of nursing faculty stress would be of interest.

REFERENCES

1. Anderson CA and Basteyns SM: Stress and the critical care nurse reaffirmed, J Nurs Adm 11:31, 1981.
2. Bailey JT and Bargagliotti LA: Stress and critical care nursing. In Holzemer W, editor: Review of research in nursing education, Thorofare, NJ, 1983, Slack, Inc.
3. Bargagliotti LA: The relationship between work-related stress, coping, and social support, doctoral dissertation, San Francisco, 1985, University of California.
4. Bullough B: Influence on role expansion, Am J Nurs 76:1476, 1976.
5. Chirboga DA, Jenkins G, and Bailey JT: Stress and coping among hospice nurses: test of an analytic model, Nurs Res 32:294, 1983.
6. Congress on stressful life events: their nature and effects, New York, 1973, John Wiley & Sons.
7. Day R: Recent direction in life stress: research from a public health perspective. In Dohrenwend BS and Dohrenwend BP, editors: Stressful life events and their contexts, New York, 1981, Prodist.
8. Dohrenwend BS and Dohrenwend BP: Life stress and illness: formation of the issues. In Dohrenwend BS and Dohrenwend BP, editors: Stressful life events and their contexts, New York, 1981, Prodist.
9. Durham JD and Hardin SB: The nurse psychotherapist in private practice, New York, 1986, Springer.
10. Elliot G and Eisdorfer C: Stress and human health, New York, 1982, Springer.
11. Fagin C: Concepts for the future: competition and substitution, J Psych Nurs MHS 21:36, 1983.
12. Foley K, Hardin SB, and Skerrett K: Dual career nursing: working and mothering, Pt View 18:17, 1981.
13. Fuller BF: Using research in practice: some beneficial effects of stress, West J Nurs Res 5(1):99, 1983.
14. Gentry WD and Foster F: Psychological responses to situational stress in intensive and nonintensive nursing, Heart Lung 1:793, 1972.
15. Hardin SB and Durham JD: First rate: structure, process, and effectiveness of nurse psychotherapy, J Psychosol Nurs MHS 23:8, 1985.
16. Hardin SB and Haack M: Preventing burnout in nursing midmanagers, unpublished manuscript, Chicago, 1983, University of Illinois.
17. Harvard School of Education, Stress and Families Project: Lives in stress: a context for depression, Cambridge, 1980, Harvard School of Education.
18. Hay P and Oken P: The psychological stress of intensive care unit nursing, Psychosom Med 34:109, 1972.
19. Hoeffer B: The private practice model: an ethical perspective, J Psych Nurs MHS 21:31, 1983.
20. Huckabay LMD and Jagla B: Nurses' stress factors in the intensive care unit, J Nurs Adm 9(2):22, 1979.
21. Hyman RB and Woog P: Stressful life events and illness onset: a review of crucial variables, Res Nurs Health 3(3):155, 1982.
22. Jacobson SF: Burnout: a hazard in nursing. In Jacobson SF and McGrath HM, editors: Nurses under stress, New York, 1973, John Wiley & Sons.
23. Jacox A: Who defines and controls nursing practice? Am J Nurs 69:977, 1969.
24. Jasmin S, Hill L, and Smith N: The art of managing stress, Nurs 81 11(6):53, 1981.
25. Kahn AM: Modifications in nursing students' attitudes as measured by the EPPS: a significant reversal from the past, Nurs Res 29:61, 1980.
26. Keelan J: Nine tips for beating stress, AORN J 30(1):138, 1979.
27. Keller N: The nurses' role: is it expanding or shrinking? Nurs Outlook 21:236, 1973.
28. Kobasa SC: Stressful life events personality and health: an inquiry into hardiness, J Pers Soc Psych 37:1, 1979.
29. Lyon BL and Werner JS: Stress. In Fitzpatrick JJ and Taunton RL, editors: Annual review of nursing research, New York, 1987, Springer.
30. McLean A: Occupational stress, Springfield, Ill, 1974, Charles C Thomas, Publisher.
31. Maloney JP: Job stress and its consequences on a group of intensive and nonintensive care nurses, Adv Nurs Sci 4:31, 1982.
32. Nursing and Nursing Education: Public policies and private actions, Washington, DC, 1973, National Academy Press.
33. Olsen M: OR nurses' perception of stress, AORN J 25(1):43, 1977.
34. Pines AM and Kanner AD: Nurses' burnout: lack of positive and presence of negative conditions as two independent sources of stress, J Psychosol Nurs MHS 20(8):30, 1982.
35. Preston CA, Ivancevich JM, and Matteson MT: Stress and the OR nurse, AORN J 33(4):662, 1981.
36. Richter JM and Sloan R: Stress: a relaxation technique, Am J Nurs 79(11):1960, 1979.
37. Scully R: Stress: in the nurse, Am J Nurs 80(5):916, 1980.
38. Selye H: The stress of life, New York, 1956, McGraw-Hill Book Co.
39. Selye H: A code for coping with stress, AORN J 25(1):35, 1977.
40. Smith MJT and Selye H: Reducing the negative effects of stress, Am J Nurs 79(11):1953, 1979.
41. Stehle JL: Critical care nursing stress: the findings revisited, Nurs Res 30(3):182, 1981.
42. Stewart BE and others: Psychological stress associated with outpatient oncology nursing, CA Nurs 5(5):383, 1982.
43. Tierney MJG and Strom LM: Stress: type A behavior in the nurse, Am J Nurs 80:915, 1980.
44. Wolff HG: Stress and disease, Springfield, Ill, 1963, Charles C Thomas, Publisher.

CHAPTER 69

Public policy issues

Will they be resolved?

MARJORIE BEYERS

Nurses as professionals have an interest in furthering the best interests of those they serve and also their own capability to serve. Allocation of scarce resources for this service takes place in complicated and often convoluted processes through public policy formation. There is an overall direction for public policy established by elected and appointed officials. Legislation determines how the nation's scarce resources are allocated. In addition to the legislative processes, regulatory actions undertaken by the administrative branch affect disbursement of funds and the parameters guiding the use of funds. *Nurses must be involved in the shaping of public policy and must win positions of influence to gain and protect their ability to serve the public.*

To fulfill this mission, *nurses must understand and participate in public policy development during the discussion, deliberation, and public input phase, before decisions are made. Using influence, persuasion, and other means to gain decisions favorable to public causes that affect nursing's ability to serve effectively are thus important.* Although the power of the vote lies with the officials, the power to influence the vote lies in the hands of the public.

Nursing has taken an increasingly active role in shaping public policy in the United States. Recommendations from national commissions have been taken seriously. The ways that nursing's involvement can be measured are in the numbers of nurses filling public offices, the numbers of nurses serving on national, state and local committees, the articles appearing in nursing's refereed journals and popular literature and in meeting agendas. Nurses through their organizations are monitoring public policy decisions. More important, nurses are bringing to the fore issues and concerns to influence public decision making on matters concerning the quality of life and health care.[1]

Nurses, as the largest group of health professionals in the United States, have reason to be involved in public policy formation. Nurses experience the problems and concerns of people with unmet health care needs.[3] They work closely with groups in the population who have chronic illnesses or AIDS and who are disabled or elderly. Nurses experience the effects of inadequate health care insurance, the problems of the uninsured, and the health care poor. They must cope with infant mortality, substance abuse, the homeless, teenage pregnancies, and other socially related health problems at the care-giver level. How can nurses, as the largest group of health professionals, translate these issues and problems into public policies and programs to help these population groups?

Nursing has three imperatives. First, nurses must accept the responsibility to influence and to become involved in public policy decisions. Second, they must develop issues and problems in meaningful positions to offer substance to deliberation and debate by the decision makers. Third, nurses must continue to develop their expertise in influencing public policy. The first imperative, accepting the responsibility to influence and become involved, is the most difficult to achieve. Considering the composition of the nursing profession and the diverse settings in which nurses practice, nursing as a profession is in a good position to represent a broad spectrum of issues and concerns relevant to public policy. Accepting the responsibility to influence and become involved means that these diverse interests must be focused in a common public policy agenda for nursing. This common public policy agenda affects all three imperatives.

Accepting the responsibility to influence and become involved in public policy agendas entails a set of activities in which nurses work together. Basic to success is that all nurses be informed about public policy issues and concerns. Attention to the public safety and welfare is a dimension of being a professional. To be informed about health policy issues is a personal responsibility of a professional. This responsibility goes beyond being informed, however, and includes caring about the outcomes of public policy decisions enough to devote time and energy to public policy processes. These processes begin with discussion and deliberation among nurses and then move into formation of a nursing public policy agenda that can be taken forward by the representatives of the profession. Those representatives are most often the elected officers of the official nursing organizations at the local, state, and national levels, appointed executives, content experts, and practice-related experts.

A nurse as an individual can become involved in public policy in many different ways. At the grassroots level, the nurse professional must be informed about public policy issues, must thoughtfully observe practice experiences to determine need and input for public policy formation, and must relate this information to the appropriate sources for action. Nurses as individuals can become involved in public policy formation by becoming members of nursing's official organizations. Membership allows the nurse to contribute financially to the organization's efforts to influence public policy, to serve on committees that deliberate and shape policy issues and agendas, to serve as an officer of the organization to represent it in the public arena, and to support the policy agendas through personal and public contacts. Giving speeches, writing informed papers, articulating positions on the issues, and exchanging views with community members are all examples of a nurse's opportunities to fulfill the dimension of professionalism related to public policy.

Nurses as individuals can also reach out into the community to extend their scope of influence. Becoming part of community groups with policy interests; seeking public office; filling positions of influence in offices engaged in legislation, policy development and analysis, regulations, and rule making; and speaking up on issues that influence and affect public health are important activities. As nurses move into these community and official sectors, they must resolve many concerns about representation. Who do they represent: the nursing profession, the community group, the interests of the institution or agency that employs them, or others?

Accepting the responsibility to influence and become involved also pertains to nursing's organizations.

In recent years, nursing organizations have begun to move together to form public policy agendas for health care that represent nursing knowledge, experience, and expertise. As the profession matures, more time can be devoted to outreach to influence public policy. Many of nursing's organizations have focused on such activities as setting standards for practice, developing certification examinations, setting qualifications for practicing individuals, and developing educational programs for maintaining and increasing competence in practice for the members. These activities are important and form the basis for outreach into activities such as influencing public policy. The organization must have an identity, a purpose, and a reason for being recognized as expert in the national "field of practice" to infuence public policy.

The perception that the organization represents an interest group is critical to use of that group in discussion and debate surrounding issues and concerns in the public policy arena. For example, a legislator who wants to represent constituency opinions and beliefs will seek information from the most valid source. Validity in this instance refers to the extent to which the information represents an official body that in turn represents large groups of people who share or support the information through their membership. It is assumed that the official stance or position of the organization is developed through formation processes that engage the members in shaping the official organizational stance or position. The individual member thus speaks out through the organizational representation.

Because nursing has numerous organizations, it is difficult to isolate one group that can be considered the valid source of opinion about public policy concerns. The greatest impact on public policy can be made if the nursing profession represents a policy agenda supported by all organizations. A policy agenda consists of priority issues the profession wishes to promote in the public sector. For each issue, information about the scope of the problem or concerns, the sectors of the population affected, the nature of the unmet or insufficiently met needs, and the solutions are developed. Solutions involve identification of programs, projects, or positions and the resources needed to implement them.

A profession's policy agenda is expected to represent the majority opinion. Individual professionals and even individual professional organizations may have different views that can be presented and that may take precedence in influencing public policy given the power and effort behind the influence. In situations in which sectors of a professional representation come forth with different positions, two major effects can occur. The first is that the profession may be viewed as lacking the power to support and sustain a position. The second is that conflicting positions are resolved not within nursing but in the public view. In decisions influenced greatly by the strength of the position as measured in numbers of people behind it, nursing would have more impact with a comprehensive nursing policy position. In situations in which the power of influence is most critical, the organization within nursing with the most influence over a particular issue prevails. Opposing or differing views from within a profession may also be used to negate the validity of any of the group's positions and may consequently weaken the ability to influence overall public policy.

The second imperative, developing issues and positions on these issues to offer substance to deliberation and debate by the decision makers, involves a number of equally important but different initiatives. At the base of these initiatives is isolation of a public need that constitutes a public policy problem or issue. Observation of patient experiences, and other observations within the care-giving processes, spoken concerns from patients, community groups, and nurses, and other informal interaction provide information for the professional about issues relevant to public policies. The seed for issue development often grows from early identification of problems at the grass-roots. When many different groups from different geographic locations are experiencing the same difficulties and when they bring the information forth at public meetings for discussion, the first test of whether the experience is an isolated event or a common need is passed. At this stage, awareness of problems and concerns is heightened, and the rudiments of a public policy position are established.

Further tests of the strength of the problem or issues occur through systematic study. Data collection is important at this stage. Research to define the problem, ways of effectively treating the problem, and the cost of treatment are also important. Epidemiologic studies, surveys of health status, and research on conditions and circumstances that contribute to or cause given problems are important. At the national level, aggregate data become important to establish the national need for action. Problems and issues relevant to a given geographic region, state, or community may

be better dealt with through state or community policy initiatives. The ability to describe a problem or issue, to relate facts and findings, and to establish a defensive posture on actions that should be taken in the public policy arena are critical at this stage of development.

Public opinion is equally important. As critical as the facts may be, public acceptance and beliefs often sway the attention to or away from problems or issues. Gaining a public audience and public support involves more than research. The information must be marketed to the general public as well as to the professional community in language that can be understood. In public policy, marketing occurs through informal and formal means. Examples of informal means are discussion at committees and public meetings or in general conversation. Formal means include providing issue papers, testimony, and public information forums to educate the public about issues.

Certain types of issues are easier than others to promote to gain public attention and support. Those that affect many or all sectors are highly visible, such as a flood or a natural disaster; ones that relate directly to a value system are easier to promote than issues related to isolated groups in which individuals have little influence. An issue such as care for the medically indigent may be an example of one that must be promoted to gain support. When solutions to a problem are or appear to be in conflict with other priorities or vested interests, gaining public attention and support requires conflict resolution, trade-offs, and compromises among the decision makers.

The third imperative, that nurses must continue to develop their expertise in influencing public policy, requires being informed about the steps required to turn an idea into legislation and to gain its passage and also knowing how to persuade, to change attitudes and beliefs, and to gain support. All of these processes are time consuming and require specialized expertise to be effective. Nurses have an interest in acquiring these skills because they are similar to ones useful in influencing policy decisions within organizations, because public policy decisions often directly affect private sector organizational initiatives and policy, and because their professional role includes acting for the public good in matters of health care.

Basic to the process of influencing public policy is the decision about whether the issue falls into the realm of public policy. Some problems pertain directly to the profession and its practice and must be dealt with there. Others are organization problems and must be dealt with in the organizational arena. Those that suit public policy action are issues that affect the public at large and that require public resources. A national shortage of nurses requires public action; adequate health care for the elderly requires public attention, which is increasingly imperative in view of the increasing numbers of elderly. Programs that are supported by public funding fit into the realm of public policy; abortion, federal health insurance, federal and state programs to support education, and programs to assist the homeless are a few such issues.

Public policy development processes are complex, partly because of the issues, conflict about how to resolve them, and competition to gain attention and action. An example of this complexity is illustrated in the issues related to poverty. Poverty is definitely a public policy issue because it affects not only the public health but the economic status and image of the nation. Even though poverty is a dominant issue, values related to poverty, its causes and effects, vary. Allocation of resources to help those in need is influenced by values about how best to deal with the problem. Consider the following questions.

What factors contribute to poverty? Are there enough people within a given community, state, or nation who have incomes below the poverty level to warrant action? Is the action best taken at the federal, state, or local levels? Is care for people with insufficient incomes the responsibility of a given community? a state? a nation? Are people who migrate across state lines, across national boundaries, eligible for help? Will policy initiatives actually result in change? What are the relative benefits of food stamp programs, work programs, health insurance? Are allocations for subsidized health care sufficient? What solutions at what cost result in the greatest amelioration of poverty? What are the effects of poverty on the community, state, or nation? Is poverty related to crime rates? to incidence of disease? to economic performance of the nation?[2]

These questions illustrate the complexity of just one public policy issue. Further study of this issue reveals that initiatives to deal with poverty have been proposed throughout history and yet poverty still exists. Programs to help the needy have not always been accessible to the most needy, have not always related to their most urgent needs, and have not always been accepted and used by those with the greatest need.

Another type of public policy issue is the prevention, treatment, and management of care for patients with AIDS. Issues surrounding AIDS are of fairly recent origin, have international impact, and directly affect the community of health care professionals. Policy issues include financing of care, funding and promotion of effective care management through demonstration projects, basic and applied research on treatments, public education, and protection of health care workers. AIDS has a direct impact on the national public health.[4] National initiatives are clearly needed to deal effectively with the issues.

Nursing's potential involvement and influence on public policy can be examined in terms of either of these issues. What experiences do nurses have that provide information useful to public policy formation? What positions can and should nursing as a profession take in the public policy arena? How does nursing engage the attention of the public to support its positions? What other professions and groups should nursing join to make an impact in public policy arenas? The three main ways to influence public policy are to identify individuals and groups who share concerns about the issues, to locate and contact persons and groups with influence to promote and achieve public policy goals, and to maneuver nurse representatives into positions of influence and decision making.

Nurses are accustomed to action, speedy decision making, clearly defined protocols and decision trees, and evaluation of results. Public policy formation and decision making is slow and deliberate, with discussion and drawn-out decision-making processes, extensive review and comment, and frequently outdated methods of evaluating results. To be effective with those who can influence public policy, nurses must take into account the differences in ways of thinking and expectations between nurses and public policy makers.

Tracing public policy through its formative stages is useful for those trying to gain influence. The processes are evolutionary. New issues are frequently raised in the literature and can be found in scholarly journals, research reports, and summaries of meetings attended by experts in a field. Articulation of a new need or a new approach to the resolution of a longstanding issue may attract the attention of motivated individuals or groups who continue to study the issue and to discuss it in the public arena. Elected officials and others in public life are approached to build support for the issue. Introduction of an issue at the legislative level usually follows study by the legislator of the extent to which the public is concerned about the issue or the extent to which public attention can be drawn to the issue. Introducing and supporting issues of known concern is as important as introducing issues the public has not yet considered.

Opportunity and timing are key ingredients in the formation of public policy. A good idea, a sound policy initiative, or even a critical public need may not receive much attention at the first introduction. Often issues are introduced several times over a period of several years before action is taken. Several events may occur. One type of event is the gradual maturation of an issue that is at first diffuse and needs to be increasingly honed to a focus that can be understood and dealt with by the public and the legislators. Another is displacement of a sound and important issue by one with greater immediate appeal that distracts attention away from other issues. Sound and important issues can be diffused in the legislative process by addition to a legislative bill of related or unrelated provisions that are controversial. The legislation may die, not because of lack of agreement on the issue, but because of the controversy on the added provisions. Some issues are not dealt with because legislative agendas are too full and sessions close before the new legislation can be introduced. Delaying tactics such as filibusters may be deliberately planned to prevent action on new legislation.

A number of factors can influence decision making throughout the formation of policy and the legislative decision-making processes. In some cases, issues are used to stimulate confrontation, and the substance and intent of the legislation may be lost in the confrontation. Some issues become negotiable, and support may be gained by trade-offs, compromises, or other means so that legislation may be delayed, defeated, or drastically revised. In some instances, legislation important to the health care community may not be considered a priority compared to issues such as the economy or national defense. Finally, some issues are gained or lost because of luck, good or bad.

Processes for implementation of legislation are as important as shaping the policies and legislation. Legislative decisions, as well as regulatory decisions, reflect the public policy directions. The substance and intent of the legislation passed can be interpreted in different ways. Thus the administrative staffers who write the regulations add to the legislative intent by defining the implementation parameters. In many

cases, the rules set forth in regulations become directives that must be followed, as in the case of Medicare and Medicaid. The regulations and rules may exceed or fail to meet the intent of the legislation.

Providing information to the persons who write the regulations, influencing their decisions, and responding to the effects of regulations published in the *Federal Register* are all important aspects of public policy formation. Likewise, there are processes for appeals to regulations, rules and directives that can be used by the public affected by the legislation. Some legislation is passed and is not enforced. In other instances, enforcement is stringent.

Transition in government after elections are held and changes in the executive staff are other variables that affect public policy and that require the attention of those wishing to influence.[5] Changeovers bring new persons with values, loyalties, and identities together with the strengths of precedent and the machinery of government that sustains implementation. The extent to which a newly appointed or elected official can change the direction of public policy is balanced by this precedent and by public opinion and expectations. In general, the bureaucracy may continue to determine implementation, whereas new policies and directions may serve to set in motion changes that may be gradual or time consuming.[6] Attending to the influential persons in the transition phases is important for those wishing to influence the direction of public policy.

Resources and support for nurses seeking to fulfill their professional responsibility to influence and become involved in public policy are increasingly available. The professional organizations and many nursing journals now contain sections on public policy initiatives. Many large institutions have a person designated to monitor the literature to keep professionals up-to-date on new issues and opportunities to influence action on all public policy directions. The strategy of developing a public policy agenda for the organization is useful for heightening awareness of priorities and opportunities to influence. In this strategy, the organization chooses its issues and focuses on gaining influence. Another important strategy is seeking willing and capable individuals who can be placed in positions of influence on committees, in elected offices, and in other groups recognized as "experts" whose opinions are sought by public officials or whose decisions influence policy directions.

In every case, the ability to influence public policy

depends on a strong constituency willing to back and support the positions being promoted. Rarely can an individual personally influence public policy without this backing. Legislators and public officials tend to listen to individuals who relate issues to them that have also been related by other groups and individuals. Frequency of mention by more than one constituency is a powerful inducement to gain the attention of those pledged to serve the public.

As nursing begins to develop a comprehensive, focused approach to influencing public policy, it will be useful to reach out and form partnerships with other influential groups with common interests. Nursing's trust—to serve the public— is an important aspect of the profession that warrants attention to the decisions made by legislators and rule makers. Nursing's capability to serve is directly affected by these decisions for several reasons. One is that the direction of public policy and legislation affects institutional de-

cision making. Federal and state initiatives reflect the general tenor of feeling of the citizens. Institutions that exist to serve the public and the nurses in them are also subject to legislation, so there is a direct influence on practice. Finally, being a professional means taking a position on meaningful issues that serve the public good.

BIBLIOGRAPHY

1. Carolyne Davis speaks out, Nurs Outlook 9(7):355, 1988.
2. Kirp and others: Poverty, welfare and workfare, Public Interest 83:34, 1986.
3. Milburn L: Medical indigency: annotated bibliography of recent research and policy documents, Nursing Economics 4(6):289, 1986.
4. Mohr RD and others: AIDS: testing, financing, insurance, Law Medicine and Health Care 15(4):178, 1987.
5. Nursing shortage: David Reed's top concern, Hospitals:44, 1988.
6. Rainey HG and Wechster B: Executive level transition: toward a conceptual framework, Public Productivity Review, 22(1):43, 1988.

CHAPTER 70

The role of the nurse executive

BARBARA A. DONAHO

INTRODUCTION

The nurse executive must provide the leadership to develop a strong nursing management team that functions effectively with the hospital management team. Being a skillful mentor for the staff will reduce dependency, increase understanding of the organization's culture, and lessen the burden of managing complex change. Only when the nursing management team is able to function with confidence will the nurse executive be able to be involved in the activities external to both the nursing department and the hospital.

VISIBILITY

Visibility is expected of the nurse executive. This is a self-imposed expectation as well as one frequently identified by staff nurses, hospital management, and medical staff.

The ability to meet this expectation is related to the degree of dependency of the nurse executive's associates. The more dependent others are on the nurse executive, the more visible the executive is expected to be. This is often reflected in remarks such as: "Oh, you're here today!" "Where are you off to next week?" "We never see you on the unit!" "Your calendar is impossible—it takes weeks to get an appointment with you!"

The expectation of visibility expressed directly and indirectly to the nurse executive can set into motion behavior that is destructive for all concerned. The literal interpretation of visibility is to be **visible.** And yet to be seen in person by a great number of staff can impose an unrealistic burden on the nurse executive.

Visibility has a much broader connotation, which must be internalized by all the in-house colleagues of the nurse executive. Representation, capable of being seen, availability—these concepts should be linked to the literal definition of visibility. The need "to see" the nurse executive suggests the existence of dependency that may interfere with the executive's desire to implement decentralized or shared governance models. The perception of visibility can be linked to the central delegation continuum (Fig. 70-1).

The narrow concept of visibility emphasizes ultimate control. If staff must seek permission prior to acting, the degree of dependence on a visible nurse executive is clearly too high, resulting in the "May I?" approach to the everyday functioning of the department. The executive in this case must be seen and heard. The broader concept of visibility suggests that the nurse executive should be visible as a result of working *through* others.

THE NURSE EXECUTIVE AND THE STAFF
Mentoring and delegation

Delegation illustrates the nurse executive's confidence in the staff: the belief that the staff can perform according to their respective job requirements. The work of the nurse executive is to *decrease* the degree of dependency, with the intention that there be greater staff participation in the decisions of the organization. To achieve this, conscious mentoring becomes a major part of the nurse executive's work (Fig. 70-2). The nurse executive must be viewed as a trusted counselor when advice is sought. The ability to exchange ideas, to share opinions, to debate are inherent in the process. However, the ability to communicate values and trust is critical, and often delicate.

The control-delegation continuum

When staff are confident in their abilities to complete their work without seeking prior approval for every task, the opportunity for visual visibility exists. The nurse executive's having communicated values and trust will be seen and understood by the staff. Balancing the control-delegation continuum mirrors the need to balance the independence-co-dependence relationship with the nurse executive. Continuous

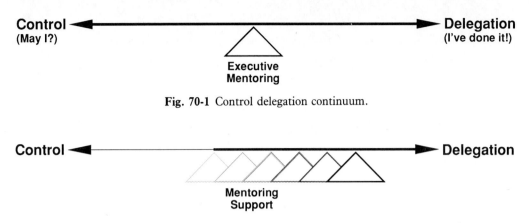

Fig. 70-1 Control delegation continuum.

Fig. 70-2 Through mentoring of staff, the nurse executive moves toward delegation.

mentoring provides the staff as well as the executive an opportunity to learn from every experience if all involved parties are willing to engage in a joint critique of an event. Analyzing the *outcome* is important, but there is probably more to be learned by analyzing the *processes* required to reach an outcome. By focusing on how another professional manager works, the analysis is directed to the components of the work and not to the personality traits of the worker. The critical issue is that being a mentor should never cease for any professional. The same techniques that nurse executives use to mentor others should also be used as learning tools for themselves. The mentoring process is a reinforcing process. Being a mentor is clearly a two-way street: the executive (as counselor) and the individual staff member (as advisee) each benefit from the other's experience, thereby creating a cohesive bond, which in some cases may blur the line between counselor and advisee. Both individuals, when communication is focused and constructive, learn and teach the other.

CLINICAL TO ORGANIZATIONAL MANAGEMENT

Research, direct clinical practice, managing, and educating are four pivotal components of the nurse's work. This work involves interaction among professional nursing colleagues, physicians, and patients and their families (Fig. 70-3). The majority of this work is accomplished in a one-on-one relationship, with the decisions affecting only one patient or family unit. When these four basic functions—research, clinical practice, managing, and educating—are integrated

and directed to collective groups, then the forces take on additional dimensions. This requires a shift from the singular concern of one nurse, one physician, and one patient, to the complex interaction of the organization and the external environment. This shift creates the potential for a much broader sphere of input and represents a move from clinical management to organizational and executive management (Fig. 70-4).

Organizational culture

Understanding the culture of an organization is the first task that must be undertaken when accepting a new position in management, which may result from a promotion or relocation to another organization. The emphasis, however, is on new position. Recognizing and understanding the complexities of a new, or changed, environment will enhance the ability of the nurse executive to develop mentoring relationships. It is also critical for the nurse executive to understand the inner workings of the organization to select decision making strategies that will be effective.

The effectiveness of these strategies depends on the depth of the nurse executive's insight, which, in turn, requires an understanding of the following elements:
- philosophy and mission
- long-range plans
- management organization
- organizational culture
  - decision-making process
  - values
  - rituals
- medical staff
- nursing staff
- support departments

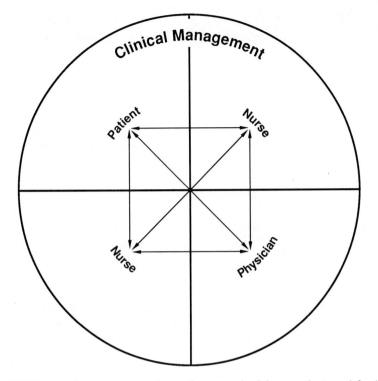

Fig. 70-3 Interactions among nursing colleagues, physicians, patients and families.

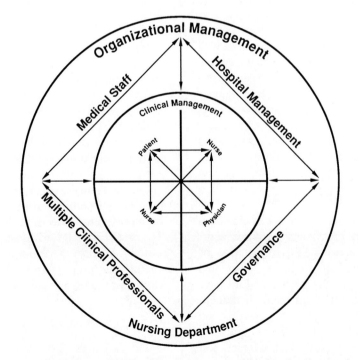

Fig. 70-4 Interactions shift from clinical management to organizational and executive management.

THE ONGOING EDUCATION OF THE NURSE EXECUTIVE
The ability to analyze

The nurse executive must maintain a familiarity with contemporary management literature, which is replete with in-depth analyses of the elements listed above. Identifying the impact of each element on the other is yet another facet of the nurse executive's role. This analysis should also include an identification of the organizational decision makers and the key influencers; the objective here is to ascertain the motivations and values of each. On completion of the initial analysis, the nurse is now equipped to function as an executive and to determine the best way to utilize an organization's strengths as well as to deal with the weaknesses within.

External environment: understanding and participating

The external environment of an institution must also be understood because of its repercussions on the organization and therefore on the work of the nurse executive (Fig. 70-5). Nearly every component included in Figure 70-5 has had a direct impact on the health care delivery system and will challenge the executive team's capacity to deal with the external environment. The opportunity to influence players in the external environment exists, but it demands a great deal of effort on the part of the organization's resources. The knowledge of political processes, as well as other complicated state and national organizational structures, can be difficult to acquire. The career employees of an organization are frequently more knowledgeable and influential than the elected officials. Consequently, the organization may take on traits more closely linked to individual staff members than to the publicly stated purpose and mission. This difference must be understood to identify the critical decision maker who must be targeted to influence an anticipated action.

The nurse executive should make a conscious decision to be involved in the external environment. Some institutions clearly articulate this expectation for the nurse executive. The external demands on personal time and energy require the nurse executive to have built a strong internal management team. If that internal strength is established, then the opportunity will be present to extend external involvement to others, building understanding of the process, the issues, and the need for this involvement. The goal of the nurse executive should be to groom as many professional staff members as possible: to advise and to work with those same people who participate internally as well as externally.

The professional nurse executive will need to integrate internal organizational activity and external environmental elements and to assess the impact of changes in both arenas. Recognizing personal biases becomes the most difficult aspect of this process. Not being able to do so may distort one's view of the environment and hinder the instigation of needed action. Nurse executives must recognize their own system of values and also must allow others their biases and values. When evaluating alternatives for action, each alternative must be considered in terms of its impact on the organization and on professional and personal values. Compromising is the result of balancing patient, institution, professional, and societal needs. Those appointing a nurse executive assume the nurse executive is able to bring objectivity to the decision-making process and is able to select alternatives that have the most positive influence on the total organization. The nurse executive's ability to define a vision for the organization's future will influence her ability to judge the potential of an alternative route in any decision-making process. That vision should be a dynamic vision with broad concepts that allow clarity to emerge as changes within and outside the organization occur.

Strategic planning

Managing change is an inherent part of the nurse executive's work. Deciding what to do is a result of sound strategic planning. Timing of the change—the "when" to do—is not so readily determined. Frequently what-when decisions may be translated as a "phase-in" process. The decisions are divided into manageable pieces of work and may result in change being perceived as evolution rather than radical redirection.

Organizational and environmental constraints may dictate implementing parts of a program, thus avoiding the all-or-nothing decision. The ability to see the fit of a partial package within the vision reflects an executive's clarity of vision: the executive recognizes whether the proposed alternative or partial program will move the organization toward its goal.

POSITIVE INFLUENCE

The nurse executive's logic regarding the what-when decision should be open and directed toward the professional-organizational match with the external environment. Skillful matching of the what decision with the when decision becomes crucial in the matter of gaining support to accomplish the stated outcome, in allowing sufficient time for implementation, and in establishing completion expectations that can be achieved. This critical sense of timing appears to be mastered as the nurse executive experiences positive reinforcement, as she takes risks in delegation. Positive reinforcement can be enhanced even if the outcome differs from what is anticipated when both failures and successes are analyzed. Seldom are failures total failures, because an unexpected consequence will often surface in some successful form within the experience. Without analyses, however, the experience will be labeled a failure, and the reinforcement will be negative, which discourages the next approach to risk.

Characteristic of the current environment are limited resources, the continuous introduction of new technology, and increasingly vocal consumer concerns about access and quality. The management challenges of tomorrow will need to revolve around similar issues. This environment demands rapid analyses and significant risk taking. The nurse executive may opt to focus on the nursing department and to deal only with today's clinical departmental issues. That decision results in relegating tomorrow's organizational decisions to other professionals. The nurse executive who operates with a vision for the profession will become a strategic player in both the organization and the external environment and will influence decisions. Only then is the nurse executive in a position to influence the future of nursing.

CHAPTER 71

Use of conflict as a positive force

MARION JOHNSON

Conflict is one of the most pervasive and significant forces influencing the professionalization of nursing today. Longstanding conflicts, such as entry into practice and doctor-nurse relationships, are receiving renewed attention. New conflicts can be anticipated as the health care system continues to adapt to a rapidly changing environment. Aydelotte[1] has identified two potential sources of conflict in the health care system: (1) conflict created by differences in economic and professional values, that is, the need to economize versus the commitment to professional behavior; and (2) conflict created by competition between and among professionals and corporate executives as roles are redefined and power redistributed. As the largest but traditionally least powerful group of workers in health care, nursing is particularly vulnerable to the conflicts that accompany change and adaptation. How nursing responds to current conflicts within the profession and with other health care professions may well determine nursing's role in tomorrow's health care system.

Nursing's traditional response to conflict—prevention at all costs[19]—is nonproductive in today's health care setting. Many of today's conflicts, if prevented or avoided, can produce results that are dysfunctional for the individual, the organization, the profession, and the consumer. Neither nursing, health care organizations, nor the consumer will benefit if conflicts about the allocation of increasingly scarce resources, the expanding role of the professional nurse, the appropriate educational preparation for entry into practice, or the reallocation of power within the health care system are avoided. It has become increasingly important for nursing to confront and manage both its internal and external conflicts if nursing is to benefit from the changes taking place in the health care arena.

The effective management of conflict requires an understanding of the dynamics of conflict and an appreciation of the benefits that can be derived from conflict. Although much has been written about the dynamics and management of conflict, there is less information about the potential benefits of conflict or how the conflict process can be used to understand the conflicts experienced by the profession and by individual nurses.

THE PROCESS OF CONFLICT

Conflict can be viewed as a process developing over time and having predictable dynamics.[24] Each conflict episode can be envisioned as consisting of five stages that need not proceed sequentially. The stages of a conflict episode include latent conflict (conditions), perceived conflict (cognition), felt conflict (affect), manifest conflict (behavior), and conflict aftermath (outcomes).[14] A modification of this model can be applied to organizational conflict or other forms of intergroup conflict and used to analyze the factors that contribute to functional or dysfunctional conflict in nursing (see Fig. 71-1).

Preference differences can occur when members of a group disagree about goals, values, or facts. They can also occur when members disagree on methods of achieving a goal. Differences in goals and values are generally more divisive and likely to result in destructive outcomes. Unfortunately, conflict that accompanies issues most significant for nursing's development often involves goal or value differences. The divisive conflict surrounding the issue of entry into practice has resulted from differences about the desirability of professional status for nursing rather than differences about how professionals are educated. Work conflicts experienced by new graduates arise from differences between practice values in the work setting and practice values learned in the educational setting.[10,20] In a study of preferences of workers in a psychiatric hospital, findings showed a high level of conflicting preferences among nurses and demonstrated little homogeneity among nurses as a group.[5] These conflicts serve

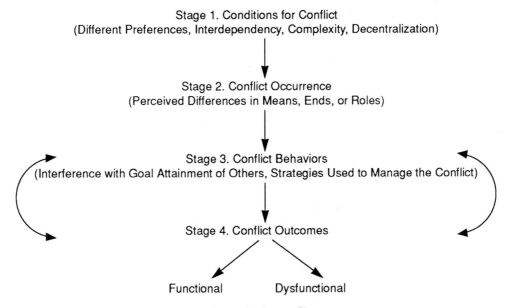

Fig. 71-1 Stages in the conflict process.

to highlight the fact that nurses as a group do not possess discipline-specific values. As hospitals become increasingly business-oriented, value conflicts may arise between nursing administrators oriented to business values and responsible for organizational goals and clinical nurses oriented to holistic patient care and responsible for patient outcomes.

Common task and resource dependencies and the need to coordinate activities are correlated with higher levels of organizational conflict.[21,26] When a high degree of task dependency is coupled with differences in autonomy the potential for conflict is increased. Nursing has been highly dependent on the cooperation of other health care professionals, particularly physicians, to carry out its work. As a knowledge base specific to nursing practice has developed, both the profession and individual nurses have sought increased autonomy. This has generated increasing role conflict within nursing and with other professions that can be expected to continue for the foreseeable future. Conflicts within nursing and with other health professionals about the allocation of resources may accelerate if economic constraints continue to be a major consideration in health care. Because nursing comprises the largest group of workers in most health care organizations, it is the group most vulnerable when organizational resources decrease.

Complex organizations characterized by nonuniform tasks, high levels of differentiation coupled with high interdependency, and greater size, experience higher levels of conflict.[4,13,26] Although health care organizations are characterized by task variability, the majority of nurses practice in organizations that use formalized rules and procedures as a method of control—practices that are inimical to the exercise of clinical judgment in settings that rely heavily on technology and in which personalized services are provided. Conflicts can arise between the policies of the organization and the actions of individual nurses in their interactions with clients and other professionals. This type of conflict can be decreased if the quality of clinical decision making is controlled by standards rather than regulations. High degrees of both horizontal (multiple levels of specialists) and vertical (multiple hierarchical levels) differentiation continue to exist in health care organizations and in many nursing departments. Either type of differentiation can be a source of role ambiguity, role conflict, and conflict about the allocation of authority and power conflicts common in nursing agencies. The introduction of clinical specialists in hospital settings created lateral role conflicts that have not been completely resolved. Varied degrees of vertical conflict exist in nursing departments and might be anticipated to escalate with the emphasis on increased productivity in an era of staff shortages. As health care organizations realign their structures, nurse administrators are moving into positions of greater responsibility. It remains to be seen if increased authority and power will accompany these changes and if nurses providing direct patient care will gain the authority necessary for autonomous practice.

Studies indicate that decentralized decision making is related to increased conflict.[26] Increasing the number of individuals involved in decision making increases the possibility that group members will become more aware of their differences. However, the long-term effects of this conflict may be positive if members are allowed to clarify their values, and agree on goals that are acceptable to all. Decentralization, if it creates less complex units, also has the potential to decrease the conflict that accompanies complexity. Despite the risks involved, decentralization of authority as well as responsibility may be the most effective long-term method of resolving conflicts about the goals, functions, and role of nursing.

Conflict begins when group members perceive interpersonal differences about issues important to them. It is not necessary that actual differences exist; it is the perception of differences that results in conflict. However, conflict will not progress to the stage of overt behavior unless the opportunity to interfere or interact with other members is present.

Conflict behaviors can include expressions of affect as well as the conflict resolution strategies employed by the group. Resolution strategies commonly identified in the literature include avoidance, accommodation, competition, compromise, and collaboration. The selection of strategies has been discussed in numerous works on the management of conflict. Most writers suggest that the strategy be chosen to match the conflict situation. However, the findings from two research studies indicate that deans of nursing schools and nurse managers in hospital settings might tend to reuse the same strategy rather than adjust behavior to the situation.[25]

Outcomes can be functional or dysfunctional for organizations. The result will depend on the type of issue, the structural components of the situation, and the strategies chosen to manage the conflict.

CONSTRUCTIVE FUNCTIONS OF CONFLICT

Various propositions explaining the function of conflict have been proposed by conflict theorists. These include:

1. Conflict is innate in all social animals, including humans.
2. Conflict is a result of the inequities in the nature and structure of certain societies.
3. Conflict is an aberration, a dysfunction.
4. Conflict is functional.
5. Conflict is a consequence of inadequate communication, misperception, and other unconscious processes.
6. Conflict is a natural process common to all societies, has predictable dynamics, and is amenable to regulation.[23]

These propositions, primarily originating in the behavioral sciences, reflect a neutral view of conflict that is popular in much of the conflict literature today. This view suggests that conflict is situational and that outcomes depend on the contexts in which conflict occurs.

Organizational conflict also is assigned a more positive role that it was in the past. The traditionalist philosophy, dominant in organizational thought until the mid 1940s, viewed conflict as a destructive force interfering with the ideal climate of stability and harmony.[3] Emphasis was placed on preventing, eliminating, or suppressing conflict. The human relations school of thought, prominent in the late 1940s and early 1950s, recognized the existence of conflict but continued to assign it a negative role in organizations.[3] Emphasis was placed on resolving conflict. For both of these positions, conflict represented a management failure. For the traditionalist, conflict was a failure in planning and controlling; for the behavioralist, conflict was a failure of leadership.[13] For both, conflict was seen as a liability with little recognition that conflict might benefit an organization.

By the 1960s, a more positive view of organizational conflict began to emerge. It was suggested that conflict could increase group cohesion and group morale,[9] improve work relations,[7] and motivate group members[21]—effects that should promote individual and group productivity. The interactionist view of conflict, proposed by Robbins[16] in 1974, was a radical departure from previous approaches to organizational conflict. Robbins identified conflict as a necessary component of organizational growth and placed emphasis on using conflict as a resource. Today the idea that conflict can promote creativity and produce change, important prerequisites of organizational growth, has gained increased recognition.[3,15] Improving the quality of problem solving in an organization has been identified as another constructive function of conflict.[17,18] By allowing divergent interests and beliefs to emerge, conflict can force decision makers to define the problem, examine conflicting opinions, and ideally arrive at more creative solutions.

Although it is recognized that conflict can be functional for an organization, there has been little research to support this perspective. However, a recent study of conflict in hospitals found that conflict can stimulate innovation and change, can motivate individuals and groups to resolve differences, and can promote the most efficient reallocation of resources.[2]

Because strategies chosen to manage conflict can influence the outcomes derived from conflict, it is important to know how nurse administrators perceive the functions of conflict. If they view conflict as having functional properties they may be more likely to seek management strategies that will produce positive outcomes. Both positive and negative effects of conflict were identified in a study of nursing administrators' perceptions of conflict.[12] In this study 51% of the responses identified positive outcomes of conflict; however, negative aspects of conflict were higher (176 responses) than positive aspects (167 responses) when considering its effects on people. From this "people" orientation, positive outcomes identified in the study included increased self-awareness, individual growth, release of tension, increased motivation, team building, and increased participation and group interaction. The major positive effect of conflict on task achievement was improved problem resolution.

I conducted a descriptive study examining nurse administrators' perceptions of the benefits of conflict in the context of individual and organizational characteristics.[6] The sample included nurse administrators in top management positions in schools of nursing in institutions of higher education (deans) and departments of nursing in teaching hospitals (directors). Questionnaires were sent to 834 nurse administrators and 480 usable questionnaires were returned, for a total response rate of 57.5%. The response rate for deans was 63% (n = 259) and for directors 57.5% (n = 221).

A summated rating scale was used to examine nurse administrators' perceptions of the benefits of conflict in their work settings. The scale was designed to measure five potential functions of conflict and their underlying causes identified in the literature:

Table 71-1 Comparisons of percentage of "agree" (A) and "disagree" (D) responses of deans, directors, and both groups by function

Function	Deans* A	Deans* D	Directors A	Directors D	Both groups A	Both groups D
Unifying	43	57	57	43	50	50
Preserving	55	45	59	41	57	43
Integrative	55	45	68	32	61.5	38.5
Growth	56	44	72	28	64	36
Problem solving	74	26	80	20	77	23

*Deans, n = 259; directors, n = 221; both groups, n = 480

1. A unifying function accomplished by increasing group cohesion;
2. A group-preserving function, accomplished by preventing the accumulation of hostility;
3. An integrative function, accomplished by promoting group and individual stability;
4. A growth function, accomplished by promoting innovation, creativity, and change; and
5. A problem-solving function, accomplished by promoting the quality of problem-solving.

Four items, also derived from the literature, were used to measure each function. All items were written as positive statements; for example, increases trust among members, prevents the accumulation of hostility, promotes accommodation between groups. Four choices were provided for each item: strongly agree, agree, disagree, and strongly disagree.

Respondents used the "agree" and "disagree" categories more frequently than the "strongly agree" or "strongly disagree" categories; therefore, the categories were collapsed to "agree" and "disagree." Responses for each of the functions appear in Table 71-1.

Only one function—the unifying function—had a higher percentage of responses in the "disagree" category, and this occurred only with deans and not with directors. The "disagree" category was chosen more frequently by deans than by directors for all the functions. When t-tests were used to test for significant differences in the responses of deans and directors, the differences were statistically significant (p < .05) for all the functions except the preserving function.

Other variables measured in this study may relate to the differences in responses. Agreement with the functions of conflict was found to be significantly greater (p < .01) in organizations with over 100 staff members, and these organizations were predominantly hospitals (n = 210) rather than colleges (n = 6). Agreement was also significantly greater (p < .05) if the administrator indicated a high degree of decisional autonomy in her or his position. Autonomy was rated higher by directors (74% was very high or high) than by deans (48% very high or high).

The findings of this study indicate that these administrators positively view outcomes of conflict related to growth and problem solving. These functions are to a large extent dependent on the creative, innovative, and analytical skills of staffs. There was less agreement with the preserving and unifying functions of conflict, functions that are more dependent on interpersonal relationships. These findings are consistent with the study of nurse administrators' perceptions of the effects of conflict[12] and indicate the need for nurse administrators to be aware of the potentially negative effects of conflict on group relations when selecting management strategies.

THE USE OF CONFLICT IN NURSING

Conflict can be a positive force for nursing if it is used to foster growth-producing change in the profession and in the organizations in which nurses work. However, nurses must know how to use conflict effectively if these benefits are to be realized. Effective use consists of more than selecting the appropriate management strategy; it means analyzing the type of issue and the situational components that help or hinder conflict resolution. Information about the steps to be taken for the effective management of conflict is readily available; therefore, the following discussion addresses other factors that I believe are important if conflict is to benefit nursing.

Nurses must develop a positive attitude toward conflict.[11] Recognizing the potential benefits to be gained from conflict should encourage nurses to develop the skills necessary to manage conflict. Conversely, recognizing the potential for destructive outcomes should alert nurses to the areas that need to be monitored when conflict occurs. Increased knowledge about the processes of conflict should encourage thoughtful selection of management strategies.

Nurses need to understand the importance of identifying the type of issue involved in a conflict situation, because conflicts about values and ends are more divisive than conflicts about means. Values are deeply held beliefs unlikely to be amenable to negotiation. If differences in values are suspected, value-clarification techniques may assist in identifying the differences. Managing value conflicts may require downgrading the conflict by defining it as a problem in means, as, for example, a resource problem or a priority problem.[22] If decisions about admissions to an intensive care unit are defined as priority problems rather than value problems, well-defined admission criteria can more readily be developed. It is also important to recognize when value conflicts cannot be resolved. In these cases, agreements must be reached about how the group will continue to function or unilateral action taken even though it may fragment the group temporarily. Change in the educational requirements for the registered nurse examination in North Dakota is an example of unilateral action taken by the board of nursing in a conflict that could not be resolved. The profession may benefit if this strategy is used more often.

Nurses need to become more astute about predicting potential conflicts if they are to be prepared to deal with them effectively. Although the method chosen by the American Medical Association (the preparation of certified care technicians) to alleviate the shortage of nurses in acute care settings could not be predicted, nursing could anticipate some action by physicians or hospitals if beds continued to close due to a shortage of nurses. Prior, less severe shortages resulted in proposals for institutional licensure, and it could be anticipated that other groups would once again devise solutions for nursing. Nurses need to become more skilled at obtaining information and at "reading" the environment if they are to foresee potential conflicts in time to prepare effective responses.

Nurses need to recognize the essential role of power in conflict. Collaboration and compromise are identified as the most effective strategies for managing conflict to achieve long-term benefits. However, collaboration is rarely used when there is a wide difference in power between the groups involved, and compromise becomes competition when the differences in power allow one group to predominate. This has been one of the major drawbacks to collaboration between nursing and medicine. As shifts in power take place in the health care arena, it will behoove nursing to be as concerned with empowering all nurses in the work setting as with empowering professional organizations and nursing leaders. Nursing will not be an autonomous profession until all professional nurses have the opportunity to control their practice. Decisional autonomy is a prerequisite to action; responses are limited if one has no authority to act.

Nursing must resolve the entry-into-practice issue. The inability of the profession to control the requirements for entry into the profession makes it impossible to define the functions of the registered nurse in a way that is meaningful to other professionals. This situation may hinder opportunities for collaboration when conflict arises. The inability to specify the behaviors expected of a professional nurse is the source of multiple conflicts in nursing. It has contributed to the rigid hierarchy and controls common in health care settings and to the role conflicts prevalent in nursing.

SUMMARY

This chapter has attempted to make the process of conflict and its potential benefits meaningful for the issues faced by nurses. It is hoped that this discussion will encourage nurses to increase their understanding of conflict. Readers may disagree with the ideas presented here; ideally, they will give rise to dissension, discussion, and more creative and effective solutions to the conflicts confronting nursing.

REFERENCES

1. Aydelotte MK: The nurse executive in 2000 AD: role and functions. In Johnson M, editor: Series on nursing administration, Vol 1, Menlo Park, Calif, 1987, Addison.
2. Cochran DS, Schnake M, and Earl R: Effect of organizational size on conflict frequency and location in hospitals, Journal of Management Studies 20(4):441, 1983.
3. Gray JL and Starke FA: Organizational behavior: concepts and applications, Columbus, Ohio, 1980, Charles E Merrill.
4. Guy ME: Interdisciplinary conflict and organizational complexity, Hospital and Health Services Administration 31(1):111, 1986.
5. Guy ME: An interorganizational analysis of interdisciplinary conflict in a psychiatric hospital, Administration in Mental Health 12(1):45, 1984.
6. Johnson M: Nurse administrators' perceptions of the utility of conflict as related to personal and organizational characteristics, Doctoral thesis, University of Iowa, Iowa City, 1986.
7. Julian JW, Bishop DW, and Fiedler FE: Quasi-therapeutic effects of intergroup competition, Journal of Personality and Social Psychology 3(3):321, 1966.
8. Kasparek AJ: Role conflict experienced and conflict strategies used by nurse managers, master's thesis, Iowa City, University of Iowa, 1984, University of Iowa.
9. Katz D and Kahn RL: The social psychology of organizations, New York, 1966, John Wiley & Sons, Inc.
10. Kramer M: Reality shock: why nurses leave nursing, St Louis, 1974, The CV Mosby Co.
11. Kramer M and Schmalenberg CE: Conflict: the cutting edge of growth, J Nurs Adm 6(8):19, 1976.
12. Myrtle RC and Glogow E: How nursing administrators view conflict, Nurs Res 27(2):103, 1978.
13. Perrow C: Complex organizations: a critical essay, ed 2, Glenview, Ill, 1979, Scott, Foresman & Co.
14. Pondy LR: Organizational conflict: concepts and models, Administrative Science Quarterly 12(2):296, 1967.
15. Rahem MA: Managing conflict in organizations, New York, 1986, Praeger.
16. Robbins SP: Managing organizational conflict: a nontraditional approach, Englewood Cliffs, NJ, 1974, Prentice-Hall.
17. Schwenk CR and Thomas H: Effects of conflicting analyses on managerial decision-making: a laboratory experiment, Decision Science 14(4):467, 1983.
18. Sexton DL: Organizational conflict: a creative or destructive force, Nursing Leadership 3(3):16, 1980.
19. Smith CG: Women, nurses, power conflict: competition and cooperative approaches. In Wieczorch RR, editor: Power, politics and policy in nursing, New York, 1985, Springer Publishing Co.
20. Snyder DL: New baccalaureate graduates' perceptions of organizational conflict, Nurs Res 31(5):300, 1982.
21. Walton RE and Dutton JM: The management of interdepartmental conflict: a model and a review, Administrative Science Quarterly 14(1):73, 1969.
22. Wax J: Solving ethical problems, AORN Journal 43(3):608, 1986.
23. Wehr P: Conflict regulation, Boulder, Colo, 1981, Westview Press.
24. Woodtli A: Conflict: insights before intervention, Nurse Educator 12(2):22, 1987.
25. Woodtli A: Deans of nursing: perceived sources of conflict and conflict handling modes, J Nurs Educ 26(7):272, 1987.
26. Zey-Ferrell M: Dimensions of organizations, Santa Monica, Calif, 1979, Goodyear.

CHAPTER 72

Traditional roles of women and nurses in the developing countries

GEORGINA DE CARRILLO

This chapter is about the traditional roles of women, their historical development, and their relationship to the primarily female nursing profession. Drawing on my own experience within a particular social context, I will limit my discussion to Ecuador and to the historical and cultural roots it shares with the Andean Pact countries (Ecuador, Columbia, Peru and Bolivia).

TRADITIONAL FEMALE ROLES

Throughout human history, the division of labor between men and women has been based on biological and sexual differences. Women as bearers and nurturers of children receive masculine protection against external dangers: nature, attacks by other groups and the everyday possibility of death.[10] Within this context men develop strength and aggressiveness and engage in combat, while women are given responsibility for maintaining the family and the home.

The Andean region was populated around 12,000 BC by nomadic tribes who subsisted by fishing, hunting, and gathering edible plants. Within these small communities there was a "natural" division of labor in which adult males did the hunting, which often involved lengthy absences from the home, and women and children gathered food. Sixty percent of the family diet consisted of vegetables; therefore the gathering of food was an essential activity. Each sex played an important role in the survival of the group.[1]

Over centuries these groups came to rely less on hunting for subsistence and more on agriculture, allowing for greater control and reliability of food sources. With the regulation of food production, people were able to settle in particular areas, leading to advances in building construction and architecture and other utilitarian products such as ceramics and textiles.

Women played an important role in agriculture during this period, attested to by the archeological discoveries of female fertility figures symbolizing the fertility of the earth.[1]

Women had a store of knowledge about gestation, pregnancy, labor, childbirth and lactation. Mothers transmitted their experiences and knowledge to their daughters, gradually resulting in a very rich empirical knowledge of pregnancy and labor. Older women, probably grandmothers, with more experience, acted as midwives, originating one of the first divisions of medical work.[5]

At about 6000 BC the shaman, or chief, appeared. Shamans created ritual calendars by observing atmospheric events, and held positions of great power in their communities through their association with magic, religion, and medicine. There is some evidence that women also acted as shamans.

With the establishment of trade around 2000 BC, women assumed new roles. The discovery of metals led to the growth of new handicraft traditions. Women became artisans, making and selling their own craftwork and thus exercising control over their labor.

About 1000 BC geographical power was centralized and assumed by the *cacicazgos*, marking the beginning of the state. The cacique ruled over a large work force and received tribute from laborers in the form of textiles, jewelry, and decorative items. Many women were thus involved in the manufacture of dye, thread, cloth, and jewelry.

Women in the pre-Columbian period were very active members of the community, occupying marginal or powerful roles according to the circumstances of the social group, not because they were women. Some women inherited positions as *cacicazgos;* sex was not important where leadership was concerned. For example, Dolores Quilago was the female cacique who led the defense of Cochasqui, a town north of Quito, Equador. She died at the hands of the enemy just like any other warrior defending her or his territory.[2]

The Spanish conquest of much of Latin America led to the imposition of European culture and its ideology of female inferiority transmitted through religion, education, and a rigid division of labor between the sexes. The subordination of women has an extensive history starting from the Aristotelian idea that woman is inferior because she lacks certain qualities; she suffers from a natural defectiveness. This notion was echoed by Thomas Aquinas, who believed that "a woman is a frustrated male." Julian Brenda said, "Man considers himself without a woman and woman does not consider herself without a man." Freud saw women as merely second-class males.[6] These traditional conceptions of women and their roles are still very influential in developing countries and have resisted the few weak efforts to overcome them.

THE CONTEMPORARY SITUATION

The subordination of women is the product of sociohistorical determinants. One prominent view holds that women's subordination is closely linked to class-based societies. The material bases of a society determine social relations, defining male-female relations and family roles that in turn become embedded in social ideology.[8]

Andean countries such as Ecuador today face complex and severe socioeconomic problems that curtail possibilities for development. Thousands of children die every year of malnutrition. Many are unable to attend school either because they must work to help support their families, or because schooling is not available for everyone. Millions of people migrate to the cities from the country because their lands have been appropriated and their cultures eroded. Large numbers of people are unemployed.

This panorama is enlarged by the numbers of illiterate women with no chance for education, training, or jobs, desperate housewives unable to fulfill basic family needs for food, and young women who have become servants, street sellers, or prostitutes because they can find no other work. On the other hand, we find paternalistic and protective laws exist on paper but are not really enforced, low salaries for women, a two-session working day, unemployment, obstacles to political participation, the heavy use of mass com-

munication media, and many other facts attesting to the realities of life for women in Latin America.[8]

THE "NATURAL" ROLE OF WOMEN

Although social structures vary in Andean countries, all women share the common denominators given by tradition: subordination and social oppression. All women have a social role and a common end—as daughters, mothers, and wives. Male dominance exists at the social and family levels. "This ancestral fact, translated to everyday machismo, has prevented women's participation in activities other than domestic matters."[11]

Education maintains tradition and perpetuates the essentially domestic role of women: A girl is a future mother and future wife and consequently is indefinitely dependent on others. Her role is to serve her husband and to make his life pleasant. She must know how to cook, wash, and clean the house. Obedience is a natural fact; women are "to obey father, husband, and male workmates."[4]

The "Latin lover" image of men promoted in films is a tacit demonstration of ancestral violence, of the superiority of men who may be physically abusive and who treat women as possessions. Submission, passivity, and vulnerability (attributes of inferior beings) are identified with beauty and femininity. It is a masculine tradition to persuade women that they are queens in order for them to forget their slave condition.[9]

Violence against women takes other forms than physical mistreatment. Family planning that involves the use of dangerous contraceptives, illegal and unsafe abortions, social punishment for sexual conduct outside marriage, rape or the fear of rape all contribute to women's lack of autonomy, in contrast to the freedom enjoyed by men. Some of these factors may be responsible for pushing women into prostitution. As Lleras Camargo, the ex-president of Colombia, has said, "If prostitution is the oldest of known professions, it is due to the fact that the treatment received by women as 'pleasure objects' is as old as man."[3]

WOMEN AND WORK

It has already been established that socio-historical determinism and tradition impose a division of labor by sex, with housework and child care allocated to women.[13] Such duties are unpaid and receive little social recognition.

The percentage of women in Quito who work solely as housewives is decreasing. In fact, according to the 1974 census, 32% of women over 12 years of age worked outside the home. By 1986 that number had increased to 36%.[13]

When women work outside the home, they increase their income but their workload is often doubled because they are still responsible for domestic tasks. In addition, most women work in low-paying, low-prestige service jobs. The main occupations include domestic service, clerical or secretarial work, teaching, business, and dressmaking. The percentage of women holding professional or technical positions is very low. Women earn between 50% and 70% of what men are paid for the same type of work. This reinforces the idea that a woman's salary merely supplements the family income and her work is secondary.[13]

Roles of rural women

Country women represent 28% of the Ecuadorian population. Like all rural people in developing countries they face hardships stemming from shortages of cultivable land, water, education, and health services, among other things. Migration to the cities is high. Yet country women share unique problems. They must undertake a number of roles and tasks that require a 16-to 18-hour workday. These roles include child care and education, housework, animal care, craftwork, the planting and cultivation of crops, and commerce or trade. Rural women cook with firewood, carry water over long distances, wash their clothes in channels and rivers and care for and feed their children, while producing artisan work, tending animals, and weeding or engaging in other agricultural activities depending on the production cycle.[12]

Rural women usually start domestic work in early youth, remaining near their mothers at home, while males attend school and later may migrate to the cities in order to find work. Men seldom return home, leaving all responsibility for the family in women's hands. Often younger women also migrate to the city, where they find work as servants, laborers, or street sellers.

Roles of suburban women

Suburban women, in addition to their traditional domestic responsibilities, have been forced by economic factors to work ouside the home as well. Because there is no organized system of child care, women often must leave their children unsupervised when they go to work. Because men have greater mobility and often must travel great distances to find work, many women must take the role of family head. Researchers have found that approximately 20% of Ecuadorian households are headed by women, usually in conditions of great poverty.[7]

ROLES OF NURSES

Nursing is affected in two major ways by the traditional position of women in Ecuador. First , it is not considered a primary role for women in this male-dominated society. A woman is seen as a housewife, wife, and mother no matter what her job. Her responsibilities center around those roles, and individual or professional development takes away from home and family.

Second, nurses are considered workers or "second-class professionals" who are not entitled to the social prestige or economic rewards of other (male) professions. Nursing is seen as a specifically female practice or technique rather than a profession. The female or feminine is always valued less than the male or masculine in patriarchal societies.[2] Perceptions of nursing as a typically feminine profession are related to the "feminine" archetypes of self-denial, sacrifice, and above all, subordination to male authority—in this case, the medical doctor. Nursing's association with caretaking and nurturance emphasizes its feminine character.

Given these powerful premises, the challenge for nursing in Ecuador is enormous. Efforts have been made on the resource-forming level to provide critical education as an effective way of looking for solutions and fostering growth for our profession and the women who are part of it. Without major efforts, the role of nursing will continue to be limited and limiting. So nurses in Ecuador face a twofold task: to tranform perceptions of nursing so that it will be valued as a profession equal to others in economic and social status; and to take on the roles of working women, mothers, and wives with the right to be complete human beings—to grow intellectually, to develop professionally, to assume responsibilities, and to make decisions as nurses and women who have the obligation to build a better world for all.

REFERENCES

1. Adam R: Mujer en el Origen, Guía de la Mujer Ecuatoriana, p 16, 1986.
2. Castañeda I and others: Enfer mería, Cadena o Camino? México, 1986, Imprenta Apaunam.
3. Chavez E: Atrocidades Sexuales en el Ecuador, Loja, Ecuador, 1985, Imprenta El Nazareno.

4. Ernest M: El Círculo Vicioso de los Roles Naturales, Cuadernos de Nueva Mujer 1:10, 1984.

5. Estrella E: Medicina y Estructura Socioeconómica, Quito Ecuador, 1977, Editorial Belén.

6. Merana A: Lan Condición Femenina, México, 1977, Editorial Grijalvo.

7. Placencia M: La Lucha de la Mujer Suburbana, Cuadernos de Nueva Mujer 1:41, 1984.

8. Rodríguez L: Una Milenaria Historia de Opresión, Cuadernos de Nueva Mujer 1:68, 1984.

9. Rodríguez M: El Machismo, Guía de la Mujer Ecuatoriana, p 70, 1986.

10. Rodríguez S: La Media Historia, Guía de la Mujer Ecuatoriana, p 12, 1986.

11. Rosero R: La Mujer Ecuatoriana a través de la Historia, Cuadernos de Nueva Mujer 1:6, 1984.

12. Rosero R: Las Mujeres Campesinas, Cuadernos de Nueva Mujer 1:36, 1984.

13. Sánches N: La Explotación Feminina en Cifras, Cuadernos de Nueva Mujer 1:28, 1984.

PART ELEVEN

CULTURAL DIVERSITY

Cultural diversity: a troublesome must for nursing

JOANNE COMI McCLOSKEY
HELEN KENNEDY GRACE

While the United States is becoming ever more culturally diverse, nursing remains remarkably homogenous. Over 90% of nurses are white. Most are from working-class or middle-class backgrounds, and enter nursing at an early age. In light of the current nursing shortage, the decline in numbers of students entering nursing educational programs, and the increased numbers of women entering other professional fields, the only way for the profession to maintain sufficient numbers to meet the demands for nursing services is to become more diverse culturally. This involves both racial and gender diversity. The following section raises some troublesome questions about the ability of nursing to incorporate concepts of cultural diversity, not only in terms of the students entering the field but also in terms of the content taught in nursing education programs.

Brink opens this section by addressing the question, "Cultural diversity in nursing: how much can we tolerate?" Starting by examining the curricular content in nursing programs, she notes that minimal attention is paid to this content in most nursing programs. She concludes that "nurses prefer formula nursing" and that they prefer to teach as if nursing care is culture free. Although three nursing education programs recognize content in transcultural nursing as an identifiable part of their curriculum, most programs integrate this content across the curriculum. This results in the content largely being ignored. Brink recommends that if the content is to be integrated, all faculty should have a background in transcultural nursing issues; continuing education for faculty is one way to address the existing deficit. Another alternative is to employ transcultural specialists to teach such content.

With respect to the student body, Brink concludes that faculty members prefer a homogeneous student body and that there are few concerted efforts to recruit students from different ethnic groups. This limits the exposure of the majority of students to diverse backgrounds and contributes to the narrow background of many nurses. Understandably, given the small percentage of nurses from ethnic minorities, the number of faculty from different cultural groups is also minimal. Whereas one approach to increasing the experiences of student nurses with ethnic minorities would be to place them in clinical practice settings where nurses from diverse ethnic groups practice, there are limited opportunities for interaction between students and health personnel from different cultural backgrounds. Brink's chapter leads readers to conclude that the answer to the question, How much cultural diversity can nursing tolerate? is, not much.

Turning specifically to the dearth of students from different cultural groups, Furuta and Lipson observe that there has been little change in the composition of the nursing student body over the past 20 years. The affirmative action programs of the 1960s have faded from view. The circular problems of few faculty role models and isolated minority students serve to reinforce and maintain the limited number of minorities entering the field. Noting that leadership begins at the top, Furuta and Lipson set forth a number of recommendations: (1) create a culturally sensitive environment, (2) enroll a cohort of minority students, (3) include cultural content in nursing, (4) implement a systematic recruitment effort that reaches out to ethnic minorities, (5) develop a minority applicant pool, (6) formalize nontraditional admissions criteria, (6) mainstream student services, and (7) recruit minority faculty.

Moving from the deficits described above, Leininger asserts that transcultural nursing forms an arching framework for all aspects of nursing.

Nurses must not only become actively involved in discovering and learning about diverse cultures and their relationships to nursing phenomena but must know how to function creatively as transcultural nurse generalists and specialists to serve many different people.

Arguing for culturally congruent care giving, Leininger identifies five major issues in transcultural nursing: (1) the lack of knowledgeable nurses prepared in transcultural nursing, (2) the limitation of current theoretical perspectives in relation to transcultural concepts, (3) the challenge of preparing nursing service personnel to provide direct community-based nursing care to culturally diverse groups, (4) the problems of exporting undergraduate and graduate programs internationally when these educational models are incongruent with other cultural contexts, and (5) the limitations of nursing research primarily oriented to quantitative measures and ignoring the qualitative issues related to cultural diversity of the population being researched.

In their chapter Reimer and Fox argue that nursing's current approach to culture is not helpful. First, they trace the historical evolution of the inclusion of cultural dimensions in nursing education and practice. They conclude that nursing uses a stereotypic approach to culture. Nurses first identify typical characteristics or categories of particular ethnic groups and then, in the rhetoric of a holistic approach, recombine these disparate parts. Reimer and Fox say that this process of breaking down into categories and recombining parts only preserves the distinctions between nurse and patient. Nurses fail to realize, the authors argue, that all categories imposed on the patient's culture arise from the nurse's culture and therefore make the patient into an object, which distances the nurse from the patient. They urge us to move from an attitude or approach that recognizes differences to one that recognizes similarities. Knowing about other cultures is desirable, but naming and categorizing differences is not. Nurses should develop an attitude of compassion, not distinction.

Turning to the issue of gender diversity, Halloran analyzes forces that have contributed to keeping men out of nursing. Ironically, although Florence Nightingale, in establishing nursing, helped to overcome social barriers excluding middle- and upper-class women from participating in nondomestic economic activity, nursing in turn has constructed social barriers. Having established nursing as a field acceptable for women to enter, nursing has had difficulty incorporating men into the field. Although increasing numbers of men are entering the profession, only 3% of nurses are men. The issue of quality of care for certain patients gave rise in the early twentieth century to the creation of specific training programs to prepare men for nursing. In the post-Nightingale period men were recruited to attend to mental patients and to provide care in certain areas such as male urology.

This early trend was disrupted by the relative paucity of men in military nursing, particularly in World War I. Men were recruited to fight the war, and women to nurse the injured. This orientation extended into World War II and resulted in a marked decrease in men entering nursing. The few men in the profession who wished to serve their country as nurses were rejected by the military. In the Vietnam War these policies were reversed, and as a result, a number of men served as military nurses. These role models influenced a number of medics and corpsmen to enter nursing and have been a factor in the increased enrollment of men in nursing programs in recent years.

Economic cycles contribute significantly to increases or decreases in the number of men entering nursing. But perhaps the most significant barrier that remains today is the definition of nursing as "woman's work." The economic effects of this gender bias are continuing low salaries for nurses. Noting the increased expenditures for educational programs in fields dominated by men, the decrease in spending for nursing education programs, and the inequity of salary and working conditions for nurses, Halloran argues that economic redistribution is the only lasting way to address the problem of the lack of men in nursing.

The American Assembly for Men in Nursing has become a vocal force in addressing questions of the role gender should play in the nursing profession, particularly in relation to entry into nursing education programs and access to employment in nursing. Halloran concludes:

Men nurses are not the answer to problems of the nursing profession, but their presence in greater numbers may well be a barometer of the economic value society affords nurses. If men in nursing are that barometer, recent trends in men's enrollment indicate that society is too slowly moving forward with its economic valuation of nurses.

Shifting discussion away from the nursing profession per se, Kus raises issues related to care of unpopular clients. Noting that defining a client as unpopular is a result of an external evaluation placed upon that person by the nurse, Kus analyzes factors contributing to this valuation. Low social value, questionable moral worth, stigmata, a perception that the individual's problem is the result of voluntary behavior, fear-inspiring conditions, negative behavior of patients, or the inability of the nurse to deal with the patient's condition, all contribute to labeling some clients as unpopular. As a result of this valuation, nurses may withdraw from care of such patients or engage in behavior expressing their hostility. Kus argues that nurses need to be honest and acknowledge that certain patients are unpopular with them, analyze the factors that contribute to this problem, and then find ways of dealing with their feelings. Arguing that nurses are nurses at all times, not just when they are officially working, and that their concerns for humankind must extend to all areas of life, Kus encourages nurses to become social activists involved in issues such as the struggle against the dehumanization of prisoners. He concludes:

The mistreatment of fellow human beings should rekindle a fire in each and every one of us nurses, a fire born of rage and fervor, a fire which will rock the very foundations of our profession in a radical social activism which will not stop until every human on Earth is treated with true dignity.

Turning to the international scene, Grace addresses issues related to international students and the importance of making graduate education relevant to the needs of this population. After describing international students from developing countries and outlining the expectations facing graduates on return to their countries, she makes recommendations for modifying graduate education to provide appropriate educational experiences.

The challenge of achieving greater cultural diversity in nursing is one of the most pressing issues of the profession today. Nursing shortage issues simply cannot be addressed unless there is greater diversity among students entering the field. Minorities cannot continue to be shut out of the profession and relegated to menial support roles. The increasing numbers of women in traditionally male fields and the corresponding decline in women entering professions such as nursing must be counterbalanced by increases in the proportion of men in nursing. Traditional college-level students are no longer an adequate pool for nursing education programs. Nursing as a second career, or as the object of mid-life career changes, must also become an accepted phenomenon.

As efforts are mounted to ensure diversity in the students entering nursing, attention must be paid to cultivating a pool of nurses from underrepresented groups to become teachers and managers in the field. It is only as the profession becomes more culturally diverse that it can attend to the culturally multifaceted dimensions of nursing practice.

CHAPTER 73

Debate

Cultural diversity in nursing

How much can we tolerate?

PAMELA J. BRINK

When nurses talk about cultural diversity, they often mean something like, "cultural diversity is how to assess the cultural variable." This definition implies that cultural diversity constitutes a database from which to derive a nursing diagnosis. One of the basic meanings of cultural diversity in nursing has to do with cultural diversity content in basic nursing education. A second meaning refers to the racial, national, and ethnic diversity of the nursing school student body. Beyond that, cultural diversity also can mean the racial, national, and ethnic diversity of the faculty, or of the staff and administration in clinical settings. In this text, cultural diversity also includes the issue of men in nursing (see Chapter 77). The answer to the question, How much cultural diversity can nursing tolerate? will differ depending on the particular type of cultural diversity referred to.

CULTURAL DIVERSITY CONTENT IN THE CURRICULUM

In the 1960s the Division of Nursing provided traineeships to nurses interested in doctoral study in anthropology (among other fields) for the express purpose of producing nurses doctorally prepared in anthropological theory and methods. The basic concept these nurses brought back to nursing was that of cultural diversity. Most were trained in cultural anthropology, some in biological anthropology, but all were convinced of the need to include cultural as well as biological diversity in nursing's armamentarium of knowledge. A number of textbooks were written (predominantly in the 1970s) to provide students and faculty with an introduction to the issue.[1-10] Today literature on cultural diversity is found primarily in chapters of clinical texts, and some articles also appear in professional nursing journals.

Beliefs about the importance of cultural diversity in the curriculum

Some schools of nursing (notably the University of Washington at Seattle, the University of Utah at Salt Lake City, and the University of Miami), have developed cultural diversity as a major component of the curriculum and devote prerequisite and required courses to the topic. In these schools not only is introductory anthropology a prerequisite to nursing, but some form of medical anthropology or transcultural nursing also is part of the undergraduate nursing curriculum. And, at the graduate level, students can specialize in transcultural nursing.

In other schools of nursing, cultural diversity is not considered a major part of the curriculum. Anthropology is not required and the only cultural diversity content occurs in introductory sociology courses that address the sociocultural problems of American ethnic groups. In these schools an advanced course in sociology (even medical sociology) is not considered necessary.

The predominant American belief system appears to view cultural diversity as relatively unimportant subject for study. I can just hear some of my colleagues saying, "I think cultural diversity is very important, and I stress to all my students that they must assess the cultural variable!" My rejoinder would be, "Good! Then in your list of curricular priorities, of what students absolutely MUST know to graduate from your school, where do you place cultural diversity? In the top 10? In the top 20? The top 30?" Then I would ask, "Other than demanding that your student assess the cultural variable, how do you assist them to learn how to do that in your clinical setting? Please tell me, step by step, what you do." Although some faculty would be able to describe specific teaching techniques, most would not.

How cultural diversity should be taught

Opinions differ as to how cultural diversity should be taught. Nurses trained in anthropology believe that both an introductory course in anthropology and an upper-division course in cultural or medical anthropology are necessary to teach the concepts of cultural relativity and biological diversity. These nurses argue that students need to understand not only how beliefs and values affect customary patterns of behavior and social mores, but also how evolution, gene pools, and environmental isolation have produced specialized biological variations that affect health and illness, and how differing economies (from horticulture and herding to a cash economy) create certain disease patterns and curing techniques that are relevant to the cultural group. Consequently, nurse-anthropologists are concerned that nursing students learn about varying human populations and their health and nursing problems, not just about health problems in their own particular communities. Cultural diversity is developed as a global theme, making it important to expose students to the world as much as to their own country.

Some schools of nursing incorporate only medical anthropology as a required or elective course, whereas others rely on introductory sociology or medical sociology to provide cultural diversity content. Sociology and anthropology, however, are separate fields in the United States, each providing different content. The theory and methods of one discipline do not substitute for the theory and methods of the other. Both content areas are important components of nursing education.

To what degree is cultural diversity actually taught?

In many schools of nursing, perhaps because it was once required by the National League for Nursing (NLN) for accreditation, cultural diversity content remains as a strand in the formal written curriculum. In reality, however, cultural diversity content is frequently ignored. Faculty often are unprepared to teach this content, passing their ignorance on to their students. In other schools of nursing faculty who are prepared to teach the content area are not asked to do so or to advise other faculty on related lecture content. In still other schools of nursing, cultural diversity is treated as an important curricular component, taught by competent, knowledgeable members of the faculty and for which students are held accountable.

Opinions differ as to whether cultural diversity is best taught through incorporation into existing courses or in separate courses. Both approaches have advantages and disadvantages. When approached as a curricular strand, cultural diversity is in danger of never being taught. For any curricular strand, someone must be able to teach the content at each level, monitor the progress of that strand, and monitor students' increasing facility with that content. In addition, lectures on cultural diversity by themselves are not sufficient. The student must be able to apply that knowledge in the clinical setting. Culturally relevant assessments and interventions cannot be supervised and evaluated by faculty who themselves are not specialists or perhaps not even knowledgeable in this area.

When cultural diversity is taught in separate courses, responsibility for the students' level of knowledge clearly falls on the individual teaching the course. The instructor is expected to be conversant with the content, and all students presumably are uniformly exposed to this content in any given term. Application of this knowledge to clinical problems, however, remains problematic. Formal course work can provide the necessary knowledge base from which to develop culturally relevant skills, but faculty who cannot apply cultural content will impede skill development in their students.

Evidence for lack of cultural diversity content in curriculum

American nurses know very little about cultural diversity and are not taught much about the topic. Evidence supporting this claim is easy to find.

One indicator of professional interest in a topic is the number of books in the area. Most of the 1970s textbooks mentioned previously are out of print, primarily because schools of nursing failed to adopt them. U.S. publishers are now reluctant to publish books on cultural diversity for nursing simply because they have not sold well in the past. Why didn't the books sell? Aside from the subject not being taught at all, the number of courses targeted to cultural diversity may well have been insufficient to support the texts. Alternatively, faculty members teaching cultural diversity as a curricular strand were not able to agree on a single text that could be used throughout the curriculum. A third possibility is that faculty relied on clinical texts featuring a chapter on cultural diversity. So one can surmise, based on the lack of cultural diversity textbooks presently available, that nurses' knowledge of cultural diversity gained from basic nursing education is very limited.

One difficulty involved in writing a nursing textbook on cultural diversity is determining what content to emphasize. The texts that have survived use the "cookbook" approach to nursing the culturally different client: "This is a black client, this is how to nurse him"; or "This is a Mexican-American client, and this is how to nurse her"; or "This is an Asian client who needs to be assessed for 1, 2, and 3. Then intervene in 2, 3, and 4." These books are much more popular than texts that provide theories of cultural diversity and allow the student to make the application to the particular client. Apparently nurses prefer formula nursing.

The problem is that in cultural diversity the emphasis is on diversity rather than homogeneity. Nurses who have studied anthropology have discovered that there is more diversity within than across cultures, and that once they try to pin down an individual in terms of cultural differences they find culture to be ephemeral. Although nurses may seek guidelines and rules to work from and generalizations to increase nursing efficiency, anthropology cannot provide such shortcut strategies. It is easy to become frustrated, therefore, with the entire concept of cultural diversity because it is so difficult to pin down. Cultural diversity remains elusive without a theoretical framework. Theories provide the base from which each nurse can develop an assessment tool that will generate for each client cultural rules and regulations that are inviolate and those that are nice but not mandatory. In other words, once the nurse is able to sort out the important rules for the client's behavior, a determination can be made about appropriate nursing care.

One of the difficulties of developing nursing care strategies is that there are so few nursing diagnoses on cultural diversity. As a result, there are even fewer nursing interventions. The lack of nursing diagnoses and interventions that reflect cultural diversity content is another indication of nursing's seeming lack of interest in this area.

Proposed remedies

One remedy for the existing weaknesses is to prepare all faculty to teach cultural diversity content in both lecture and clinical settings. Not everyone needs to be a nurse-anthropologist, nor does everyone need to have a doctoral degree in transcultural nursing; however, exposing every nursing faculty member to this content through continuing education courses could increase both their enthusiasm and their knowledge about this important area of nursing. Another remedy could be to designate at least one member of the faculty as a transcultural nursing authority, to be held responsible for developing and teaching the cultural diversity content in the curriculum. That individual would have as much credence as the critical care specialist and would be given as much respect for their particular knowledge base as for any other clinical area. Such faculty members will need advanced preparation to teach this content if they have not received training in anthropology or transcultural nursing previously. Continuing education courses and workshops on cultural diversity could be developed to prepare that individual.

Cultural diversity content can be presented to students in a number of ways. The two most frequently used approaches have been to develop required or elective courses in the basic curriculum or to weave a curricular strand that runs through all courses. In addition, students deliberately can be given clinical placements in culturally diverse neighborhoods and be required to include cultural diagnoses and interventions in their care plans. For schools of nursing that are not in culturally diverse neighborhoods, appropriate clinical placements might require busing students out of the local area. For example, a school in Iowa might send its students to Chicago, Minneapolis, or Kansas City, or provide for optional study-abroad experiences. Some undergraduate students have negotiated for experiences on American Indian reservations, clinics in migrant workers' camps, a year of study in Nigeria, and so on. Another alternative is to invite students or clients from other cultures or ethnic groups to talk to students about their experiences with health and illness at home. If every clinical course contained a panel of experts (clients from different ethnic and cultural backgrounds) who talked about their experience with that particular clinical area, allowing for student-client interaction and questions afterwards, at least some exposure to cultural diversity could be achieved. In addition, the expert panel approach may be less costly than sending students away.

All these solutions need support by the designated head of the school or department of nursing. Cultural diversity will not be taught if the dean or department chair does not think it is important. Conversely, cultural diversity will be taught and taught well if made a priority by the chief executive officer. Just as in any other organizational structure, the leader both sets the tone of the school or department and strongly influences faculty response. Cultural diversity, as with any other decision, has budgetary implications.

CULTURAL DIVERSITY IN THE STUDENT BODY

A second major area of cultural diversity is the diversity of the student population. For the most part, faculties prefer a homogeneous student body. Homogeneity makes the task of teaching easier. One can better determine the appropriate content, pace, clinical experiences, examinations, and level of reading assignments when students share common backgrounds and ability levels. Indeed, one duty of selection committees is to provide a fairly homogeneous student group. Too much diversity impedes efficiency as content, pace, experience, and readings must expand to take into account a broader range of student abilities and backgrounds. When faculty have been accustomed to teaching students with a mean grade point average (GPA) of 3.5, they will complain bitterly when the mean GPA drops to 3.0. If faculty complain that it is harder to teach a fairly homogeneous group with a lower mean GPA, how much more will they complain when a lower mean GPA occurs in conjunction with an increase in heterogeneity and a wider range of abilities? How many faculty prefer not to teach foreign students to whom English is a second language because "they take too much time"? And time is indeed the issue, especially when classes are large, teacher-student contact hours are long, and faculty are pressed into other duties besides teaching. An added hardship is the expectation that students from other cultures will graduate with their peers rather than progressing more slowly through the program.

But a culturally diverse student population, although requiring more faculty time and effort, provides a breadth of experience for the American student who may not have had prior exposure to other cultures. Associating with people different from themselves ex-

poses students to different values and beliefs and provides them with the chance to know, like, and learn to respect people with diametrically opposed views and customs. Because American nurses are working more and more alongside nurses from other countries, it seems sensible to have them learn alongside students from other countries. In fact, international students can be used as informants about differential cultural beliefs, values, and health care practices, thus offering an educational resource not otherwise available. If this experience is valued, it will be given time and effort; if not, faculty will continue to complain of excess work loads.

One of the major tenets of Branch and Paxton's book[2] was that the ethnically diverse population of the United States deserves to be nursed by people who are not just knowledgeable about the special problems of particular subgroups but are themselves members of those groups. Branch and Paxton made a plea for more schools and departments to "open their doors wider"* to ethnic students of color and provide them with the chance for a nursing education even if it takes them longer to complete the program.

Although Branch and Paxton were referring specifically to the highly visible disadvantaged ethnic populations in the United States, their plea is easily extended to disadvantaged students from developing countries. Schools of nursing might consider sponsoring one student a year from a disadvantaged U.S. minority group or a Third World country to increase cultural awareness of students and faculty. Such sponsorship might be affected through institutional linkages, sister schools, or church affiliations. Students and faculty might raise the money for tuition and fees by providing services through fee-for-service nursing clinics. If a culturally diverse student body is desired, means of achieving that goal can be found.

CULTURAL DIVERSITY OF THE FACULTY

A third, rarely discussed, area of cultural diversity is the need for culturally diverse faculty to teach nursing students. This diversity can be achieved simply by hiring qualified faculty from American ethnic groups (an expedient approach), by recruiting faculty from other countries, or by seeking out faculty who have extensive experience with or knowledge of other cul-

*This concept derives from Boston University's seminal program of the early 1960s, ODWIN (Opening the Doors Wider in Nursing).

tures and countries. All three approaches would enhance the quality of the educational experience.

There are educationally prepared and doctorally trained "ethnic nurses of color" (in Branch and Paxton[2] terminology) competing for faculty positions. I still believe that when two applicants are equally qualified, the ethnic person of color should be given a slight edge in hiring to increase the numbers of culturally diverse faculty. When an ethnic minority nurse is available to lecture to students but is ineligible for a permanent faculty position (for whatever reasons), that nurse's expertise and experience should be used in whatever way possible. The relationship with the school may be formalized through the use of the "lecturer" title. Here, the sought-for expertise is in the form of nursing diagnoses and interventions specific to that individual's experience. These nurses would not be expected to teach courses on medical anthropology or transcultural nursing but rather would serve as guest lecturers for the cultural diversity strand in the curriculum.

A second resource for cultural diversity content is faculty members who have been Fulbright scholars, Peace Corps volunteers, missionaries, World Health Organization employees, or have conducted research on American, Third World, or other national populations. These faculty need to be part of the cultural diversity pool of expertise developed to lecture on cultural diversity content to provide clinical examples from their experience. The wealth of experience provided by our own faculties is frequently wasted.

A third resource for cultural diversity content is faculty from other schools of nursing around the world. There are a variety of ways to solicit their lecture services on a temporary or permanent basis. Formal university linkages can facilitate faculty and student exchanges for varying periods of time. Foreign faculty who come to a U.S. university to complete requirements for a degree can serve as faculty lecturers during that time. If these faculty were to provide an occasional lecture in every course during the period of the stay, each student in the school would have at least one contact with a person from that country. A lecture beginning with, "In my country when a person has an automobile accident . . ." could finish with a reconstruction of emergency services, orthopedics, or surgery. A lecture beginning, "In my country when a woman becomes pregnant . . ." could move through household and family customs, compare traditional birthing methods to those of the Western health care delivery system, and provide anecdotal data from personal experiences with childbirth. Other lectures might begin, "In my country, nursing administrators are . . ." or "nurses become faculty by . . ." The ideas for such lectures are limited only by one's imagination.

Nurses from other countries also frequently visit the United States on an informal basis. Many would be delighted to deliver a lecture for a small honorarium. Any school interested in having a guest lecture by a foreign nurse can contact the International Council of Nurses or the World Health Organization for information.

Increasingly, the cultural diversity of the faculty will expand the range of cultural experiences to which students are exposed. Such expansion of cultural experiences is not merely desirable but necessary. How can nurses care for culturally, ethnically, and nationally diverse patients with any sense of familiarity if they have never met anyone from that or a similar culture?

Unfortunately, several barriers make such faculty expansion difficult to accomplish. All faculty members of schools of nursing are required to hold a valid state license to practice nursing. This requirement is held as sacred by those who do not want foreign nurses in their schools. The requirement of licensure is upheld by state boards of nursing to prevent unscrupulous, poorly trained nurses to practice bad nursing. Some nurses believe that faculty from Third World countries are so lacking in technological familiarity that they have nothing to offer our students. Others see European nurse researchers as conducting simplistic research with little to offer advanced U.S. students. For these reasons nurse faculty and deans are hesitant to invite foreign nurses to their schools, and support rigid state board regulations that prevent these nurses from teaching in the United States. I believe these practices and excuses should change.

CULTURAL DIVERSITY OF CLINICAL STAFF

The last area of cultural diversity I want to mention is rarely discussed in the literature. For some reason the cultural mix of staff in clinical settings is rarely seen as an educational advantage for students. Yet many clinical agencies are staffed by nurses from other countries who could provide clinical preceptorships in cultural content. When students present their cases these nurses could offer valuable advice on cultural differences, particularly if the patient is from the same country as the nurse. Third World physicians, who frequently come to the United States for residencies, could be tapped as resources for the health beliefs and practices in their own countries. Very little use is made of foreign staff members' expertise about their own countries. Our profession relies on educational degrees to validate an individual's expertise, giving little credence to experience as an avenue to such expertise. Yet many nationals in the United States have clinical experiences that could enhance students' learning.

Again, however, a culturally homogeneous staff is often easier to work with. Faculty understand staff members who share their background and experience and speak the same language. Working with staff of another country is time consuming and beset with communication problems. These difficulties in themselves are worthy of discussion; entire clinical conferences could be devoted to this issue. Patients are confronted with these cultural variations daily, yet no one talks about them. How does the American patient cope with nursing and medical staff from different countries who may have different expectations of the patient? How do students learn from foreign nationals? What is common and what is different? Again, such discussion assumes a knowledgeable moderator. And knowledge can come from experience as well as from short in-service courses.

Cultural diversity of clinical staff is not a choice but a reality. Nurses' abilities to work with a culturally diverse staff could be enhanced by exposing them to such environments as students. A knowledgeable teacher will lead discussions about the difficulties of working with people from different cultures and strategies for overcoming those difficulties. For example, foreign nurses are expected to make all the adjustments, and rather rapidly, with few American nurses seeking them out for what they can give.

WHAT MORE IS NEEDED?

American nurses need to respect cultural diversity in all four areas: educational content, students, faculty, and clinical staff. This respect can be demonstrated in a variety of ways other than those described above. First and foremost, state boards of nursing can improve nursing's relationship with other countries by relaxing the rules and regulations for foreign students, enabling them to obtain temporary licensure. This temporary licensure could be extended as a courtesy to foreign nurse faculty who come to the United States

to teach for brief periods. So long as they are employed as faculty, they could be granted a license to practice. In both instances, these nurses should work in U.S. institutions to learn how things are done and to take with them a better notion of what American nursing is really like. American nursing would not be contributing to the "brain drain" by mandating that foreign nurses have a regular license but would instead acknowledge that their presence, although temporary, is still valuable.

Second, American nurses can present more papers at conferences abroad and bring back with them the work done by other nurses to share with their students. Conversely, when an international conference is held near a school, faculty may find some of the participants willing to stay on an extra day or two to talk to their students.

In addition, nursing journals from other countries can be placed regularly on reading lists. U.S. nurses tend to read and refer only to their own journals, even though nurses in other countries are conducting valuable research in important areas. Reading foreign journals should be reciprocal—nurses in other countries are expected to keep up with research in the United States.

Finally, work groups or open forums at international meetings can facilitate exchange programs and linkages among faculties. Schools looking for particular persons with specific expertise can advertise through these organizations and interview applicants at meetings. Schools desiring to form linkages can advertise their particular interests at meetings. Such an open exchange of interest would be exciting and refreshing. European schools of nursing are beginning to request Fulbright scholars on a regular basis, seeking particular expertise for their new programs. American nurses need to know both that Fulbright awards exist and that several exchange programs are available for nurses.

How can we tolerate so much cultural diversity?

The United States' greatness rests in its enormous cultural diversity, its tolerance for a wide variety of ways of doing things. American nurses also can benefit from this diversity. Rather than seeking uniformity, homogeneity, and efficiency, cultural diversity in educational content, student populations, faculty, and clinical settings can be used to advantage.

Schools of nursing may have to allocate specific funds at the expense of other needs until cultural diversity is an accepted part of nursing education. To nourish cultural diversity, nurses will have to focus on it, give it our attention, and make it work. Without this attention, cultural diversity will remain a dream rather than a goal, and will never be a reality.

Cultural diversity does not happen peacefully, without struggle and strain. The United States has had numerous difficulties in coming to terms with its diverse population, in ensuring everyone the same freedoms and same opportunities. How then can we in nursing expect that our efforts to promote cultural diversity will go smoothly? Without conflict or pain, change and growth remain unattainable.

REFERENCES

1. Bauens EE, editor: The anthropology of health, St Louis, 1978, The CV Mosby Co.
2. Branch M and Paxton PP: Providing safe nursing care for ethnic people of color, New York, 1976, Appleton-Century-Crofts.
3. Brink PJ, editor: Transcultural nursing: a book of readings, Englewood Cliffs, NJ, 1976, Prentice Hall, Inc.
4. Clark AL, editor: Culture childbearing health professionals, Philadelphia, 1978, FA Davis Co.
5. Henderson G and Primeaux M, editors: Transcultural health care, Reading, Mass, 1981, Addison-Wesley Publishing Co, Inc.
6. Kay M, editor: The anthropology of birth, Philadelphia, 1980, FA Davis Co.
7. Leininger MM: Nursing and anthropology: two worlds to blend, New York, 1970, John Wiley & Sons, Inc.
8. Leininger M, editor: Transcultural nursing: concepts, theories, and practices, New York, 1978, John Wiley & Sons, Inc.
9. Orque MS, Block B, and Monrray LS: Ethnic nursing care: a multicultural approach, St Louis, 1983, The CV Mosby Co.
10. Spector RE: Cultural diversity in health and illness, New York, 1979, Appleton-Century-Crofts.

CHAPTER 74

Viewpoints

Where is cultural diversity in the student body?

BETTY S. FURUTA
JULIENE G. LIPSON

Twenty years ago, students in American schools of nursing were predominantly young, white, middle-class women. Nursing is much the same today. Proportionally, there are a few more ethnic students, but their numbers remain small. The multicultural expansion that has taken place in so many other areas of society has not occurred in professional nursing. Branch[2] has characterized this problem of ethnic underrepresentation as follows:

It is safe to say that the momentum of the 1960s and early 1970s has almost disappeared. Ethnic recruitment and retention programs have dropped in number and intensity. . . . This mood in nursing echoes the mood in the nation as a whole and it is a dismal prospect for both.

ISSUES

It is important that nursing recapture the lost momentum—important for the profession, its clients, and its practitioners. Nursing, caring for a culturally diverse population, must be equally diverse itself.

Cultural Diversity

In 1987, approximately 10.9% of students enrolled in registered nurse (RN) programs were black, 2.9% Hispanic, 2.0% Asian, and 0.7% Native American. These are not encouraging figures. Although there has been an increase in the enrollment of minority students in basic RN programs within the last decade, the percentage of those students admitted in 1987 (the most recent figures available) is only a few tenths of a percent different than in 1981. Only for blacks has there been an actual increase.[8]

In every case, too, the figures are not proportional to their respective populations, that is, far fewer minorities are nurses than would be expected from the size of their population groups. If nursing schools are not now representative of the ethnic population, they are even less likely to be so in the future. Immigration and a changing domestic population forecast a profound demographic shift in the United States. By the year 2000, one of every three Americans is projected to be an ethnic minority. Unless nursing can draw from this resource, it risks not serving the changing society of which it is a part.

Minority admissions

From the onset of federal regulations, affirmative action was to be voluntarily implemented in higher education but mandated in employment. And, in fact, student admissions did receive serious affirmative action attention at most schools, which meant accepting a minority applicant before a white one when both met the minimum requirements for admission. Still, few minorities were admitted. This raises the question of whether admission standards should be lowered for the sake of diversifying the student body. Perhaps a better question is whether standards are appropriate and valid for underrepresented groups.

The traditional indicators of academic achievement and capability—grade point average and standardized test scores—generally have been effective measures for applicants from the dominant society.[1] However, data also show that scores on standardized tests such as the Scholastic Aptitude Test (SAT) and Graduate Record Examination (GRE) are more often lowest for those from lower socioeconomic groups. Thus, the poor performance of this group might reflect educational deprivation rather than intellectual or academic capability.

Solo and token phenomena

After gaining admission even emotionally strong, academically superior minority students may experience occasional assaults on their self-esteem. One of the most common stressors is the "solo phenomenon," that is, being one of a kind or one of very few. Pettigrew[9] has stated that this phenomenon creates repeated experiences in which the individual feels self-consciously visible. Such persons cannot temporarily retreat into the anonymity of the group, which is a refuge for most others; nor does their situation allow opportunity to relax with their own kind. Minorities (men in nursing are another example) often feel the need to ascertain whether others are reacting to them as individuals or to their being different.

As a result, the expression of one's ethnic identity— being able to converse in one's native tongue or to share an ethnic insight—tends to be diluted. It may become too threatening or require too much effort to maintain one's ethnic face.[3] Students might opt to leave school rather than endure the continual tension that accompanies such self-consciousness. The solo phenomenon might manifest itself until the cultural diversity of the student body approaches 20%.[9]

The "token phenomenon" is a companion to the solo experience. Tokenism occurs when an institution makes a minimal but visible gesture of compliance to a policy or practice. A consequence of tokenism in affirmative action is the persistent question usually unvoiced both by the ethnic student and others, as to whether admission was earned on academic merit or represented institutional tokenism. Being ethnically identifiable, even outstanding students may occasionally wonder whether they are tokens. Also, majority students may raise the same question and unfairly communicate that the person should not have been admitted.

Minority faculty

A major constraint to increasing cultural diversity in the student body is its absence among faculty. Nursing schools are confronted with a paradox in their quest to substantially increase minority faculty: an institution may find it easier to appoint underrepresented faculty to clinical or other nontenured positions, that do not require the rigor of an academic-ladder appointment. Because such positions are likely to be funded by grants or other less stable resources, these same faculty are vulnerable to termination.

Besides customary assignments and responsibilities, ethnic faculty also may inherit some tasks not shared by others. These may include being assigned as an adviser to most, if not all, minority students; being appointed the ethnic member to committees; and being asked to serve as the institution's ethnic representative at events. At best, such faculty members can become overburdened with too much to do and too little time in which to do it. At worst, they slip into institutional jeopardy due to inadequate productivity in research, publication, teaching, and professional or clinical activity—the important criteria for tenure. The net result is loss of minority faculty.

SUGGESTIONS

There is no question that nursing must attend to diversifying the student body and so regain the momentum that the profession once enjoyed. Leadership does begin at the top. The deans and directors of schools of nursing, together with their faculties, need to reaffirm their commitment to cultural diversity and give it high priority. There is ample evidence of previous actions that have resulted in the successful enrollment of more minority students into nursing schools, but they require *systematic*, *sustained*, *and organized* effort. The following are a few suggestions for how to realize such an effort.

Create a culturally sensitive learning environment

Serious improvement in cultural diversity requires shared responsibility between administration and faculty; both play a critical role in building a diverse student body and maintaining a culturally sensitive environment. Faculty commitment means a willingness to modify ineffective teaching and evaluation methods and a willingness to explore one's racial attitudes.[11] Minority students are apt to withdraw from nursing school if they repeatedly encounter what they perceive as bias, cultural naiveté, or entrenched ethnocentrism in insensitive faculty members.

Careful assignment of a faculty advise or mentor is indicated. It is useful to assign fewer advisees to those faculty members who are culturally sensitive and committed to helping underrepresented students succeed, so as to allow extra time for them to function as advisers and advocates. With regard to the psychological hazards of being a solo student, faculty members can be instrumental in helping minority students meet one another. Advisers should learn whether ethnic organizations exist on campus or nearby, and encourage newcomers to join.

Some programs make a deliberate attempt to group underrepresented students into a particular section of some required course. This provides ethnic students with an opportunity to engage one another directly on substantive nursing content and to learn about its cultural relevance.

Enroll a cohort of minority students

In a given admissions cycle, schools should admit as large a cohort of minority students as possible so that there is an opportunity for ethnic social support. To do otherwise is to make minority students vulnerable to the solo phenomenon and all that it implies. Attrition of ethnic students has been a problem in schools of nursing, particularly where they were few in number to begin with. The presence of a critical mass could provide not only peer support but also rich opportunities for cross-cultural learning for students in both the dominant and minority cultures.

Include cultural content in nursing

Since the mid-1970s nursing organizations have acknowledged the importance of cultural content in the curriculum (e.g., the American Nurses' Association's 1976 Code for Nurses; the National League for Nursing's 1977 mandate to include cultural content for accreditation). But implementation has been uneven, and the content in nursing education still places emphasis on the dominant culture. However, a diverse student body and the inclusion of cultural content in a nursing curriculum are mutually enhancing. An example was the Western Interstate Commission on Higher Education in Nursing project of the 1970s that aimed to help schools increase the number of students from underrepresented groups. It soon broadened its mission to encourage faculty to improve their cultural knowledge and awareness for more effective teaching.

With little diversity among faculty and students, misinformation and misunderstanding about various ethnicities may result in stereotyping. Direct experience allows the meaning of cultural differences to come alive and to be consensually validated. Ethnic and immigrant students can enrich the experiences of their peers by helping them understand what they have observed, read about, and inadvertently overlooked, and

by offering practical suggestions. Obviously, more bilingual nurses also would improve health care delivery to minorities: for example, Hispanics represent 19% of California's population, but only 0.5% of its nurses are bilingual in Spanish.[4]

Implement a systematic recruitment effort

Recruiting sufficient numbers of nursing students from a shrinking applicant pool is vexing enough, but locating qualified ethnic students is doubly vexing. Nursing needs to restore effective recruitment efforts, to institute change where needed, and to introduce new strategies. These are not easy to accomplish, but some important lessons have been learned from the past.

For instance, sustained personal contact with prospective applicants, wherever one might find them, can make a difference. Every qualified undergraduate minority who has expressed interest in the health sciences or professions should be regarded as a prospective nursing student and entered into the institutional recruitment file. At the least, that person should be personally contacted with information on current application deadlines and assistance on admission requirements. Not surprisingly, many matriculated students reveal that the reason for choosing to enroll at an institution was personal contact with an enrolled student, a faculty member, or an alumna. Students make the best recruiters, especially if they themselves are from ethnic minority groups.[6]

More individually tailored approaches are needed. Although recruiters may discuss topics (program planning, research, degree requirements, class schedules, part-time study options, availability of financial aid) germane to any student considering graduate study, the ethnic applicant might have specific additional concerns. For example, what is the attitude and receptiveness of the school toward ethnic minorities? What are the tangible and intangible costs to the family if a member attends graduate school? How will another degree materially help nursing practice in the ethnic community? These questions can be as varied as the needs of the individual.

Recruiting stellar minority graduate student applicants, particularly at the doctoral level, requires competitive effort. This might mean subsidizing a prospective student's travel and per diem to visit the campus and meet potential faculty mentors and matriculated students. In the current context of hospitals offering bounties and businesses paying headhunters to help recruit personnel, nursing schools also might provide honoraria and special recognition to alumnae for successfully recruiting and mentoring prospective ethnic applicants.

Develop a minority applicant pool

Some nursing schools have concluded that the way to increase minority enrollment is to develop their own applicant pool; that is, to create their own "pipeline." This can be done by structuring and maintaining linkages with schools and programs that have the potential to provide prospective applicants over time. One approach is for a nursing school to establish formal or semiformal "feeder school" arrangements with an obligation to sponsor recruitment activities. Examples include conducting recruitment presentations, inviting potential students to visit classes at the nursing school, offering regular counseling sessions with assigned advisers providing specialized help, and participating in preadmission or remediation courses. Able ethnic students would be identified and placed in the institutional pipeline, ideally with a mentor assigned to them. Thereafter the student would receive careful guidance for advancement into the next academic degree program, culminating, for some, in a doctorate.

Another approach to developing a minority pool is to create specific mentorship programs that engage promising students in some facet of nursing. An example is a univeristy school of nursing that offers undergraduates the opportunity to compete for one of several 10-week minority student summer research residencies. They would be awarded a modest stipend, mentored by recognized faculty researchers, and integrated into the research team during their residency. This model effectively immerses potential students in nursing research, which is a major focus of graduate study, and accords them some prestige as well. Another example involves mentorships in certain nursing specialties for preprofessional students during a 6-week summer program. The intention is to pique the interest of academically able minority students early in their careers by directly engaging them in the complexity and array of nursing activities that require advanced educational preparation.

One university has instituted formal mentorship programs for underrepresented doctoral students that include dissertation-year funding and eventual postdoctoral fellowships to prepare them for research and academic careers. In addition to the obvious pedagogical benefits that accrue from such mentor relationships, these doctoral nurses learn to present research papers at conferences, write grant proposals, and undergo the rigor of external peer review, all invaluable experiences. There are often social or media events to publicize these mentorships. A dividend of such public recognition is that faculty mentors are tacitly held accountable to help these promising students succeed.

Formalize nontraditional admissions criteria

Applicants from underrepresented groups, particularly those raised in disadvantaged socioeconomic circumstances or with problematic educational preparation, typically score lower on tests and may apply with marginal grade point averages. Carefully screened and given the opportunity to succeed in higher education, many of them do so. Supplemental criteria by which to evaluate these applicants usually are already requested by most nursing schools: employment records, including promotions; evidence of leadership and creative behavior wherever manifested; a personal interview to validate or clarify ambiguous details or elicit other information that might be helpful.

A school's commitment to cultural diversity should also be reflected in its willingness to admit applicants for whom English is a second language and whose culture, habits, and appearance may differ from that of other students. If much of their schooling was obtained elsewhere and English is their second language, immigrants can be faced with some difficult admissions problems. They may score poorly because of language problems or the unfamiliar construction of tests (multiple choice questions are unknown in many other cultures), and not because of a lack of aptitude. Nursing students from non-Western societies also may encounter difficulties with a different mode of reasoning and conceptualization because of a lack of knowledge of certain required subjects, typically the social and behavioral sciences, or because of an emphasis on unfamiliar interpersonal skills.

The challenge to admission committees is to stipulate what the nontraditional criteria are and then to formally standardize how they will be considered in lieu of grade point averages and test scores. Weekes[10] has suggested that institutions develop a profile of minority applicants who have a reasonable chance of succeeding, including those for whom English is a second language. This is determined by reviewing the applications and academic and clinical performances of students for whom the school has acted affirmatively in the past. Such data would provide qualitative support for an admissions decision when, by traditional indicators, an applicant's quantitative profile is marginal. Higher education needs to continue its search for better criteria to evaluate minority applicants' academic potential.

Mainstream student services

Success is measured both by increased ethnic student enrollment *and* by retention. It is important that programs and academic services for these students be integral to the institution. With worthy intent, institutions in the 1960s and 1970s frequently created separate services for underrepresented students that paralleled those already existing on campus. Yet if they became identified as remediation centers for poorly prepared affirmative action students, they were doomed to failure because of the stigma. Majority faculty and students also tended to deny any responsibility to assist underrepresented students when a special service and staff existed for that purpose. Furthermore, the services were usually funded by federal or state grants subject to political and economic vicissitudes. When monies were terminated, so were the services.

It is far better to cluster minorities within the mainstream of services established for all students, such as the learning resources center, tutoring center, financial aid office, and counseling service. Past experience has shown that ethnic students need more financial assistance earlier in their education and for longer periods than do other students. Family responsibilities and problems in adjustment can jeopardize the success of these students just as surely as any academic difficulty. Admittedly, minority students may be reluctant to resort to these support services and need to be taught how best to use them.

Intensive social and academic enculturation that is structured on admission can greatly facilitate the adjustment and educational competence of students over the entire course of their education. Although such an orientation program is expensive in terms of personnel and resources, it is ultimately worth the expense. Clustering underrepresented students, or placing several of them in a mixed group, provides necessary peer support and mitigates the solo phenomenon that may otherwise surface. Peer support, coupled with sustained and supervised small-group studying, also can help to attenuate attrition.

Every underrepresented newcomer should have a "buddy," a continuing student who can be supportive, a role model, and a friend. This arrangement works best when it is structured as a course and is assigned credit, perhaps one unit graded as pass or fail. In addition to each pair meeting regularly, the faculty member may schedule a group seminar with all the students once or twice during the term. This minimal course structure obligates students to develop learning objectives that relate to their buddy arrangement as a basis for learning about cultural diversity, and to maintain a coequal relationship for a reasonable period.

Recruit minority faculty

Nurse educators need to be recruited from underrepresented groups and their development nurtured once they are appointed. A homogeneous faculty tends to perpetuate its own kind, and this needs to change. Several of the ideas suggested previously in this chapter and many others concerning recruiting, retaining, and mentoring minority undergraduate and graduate students also must be aggressively implemented with minority faculty.

Probably the most promising long-term strategy is to groom the best and brightest minority doctoral students and postdoctoral fellows for faculty careers. But this will take time. For now, nursing schools need to compete in the marketplace for the few doctorally prepared ethnic faculty, who already are highly recruited or in well-established positions. A school courting such people needs time, energy, resources, imagination, persistence, and luck.

As difficult as it may seem, institutions might consider hiring several minority faculty concurrently, to lessen solo experiences and attrition. Some university administrations have set aside academic-ladder positions for which departments can compete by recruiting top ethnic faculty. Salary savings from unfilled positions also can be used to support recruitment efforts. Following their appointments, minority faculty members should be offered senior faculty mentors and encouraged to structure scholarly work and faculty assignments to ensure exemplary productivity for eventual promotion to tenure.

CONCLUSION

Nursing education needs to make a stronger effort to represent the kaleidoscope of American society in its student body. But recruiting adequate numbers of diverse students is not enough. Administrators must actively commit their schools to nurturing minority students so they can complete their programs and contribute to the profession. This means providing them with genuine institutional commitment to cultural diversity, a curriculum that includes cultural content in nursing care, and a culturally diverse faculty. Nursing cannot solve the problems of society in general, but it can provide a model for increasing opportunities for students from underrepresented groups.

Nursing has a moral and professional obligation to reaffirm its commitment to the education of nurses from all parts of society. Unless this is done, nursing risks becoming isolated from the communities it seeks to serve. Ultimately, the issue is not about affirmative action for the improvement of cultural diversity in the student body but about nursing's own humanity. It needs to attend to this moral imperative, for otherwise both the profession and those excluded from it will suffer.

REFERENCES

1. Boyle KK: Predicting the success of minority students in a baccalaureate nursing program, J Nurs Educ 25(5):186, 1986.
2. Branch MF: Ethnicity and cultural diversity in the nursing profession. In McCloskey JC and Grace HK, editors: Current issues in nursing, ed 2, Boston, 1985, Blackwell Scientific Publications, Inc.
3. Clark MM, Kaufman S, and Pierce RC: Explorations of acculturation: toward a model of ethnic identity, Human Organization 35(3):231, 1976.
4. CNA expands outreach to Hispanic students with innovative program, California Nurse 84(5):8, 1988.
5. DeVos G: Ethnic pluralism: conflict and accommodation. In DeVos G and Romanucci-Ross L, editor: Ethnic identity, Palo Alto; Calif, 1975, Mayfield Publishing Co.
6. Gaona T: Entering Hispanic freshman outnumber blacks for fourth straight year, Hispanic Times p 42, August 1986.
7. Harvey WB: Where are the black faculty members? Chronicle of Higher Education, p 96, January 22, 1988.
8. National League for Nursing Division of Research: Nursing data review, 1988 (Publication No 19-2290) New York, 1987, NLN.
9. Pettigrew C: Proceedings of colloquium on affirmative action in higher education, University of California at San Francisco, February 22, 1984.
10. Weekes D: Personal communication, 1988.
11. Wong S and Wong J: Problems in teaching ethnic minority nursing students, J Nurs 7:255, 1982.

CHAPTER 75

Transcultural nursing

A worldwide necessity to advance nursing knowledge and practice

MADELEINE M. LEININGER

Almost three decades have passed since transcultural nursing was established as a formal area of study in nursing and as essential to the provision of culturally based nursing care services to clients and institutions in a multicultural world.[2,3,4] Although significant progress has been made, many issues and viewpoints still prevail and much work lies ahead. Indeed, much work remains to help 4.5 million nurses around the world discover and value transcultural nursing as the arching framework for all nursing and as a specific knowledge to guide nursing education, consultation, research, and clinical practices. Transcultural knowledge and skills are essential for the nursing care of clients, families, and community groups in our pluralistic world. Given the critical importance of transcultural nursing today and in the future, it is a major challenge for the nursing profession to educate nurses and help them develop skills in transcultural nursing to serve people of diverse cultures and to function in different sociocultural institutions and settings worldwide.

In this chapter I will present essential conceptualizations, critical issues, and major viewpoints of transcultural nursing to stimulate readers to think anew about the evolving field. These perspectives should help to advance nursing's views about transcultural nursing education, practice, and research. Ideally, these ideas will generate additional thoughts and actions as nurses find themselves becoming more involved in transcultural nursing and part of one of the most important and rewarding areas of nursing education and practice.

As founder and central leader of the field, I contend that until the diverse and universal dimensions of transcultural nursing care and health phenomena are identified and systematically studied, it will be extremely difficult to establish a sound and reliable epistemological or fundamental base of nursing knowledge. Nursing is foremost a culturally based profession, with its roots of knowledge and practice grounded in culture. Moreover, advancing nursing as a discipline and profession requires the development of transcultural nursing knowledge to meet its claim of serving all people and health institutions. Thus nurses must fully respect the importance of transcultural nursing and work toward establishing and explaining diverse and common features of nursing phenomena.

This knowledge base will then be the most powerful and helpful means for the profession and discipline. I further argue that no nurse can truly be competent, knowledgeable, and effective unless she or he knows and can use transcultural knowledge in a skilled and creative way. This posture can be sustained because the people nurses serve are born, live, and die within a cultural framework. Hence transcultural nursing concepts, principles, and research findings are essential to help nurses care for clients, families, and communities of diverse and similar cultures.

Transcultural nursing knowledge is essential to function effectively in international situations and institutions and to develop worldwide nursing and health care policies and practices. Nurses live in pluralistic societies and a multicultural world, and so they must become knowledgeable, sensitive, and compassionate to accommodate and work with cultural variabilities. The nurse's world will become even more pluralistic in the future as people migrate from virtually every place in the world and expect nurses to care for them with respect to their values and lifeways. To some nurses who have never considered these issues, my persistent stance that transcultural nursing is the arching framework of all aspects of nursing and a highly specialized field of formal study and practice is thought-provoking and perhaps disquieting. Nurses must also not only become actively involved in discovering and learning about diverse cultures and their relationships to nursing phenomena but must know how to function creatively as transcultural nurse generalists and specialists to serve many different people. How to reach this goal is unquestionably one of the greatest and most important nursing challenges today and in the future.

UNDERSTANDING THE NATURE AND SCOPE OF TRANSCULTURAL NURSING

A major issue in transcultural nursing is helping nurses understand its nature, scope, and general features. In conceptualizing the nature and scope of transcultural nursing in the mid-1950s, I envisioned transcultural nursing as a worldwide phenomenon. The field as an area of study and practice incorporates the broadest worldwide view of nursing. It includes all cultures and cultural institutions of nations and nonnations. Transcultural nursing was conceptualized from a macro perspective and also with respect to specific cultures and their lifeways (a micro view). Hence transcultural nursing has a global view as well as more specific views of individuals, families, and cultural groups. Institutions, societies, and other macro features of transcultural nursing were identified and discussed in the first and second and earliest transcultural nursing publications as important knowledge domains.[2,3] Contrary to a recent viewpoint and false dichotomy about transcultural nursing and international nursing propounded by DeSantis,[1] transcultural nursing is by far a much broader and more comprehensive viewpoint than international nursing. Although international nursing is a part of transcultural nursing it is more limited and linguistically refers by definition to a focus between two or more nations. Transcultural nursing includes not only nations but nonnations or any actual or potential cultural entities related to comparative nursing phenomena. Thus transcultural nurses are (and have been since the beginning of the field) interested and involved in worldwide cultural and societal policies, concerns, actions, and practices ranging from micro or macro levels, including international matters. Hence DeSantis gives a misleading picture and holds an opposite viewpoint to that of the founder and other leaders in the field, because transcultural nursing has from the beginning been conceptualized as the broadest depiction of nursing and

of all human cultures at micro and macro levels of knowing.

Discovering what might constitute worldwide or universal nursing phenomena, as well as the diverse or special features and components of nursing, was an exciting idea to me. Transcultural nurses imbued with this philosophy and goal were eager to discover what characterizes the unique and diverse features of nursing. I took a position in the early 1950s that human care is the essence of nursing, and so discovery of this major component of nursing has been the focus of my research.[5,10,11] Accordingly, my theory of "cultural care diversity and universality" was developed in the early 1960s to study systematically the commonalities and diverse forms and expressions of human care transculturally.[8] This theoretical interest has led to the discovery over the past 30 years of 95 different cultural concepts and meanings of care in different cultures.[5,9,10,11] Most importantly, the theory has included not only cultures but subcultures, with documentation and explanations of universal and specific features of care and health in diverse environmental contexts. Such a worldwide viewpoint and theoretical posture may seem overwhelming to some nurses who have never studied anthropology or thought about commonalities and differences in nursing care phenomena among all cultures of the world. Moreover, no other branch or philosophy of nursing is so broad and comprehensive as transcultural nursing. This is the major reason for viewing transcultural nursing as the arching structural and theoretical framework for all aspects of nursing.

This perspective provides great potential power to know and explain nursing. But to grasp the scope of transcultural nursing requires that one understand the meaning, nature and scope of culture. Culture includes all human activities taking material and nonmaterial forms and expressions. Culture includes the political, economic, social, religious, educational, philosophical, technological, and environmental contexts in which human beings live and function. This broad conceptualization of culture can move nurses beyond a narrow individual, particularistic or local view to a holistic view of the scope and nature of nursing. Indeed, nursing as a culturally based discipline and profession means searching for and documenting the structural features and functions of nursing with its cultural values and institutional expressions worldwide. Transcultural nursing includes these broad dimensions to know and establish accurate and unique interpretations of cultural care and health components of nursing phenomena.

A critical issue remains: how to help nurses expand their worldview of nursing to a broad conceptualization of transcultural nursing with its universal and diverse expressions, forms, structures, and meanings of nursing phenomena. This viewpoint is not only essential for modern nursing theory and practice but is imperative to help nurses move beyond the prevailing focus on individuals, small groups, particular nursing tasks, activities and problems. It is the transcultural comparative knowledge that is so valuable to help nurses understand human beings, care and health expressions, changes in cultures, and other universal and specific aspects of nursing. Transcultural knowledge is the true epistemological base from which to advance nursing knowledge as a discipline and profession. Establishing this knowledge will be the powerhouse for explaining nursing practices as the basis for cultural healing, health, and well-being of clients. Transcultural nursing with a comparative and holistic cultural viewpoint, transcends common views of most nurse practitioners, educators, researchers and theoreticians today. At the same time, transcultural nursing takes into account culture specific needs and concerns of individuals, families, and groups of particular cultures.

DEFINITION OF TRANSCULTURAL NURSING

For nurses who may be unfamiliar with transcultural nursing, the following definition is well established. *Transcultural nursing is a formal area of study and practice focused on a comparative study of human cultures with respect to discovering universalities (similarities) and diversities (differences) as related to nursing phenomena of care (caring), health (wellness), or illness patterns within a cultural context and with a focus on cultural values, beliefs, and lifeways of people and institutions, and using this knowledge to provide culture-specific or universal care practices.*[3,5,6]

In order to explain the full meaning of this definition and the dominant features of transcultural nursing, it is necessary to highlight a few ideas. First, transcultural nursing requires that nurses formally study the nature, scope, concepts, theories, research methods, and knowledge domains related to the field. This position is essential, because transcultural nursing phenomena and cultures are very complex, diverse,

and changing, and most human cultures have a long cultural history. A study of transcultural nursing with a focus on care, health, other environmental contexts, and related nursing phenomena that are unique or common to cultures requires the study of vague and complex ideas of diverse lifeways of people.

The field of transcultural nursing is still a relatively new area of study and practice. Students will, therefore, be expected to study new and strange cultures with a focus on the cultural lifeways, values, and practices that bear on nursing phenomena. And the more one studies cultures, the more one realizes how important they are in understanding the nature of care, healing practices, and wellness patterns of cultures, as well as their illness expressions. The student soon learns that transcultural nursing has its roots in anthropology (the oldest and the major discipline focused on cultures over time and across geographic areas) and that transcultural nurses must identify and develop ideas unique to the discipline of nursing. Thus transcultural nursing students are challenged to identify, describe, document, and use nursing knowledge that has a cultural base in anthropology—but which has been transformed to become relevant to nursing.

A major problem in transcultural nursing is helping nursing students, practicing nurses, and faculty to understand cultural aspects when they have no fundamental knowledge of diverse cultures. As a consequence, transcultural nursing faculty often have to spend considerable time explaining basic concepts of anthropology. This problem needs to be addressed by nursing educators. I contend that all nursing students should be required to take foundation courses in anthropology, just as they are required to study anatomy and physiology. Transcultural nursing and anthropology are very interesting and mind-expanding to graduate and undergraduate students in that they discover new and different views and values about themselves and the cultures they never knew. The more nurses study transcultural nursing the more they become aware of their own ethnocentrism, cultural biases, and cultural imposition practices. This discovery is often a cultural shock and may be quite disturbing to some nursing students and registered nurses, who always thought they knew the "correct" way to live. Suddenly they find that their beliefs and values are inaccurate, or biased.

How to deal with cultural differences, cultural shock experiences, and cultural prejudices remains a major and unresolved problem in nursing. Similarly, learning from clients and learning not to impose unduly one's professional and personal cultural knowledge is often most difficult to overcome, and especially if nurses have been practicing nursing for some time. Altering one's prejudices or making drastic changes in what one has already learned at home or in previous nursing courses requires time and thoughtful reflections. Often nursing content and values learned earlier in nursing, and without a transcultural nursing perspective tends to be unicultural or culture-bound knowledge specific to nursing's ideological beliefs. Only very recently are nursing faculty beginning to recognize this problem. But students who immerse themselves in transcultural nursing and anthropology are quick to want to deal with the problem. Then, these students tend to challenge faculty and nursing service personnel with their newly found knowledge. Much more work needs to be done soon to educate faculty and nursing service personnel who have had no preparation in transcultural nursing.

Second, transcultural nursing is quite different from the traditional areas of nursing in that its theoreticians, researchers, and practitioners explicitly focus on the discovery of *comparative cultural nursing knowledge of people and institutions that are culturally different or alike.* Most importantly, transcultural nursing involves the identification, documentation, and interpretation of the *people's* viewpoints (or emic local perspective) related to human care, health, and other related nursing phenomena. This approach contrasts with the etic, or more universal, professional view of nurses or health professionals. Discovering and using comparative emic and etic knowledge domains characterize the transcultural nursing field.[3,6,13] Accordingly, getting nursing staff and faculty to value and use the emic and etic approaches to knowledge generation is just beginning to be realized.

Comparative data about people's cultural assets and values and the cultural institutions that have supported health care over time are important areas of studying and use in transcultural nursing. Identifying comparative patterns of cultures with respect to care and health contrasts sharply with schools of nursing that still focus on studying medical symptoms and disease entities, or pathological conditions of patients. Providing culturally congruent care, that is, care that is beneficial and meaningful to clients and institutions, is another major emphases in transcultural nursing, and an integral part of my theory.[12] The comparative approach as a dominant feature of transcultural nursing is used to challenge nurses to think about and act appropriately toward people with different cultural practices and understandings. This approach requires considerable knowledge, flexibility and creativity, and is often difficult for staff nurses or students who have learned rigid or "one way" unicultural responses. The comparative approach is extremely valuable to stimulate the generation of new knowledge about people and institutions of different cultures. For example, in my use of the comparative approach and my cultural care theory, I have generated data about 95 different care constructs that contrast significantly with 40 different cultures.[9,12] These comparative transcultural nursing findings are leading to new approaches to nursing practices. Still today there are only a few nurse clinicians and nursing service administrators who are using these culture-specific care concepts as central guides to therapeutic nursing practices.

Third, this definition of transcultural nursing has its major goal to help nurses give culturally specific or culturally congruent care to individuals, families, and community groups for beneficial outcomes. I have predicted that if nurses provided culturally congruent client care to individuals and groups, one will see positive signs of healing or well-being and will help clients to face meaningful or peaceful death experiences.[8,12] Culturally congruent care practices should provide satisfying, meaningful and effective care that can be identified in terms of short-term or long-term benefits to clients. But to witness the effects of culturally congruent care as a powerful healing outcome, nurses need to understand and apply transcultural nursing principles with creative strategies to promote positive healing care practices. These practices should include the appropriate use of folk and professional practices to benefit clients. Providing culturally congruent care often requires nurses to modify drastically many past nursing beliefs and practices that fail to fit the client or family health care needs. Changing dysfunctional or traditional values, rules, policies, or practices in nursing is not particularly easy.

Transcultural nursing means that nurses must often preserve cultural values and beliefs that are meaningful or beneficial for clients, families, and institutions. In my theory there are three modes of transcultural nursing decisions and actions namely; cultural care preservation or maintenance; cultural care accommodation; and cultural care repatterning.[12] These three modes of action are designed to provide culturally congruent care.

In general, transcultural nurses have the goal to provide culturally relevant care to human groups and institutions in a changing and rapidly growing multicultural world. Transcultural nursing is the broadest way to conceptualize nursing and it can offer the greatest potential to generate grass-root comparative knowledge in nursing in order to expand or modify present-day knowledge in nursing. As a comparative science, transcultural nursing scholars and theoreticians have tremendous capabilities to explain, interpret, and understand people worldwide in relation to care, health and environmental context—the three major concepts in the metaparadigms of nursing. Transcultural nursing has a refreshing and liberating approach to nursing knowledge and practices with far-reaching implications for new ways to develop and implement nursing education and practice in the future. But considerable more work is needed to reduce the barriers that inhibit the full implementation of transcultural nursing. It is, indeed, a futuristic challenge for nurses with many unresolved issues.

SELECTED QUESTIONS AND ISSUES IN TRANSCULTURAL NURSING

Granted, considerable progress has been made during the past three decades to establish transcultural nursing as a formal area of study and practice, but there are major issues and a number of provocative questions yet to be addressed as nursing enters the next century. Only a few of these questions will be identified and briefly discussed in the following section.

What steps can be taken to increase markedly transcultural nursing education and practice for the nearly 5 million nurses in the world who are expected to be knowledgeable about cultural care and provide services to clients and institutions in multicultural settings?

Currently there are still too few nurses culturally knowledgeable and skilled enough to serve clients and institutions worldwide in a culture-specific way. Today in the United States (the birthplace of transcultural nursing) fewer than 15% of graduate nursing students have had one substantive course in transcultural nursing, and even fewer have had mentored clinical or direct transcultural field experiences.[6,9] In other countries these percentages are lower, because these countries are just beginning to recognize the need for formal course instruction in transcultural nursing. In my view, the nursing professional is moving too slow to

meet the increasing consumer demand for culturally congruent care or nursing care in which nurses respect, understand, and can skillfully use transcultural knowledge. This is a critical and major problem that will become even more apparent by the year 2000, when transcultural nursing and health care is in greater demand by many different cultural groups within and outside one's homeland.

One must also be aware of the related issue that there are too few graduate programs in transcultural nursing to prepare transcultural nurse specialists and generalists to serve people worldwide.[13] Similarly, there are too few qualified nursing faculty prepared in transcultural nursing to provide highly knowledgeable instruction in schools of nursing, with field research and clinical experiences. The four or five graduate programs in transcultural nursing in the United States are not sufficient to meet current and future needs of schools of nursing and clinical service agencies. And in 1988, with the certification of transcultural nurses by the Transcultural Nursing Society to protect the public from cultural negligence and harmful acts, there are already greater numbers of nurses who desire preparation in the field. In countries other than the United States transcultural nursing is beginning to be recognized as a societal imperative, and it is predicted that nursing schools will develop similar education and service programs to meet the cultural needs of clients, community groups, and institutions. Furthermore, the role of the transcultural nurse generalist and specialist is taking hold, with a division of role expectations based on educational preparation and experiences.[13] Thus a critical need remains for more human and financial resources to develop educational programs and to prepare faculty to teach and guide more students in transcultural nursing. It is an urgent need worldwide in education, research and service. Until more nursing schools focus on cultural values, beliefs, and practices of different cultures and weave this content directly into nursing curricula, it will be difficult to ensure that nurses can function with multicultural clients and contexts. Concomitantly, many nurse researchers are still not taking into account cultural factors in their research problems, designs, and tools they use. An accurate interpretation of research findings, necessitates in-depth, knowledge about the people under study. This knowledge base in nursing research is often missing.

What theories or theoretical perspectives should be used to study transcultural nursing phenomena worldwide?

As nurses continue to develop and test theories to establish nursing knowledge, thoughtful and critical consideration needs be given to theories that tend to be culture bound, and thus greatly limit their understanding of phenomena. Currently, many nursing theories are quite culture bound or too limited in their conceptualizations to be useful to study transcultural factors within a particular cultural frame of reference. How can these theories be justified or ethically used to advance nursing knowledge when they are culture-bound? As nurse theorists and researchers become knowledgeable about the beliefs, lifeways, and practices of diverse cultures, many will need to reformulate their theories to include cultural values and concepts previously unknown to them, yet important to explain or predict behavior. This will help to reduce theory imposition and ethnocentric practices in which theorists inappropriately or inaccurately interpret phenomena that fits their particular culture or belief system. For example, self-care theories are largely Western conceptualizations that primarily fit with Anglo-American or European values of self-reliance, independence, autonomy, and self-control. Such theories are difficult to use in many non-Western cultures that emphasize values related to interdependence, reliance on others, and sociocultural solidarity. Self-care is but one example of several theories now receiving attention in the United States that limit getting to the heart of care, health, and illness meanings, expressions and uses by informants. Currently, my theory of cultural care diversity and universality remains one of the few and most comprehensive theories to focus on transcultural variabilities of the major concepts of human care, health, and environmental contexts. The theory is essential to build an epistemological and emically derived base and structure of nursing knowledge. Theories also influence ethical discoveries, and they, too, should have a transcultural nursing perspective. Hence ethical cultural implications must be considered as nurse theorists test or examine their theories in Western and non-Western cultures.

With the future shift to develop and provide direct community-based nursing care and less hospitalized care services, how can the profession prepare nursing service personnel to provide culturally relevant care that reflects cultural knowledge of diverse individuals and communities.

With worldwide immigration trends, population shifts due to wars and oppressive political behaviors, health services must be responsive to the needs of different cultural groups. Nursing service personnel will need to move from the hospital culture to communities with many different cultural groups and individuals wanting culturally based care. The critical issue is how nursing service personnel can be prepared to respond effectively to several different cultural groups in rural, suburban and large urban communities. How can these nurses be prepared soon in preventing unnecessary cultural illnesses or conflicts?

Still today, many health policies and practices reflect incongruencies among different cultural group values and beliefs in receiving nursing care services. It is, therefore, essential that nursing service and education begin to address differential cultural care of present and future cultural groups in different communities. How can these nurse administrators shift their focus to provide care to culturally diverse populations? This is a major issue and an urgent administrative challenge that needs to be addressed nationally and internationally. "Sensitivity training" or "cultural awareness" will not be adequate for these administrators, because they need substantive cultural knowledge equivalent to advanced preparation in management, computer science, or business skills, to develop transcultural nursing practices. Predoctoral and postdoctoral transcultural nursing with community-based field studies is essential to prepare these nurses for future cultural management and leadership roles. I believe transcultural and anthropological knowledge will be even more in demand than many of the business management and computer science courses that nurses are taking today. (It should be noted that students in those disciplines are now enrolling in anthropological courses to help them understand and work with diverse cultures related to business matters within and outside one's home culture.) Transcultural nurse leaders have been active for three decades and there still is only a handful of nurse administrators and educators in these courses. Of major concern are nurse administrators in hospitals who are unable to manage clients and personnel with different cultural backgrounds and values and have limited effectiveness in dealing with intracultural or intercultural administrative problems. For example, Anglo-American nurse administrators in a large urban hospital located in a large Arab and Hispanic community were "most frustrated with these people, as they never comply with our hospital policies."[14] These administrators were not aware of Hispanic and Arab cultural behavior or how to work with these people. They also assumed all Arabs and Hispanics were alike, not realizing the many cultural differences between these people in beliefs and values. They were attempting to serve them like European-Americans. As a consequence, the clients and families of these cultures were frustrated and angry with the nursing staff. Most of the mothers stayed away from the hospital and did not come for prenatal services; instead used their own folk health practices. A transcultural nurse specialist began to work with the nursing hospital administrators, and gradually a different attitude with culture-specific care were provided to the patients, and tailored to their particular cultural backgrounds, values, and beliefs. The Arab and Hispanic community slowly gained trust in the hospital, but not for several years.[9]

To what extent should deans and faculty of USA schools of nursing be "exporting their wares," to other foreign countries with curricular philosophies, theories, and models, when such ideas are often incongruent and against the dominant cultural values, beliefs, and practices of the host country?

For some years, and as the first doctorally prepared nurse-anthropologist, I have been observing and listening to nursing educators and administrators from the United States who are eager to "export" their ideas, models, and practices to non-Western schools of nursing. After the exporters leave a country, I have often heard about the difficulties experienced by the host cultures in using American nursing education ideas and practices. The host nurse leaders very cautiously make statements such as "They don't really fit our political, economic and cultural lifeways"; "These ideas are very difficult to implement in our country, but we remained polite and acted as if they might fit our needs"; "We often have difficulty with the government to implement the ideas." Most nursing education exporters seldom stay in the country long enough to see the consequences of their ideas. Of course, some foreign leaders who respond favorably to American ideas, but sometimes out of respect for or deference to U.S. nurse leaders. The larger nursing population that has to live with the new Western ideas and make them work may suffer from cultural frustrations and political repercussions by their government or political groups. Nursing experts who are knowledgeable about the culture, including transcultural nurses, are generally cautious about imposing such ideologies and practices on a foreign culture unless they fully understand what they are doing and work through agreed aspects to fit their traditional cultural values. I find that cultural imposition or cul-

tural exportation practices in some countries are already leading to "cultural backlash"—unfavorable short-term and long-term consequences—in several cultures. It is time to rethink and reassess what Western nurse exporters are doing in other countries, and the short-term and long-term consequences of their practices. This requires knowledge of the past history of that culture and careful appraisal of what is being introduced into the host culture.

There are also ethical and moral dimensions to foreign nurses exporting their ideas and values that need to be identified and understood in nursing arenas. Transcultural nursing ethical policies and practices need to be established to prevent future problems. From an anthropological perspective, some nurse exporters employing commercial seminars and courses may be setting up some cultures for political unrest and educational problems. Moreover, some exporter practices hark of neocolonialism, with consequences that have been well documented by anthropologists for more than 100 years. Are nurse leaders in the United States, Canada and other countries following a naive neocolonialist course without full awareness of what they are doing and the consequences of their actions?

How can nurse researchers accurately and reliably study nursing problems and include diverse cultures in their samples, and yet use research instruments and designs that are highly culture-bound?

This question must be taken seriously today with diverse cultures in any country. It raises another question of how nurse researchers can make accurate interpretations of their findings when they know virtually nothing about the cultures they include in their quantitative samples or populations. Although many sampling strategists claim they can get a discriminatory analysis, often strange interpretations of data may result when one lumps together many diverse cultures in one population sample. Using small sampled results about cultures that "happen to come forth" from quantitative studies are highly questionable. It is time that nurse researchers know more about the cultures or subcultures included in any research study so that cultural minority groups receive accurate interpretations of their lifeways or behaviour.

As a leader in developing and encouraging the use of qualitative methods to study largely unknown diverse cultures, I believe it is time to use these methods more and in a knowledgeable way. For example, nurse researchers need to be aware of the serious problems in mixing qualitative and quantitative paradigms when the research goals and purposes are very different.[7] Nurse researchers also need to reconsider tendencies to reduce qualitative cultural expressions, norms, and values to meaningless statistics or measurement outcomes—a problematic feature of quantitative studies today. Transcultural nurse researchers are keenly aware of the consequences of numerical reduction data on culture groups, but there are many quantitatively oriented nurse researchers still believing that they get an accurate picture of cultures through traditional modes of reduction analyses, inadequate sampling and generalized interpretations of culture. A larger and pressing issue remains: namely, how to reeducate many doctorally prepared nurses who have had no educational preparation in transcultural nursing and qualitative methods and yet these nurses often make claim of doing "cultural studies." This critical area must be addressed in the near future as part of attempts to reduce ethnocentric and questionable findings that fail to take into account cultural variabilities and qualitative cultural interpretations of findings.

In this chapter I have identified and briefly discussed a few provocative trends, questions and issues related to transcultural nursing and nursing in general. Unquestionably there are many more issues that could be addressed. As a pioneer leader to establish educational and research programs in transcultural nursing, sites, I can identify many noteworthy areas of progress along with the areas yet to be developed. Nonetheless, it has been encouraging to see how transcultural nursing research and education begin to take hold in the United States, Canada and in a few other places in the world. Nurses are beginning to realize the importance of this field to advance nursing knowledge and practice. One can say that we are at the threshold of educating a new generation of nurses who are valuing and developing transcultural nursing knowledge and practices worldwide. This is most rewarding and encouraging to realize. It is a major achievement of a small cadre of dedicated transcultural nursing leaders

and followers who spearheaded the cultural movement more than 35 years ago. But the greatest reward will be realized when nurses worldwide are prepared and sufficiently skilled to practice transcultural nursing and to serve all minority and majority cultures and their cultural institutions. This goal will require an active and vigorous posture by nurse educators, administrators, and clinicians. It will also require financial support and open dialog to resolve the issues and critical questions identified in this chapter.

REFERENCES

1. DeSantis L: The relevance of transcultural nursing to international nursing, International Nursing Review 35(4):110-112, 1988.
2. Leininger M: Nursing and anthropology: two worlds to blend, New York, 1970, John Wiley & Sons, Inc.
3. Leininger M: Transcultural nursing concepts, theories and practices, New York, 1978, John Wiley & Sons, Inc.
4. Leininger M: Transcultural nursing, New York, 1979, Masson Publishing, Inc.
5. Leininger M: Cultural care: an essential goal for nursing and health care, American Association of Nephrology Nurses and Technicians (AANNT) Journal, 10(5):11-17, 1983.
6. Leininger M: Transcultural nursing: an essential knowledge and practice field for today, Canadian Nurse, p 41-45, Dec 1984.
7. Leininger M: Qualitative research methods in nursing, Orlando, Fla, 1985, Grune & Stratton, Inc.
8. Leininger M: Transcultural nursing care diversity and universality: a theory of nursing, Nursing and Health Care 16(4):209, 1985.
9. Leininger M: Care: discovery and uses in clinical-community nursing, Detroit, 1988, Wayne State University Press.
10. Leininger M: Care: the essence of nursing and health, Detroit, 1988, Wayne State University Press, reprinted in 1988 (First published by Charles B. Slack, Inc., 1984).
11. Leininger M: Caring: an essential human need, Detroit, 1988, Wayne State University Press, reprinted in 1988 (First published by Charles B. Slack, Inc., 1981).
12. Leininger M: Leininger's theory of transcultural care diversity and universality, Nursing Science Quarterly, Baltimore: Williams & Wilkens Pub., Vol 3, Nov 1988, p. 152-160.
13. Leininger M: The transcultural nurse specialist: Imperative in today's world, Nursing and Health Care, New York: National League for Nursing, Vol 10, No 5, May 1989.
14. Leininger M: Study of Arab and Hispanic ethnocare and ethnohealth needs in an urban community, Detroit, Wayne State University: Unpublished Report 1988.

CHAPTER 76

Beyond the concept of culture

Or, how knowing the cultural formula does not predict clinical success

TONI TRIPP-REIMER
STEPHEN S. FOX

In the nineteenth century concepts from the biological sciences were introduced into nursing and were followed by contributions from psychology and sociology. More recently concepts from anthropology have been introduced into the mainstream of nursing education and practice. However, the incorporation of cultural concepts into the discipline of nursing has not generally occurred in such a way as to optimize the relationship between professional and layperson. Specifically, an overemphasis on units of culture and cultural differences fosters the alienation of nurse and patient.

In this chapter we briefly trace the historical evolution of the inclusion of cultural dimensions within nursing education and practice. We point out how this approach could be assistive, but how it is generally misapplied. Specifically, we contend that nursing approaches to cultural dimensions have tended to foster ethnic stereotypes. The assessment and treatment of patients based on specified characteristics of their culture emphasizes the differences between nurse and patient and promotes a separation from the patient. We further propose that the intent underlying this approach stems from an agenda in which concern for therapeutic compliance, rather than for the person, holds primacy. Finally, we propose an approach that transcends cultural distinctiveness or categories.

THE EVOLUTION OF A CULTURAL APPROACH IN NURSING

In the discipline of nursing, concern with the culture of the client dates at least to the beginning of the twentieth century. This early interest is particularly evident in public health nursing, where a major impetus for considering the client's cultural context was the need to work with immigrant groups. Early in the century a series of articles appearing in the *Public Health Nursing Quarterly* gave cultural overviews of various immigrant groups such as Italians, Russians, and Portuguese. However, the majority of this early literature was parochial in its intent to homogenize (assimilate) the immigrant groups. That is, different European nationalities were described not for the purpose of tailoring culturally sensitive care, but to assist nurses and social workers in transforming foreign beliefs and customs so that the group could be blended in the proverbial "melting pot."

In areas of nursing other than public health, the cultural dimension was generally ignored until World War II. At that time anthropologists and other social scientists, national organizations and foundations, and the educational reform movement were instrumental in moving cultural content into nursing. For example, the National Nursing Council commissioned the anthropologist Esther Lucille Brown to conduct a study of nursing education. Her findings, containing recommendations for nursing education, were published in the 1948 book *Nursing for the Future*,[3] which spearheaded the movement for midcentury educational reform in nursing.

As a consequence, schools of nursing were progressively integrated into university settings where there was a closer relationship between nursing faculty and social scientists. The content of nursing education in its new collegiate setting was characterized by increased attention to content from the social sciences.[2,6] The social sciences (specifically psychology and sociology) provided a theoretical base for what nursing had previously done intuitively.

Addressing the National League of Nursing Education in 1949, Birdwhistell[1] identified some of the uses of the anthropological approach to the problems of nursing. Other national nursing groups invited speakers such as Brown, Margaret Mead, and Lyle Saunders to address their organizations.

An example of the interplay among anthropologists, nurses, and national foundations may be seen in the 3-year experimental project on the application of the social sciences to nursing conducted at the Cornell University School of Nursing from 1954 to 1957 and supported by the Russell Sage Foundation. In this course a number of anthropologists and sociologists (Mead, Renee Fox, Rhoda Metraux, August Hollingshead, and others) presented lectures highlighting the importance of cultural and social concepts in the practice of nursing.[5]

As nursing became concerned with its professional definition, there was increasing appreciation that nurses deal primarily with those aspects of a person's life shaped by cultural practices such as diet, family patterns, communication styles, and rituals. Subsequently there was greater interest in the influence of the patient's culture. In 1949 Margaret Huger initiated the first nursing research project concerned with the cultural component in the delivery of health care. She conducted a year-long hospital field study of Italian-American patients' responses to the nursing situation.[8]

Similarly, in 1954 the University of North Carolina School of Nursing received a training grant from the National Institute of Mental Health (NIMH) to incorporate concepts from social science into the undergraduate program in nursing. Gracia McCabe, a psychiatric nurse and research assistant, conducted a subproject for the grant by investigating cultural factors to be considered when providing nursing care to African-American patients.[7]

The National League for Nursing (NLN) was also instrumental in the incorporation of culture content into nursing. In 1927 the NLN recommended that social sciences be included in nursing curricula; this recommendation was strengthened in 1937 when the NLN suggested that nursing students enroll in at least 10 semester hours in the social sciences. Movement toward inclusion of the social sciences was furthered by the 1942 organization of the Joint Commission on Integration of Social and Health Aspects of Nursing

in the Basic Curriculum by the NLN and the National Organization for Public Health Nursing. Finally, in 1977 the NLN mandated for accreditation the inclusion of cultural content in nursing curricula.

With the advent of the federally funded Nurse Scientist Program, nurses began to obtain doctoral degrees in increasing numbers, and several nurses obtained doctoral preparation in anthropology. In 1968 sufficient interest had developed to form the Council on Nursing and Anthropology in relation with the Society for Medical Anthropology. Subsequently other organizations were formed: the Transcultural Nursing Society, in 1974, and the American Nurses' Association's Council on Inter-Cultural Diversity (later called the Council on Cultural Diversity in Nursing Practice) in 1980.

In part these events may be seen as stemming from the work of nurses, anthropologists, and organizations. In part they also stemmed from the civil rights and affirmative action movements of the 1960s and 1970s, in which some groups of minority nurses emphasized minority rights and nursing care for "ethnic people of color."

Since that time the cultural aspects of clinical care have experienced an explosion of interest. Several special issues in nursing journals have been devoted to cultural considerations in clinical practice and research. Amplification of this history may be found in Dougherty and Tripp-Reimer.[4]

Nursing seldom acknowledges any specific culturally based theoretical orientation, even though a wide array of theoretical orientations are available from anthropology (including cultural evolutionism, functionalism, cultural materialism, neoevolutionism, culture ecology, and structuralism). On the few occasions in which theory is invoked, it is generally a narrowly applied functionalist approach that errs by stressing the specifics of individual cultural components rather than their interrelationships. Stripped of cultural theory, nursing is left with only a set of atheoretical components (primarily in the form of customs or beliefs such as dietary habits or health beliefs and practices). Nursing has moved as if an understanding of the workings of the whole culture can be revealed by the progressively evolving distinction of cultural components. As a consequence nursing is left with culture lists, for example, with typologies of "folk" illness beliefs (witchcraft, spirit possession, object intrusion, breach of taboo).

The rich matrix encountered when a whole culture is embraced has little in common with the fragments left as a result of viewing the concept of culture through a narrow focus on discrete components. Although nursing attempts to deemphasize this discrepancy by invoking the concept of holism, it contradictorily emphasizes distinctions among cultural components and treats these distinctions as if they, not the patient, were important.

It is commonly proposed that by knowing cultural characteristics, nurses will be able to provide more culturally sensitive approaches to health care. However, if notions of culture arising from the integration of nursing and anthropology are conceptually restrictive, a stereotypic or inauthentic approach to patients is fostered. This designation by category emphasizes differences and promotes a separation from the patient.

Nursing education reflects this stereotypic approach, evidenced by the routine textbook inclusion of transcultural concepts as a means to identifying "typical" characteristics of particular ethnic groups. The underlying assumption is that if only the "right" formula or recipe were known to nursing, it would be possible to tailor interventions to maximize patient compliance. Texts often contain lists of characteristics of African-Americans, Hispanics, Native Americans, Asians, and Euro-Americans—as if cultural traits are held uniformly and are static. This approach may be likened to the pathogenic analogy from microbiology where clinicians, in an attempt to identify pathogenic organisms and the most effective therapy, order "culture and sensitivity" laboratory tests.

Nursing has been exhorted to treat the client, not the disease. That is, we have come to appreciate the difference between treating "the cholysystectomy in Room 407" and treating Mrs. Golden. However, treating Mrs. Golden as an Indian (or African-American or Hispanic) is just as depersonalizing. Nursing may wish to transcend this static stereotypic view of culture.

THE PROBLEM OF CATEGORIES

Thus far we have presented the history of the evolution of a cultural perspective in nursing and have discussed ways that this cultural perspective has been incorrectly adapted by the profession. There is, however, an even broader problem that goes beyond those incurred by a stereotypic approach. The broader problem is that, without caution, *any* categories that nursing creates may serve to objectify the patient.

In Western science a tradition holds that understanding can be derived from distinction and categorization. Scientists create scales of difference through objectification and categorization, and often fail to realize that the process of producing categories is structured and therefore limited by specific assumptions. Understanding through distinction by difference requires methods for the detection of differences; in the end, these are only projections from the standpoint of the observer's own culture.

The process of producing categories reflects the desire to struggle against all others, to understand the self (as distinct from the other) in the guise of understanding the other. Such a paradigm of understanding by delineation of categories of difference does not unify conceptions of human diversity. While it attempts to exhaust that diversity, it fails to take into account the separating and alienating effects of the method, and is therefore a paradigm of distance.

The problem is not a matter of an ill-defined category but a matter of the origin of the category. We propose that stereotypy results not merely from the imposition of too general or imprecise categories. Rather, stereotypy resides in the imposition of the category itself, regardless of how detailed or refined such categories may become. This point of view implies that stereotypy is not overcome by the proliferation of additional appropriate categories, but rather that all categories imposed on the patient's culture are simply statements arising from the nurse's culture and are therefore inherently objectifying.

Nursing may advocate advancing beyond stereotypes. However, there is not a clear understanding of what form this advancement might take. The elimination of stereotypes does not occur through the proliferation of differences. For example, the few nursing texts that advocate cultural sensitivity without stereotypic response usually illustrate the necessity of doing so by describing the diversity within minority groups. For example, the broader category "Hispanic" is broken into populations of Mexican-Americans, Puerto Ricans, Cubans, and others. Further distinction is made between new immigrants and those who have lived in the United States for several generations. Additional distinctions are made between characteristics of urban and rural Hispanics as well as those who are Catholic, Protestant, or other. Emphasis is also placed on the importance of characteristics that correlate with income levels (the difference between Hispanics of the lower and middle classes). If these distinctions are pursued to their logical conclusion, nursing would prescribe different nursing actions if the patient is low income, urban, Catholic, and Puerto Rican than if the patient is middle income, urban, agnostic, and Cuban.

However, in making these finer distinctions nurses fail to see the error inherent in the entire process. The problem is that all these distinctions arise from the point of view of the nurse's culture. These are distinctions that nurses think have meaning. They fail to understand that these even finer distinctions do not allow greater access to the patient. All distinctions are just that: facets that separate the patient from the nurse, facets that allow the nurse the illusion that the patient is other (not related to self), is an object.

Nurses must confront not merely the fact that they make such cultural distinctions, but also that the disposition to differentiate is part of the attempt to create the self, using the products of such distinctions. This is the unexamined and unconscious agenda of the ontological use of cultural difference. The prediction of effective care on an understanding of categories of difference has given rise historically to the dilution of the concept of care through emergent theories of distinction.

Attempts have been made to recognize and reverse this trend by a reconstruction of "holistic nursing care." However, the recombination of the disparate parts into larger cognitive units effectively preserves the process of distinction. Identification as division and recombination does not enhance patient acceptance. Rather, this reduces the patient to a set of categories that ultimately objectifies and alienates patient from nurse, nurse from patient, and nurse from self.

Nursing's concern for human respect and its recognition of the creative implications of diversity mean that it is naturally drawn to a discipline such as anthropology, which, on the surface, has done much to support and preserve human diversity in a world of progressive homogenization and under the undue influence of dominant cultures. However, diversity as defined by the categories imposed by the dominant observer culture at the same time undermines recognition of diversity's value and positions the observer culture as the "namer" or "definer" of the object culture. By breaking down and superimposing their categories, nurses disembody the patient's culture.

TRANSCENDING CATEGORIES OF DIFFERENCES

Nursing is faced with the option of predicating care on categories of difference or, alternatively, on those that address the core of all humanity, independent of form. This latter approach, that of convergence, implies not the naive elimination or disregard of difference but the displacement of the locus of difference from the object to the observer. Individuals are cared for beyond and within the expression of difference, since they exist differently only as manifestations of their sameness and commonality.

Cultural specificity is not excluded and cultural sensitivity is not devalued. They are lived contextually within the life of the nurse; they are not means to particular ends. Nursing now must choose between these two approaches: that of understanding others through the analysis of categories of difference, or that of unconditional acceptance, regardless of form. Nurses may consider, for example, whether the objectification of African-American culture has created greater limitations or greater access to patients?

We propose a recognition of diversity of different forms without the subsequent formulation of a set of fixed categories that predict at the level of the individual. With this approach nurses could come to see that all people face the same human dilemmas; the specifics vary and their consideration is important, but the human dilemmas remain the same. Cultural expression is not ignored or excluded, but is elevated beyond any formulated objectification of cultures. The caveat is not to allow differences in form to be misinterpreted as differences among people. We remember that the relation that we have with anyone who we perceive as culturally distinct will be just that: distinct, objectified and separate. Alternatively, difference may be recognized but remains unknown and unknowable in its separateness.

A different relationship thus transpires: an unconditional concern for and affirmation of that which is universally human. This formulation is more consistent with nursing than that of distance and differentiation. Although nurses can consider cultural form a relevant dimension of treatment, we must also recognize that an understanding of *no* difference is the true basis for care. Nursing's attitude toward cultural diversity can be an attitude of compassion, not distinction.

REFERENCES

1. Birdwhistell R: Social science and nursing education, Annual Report of the National League for Nursing Education, New York, 1949, National League for Nursing.
2. Bridgeman M: Collegiate education for nursing, New York, 1953, Sage Foundation.
3. Brown EL: Nursing for the future, New York, 1948, Sage Foundation.
4. Dougherty MC and Tripp-Reimer T: The interface of nursing and anthropology, Annual Review of Anthropology, 14:219, 1985.
5. MacGregor FC: Social science in nursing: applications for the improvement of patient care, New York, 1960, Sage Foundation.
6. Martin HW: The behavioral sciences and nursing education: some problems and prospects, Social Forces 37:61, 1958.
7. McCabe GS: Cultural influences on patient behavior, Am J Nurs 60(8):1101, 1960.
8. Mead M: Understanding cultural patterns, Nurs Outlook 4(3):260, 1956.

CHAPTER 77

Men in nursing

EDWARD J HALLORAN

Florence Nightingale's achievement in establishing modern nursing was remarkable for two reasons. She established the science of nursing, and she overcame extreme societal pressure for women to conform to Victorian mores that segregated the sexes. Nightingale confronted, and successfully overcame, social barriers that excluded women of class from participating in nondomestic economic activity. Contemporary American society is now challenging some of these same sex-role stereotypical beliefs about roles for men and women. More women than ever are joining the workforce, and many are entering professions like business, engineering, accounting, law, and medicine that in the recent past practically excluded them. Men, too, are telephone operators, elementary school teachers, librarians, and secretaries in increasing numbers. It is perplexing, however, that the nursing profession, established by a pioneer who facilitated the entry of women into a man's world, is behind other fields in changing its gender mix. This chapter explores some reasons why some men are nurses and why more men are not.

There were an estimated 57,199 male nurses in the United States in 1984, which represented 3% of the country's 1,887,697 registered nurses (Table 77-1). Although the proportion remains insignificant, the number of nurses who are men continues to increase at a rate exceeding the growth rate of all nurses. In 1980 the number was 2.7% of nurses—a 4-year growth rate of 29% compared with a growth rate for all nurses of 17%.

The proportion of men in nursing is now showing a gain. From 1930 through 1977 the proportion was constant, just under 2%. It is interesting to note, however, that in the early decades of this century the proportion of men in the field was considerably higher. In 1910 that proportion was 7.6%, and in 1920 it was 3.8% According to American Nurses' Association (ANA) statistics, the number of male nurses remained constant from 1910 through 1930 at approximately 5500. In the same two decades, however, the number of female nurses grew by a factor of four, from 76,000 to 288,000. Nursing schools, which experienced phenomenal growth in number and in the number of enrolees from 1910 to 1930, largely excluded men.

Four issues emerge in the history of men in modern American nursing. They are (1) quality care for selected patients, which gave rise to men in modern nursing; (2) the selective service and the military, which nearly eliminated men from the field; (3) economic circumstances, which alternately have led men to enter nursing and also have served as a disincentive; and (4) the economic implications of nursing as a gender-stereotyped profession for women. A recent development has been the founding of the American Assembly for Men in Nursing.

QUALITY CARE FOR SELECTED PATIENTS

Barely 10 years after the first American nursing school graduated its first nurse, the Mills School of Nursing for Men at Bellevue Hospital in New York was established. The school was founded on the premise that men as well as women could provide care.* The men who were the earliest graduates of nursing schools in this country were educated for the same reasons as were women. To quote Nightingale, they were to "place patients in the best possible condition for nature to act favorably upon them."

---

*Nightingale equated "nursing" with "female" for several reasons. Her pre-Crimean search for a career in helping the sick took her through Europe, where religious and lay sisters had a long tradition of caring for those suffering from illness. Nightingale was greatly influenced by this. Victorian women of privilege had no opportunity for meaningful contribution beyond the home in English society. Her essay "Cassandra,"[14] written just before her Kaiserworth nurse training, details and laments the role of high-class women in Vic-

Table 77-1 Men in nursing*

Year	Total Number of Nurses†	Number of Male Nurses†	%
1910	83,327	5,819	7.06
1920	149,128	5,464	3.66
1930	294,189	5,452	1.85
1940	369,287	8,072	2.18
1950	374,584	9,613	2.56
1960‡	504,000	4,587	.91†‡
1970	1,127,657	14,625	1.29
1980	1,615,846	44,237	2.74
1984	1,887,697	57,199	3.03

*Data from references 6, 19, and 20.
†Figures for years before 1955 include students as well as graduates.
‡1960 figures include nurses (men and women) employed in nursing.

Very early on in the history of the nursing profession, technological advances in anesthesia and infection control created a shift in the provision of nursing care from the home to the hospital. Care in the home was provided in the main by families, and to some extent by graduate nurses, and care in the hospital was increasingly provided by students and graduate nurses. Conflict emerged during the first few decades of organized nursing over whether the objective of nurse training was the education of students or the provision of service for patients.[10] As the service orientation prevailed (largely because of the training schools' loss of independence from hospitals), specialty institutions providing care to the mentally ill actively recruited men into their training programs. This early

division of labor was consistent with the social prejudice against women caring for patients who might become violent. Similarly, those having conditions requiring privacy, like patients with urological disorders, could be more discretely cared for by men. Thus, concern for quality patient care for selected categories of patients led to the earliest involvement of men in post-Nightingale nursing.

SELECTIVE SERVICE AND THE MILITARY

A major cause of the relative dearth of men in nursing was the demands of the military. During World War I it was apparent that available nurses could not meet the needs of both civilian and military patients. Because men were combatants in the war, the major recruitment of nurses during that period involved women. In 1918 alone there was a 25% increase in the entrants in American nursing schools.[11] Even men who were nursing students at the time were vulnerable to the draft and participated in the war as soldiers in the trenches rather than as nurses. Parenthetically, when the Army Nurse Corps was established in 1901, the law describing it read, "Army Nurse Corps, Female." As Kalish and Kalish write, "The effect of the war and of selective service was practically to wipe out the enrollment of men in schools of nursing."

The situation for men during World War I was identical at the outbreak of World War II. Men who were nurses found themselves bearing arms and driving earth movers rather than caring for the sick and injured.[17] Men in nursing were very well served by Leroy Craig, R.N., director of the School of Nursing for Men in Pennsylvania Hospital, Department of Mental and Nervous Diseases. Concerned about the

torian society. She was determined to care for the sick and accepted a post as a hospital matron. The British war with Russia intervened. After organizing and leading a group of 38 women (independently organized but sanctioned by the British government) to the Crimea to nurse the wounded, she was stymied by military and medical bureaucracy, which were controlled by men. The men caring for the wounded were neglectful or unfit for other duty. Nightingale, due to her perseverance and her independence of the military, was able to reform the Barrack Hospital at Scutari and significantly reduce the hospital mortality rates. One strategy she seemed to use to ensure the success of nursing was to organize it separately from the hospital (as was the first nursing school at St. Thomas Hospital) and limit the school's enrolees to women. In promoting a separate organization for the nursing school, Nightingale defined nurses as female and used societal prohibitions on integrating the sexes to maintain independence for nurses. Describing nursing as a field for women accomplished two of Nightingale's objectives: to create an opportunity for women outside the home, and to have a measure of independence from men in the medical/hospital bureaucracy. These matters are thoroughly covered by Nightingale in "Subsidary Notes as to the Introduction of Female Nursing into Military Hospitals."[15]

possible repetition of events that affected male nurses during World War I, Craig and other men at the 1940 American Nurses' Association convention petitioned for recognition. The following January the ANA board of directors created the Men Nurses' Section of the ANA. The initial objectives of this section were the improvement of patient care, but soon the concerns gravitated toward the treatment of men nurses in the military and the inadequate salaries for nurses.

Another nurse, Luther Christman, as a 1939 graduate of the Pennsylvania Hospital School of Nursing for Men, found he could not enlist in the Army Nurse Corps at the outset of World War II. Men nurses were not even given priority enrollment in Medical Corpsmen schools because their knowledge often intimidated less well-educated teachers. Christman enlisted in the Merchant Marine as a Medical Corpsman and then petitioned the ranking Army medical officer for appointment to the Army Nurse Corps and assignment to the front, where women (and nurses) were not assigned. His request was rejected in a terse letter from the general. Christman sent his correspondence with the general to all members of the U.S. Senate and to two thirds of the House of Representatives. The stir Christman created subsided only after the Allies won the Battle of the Bulge, obviating the need to draft women nurses.

According to Olga Benderoff, Chief Nurse of the 4th General Hospital, who served in the South Pacific during World War II, Army nurses received less pay than their counterparts of equal rank in the medical corps. She remembers receiving a substantial pay raise while serving in New Guinea. Frances Payne Bolton was responsible for the raise, having introduced Congressional legislation giving Army nurses pay parity with other Army officers.

For nearly all of its 12-year history the Men Nurses' Section was concerned with equal treatment and adequate salaries for men and women nurses in the U.S. armed forces. Equal treatment did not become a reality during the life of the Men Nurses' Section, but the men were sufficiently involved in the mainstream of the professional nursing organization that they did not disappear, as they had shortly after World War I. The ANA reorganized in 1952, and the Men Nurses' Section, in support of the reorganization, voted itself out of existence. Edward Lyon became the first registered nurse commissioned a reserve officer in the Army Nurse Corps on October 6, 1955. The legislation facilitating his commission was again introduced by the

representative from Ohio, Frances Payne Bolton. More than a decade later men were given the first commissions as regular officers in the Army Nurse Corps. During the conflict in Vietnam, more than 500 men nurses were drafted, provided commissions in the Military Nurse Corps, and, at last, cared for the injured as registered nurses. The role of the selective service and the military is now positive. More than 30% of the registered nurses in the Military Nurse Corps are men. Many of the more recent male recruits to the nursing profession are former medics and corpsmen who saw, and see, men nurses on active duty.

ECONOMIC CYCLES

Another major force having an impact on men in the nursing profession was the economy. After World War I, the number of men admitted to nursing schools was slow to increase. During the 1920s the salaries for nurses were not competitive with those for teachers, union laborers, or municipal workers. Most graduate nurses worked in private duty, a particularly unstable source of income. As a consequence, in a growing economy there was no economic incentive for a man to become a nurse. Male recruits to nursing increased considerably during the depression. Nursing schools became one of the few places in which an education could be obtained, along with room, board, and a small stipend. The pattern of specialization established earlier continued. Men tended to be admitted to training programs in hospitals that specialized in the care of mental illness. But because American nurses at the entry level were generalists, all of them had to have experience in the care of maternity patients, children, and acutely ill adults in general hospitals.

The low salary levels for nurses between World War II and 1970 continued to discourage men from entering nursing, as America was in the midst of a growth economy. When the passage of Medicare legislation began to infuse money into hospitals, salaries for high-demand positions began to rise. Entry-level nurse salaries increased during this post-Medicare period. Secondary effects of the post-Medicare increase in money for health care have been both the increase in the number of nurses being trained and the increase in the number of nurses in the workforce. Since the oil embargo of 1973, economic cycles have produced intermittent unemployment and the loss of job security. Both the salary changes and depressed economy in manufacturing and in government employment produced the economic conditions necessary to increase the rate of men entering nursing. The prospective payment system and decreased availability of nurses are likely to contribute to increased wages and therefore contribute to increased enrollment of men, if the number of men in nursing serves as an index of economic well-being of nurses. However, general economic prosperity, experienced during the late 1980s, has slowed the high rate of growth in men entering nursing. The growth rate for 1977-1980 was 63% and half that, at 29%, since then.

NURSING AS WOMEN'S WORK

In our culture most people see human behavioral characteristics as being either feminine or masculine; further, women who display masculine characteristics and men who display feminine characteristics are seen as being unusual. Cultural tolerance of these abberations varies with gender. The young woman who acts like a tomboy is, by and large, more acceptable than the young man who acts like a sissy. It is no wonder, then, that nursing, a profession that Nightingale and other Victorians identified as being femine, is not even considered a possibility for most boys.[13] These sex-role stereotypes are common throughout life but tend to moderate somewhat with age. Cultural predispositions tend to reinforce sex-role stereotypical entry into the professions. Sex-role stereotypical behaviors are at least in part responsible for the relative scarcity of men in nursing and for the age of those men who do enter the nursing profession.[9] Holtzclaw[8] concluded that men who succeed in nursing are apt to be better accepted if they retain personality attributes associated with masculinity.

Nuttal,[16] in a study of British nursing, expressed concern that half of the top posts in nursing within the National Health Service were held by men, who account for less than 10% of the total state registered nurses. When Nuttall examined the Council of the Royal College of Nursing, she found that 15 of the 31 elected members were men. Nuttall suggested that rather than men nurses taking over these leadership positions in British nursing, women nurses seemed to be giving them away. If both men and women agree on appropriate leadership qualities and they seem to be consistent with masculine characteristics, then men nurses exhibiting these traits will continue to be identified by nurses as leaders.

The picture in the United States is complicated by a rigid educational hierarchy among registered nurses. In America, unlike Britain, the top posts tend to have experience and high (master's and above) educational qualifications as prerequisites. The paucity of American men in nursing, educated at those levels, will prevent a repetition of the British situation Nuttal describes, but London[12] urges caution.

The recent and rather remarkable changes in sex-role stereotyping, especially among the professionals in America, has given researchers pause to question some of the assumptions underlying the dichotomization of masculine versus feminine characteristics. Considering masculinity and feminity as a polar opposites has outlived its usefulness.[18] Well-adjusted adults are increasingly being recognized as people who have both male and female characteristics, that is, they are androgenous.[2] In fact, Holtzclaw, who studied a panel of men and women nurses, found them equally androgenous.

A noteworthy finding of the Holtzclaw study was that men and women nurses are highly supportive of their sons and daughters entering the nursing profession. Holtzclaw described as sex-typed occupations that have a majority of people of one sex when there is no logical reason for the disparity. When nursing was one of the few professions in which women could participate, it benefited from having a disproportionate number of members who were essentially barred from other fields of endeavor. The last several years have seen changes in opportunities for women to enter non-traditional fields. This will have an effect on the talent pool for nursing unless talented men can be attracted. Research on men in nursing indicates that most men nurses have been influenced by a living role model who encouraged their entry into the nursing profession.[3,8] Most men nurses could identify a nurse (woman or man)—frequently a spouse, other close relative, or co-worker—who encouraged them to study nursing.

THE ECONOMIC EFFECTS OF GENDER BIAS

Gender bias has contributed in two ways to the current economic status of nursing in America. Neither women's pay nor women's educational programs have reached parity with men's pay and with programs that educate mostly men. In general, it still seems acceptable to pay women 59 cents for every dollar earned by a man. Similarly, there is not much investment in educating women except, of course, as women enter fields in which men predominate. Molly Yard, president of the National Organization for Women, stated in a speech at the Cleveland City Club that the admission of women to law, medical, business, and theological schools is related less to fundamental changes and beliefs about women than to the receipt of federal funds to comply with Title IX of the Civil Rights Act. Those places that have a long history of educating women—schools of nursing, social work, education, and library science—are all experiencing economic difficulties. Case Western Reserve University closed its schools of education and library science, changed the name and focus of the School of Applied Social Service, and shrunk the size of the nursing school to half what it was 15 years ago.

In contrast, the costs of legal, business, and medical education have skyrocketed. The CWRU medical school has doubled in size over the last 15 years, and support for medical education now comes from patient charges through the hospital, federal grant funds, tuition, and state subsidies. These economic realities are the only plausible explanation for the current concern over lower nursing school enrollments and future nurse shortages.

The per-graduate registered nurse education expense in the United States is actually shrinking, and at an alarming rate. As a hospital takes a diploma nursing school out of service, the dollar expenditures for capital (school of nursing building and expenses of operating it) administrative overhead, and generally low student-faculty ratio (one faculty to 3.9 students for diploma programs, versus one faculty to 6.3 students for associate degree programs) evaporate. More than 540 such hospital schools have been closed since 1965.[21] Local governments have replaced hospital schools with community college programs (605 associate degree schools have been added since 1965). The A.D. programs graduated 57 students per school in 1984, versus 35 per school in diploma programs.[21] There are many controversial issues surrounding this shift in education from hospital to community college about which nurses do not agree. Yet all those familiar with contemporary patient care would agree that more, not less, money should be spent on the education of tomorrow's nurse.

When salary benefits, and working conditions for nurses become competitive economically, then nurses will have achieved their appropriate valuation. Such valuation may not necessarily mean much more money

for women, but rather a redistribution, or even less money for men. Another, perhaps even more desirable, redistribution process can involve the development of a national health scheme that would cut the disparity between the incomes of doctors and nurses, now at a 5:1 ratio, and, at the same time lower the cost of health care and provide greater access to care. When such revaluation occurs, there will be a noticeable shift in the gender mix of nurses. It is now 97% female; and in equatorial Africa, where there are not the economic disincentives mentioned, half the nurses are male.

Support for nursing education in America is dwindling. The per-graduate costs of nursing education are low and are dropping. That this is the case is somewhat ironic when one considers what nurses are increasingly called on to do. This lack of investment in the education of the nurse seems to me to be fundamentally related to the absence of much investment in the education of women. If women are to be well educated in our present society, they must now enter a field once the exclusive domain of men. For the health and well-being of all, greater investments must be made in the education of nurses for them to meet demands reasonably placed on them as society proceeds toward the economic, epidemiologic, and demographic realities to occur in our aging society in the early decades of the next century.

The effects of economic gender bias are pervasive. Women nurses must take the lead in redressing economic wrongs because men nurses cannot claim gender discrimination even if they are affected by wage discrimination. As a nurse executive, my salary has been ample by any measure, save one. In my experience, men in similar positions, with the same or less responsibility than the chief nurse (like the chief of staff or the chief financial officer), earn half again as much money. The annual salary surveys reported in *Hospitals JAHA* and *Modern Healthcare* graphically illustrate this point. In the case of the nurse executive, the market external to the hospital is most often invoked to establish starting salaries using the premise that "you can't make more than the nursing director at Mass General." Because the wage is established using women nurse executives as the reference point, the wage tends to be less than their male co-workers. Because men are not protected, they cannot claim gender discrimination.

Three women nurses who have sought and won redress for gender bias are Rozella Schlotfeldt, Ada

Jacox, and Virginia Cleland. At some personal expense (Schlotfield, for example, was chastised by her university president) and at the urging of the American Nurses' Association these determined women, all university professors, filed a sex discrimination complaint against their universities and the Teachers Insurance and Annuity Association (TIAA) for paying women less than men in monthly retirement income benefits. TIAA justified the practice by arguing that women live longer. Schlotfeldt, anticipating their response, argued that differential benefits were not paid to African Americans who actuarially had even shorter life spans. Retirement benefits are now equal for men and women, black or white.

Denver nurses unsuccessfully pursued redress for wage discrimination to the U.S. Supreme Court on the basis of comparable worth. Economists have asserted that nurse salaries would improve by between 10% to 15% if comparable worth became the law of the land.[1]

AMERICAN ASSEMBLY FOR MEN IN NURSING

One way to increase the proportion of men nurses in America is to be visible and to support nursing as a satisfying and rewarding profession. To achieve visibility, the American Assembly for Men in Nursing (AAMN) was organized in 1971 by Dennis Martin of Michigan. The independent group of nurses, formerly know as the National Male Nurse Association, has several hundred members in nearly every state of the union. The objectives of the organization were restated in 1981 when the association was renamed.

1. Men and boys in the United States are encouraged to become nurses and join together with all nurses in strengthening and humanizing health care for Americans.
2. Men who are now nurses are encouraged to grow professionally and to demonstrate to each other and to society the increasing contributions made by men within the nursing profession.
3. The American Assembly for Men in Nursing intends that its members be full participants in the nursing profession and its organizations and use this association to achieve the limited goals stated above.

The work of the AAMN is carried on by voluntary officers who organize and conduct an annual meeting and through local chapters located in Philadelphia, Chicago, Indianapolis, Los Angeles, San Francisco, New York, and Cleveland.

In the interest of promoting the objectives of the AAMN, two men nurses appeared on a Cleveland television talk show. This was one in a series of media interviews the organization solicited to alter common misconceptions about nursing. The format for the show was an interview with the show's host, followed by a period of responding to telephone calls from home viewers. During the 15-minute segment two phone calls were answered. The first was from an irate registered nurse who complained that men were taking over the administrative posts and were not involved in caring for patients. The nurses responded that the overwhelming majority of administrative positions in nursing were held by women and that most men nurses are involved in clinical practice. The second comment came from a caller whose mother had recently been a patient in the hospital. She said it was unreasonable for either her mother or her 12-year old daughter to be cared for by men nurses. The nurses cited a study by D'Amelio[5] at Adelphi University, who found that women patients, when they were in real need of nursing care, had no preference for the gender of the nurse providing the care. Further, it was stated that if patients' privacy and modesty needs exceeded their needs for assistance with hygiene, then nurses would enlist the patients' assistance thus becoming free of the nurses' help as soon as possible.[7] The show moderator asked the caller if her mother's doctor was a man. When she replied in the affirmative, the moderator asked why a male nurse was unacceptable but a male doctor was not. Both questions reflected the emotion-laden issues confronting men in the nursing profession.

There have been two court cases of interest to men in nursing. The first was a Supreme Court decision issued by Justice Sandra Day O'Connor. The case involved the Mississippi Women's University practice of limiting enrollment to women and denying otherwise qualified men the right to enroll for credits in its school of nursing. Speaking for the court, Justice O'Connor held that the practice was in violation of the equal protection clause of the Fourteenth Amendment. To quote O'Connor: "Rather than compensate for discriminatory barriers faced by women, Mississippi Women's University policy of excluding men from admission to its School of Nursing, tends to perpetuate the stereotype of nursing as an exclusively women's job."

In the second case, *Backus v Baptist Medical Center,* nurse Gregory Backus was rejected in his repeated attempts to obtain employment in the Baptist Medical Center obstetrical and gynecology unit. After being refused this position, he resigned from the hospital and, in October of 1979, sued Baptist Medical Center, charging discrimination based on sex. A lower court agreed with the Baptist Medical Center's position that having a male nurse work in the obstetrical unit violated the patient's right to privacy. On appeal to the U.S. Court of Appeals for the Eighth Circuit, the judge refused to hear the case because Backus had quit his job at the Baptist Medical Center voluntarily. It is not clear how the case would have been decided had the court not determined that the point was moot. In light of both these cases and the issues they represent, the American Assembly for Men in Nursing has developed a position statement on the role gender should play in the nursing profession in terms of entry into nursing education programs and access to employment in nursing. Members of the AAMN believe that "Every professional nurse position and every nursing educational opportunity shall be equally available to those meeting the entry qualifications regardless of gender."

The argument is not that the wholesale addition of men nurses will make the nursing profession a better one. In fact, past sex-role stereotyping has funneled a disproportionate number of highly intelligent, well-motivated women into nursing. Men in nursing may contribute to a decrease in the economic bias associated with women's work and women's education. Increasing the number of men nurses will, however, make the profession different. The difference will enable our patients to experience a fuller range of professional interventions for their human response to actual or potential health problems. Men nurses are not the answer to all the problems of the nursing profession, but their presence in greater numbers may well be a barometer of the economic value society affords nurses. If men in nursing are that barometer, recent trends in men's enrollment indicate that society is moving forward too slowly in its economic valuation of nurses.

REFERENCES

1. Aldrich M and Buchele R: The economics of comparable worth. Cambridge, Mass, 1986, Ballinger.
2. Beere C: Women and women's issues: a handbook of tests and measures, San Francisco, 1979, Jossey-Bass.
3. Brown R and Stones R: The male nurse. Occassional Papers on Social Administration, Number 52. London, 1973, Social Administration Research Trust at the London School of Economics.
4. Christman L: Men in nursing. In Fitzpatrick J, Taunton R, and Benoliel J, editors: Annual review of nursing research, vol 6, New York, 1988, Springer.
5. D'Amelio R: Patients response to intimate nursing care provided by male or female nurses. Paper presented at the annual meeting of the American Assembly for Men in Nursing, Chicago, Dec 1983.
6. Facts about Nursing, 1942, 1957, 1960, 1961, 1962-1963, 1964, 1966, 1972-1973, 1982-1983, 1984-1985, 1986-1987, Kansas City Mo, American Nurses' Association.
7. Henderson V: The nature of nursing. New York, 1966, Macmillan Co.
8. Holtzclaw B: The man in nursing: relationships between sex-typed perceptions and focus of control. Diss Abstr Int 42(02):Sec. A:P0562, 1981.
9. Hudson H: Source book: nursing personnel, DHEW Pub No (HRA) 75-43, Washington, DC, 1974, Department of Health, Education and Welfare.
10. The Johns Hopkins Hospital: Hospital construction and organization: five essays relating to the construction, organization and management of hospitals, New York, 1875, William Wood.
11. Kalish P and Kalish B: The advance of American nursing, ed 2, Boston, 1986, Little, Brown & Co.
12. London F: Should men be actively recruited into nursing? Nursing Administration Quarterly 12(1):75, 1987.
13. Nemerowicz G: Children's perceptions of gender and work roles, New York, 1979, Praeger.
14. Nightingale F: Cassandra. In Stark M, editor: Cassandra, Old Westbury, NY, 1979, The Feminist Press (originally published in 1852).
15. Nightingale F: Subsidiary notes as to the introduction of female nursing into military hospitals. Reprinted in Seymer LR, editor: Selected writings of Florence Nightingale, New York, 1954, Macmillan (orginally published in 1858).
16. Nuttall P: British nursing: beginning of a power struggle, Nurs Outlook 31(3):184, 1983.
17. Rose J: Men nurses in the military service, AM J Nurs 47:3, 1947.
18. Rossi A: Equality between the sexes: an immodest proposal, Daedalus 93:607, 1964.
19. Some facts about nursing, New York, 1935, American Nurses' Association.
20. The registered nurse population: findings for the national sample survey of registered nurses, November 1984, NTIS #HRP-0906938, Washington, DC, 1986, US Department of Health and Human Services.
21. Rosenfeld P: Nursing data review 1986, New York, 1987, National League for Nursing.

CHAPTER 78

Nurses and unpopular clients

ROBERT J. KUS

INTRODUCTION

Once a visitor watched Mother Theresa, founder of the Missionaries of Charity, care for a dying street person. Because the dying person was dirty, smelly, and had open lesions, the visitor turned to Mother Theresa and said, "I wouldn't do what you do for all the money in the world." Mother Theresa turned to him and said, "I wouldn't either!"

Few of us in nursing would dare compare our sanctity with that of Mother Theresa, yet I believe most of us would agree that our own motivation for caring for clients cannot be explained by money alone. For one thing, no amount of money could adequately compensate us for doing what we do. But more important, most of us in nursing see our work as transcending ordinary toil; it is, rather, a reflection of the human spirit, spirituality at its very best.

All nurses at some time have patients they do not like. Such encounters often make life miserable for the nurse and can actually harm the patient. Understanding the nature of unpopularity in clients can help nurses recognize the roots of their feelings and combat negative behaviors in themselves that can be harmful for patients they do not like. This will improve their own mental health as well as the care of their patients.

This chapter, then, examines the concept of *unpopularity* as it refers to nurses' patients, identifies the roots of unpopularity, and offers some ideas on how to prevent our negative views of clients from becoming destructive to ourselves and to them. Finally, one unpopular, vulnerable, and mistreated population in our society will be examined—prisoners—and some suggestions will be made concerning how nurses can intervene as nurses and citizens to combat the everyday antihuman treatment that prisoners endure.

THE CONCEPT OF UNPOPULARITY

Popularity comes from the Latin word populus, meaning "people." It refers to the state of something being liked or accepted by the population at large. *Unpopularity*, then, refers to a person, place, or thing being seen as not likeable or acceptable by most people. When we say patients are unpopular, it is important to note that there is nothing intrinsic to any patient making that person unpopular or popular. Unpopularity can only exist when an external evaluation is placed on a person, place, or thing by people, in this case by nurses. Another important point is that there is often broad agreement among nurses about who is unpopular, whereas at other times defining a patient as unpopular is specific to a single nurse. An example of the former would be clients who are obnoxious toward nurses; an example of the latter is the client who looks like a nurse's despised ex-spouse.

THE ROOTS OF UNPOPULARITY

Why are some patients unpopular with nurses? This section explores some of the roots of unpopularity.

Low social value. Some persons are seen by nurses and other helping professionals as having less social value than others. This has been well documented by sociologists Glaser and Strauss,[1] among others. Social value is determined by demographic characteristics such as age, marital status, income, and the like. For example, a 98-year-old person is often seen as having less social value than a 20-year-old person. As a result, the heroic measures used to save the 20-year-old will often be withheld from the 98-year-old. Likewise, married persons—especially those with small children—are often seen as having higher social worth than single persons or married persons with no children. Nurses, being human, often see clients with low social value as being less desirable—unpopular—than those with high social value.

Low moral worth. Sometimes nurses classify persons as moral or immoral. Those deemed to be immoral become unpopular and thus may receive inferior nursing care to those deemed to be moral. For example, nurses may see a prostitute as immoral and a priest as moral because of the moral implications of their careers. Or the nurse may define as immoral clients who use physical violence to discipline their children. In short, when a client behaves in ways that go against our own value systems, we may define that person as immoral and unpopular.

Unchosen stigmata. Certain persons carry with them one or more stigmata that they did not choose, which make them unpopular with large numbers of people. Examples of such stigmata include gay or lesbian sexual orientation, gender (either male or female), and race or ethnicity. If the nurse is antimale or antiblack, chances are that male or black patients will be unpopular with that nurse.

"Own fault" diagnoses. Sometimes the root of unpopularity is the medical diagnosis the patient carries. If nurses perceive the disease or condition to be the result of behaviors chosen by the clients, they often find such patients unpopular. Typical examples of such patients are alcoholics, heavy smokers who have lung cancer, adults who contracted AIDS from having unsafe sex or from HIV-contaminated needles, and suicidal patients. Often nurses want to care for "innocent" persons who "deserve" their care rather than those whom they feel are "getting what they deserve."

Fear-causing conditions. Some patients' behaviors or medical diagnoses are frightening to nurses, which makes such patients unpopular. The person with a highly contagious, incurable disease or the violent patient are two common examples. Fear of contracting a disease, however, is often a cover-up for bigotry, as when a truly homophobic nurse claims that a fear of catching the disease is the reason for refusing to care for a gay man with AIDS.

Clients who behave negatively. In addition to violent clients who frighten nurses, certain clients behave in ways that are generally perceived by nurses to be negative. These include clients who are seen as ungrateful, "spoiled brats," hostile, staff-splitters, manipulators, eager to sue, constant complainers, and noncompliant. In addition, people who seem to be "professional patients" (hypochondriacs) and those who overuse their call lights are often unpopular with many nurses.

Incompetence on the nurse's part. Sometimes clients are unpopular with nurses simply because the nurses do not feel competent to care for them. It is frightening and dangerous to care for clients about whom you know little. For example, child-health nurses floated to a coronary care unit might see their new clients as having needs far beyond their ability to meet.

THE CONSEQUENCES OF UNPOPULARITY

When clients are defined as unpopular by their nurses, there are potential consequences for both clients and nurses. For nurses, caring for unpopular patients may lead to job dissatisfaction, which, in turn, may lead to diminished health—physical, mental, and spiritual. Nurses may increasingly call in sick; suffer from insomnia, anorexia, or other compulsive behaviors; withdraw from their peers; criticize the profession or the institution; or exhibit a lack of energy on the job. If nurses begin to put all or most of their patients in the unpopular category—as might nurses who cannot find work in their field of expertise—quitting the job or the profession might result.

Nurses may also take out their negative feelings toward unpopular patients by engaging in behaviors based on hostility or frustration. They can withhold pain medications, ignore call lights, act cool and detached instead of warm and sensitive, ignore basic psychosocial needs, and turn other staff against such patients. These behaviors harm the unpopular patient, certainly, yet they also may harm the nurse. For example, although it might give the nurse immediate gratification to get back at an obnoxious patient, in the long run it might (and should) produce feelings of guilt. On the other hand, wise nurses may engage in hyperpositive behaviors toward their unpopular clients to counteract their inclinations to treat them unkindly.

COMBATTING NEGATIVE EFFECTS OF UNPOPULARITY

Because defining certain clients as unpopular often leads to negative feelings and behavior on the part of the nurse, and because this labeling often leads to negative nursing behavior directed toward such clients, it is wise to explore how nurses can minimize these negatives.

First, nurses need to admit to their negative feelings toward certain clients. They need to identify those patients who make them feel uncomfortable, angry, self-righteous, and the like. Second, they need to make a list of unpopular patients. Writing down the characteristics of such patients is most helpful, as this will help nurses identify more easily the categories that emerge. Nurses should analyze this list to determine exactly what it is about such patients that makes them unpopular. In other words, what are the "negativity generators." Negativity generators will be defined here as those client characteristics that generate negative feelings in nurses and, therefore, make such clients unpopular. Are they skin color? Religion? Obnoxious or seductive behavior? Legal status, as in the case of prisoners?

After examining the categories of persons on their lists, nurses can ask themselves whether the negativity generators are changeable or unchangeable. Negativity generators are considered unchangeable if the client has no control over their existence. These would include such characteristics as gender (transsexuals excluded), race, ethnicity, sexual orientation, age, and often various disease conditions such as cerebral palsy. Likewise, the client may have done something in the past and received a label that generates negative feelings in the nurse. Examples of these include heavy smokers who now have lung cancer or prisoners. Although prisoners may have been responsible for doing something negative that led to their being incarcerated, they are not able to change their current status.

In contrast to the unchangeable generators, there are two types that are clearly changeable. One type includes characteristics that nurses would usually be reluctant to try to change. Examples of these include religion or marital status. A second type are characteristics that nurses generally feel require nursing intervention to change to make the client a more fulfilled person. Examples of these would be behaviors that are nonassertive, manipulative, seductive, violent, hostile, noncompliant, or generally obnoxious.

Third, nurses must examine how they treat those clients they see as unpopular. Do they give such patients less time than they do other patients? Do they avoid them? Talk negatively about them to other staff? Withhold pain medication? Neglect their psychosocial needs? If nurses find that they care for each client in a caring, sensitive, and professional manner no matter what the circumstances, then they need go no further. But if nurses realize they are treating certain patients negatively either directly (e.g., by withholding pain medication or by being unfriendly) or indirectly (e.g.,

by turning other staff against them or by allowing staff to treat such patients negatively), they must then make a decision to change any negative behaviors they are engaging in toward unpopular clients. This requires reminding themselves of the lofty nursing ideals that all humans, by virtue of their humanity, are worthy of total respect, care, and compassion regardless of their various life circumstances or past or present behaviors.

If nurses find that their negative patient list includes people who have unchangeable personal characteristics, nurses can do one of three things: (1) stay clear of such patients, (2) change their attitudes, or (3) keep their attitudes but change any behavior that would reflect their negativity toward the client.

Staying clear of such patients is a relatively straightforward prospect. A nurse who cannot stand children might quit a hospital job on a pediatric unit to become a medical nurse, or a psychiatric nurse might leave a medical-surgical unit to work in a mental health center. Changing negative attitudes is more difficult. It requires work and a great willingness to change. If nurses find they are antiwhite or antigay, for example, they must be willing to confront white people or gay people to change their feelings. If they cannot change, they must simply adopt the third strategy of keeping their attitudes but changing any negative behaviors they may use toward such clients.

If nurses find their unpopular patient list is composed of persons whose negativity generators are changeable, they need to ask themselves whether helping the client to change these characteristics is ethical or not. For example, a person's religion is usually not something a nurse tries to change unless it is a cult generally seen as dangerous by society at large. On the other hand, if a client has a pattern of violence or seductive behavior, the nurse would be helping the patient by encouraging such a change in behavior. Such change would not only eliminate negativity on the part of the nurse, it would also benefit the patient in the long run.

Fourth, nurses can combat the negative effects of unpopularity in patients by seeing nursing as a way of life, not merely a job having relevance when the nurse is on duty. When nurses do this, they not only focus on their particular patients or believe in taking action only in their work setting, but also see themselves and their profession as holding the key to radically changing negative actions toward all humans, in all settings, at all times. Thus, no policy that degrades any human is deemed outside the province of nursing. Let us look at one such example.

THE PRISONER AND NURSING

Having read this far, most nurses, I am sure, feel pretty confident that they are not too far off the mark in treating all patients with the dignity they deserve simply because of their humanity. After all, nurses are pretty decent folk. Those readers who have identified some clients whom they have treated negatively are probably willing to change.

But before becoming too smug and complacent, we nurses need to ask ourselves some difficult questions. One is, when are we nurses? Only when officially on duty or at all times? If we answer only when on duty, then we may indeed pat ourselves on the back if we strive to treat all patients, even the most unpopular ones, with great compassion, sensitivity, and care. On the other hand, if we see ourselves as being nurses at all times, then we will be less smug.

The second question we must ask is who are our clients? If we believe our clients are only those persons to whom we are legally responsible while on duty, then we probably can be comfortable in examining our care. On the other hand, if we believe that all humanity is our client, then we have to realize that nursing has just begun to be practiced.

The third question is what is nursing? For some nurses it is traditional functions such as one-to-one counseling, patient teaching, and performing technical procedures. For others it is a radical social activism designed to elevate humanity to its highest level by eliminating the suffering of *all* humans and destroying the roots of suffering of *all* humans. I believe nurses must make every attempt to ensure that the Golden Rule—"Do unto others as you would have them do unto you"—be followed for *all* humans, not just those who are popular.

This brings us to prisoners. No persons in our society are more vulnerable to the hatred and truly dark, punitive side of human nature. Nurses are certainly not immune; they have been shown to be followers, rather than leaders, in prison reform and the general treatment of prisoners.

But talking about prisoners often generates intense feelings in some individuals. Many argue that prisoners "deserve" to be punished. Thus they are not merely content to see police, prison guards, judges, and others mistreat prisoners; they often encourage it. Nurses have proved time and again to be a reflection of the larger society—followers rather than leaders or social activists.

From my perspective, all actions that counteract the Golden Rule are acts of antilove. All antilove acts are against the dignity of humanity. All acts against human dignity are morally wrong. All such acts are, then, against the very core of nursing. And as long as such acts continue, nurses must fight to eliminate them.

So it is not okay to chain human beings to beds. It is not okay to parade human beings around hospitals or anywhere else in identifiable prison garb and chains and handcuffs. It is not okay to allow prisoners to be raped. It is not okay to lock persons up in prisons *as they exist today*.

If nurses believe these things are violations of human dignity, what can they do? They can oppose all policies that permit prisoners to be chained to beds or paraded around in prison garb and chains. These disgusting practices offend the sensibilities of any person who has an ounce of decency. True, there must be a way to prevent escape or, more accurately, to prevent police from harming prisoners under the guise of "preventing attempted escape." But could we not invent a device to be worn under clothing that would prevent a person from running? Could we not have nonuniformed guards by clients' beds instead of chaining them to a bed? Of course we can. The question is not whether we can but whether we value human life and human dignity enough to do so.

Nurses need to fight for prison reform, or rather for the elimination of virtually all prisons except for a limited number to house those who are truly dangerous. Some people need to be out of society. But they do not need to be treated like rabid animals as they are today, and certainly they do not need to be confined in the antihuman institutions that many prisons are today. Prison architecture and programs must be designed to provide the prisoner with the highest quality of life possible. It seems to me that being locked away from loved ones, denied basic freedoms, stigmatized for life, and forced to associate with people who have devoted much of their lives to degrading human beings—judges, probation and parole officers, police, prison guards, and the like—is truly enough punishment. Nurses must also fight against the rape of prisoners, most of whom are males, just as hard as they fight against the rape of nonincarcerated females. To do otherwise is incredibly sexist.

From my perspective, a nurse is always a nurse. Our clients are all humanity. However, although all people are our clients in a moral sense, those who suffer—especially the disadvantaged—deserve our most fervent and compassionate attention. And nursing is for me a radical social activism designed to protect the dignity of *all* humans and destroy *all* things that lead to a person's mental, physical, and spiritual distress. The mistreatment of fellow humans should rekindle a fire in every nurse, a fire born of rage and fervor, a fire that will rock the very foundations of our profession in a radical social activism that will not stop until every human on earth is treated with true dignity.

REFERENCES

1. Glaser BG and Strauss AL: (1968) Time for Dying, Chicago: Aldine.

CHAPTER 79

Cultural diversity

The international student

HELEN K. GRACE

Increasingly nurses throughout the developing world are looking to the United States for educational preparation for their nursing educators and leaders. In most instances, nurses from other countries enter undergraduate and graduate educational programs, complete the prescribed program of study, and return to their own countries to grapple with the applicability of their educational preparation within the context of their home country. U.S. nursing educational programs frequently have little understanding of the background of these nurses, both educationally and experientially, and little appreciation of the expectations for this nurse when she returns to her home country. Although the experiences of faculty and other students could be enriched by learning about health care in other countries, foreign students are rarely called on to share their rich background with others. In this paper, the international student will be described. Future roles of nurses with advanced preparation will be outlined. Finally, some suggestions for educational innovations to modify programs of study for international students will be made. The ideas expressed in this chapter are drawn from observations of nursing practice and education in Bahrain, an Arab country, Latin America, and southern Africa.

THE INTERNATIONAL NURSING STUDENT

The international student coming from a developing country is usually coming from a culture that is male dominated and one in which roles for women are tightly circumscribed. Issues related to nursing and nursing education are intertwined with broader concerns related to the roles of women in these societies. In most instances women in developing countries are responsible for most of the functions related to maintaining the family. They are responsible for bearing and nurturing children and, to varying degrees, for providing basic sustenance for the family. Within such a cultural context, the entrance into nursing as a profession may be for some an acceptable way of gaining social mobility. For example, when asked why she had become a nurse, a woman from a rural area in Botswana replied: "I always did well in school. After completing my secondary school study at the mission school, I was sent to (the city) to do my Cambridge level study (to qualify for entrance to advanced study). I saw the nurses in their white uniforms and carrying lots of books. I thought that nurses were very smart people, and that was one thing that I could become that would be acceptable." In contrast, in Bahrain, a woman from a social class in which education is encouraged would be pressured by her family to become educated in a field that has prestige, such as banking or business. Nursing is associated with servitude. For women to enter nursing, they frequently have to overcome the opposition of family, who see this as a demeaning profession. In this context, educated Bahraini nurses have an image problem to overcome in pursuing a nursing career. Nurses from the male-dominated cultures of Latin America also face varying degrees of stigmatization. Those who are educated within the universities have completed a program of study equivalent in length to that for other professions such as medicine or dentistry. Yet when they enter the workforce they are paid less than half of the salary earned by beginning physicians. Medicine, dentistry, law, and other professional fields are socially more acceptable, and educated nurses have to deal with considerable bias within their societies.

Once nursees are in practice they also face some unique problems. In some instances, nurses are treated as if they are married to their profession. For example, in southern African countries, upon completion of basic preparation, nurses are posted by the Ministry of Health to remote areas of the country, where they staff rural health clinics. In some of these settings they live in a house adjacent to the clinic and are responsible 24 hours a day, 7 days a week for managing the health problems of the village and the community in which the clinic is located. They manage deliveries of babies, handle emergency care of all types, prescribe and administer medications, and educate the people. If they are fortunate, a physician from a neighboring mission hospital visits once a month to provide consultation on specific cases. Advancement within the system is to be assigned to a post nearer to the city when there is a vacancy. Within this system a nurse who is married is separated from her husband for long periods of time. In contrast, in Latin America, a nurse who is married is expected to manage her career while simultaneously meeting the expectations for a married woman in that culture. This means that nurses rarely have the opportunity to travel beyond their home communities, and opportunities for educational and career advancement, particularly for married women, are extremely limited.

A nurse who has advanced to a position to be considered for educational programs abroad, has had to overcome a large number of obstacles related to expectations for women within their societies. They are achievers and leaders. However, because of the educational programs available within their countries there may be deficits in their theoretical knowledge compared with students who have come through U.S. educational programs. On the practical side, they have had worlds of experience but of a much different order than that of U.S. students. Imagine how bizarre some of the debates of scope on practice must seem to nurses who have been sole providers of care for large numbers of people in remote areas. Yet because of theoretical knowledge deficits, compounded in some instances by language difficulties, the nurse from another culture is frequently treated as though she were "not too bright," certainly not on a par with U.S. students. The international student, in this unfamiliar environment where her leadership and skills are not recognized, frequently becomes unsure of herself and begins

to fulfill the expectations that she is less than her fellow classmates.

FUTURE ROLE EXPECTATIONS

Although within the U.S. educational program the nurse from a developing country may be treated as not up to par with the more articulate U.S. student, particularly in theoretical discourse, once that nurse returns to her country she is immediately placed in a major leadership role. Most nurses educated outside of the country return to a faculty position. In many instances, particularly in countries in which nursing education is organized on the British system, these educational programs are located within the ministry of health and in terms of content are quite similar to our hospital-based nursing programs of the past. Students who have completed the equivalent of high school are admitted into programs that are 3 years in length and disassociated from university education. Following completion of the 3-year basic program, nurses have an additional year of preparation as a midwife, which is recognized by certification. In many countries nurses complete additional specialization programs, such as community nursing, which require yet another year of study. The faculty in such programs frequently teach both the basic content of a field in the general program and also specific subjects for the specialization programs.

As university education is beginning to develop in some countries, nursing faculty may also fill university positions. In this role the expectations for them are similar to those for faculty in the United States. In Latin America there are a number of university-based basic programs that combine characteristics of nursing education similar to those described in the ministry of health programs combined with characteristics of university-based education in the United States. The pattern of specialty certification, postbasic nursing education is similar in both types of program arrangements.

Although the majority of international nursing students returning to developing countries will have faculty positions, the types of challenges facing them as faculty are quite different from those faced by U.S. nursing faculties. First, they must address the question of suitable educational materials for their students. In the United States we assume that there are a variety of textbooks available to students and that libraries have significant holdings of nursing journals and books that can be drawn on to provide a rich educational experience. Faculty members are responsible for setting the learning objectives for a particular class, identifying textbooks from a large number of choices, and compiling a reading list of relevant material. The student is responsible for synthesizing this material. It is assumed that the available literature covers content appropriate to the context of nursing in the United States.

For a nurse faculty member in a developing country, few of these assumptions hold true. Faculty members are called on to "write their own books" as course syllabi for the students. Limited resource materials are available to them. The resource materials available are frequently too broad in scope for basic learning materials for students. At best there is a limited library available for student use, and there are few, if any, textbooks written by native authors, so that all material requires considerable adaptation to be culturally relevant. Faculty in developing countries spend hours developing course syllabi, which become the sole reference source for students. Because of the scope of practice of nurses who graduate from their programs, knowledge of pharmacology, for example, has to be an entirely different order from that of programs in the United States. In some instances nurse faculty need much more extensive knowledge, and in other areas, generalist perspectives are appropriate.

Of the numbers of nurses from developing countries returning to faculty positions, some will return to become the directors of educational programs either within a ministry of health setting or in a basic university program. They need knowledge of both education and administration in addition to their knowledge base in nursing. Other nurses return to managerial positions in the ministry of health, and in this area they need depth of knowledge of management, planning, and public policy formulation.

As for the knowledge base in nursing, much of the focus of attention around the world is on primary health care and community nursing. Educational programs for preparation of nurses in developing countries remain heavily focused on acute-care nursing issues and hospital-based practice. Nurses in leadership roles are responsible for shifting this emphasis both in education and practice. The few nurses who have advanced preparation in these countries have varying degrees of responsibility for managing others,

such as community health workers and auxiliary nurses and nurses' aides. Unlike the nurse in the United States with master's-level practice who is being prepared either as an expert clinical practitioner or as a teacher of a nursing specialty area, the nurse with advanced preparation from a developing country will be called on to provide a much different type of leadership in both the educational and practice domains.

MAKING THE EDUCATIONAL EXPERIENCE RELEVANT

Given differences in backgrounds of the students coming to the United States for advanced educational preparation and the role expectations for them when they return to their countries, it is important to give specialized attention to modification of nursing educational programs to address these needs. Two approaches, or a combination of the two, might be employed to assure the relevance of the educational program for the advanced student: (1) to modify graduate education in the United States to accommodate the student or (2) to deliver educational programs off site to international settings.

Program modifications

Modifications in both the clinical and functional content of graduate programs are needed to accommodate the specialized needs of international students. In the clinical area, the international student requires a more generalist approach to clinical nursing than does the typical U.S. graduate student. In planning for a student program it is important for both the prospective student and the faculty to have a shared understanding of the planned content of the program. For example, a prospective student from Botswana registered for the intensive-care specialty program in a well-regarded master's program in the United States. In an interview with the faculty adviser, the student described her experiences working in a remote area, where she had to provide primary health care and attend to all of the injuries that came to the clinic door. She was seeking to expand her expertise in caring for such patients. Had she enrolled in the graduate program without the faculty understanding her background and interests, the clinical content and experience would have focused on the high degree of specialization specific to hospital care in the United States. After sitting down with advisers, a modified program of study was worked out that was a mix of community and primary health care nursing with time in emergency rooms for the clinical practicum components.

The majority of nurses from developing countries who seek advanced study require a community or primary health care specialization. Over the past several decades, this area of study has been deemphasized in U.S. programs, and a large number of acute-care specialty areas have developed. Similarly, the clinical component of these programs in highly specialized acute-care settings is inappropriate for nurses from developing countries. Modification of the curriculum would be to the advantage not only of the international student, but also the U.S. students seeking to work with a wide variety of patients in community settings.

In addition to modifying the clinical component of the curriculum, most international students need increased content in either the teaching component or the administrative component of the curriculum. Both of these areas also could be more useful by modifying the content to address the specialized problems these nurses will face on return to their countries. Development of appropriate learning materials for use in their home countries and health planning experiences in a public health program are examples of areas that could be modified to make the learning experience more relevant.

The research component of graduate programs could also be much more relevant if provision were made for the student to return to their home country to conduct their research. This approach generally involves added cost of travel, but the advantages to doing research in the home country far outweigh the costs of this added expense.

One difficulty in making modifications such as those described above is that U.S. faculty frequently have little understanding of the setting from which the student comes and the responsibilities to which she will return. Exchange programs in which faculty teach or practice in foreign countries would do much to build awareness of the types of modifications important to the international nursing student.

Delivery of educational programs to other countries

In some instances in which there is a comprehensive plan for development of human resources for nursing education and practice it would be preferable for U.S. programs to deliver their educational programs within the foreign country. To do so may require adult learning approaches in which students from a region come together for short periods of intensive study and then return to their home setting to apply the knowledge gained in the clinical setting of their home country. Particularly in cultures that are male dominated, a program delivered to the area that allows the nursing student to fulfill obligations to the family while also gaining advanced preparation would allow many more nurses to pursue additional study. Once a critical mass of nurses prepared at advanced levels is reached in a country, these nurses can provide leadership to nursing education programs adequate for preparation of nurses for the years ahead.

Faculty from U.S programs who teach in such exported educational programs would have a unique opportunity for their own professional development, first in understanding other cultures and also in modifying approaches to graduate education. This in turn would contribute to needed modifications in graduate education in the United States to provide a much more relevant type of graduate program to meet the needs for community-based primary care in the United States.

SUMMARY

The United States is a major resource for educational preparation of nursing leadership throughout the world. To provide appropriate educational experiences, it is important to understand the setting from which students come and to which they will return. Educational programs that accommodate to the specialized needs of the international student not only will serve the developing world, but also will provide the needed stimulus to change our own educational programs to prepare nurses for community-based primary health care in the United States.

PART TWELVE

ETHICS

Complex ethical dilemmas for nurses and nursing

JOANNE COMI McCLOSKEY
HELEN KENNEDY GRACE

Ethical issues confronting nursing reflect a number of themes addressed throughout this book. The capability of the health technologies currently available to deal with complex diseases and prolong life, the increased numbers of elderly in our society requiring services, the shortage of nurses, increasing costs, and the numbers of persons experiencing difficulty in gaining access to needed health services all combine to create ethical dilemmas for individual nurses and for nursing collectively.

Part 12 opens with a debate chapter focusing on the individual patient-nurse dilemma of truth telling. The second chapter provides an overview of the broad range of ethical dilemmas. The three succeeding chapters focus on ethical issues that have arisen because of the increasing use of advanced technology. Turning to more specific issues, ethical dilemmas surrounding indigent care, care for AIDS victims, and in vitro fertilization are addressed. The final chapter turns to ethical issues in the international domain.

Posing the question of "under what circumstances, if any, and for what reason, if any, is a nurse justified in deceiving a patient through silence, nonverbal pretense, or withholding relevant information, or outright lying?" Freel addresses the issues related to truth telling. Having established a framework for understanding basic human rights and having presented the four basic methods for establishing ethical arguments, Freel then argues that the three basic principles of autonomy, beneficence, and justice form the foundation for understanding the arguments for and against truth telling. Six major reasons are cited for truth telling: "It is essential to trust in the nurse-patient relationship, patients have the right to know, it is the moral thing to do, it alleviates anxiety and suffering, it is necessary to achieve patient and family cooperation, and it can meet the need of the nurse." Four arguments are marshalled against truth telling: "Truthfulness is impossible to achieve, patients may not want to know the truth if it unpleasant, professionals have a duty to do no harm, and deception may be a means of gaining cooperation to facilitate a therapeutic situation." Nursing does not operate in a vacuum, and Freel notes the need for ethical committees and guidelines to help nurses deal in a rational and reasoned manner with the complex patient care issues they are confronting.

Noting the current preoccupation with principles of ethics, Donahue cautions that "The tyranny of ethics is rapidly becoming a reality, in the sense of ethics becoming an absolute power that may ultimately oppress." She argues for "the translation to real-life situations in which a balance must be achieved between moral principles and individual, social, and cultural differences." Drawing the parallel between contagious diseases of the past and the current problem of AIDS, the author notes the inconsistency of nursing's ethical positions. Donahue cautions against reliance on codes of ethics to guide decision making and instead argues for teaching nurses critical thinking "in order that they may develop confidence to act on their analyses."

One way to deal with problems of equity in health care services is through rationing. Implications of varying forms of health care rationing for nursing are outlined in the chapter by Fry. She notes first that, whether we acknowledge it or not, a rationing system is already in place. The fee-for-service system limits services to those who can pay, either directly or through insurance. Cost sharing for health care through coinsurance is also another form of rationing. The basic strategy for containing costs under HMO arrangements is yet another form. In contrast to these implicit approaches to rationing, explicit rationing is based on administrative decisions about such things as extent of coverage within health care plans, limitation of health care services, and setting of intervals between care episodes. Noting that the above strategies have not done much to control costs, Fry turns to a discussion of rationing services to a segment of the population, the elderly. Instead of rationing care to certain segments of the population, Fry argues instead for focusing on a philosophy of caring. Reducing the use of high-technology interventions and instead providing humane care as a means of ameliorating the ethical dilemmas posed by rationing strategies.

Continuing this theme, Murphy addresses the increasing conflicts created by the interaction among science, technology, and institutional interests. With the almost limitless capacity of technology to keep patients alive and the countervailing interest of institutions in cost-effectiveness, "the challenge for the nursing profession is how to continue to render humane and moral care that gives life, health, and death its meaning."

Turning to knowledge technology, Amos and Graves address the subject of how computer capabilities can be used as an aid to nurse decision making. Creation of expert systems holds the promise of assisting nurses in clincal management. However, the use of such expert systems brings with it another set of ethical problems, in particular the question of whether individual judgment will be abandoned and thus further diminish the role of nurses. Cost-benefit issues in establishing expert knowledge systems in clincal practice are another consideration. The authors conclude that "although the costs of initial investment . . . may be considerable, we cannot afford not to take advantage of this significant opportunity to mainstream nursing so that significant strides can be made in the quality of care delivered and the expansion of the profession's knowledge base."

Continuing the discussion of computer technology, Delaney argues for a balance between high-technology computers and high-touch caring. Using computers to do some of the work that nurses traditionally have done provides an opportunity to focus on the caring dimensions of clinical practice. Noting the potential for negative effects from overreliance on computer technology, nurses are charged with the responsibility for safeguarding the interests of the patient. "Nurses' abilities to achieve a balance between the technology and the humanness of nursing practice will be measured by the degree to which human dignity is protected, preserved, and enhanced."

Turning to more specific problems, Malloy addresses issues related to indigent care. Characterizing the change as one of moving from an idea of the Great Society of the 1960s to corporatization in the 1980s, the lack of access to care of large segments of our society challenges our view of living in a humane democracy. Malloy reduces the debate to two basic questions: "Who receives care?" and "Who pays?" Noting that nurses have traditionally championed the cause of health care for the poor and vulnerable, the author calls for a "modern-day Lillian Wald, a mover and shaker of society's purse strings and conscience."

The rise in the numbers of patients with AIDS constitutes a further challenge to nurses' concerns for humane care for all people. Stigmatization of persons with AIDS (PWAs) extends to the health professions. Concerns for personal safety in providing care for AIDS patients, personal and professional values, and concerns for patient autonomy become part of the broader ethical issues involved in providing care. Forrester concludes that an appropriate nursing response to the AIDS epidemic should have three components: (1) to prevent HIV infection, (2) to provide care for those already infected, and (3) to participate in national and international efforts to fight AIDS and its associated stigma.

Shifting to a discussion of ethical dilemmas associated with reproductive technology, Oshansky focuses on three concepts: (1) choice, (2) control, and (3) the meaning of parenthood. Although some argue that women who are infertile should have the choice of in vitro fertilization, the author points out that only those women who can pay or who are considered appropriate for the procedure by the medical profession have this choice. Thus the concept of choice becomes intertwined with that of control and the meaning of parenthood in our society. The nurse has responsibility for counseling patients so that they are informed and knowledgeable and can make appropriate decisions for themselves.

Arguing first that ethical values hold across cultures, Halloran notes some key concerns and encourages nurses to become informed about international issues and to speak out against ethical abuses. The export of outdated drugs, the export of drugs not yet certified as safe, and the promotion and aggressive sale of nonessential drugs are questionable practices. The promotion of commercially prepared baby formula is another practice of concern to many. Policies regarding AIDS testing, questionable practices associated with organ transplants, the jailing of health workers because they provided emergency care to political dissidents are all areas of concern for nurses. The challenge is for nurses to be informed and to be activists on behalf of equity and justice for all.

The issues confronting nurses throughout the world are complex. Maintaining a focus on the needs of people for health care services and the responsibility of nurses to see that equitable health care services are provided for all is a major challenge as we move into the last decade of the century.

CHAPTER 80

Debate

Truth telling

MILDRED I. FREEL

The issue of whether patients should be told the truth raises a number of questions. Which patient, what truth, and who should or should not do the telling? Who has the right and obligation to tell? How should the patient be told, what method or sequence should be used? Should the disclosure result from action, words, or both? Should the patient be told when questions are asked or when the care giver deems that the patient is ready to handle the information?

When providing care for the terminally ill the nurse is often faced with a number of legal and ethical issues for which she or he may not be prepared. The critical ethical question regarding truth telling is under what circumstance, if any, and for what reason, if any, is a nurse justified in deceiving a patient through silence, nonverbal pretense, withholding relevant information, or outright lying?

One of the major areas of ethical dilemma that confronts the health care worker today evolves from the effects of scientific progress, the advancement of knowledge, and technical developments. Dilemmas in this category include issues such as whether resuscitation technology should be used for the terminally ill, or whether the use of life support equipment ought to be discontinued. The second major category of dilemma relates to communication among health workers and between health workers and their patients. This interpersonal, interprofessional relationship area includes the issue of whether to tell the patient the truth and what information should be disclosed.

To make sound decisions regarding disclosure, the care giver needs to understand the basic elements that relate to ethical or moral choices. Curtin[7] has identified three characteristics or criteria of an ethical problem. First, the resolution of an ethical problem does not evolve from empirical data. Second, the problem is inherently perplexing, making it difficult to determine what database should be utilized in the decision-making process. Third, the answer to an ethical problem affects more than the specific situation; it has a profound and far-reaching effect on one's perception of human beings and their relationship to one another and the world. Curtin defines an ethical dilemma as "a choice between equally undesirable alternatives."[7] To resolve an ethical dilemma one must try to make the right choice among equally unfavorable alternatives.

The way a moral or ethical question is addressed is partially determined by one's role in society. When the role rapidly changes, as currently is occurring for both patients and health care givers, confusion concerning the scope of responsibility, obligation, and duties often results.

This chapter attempts to identify the scope of truth telling and debates this issue. Human rights, the nature of ethical inquiry, the principles of ethics related to truth telling, the espoused views of laypersons and health care professionals regarding truth telling, and professional ethics are first discussed. This is followed by a presentation of arguments for and against telling the patient the truth. The conclusion discusses how working from an ethical framework can help prevent problems with truth telling from becoming ethical dilemmas.

HUMAN RIGHTS

Basic and universal human needs are the core of the concept of human rights. A right is a rational claim that comes from interpreting the consequences and practicality of a situation. Rights exist regardless of whether they are acknowledged, respected, or abridged. To be human is to be rational and dependent on other humans. Therefore, the welfare of a human being is the concern of all other human beings. All people have certain human rights that may be referred to as natural rights, primary among them the right to be respected as a human being.

Every right has a corresponding duty. Health care givers need to determine what are patient rights in a given situation, both legally and morally, and then determine who has a duty or obligation to fulfill or respect those rights. It must also be determined if a higher duty or a prior claim exists, as well as whether the fulfillment of these obligations would violate the rights of another.

Two major ideas underlie the patient rights movement. The first is the acknowledgment that a patient is a person who has the same rights people have in general; the second is that a patient does not forfeit these rights by the fact of illness, injury, or entry into the health care system. Since the early 1970s there has been a weakening of the professional-dominance model of health care and a movement toward a partnership model with more emphasis on the development of mechanisms for protecting patient rights. One of the initial mechanisms was the publication of a Patient Bill of Rights by the American Hospital Association (AHA) in 1972. This bill, by identifying the existing legal and ethical rights of patients, gave impetus for moving toward a more universal recognition and protection of these rights. In addition, there exists the right not to exercise a right. Therefore if a patient indicates that disclosure of information is not desired, the duty to disclose is not present.

THE NATURE OF ETHICS

Ethics is the philosophical inquiry into the principles of morality, of right and wrong conduct, or of good and evil as they relate to conduct. Philosophy often uses the terms *ethics* and *morality* synonymously. Ethics comprises principles and rules that can be used to critique and evaluate the norms of law, custom, institutional practice, and positive morality. However, ethics is not directly concerned with what these norms are, but rather with what ought to be. The nature of ethics can of itself produce controversy. Reasonable but opposing positions can evolve from different in-

terpretations of ethical principles and their rules or directed actions.

The field of ethics may be divided into "normative ethics" and "metaethics." Normative ethics is concerned with questions of right and wrong action, good and evil, or moral conduct. Metaethics is concerned with the nature of ethical discourse.

Ethical discussions use four major methods of argument.[14] One method uses appeals to authority. This method establishes a proposition on the grounds that a particular authority declares it to be so. The authority may be a human or a supernatural being, a group of persons, or an institution such as a church or government. In this method it is necessary to show why the reported authority is an authority and the authenticity of the report of its pronouncements. Use of this method is limited as its appeal is only for the believer. A second method of argument is the appeal to *consensum hominum*, that is, using an argument based on the alleged agreement of people in general or of a particular group of people concerning an issue. Underlying this method is the belief that those cited are wise and ethically competent and that they in fact subscribe to the belief being attributed to them. A third method is an appeal to intuition or self-evidence. The intuitionist philosophers ultimately base their ethical positions on what they identify as the technical concept of intuition. This method of appeal is limited mainly to those who have had the intuition. The fourth method is called the method of argumentation, or the dilectical or Socratic method. This method uses the approach of asking questions and looking for answers that are backed up by sound reason. This analytical method, which draws on theory, principles, and rules, is the primary method used to gain an understanding of ethical phenomena.

Various rules, principles, and theories are used in the process of making moral decisions. Rules state that certain actions should or should not be performed because they are right or wrong. An example is that one ought to tell the truth. Frankena[9] identified two major difficulties or limits of rules. The first is that the ethical rules of society are often vague, imprecise, allowing for exceptions, and in conflict with one another. The second is that rules are usually developed from a negative or conservative position which does not allow constructive creativity for adaptation to new or changed situations.

Rules are derived from principles. Principles are more abstract than rules and are used as guides to action. They are presuppositions about what is ultimately good or right. They are expressions of human ideas that are stated as generalized universal truths. For example, the ethical principle of autonomy addresses the right of self-determination and is the basis for rules related to informed consent, patient privacy, and truth telling.

It is out of theories that principles and rules evolve. Theories both explain and provide the bases for decisions when principles or rules are in conflict. Moral philosophers have developed several ethical theories; however, most can be classified as either deontological or teleological theories.[2,9]

Teleological theories (from the Greek *telos*, meaning "end") seek to justify moral principles in terms of some overall goal or purpose in nature or human experience. Theories that interpret the pursuit of happiness as a chosen rational goal of the human society have been called utilitarian. In utilitarianism the usefulness or value of an action or policy is determined by whether it adds to the sum total of human happiness. Utilitarian theories tend to emphasize the importance of rational choice and convention. They can be categorized as addressing either rule utilitarianism or act utilitarianism. Rule utilitarianism holds that the utility or value of an action depends on whether it contributes to greater happiness for all. The major rule related to this theory is that an action or principle is good if and only if it is conducive to the greater happiness for the greatest number. Act utilitarianism is more restrictive; it does not involve a universal rule but tries to determine, for a particular situation, with regard to particular acts, what course of action will bring the most happiness or the least harm or suffering to individuals. Thus teleological utilitarian theories have been characterized by the principle of the greatest good or the greatest happiness. In teleological theories it is the outcome, consequences, or end that is paramount in the decision.

Deontological theories (from the Greek *deon*, meaning "duty") are concerned with action. Kant, a proponent of this theory, argues that is is not the end or consequences of an act that make it right or wrong, but the moral intention of the agent.[12] It is the good intention, the intention to do one's moral duty, that determines whether an action is morally correct or not. Kant argues that for a principle to be moral or binding as a duty it must be universal, unconditional, and imperative. The concept of duty follows as a logical consequence from the nature of rational practice. Kant believed human action could not be consistently rational unless the rules obeyed were universal, unconditional, and imperative. The following are two such rules that Kant formulated: Man should always act so that the rule on which he bases his action could become a universal moral law. This is called the law of universalizability. Second, man should never treat another person simply as a means, but always as an end in himself.[12]

Deontological ethics has also been developed in rule and act form. Rule deontology is the view that emphasizes the objective character of moral principles in terms of the universal, unconditional, and imperative character of duties. This view is based on the claim that a universal structure governs human reason. Act deontology is based on a more personal and subjective view of duty. It is based on intuition and attempts to determine whether a particular action is right or wrong on the basis of whether one's intention conforms to what one believes to be one's duty. Act deontology is a form of intuitionism and does not make any claims about the necessary universality of moral laws.

AUTONOMY, BENEFICENCE, AND JUSTICE

Principles related to autonomy, beneficence, and justice, which directly relate to the issue of truth telling, evolve out of both the teleological and deontological theories of ethics. Autonomy relates to an individual's independence in making choices and implementing them. Autonomy is a form of personal liberty of action where the individual determines his or her own course of action in accordance with the plan chosen. Philosophers have espoused various themes associated with autonomy such as freedom of choice, creating one's own moral practices, and accepting ultimate responsibility for one's moral view. To honor this principle infers respect for persons and acknowledges their personal right to make choices and to act in accordance with their wishes. This moral principle is also supported by the legal right of self-determination.

The principle of beneficence states that people ought to do good and avoid doing harm.[9] It includes the ideas that one ought to prevent evil or harm and promote good. The principle of beneficence requires individuals to respect the liberty and freedom of others. The concept of nonmaleficence is associated with the maxim *primum non nocere*—above all do no harm—which is part of the Hippocratic oath.[2] The principle of beneficence is broader than this, because it requires positive steps to help others. It is a duty to help others further their important interests when one can do so with minimal risk to oneself. This principle also carries the idea of a duty to balance the good it is possible to do with the harm that might result from doing or not doing the good. This balance of benefit and harm has been labeled positive beneficence and is the principle of utility.

The concept of paternalism relates to both positive beneficence and the principle of utility. In ethics, paternalism refers to practices that restrict the liberty of individuals without their consent.[3] The paternalistic principle says that limiting a person's liberty is justified if the individual's actions would result in serious harm or would fail to produce an important benefit. The question of whether patients should be told the truth is paternalistic because it implies that others will decide, thus limiting the individual's freedom of choice. Paternalism is the principle most often used to justify not telling a patient of a poor prognosis.

The principle of justice states that equals should be treated equally and that those who are unequal should be treated differently according to their difference.[2,9] Equal treatment is not necessarily identical. Equality means the same relative contribution to the goodness of people's lives, such as the equal opportunity to achieve a virtue or benefit. This has also been referred to as the principle of formal equality. Principles of distributive justice apply when there is both a scarcity and competition for benefits. Just distribution can be according to equal shares, individual need, individual effort or merit, or societal contribution.

Moral rules and principles are arranged according to their importance or justifiability in the context of specific theories. In teleological theory the principle of beneficence carries more weight than the ethical principle of autonomy or justice. However, the principle of beneficence can be overridden by either of the other principles in given circumstances. In deontological theories the ethical principle of autonomy usually carries the most weight but may be overridden by the principles of beneficence or justice. An ethical principle is always morally significant but may not always be acknowledged when it is in conflict with other principles. Ethical theories help interpret what principle will most likely prevail in a given situation of moral decision making.

ESPOUSED VIEWS

The validity of research regarding beliefs and attitudes about medical disclosure must always be questioned because of the difficulty of eliciting true beliefs when the individual is not responding to a real-life, personally involving situation.

Kelly and Friesen,[13] in a 1950 survey of 100 persons with cancer, found that 73% believed that a person should be told of their diagnosis. Only four persons felt they should not be told; the others were undecided. In a second group of 100 persons who did not have cancer, they found that 82% wanted to be told; 14% did not. In a third group of 740 persons who were being examined at a cancer detection center, 98.5% wanted to know if they had a diagnosis of cancer.

Branch[5] and Samp and Curreri[21] found similar results in groups they surveyed, with over 80% of these lay groups feeling that patients should be told of a diagnosis of cancer. Most surveys have dealt with the question of medical disclosure of a diagnosis of cancer rather than of other terminal or debilitating illnesses. However, with the recent activity and public education regarding patient involvement in decision making as a result of the patient rights, hospice, holistic health, and self-care movements, it could be speculated that current lay opinion would be at least at this level of belief regarding disclosure.

An issue pertinent to these health care movements is whether the lay public and professional care givers have similar perspectives about disclosure. Traditionally physicians have been committed to professional secrecy, in the belief that this was in the best interest of the patient and family. In 1953 Fitts and Ravdin[8] surveyed 444 Philadelphia physicians as to their practice of disclosure of the diagnosis of cancer. Of this group, 57% reported that they usually did not disclose this diagnosis; 12% stated they never did. In a 1961 study of 219 physicians by Oken,[17] 88% had a policy of not disclosing to a patient a cancer diagnosis. However, by the 1970s a considerable change was found in physician practices regarding disclosure. In a 1970 survey by Friedman,[10] only 9% of a group of 178 physicians indicated that they never told the patient about a cancer diagnosis. In a 1976 study by Rea, Greenspoon, and Spilka[20] only 22% of a group of 191 physicians indicated they would not tell a terminal patient about that person's condition. They also found that 37% of the group would honor the wishes of the family, while 9% would inform the patient regardless of family wishes. In a 1979 replication of the Oken study with 264 medical staff at a university hospital, 97% of the group indicated that they preferred to disclose a cancer diagnosis to the patient.[16]

Other health care personnel, including nurses, traditionally have been trained to leave the responsibility of information transmission to the physician. However, in a 1975 survey by the journal *Nursing*, 60% of the 15,430 nurses responding indicated that they believed a patient with a terminal diagnosis should be informed about this state as soon as possible after the diagnosis is made.[18] Twenty-one percent indicated this should only be done when the patent asks. In response to the question of what they would do if a patient asked if he or she was dying and the physician did not want the patient to know, only 1% indicated they would tell the patient. The majority, 81%, indicated that they would collect more data about the patient's feelings and why the question was being asked.

Differences in attitudes regarding disclosure of information about a patient's medical condition often evolve out of differences in roles, in emphasis regarding the consequences of the disclosure, and individual preferences for direct or indirect approaches to problems. However, when the patient, family, physician, and other health care givers hold differing attitudes and beliefs about disclosure, moral issues and ethical dilemmas can evolve.

PROFESSIONAL ETHICS

In addition to ethical theories and principles, professional conduct is also guided by rules that evolve from the professional's helper role and from intraprofessional relationships. These professional responsibilities and conduct rules flow from professional codes of ethics, societal expectations, and intraprofessional responsibilities.

Professional codes of ethics are statements encompassing rules that apply to persons in professional roles. Rules contained in the professional code of ethics for nurses are basically specific applications of more universal moral principles. These rules essentially are applied ethics. Some of these rules are also defined legally in nurse practice acts. Professional ethics that address the four major concepts of confidentiality, accountability, patient advocacy, and informed consent affect the moral choices of professionals.

The rule of confidentiality flows from the right to privacy. This recognized human right evolves from the ethical principle that persons are self-determining moral agents. In respect for this right nurses maintain patient privacy under the rule of confidentiality. The ethical code for nurses defines accountability as being answerable to someone for something one has done. This obligation is both moral and legal: being account-

able in a care situation involves a contractual agreement as well as a moral duty to safeguard a patient's rights. The duty of advocacy referred to in the code is derived from the ethical principle of beneficence. It is the duty of the nurse to protect patients from harm. The moral duty to obtain a valid, informed consent flows from the ethical principle of autonomy and the right of self-determination. In light of current malpractice problems, this duty also relates to the ethical principle of utility. The action of obtaining informed consent benefits all involved—the patient, the professional care giver, and the institution in which the care is being provided.

Most professional codes also address rules related to relationships between and among professionals. According to Curtin[7] the sources underlying the formulation of rules related to professional relationships are derived from the principles of human rights, the obligation to promote the public's welfare, and the bond that results from regarding professional colleagues as brothers and sisters and applying the ethics of fraternal loyalty.

THE DUTY TO TELL THE TRUTH—THE PRO POSITION

Deception comes from the word *deceive*, to make a person believe what is not true, to delude, or to mislead. To deceive implies deliberate misrepresentation by words or actions to generally further one's ends. Deception can include outright lying, understatement or exaggeration, withholding information, dodging questions by providing an answer to a different question or simply remaining silent when information is asked for.

Deception is a form of manipulation; deceptive behavior, verbal or nonverbal, is intended to mislead or control another's actions or thoughts. It is dishonest and bypasses the deceived individual's rational capacity. Lying is the most dramatic illustration of deception, because one states what is believed to be false with the aim of having another believe it is true. However, deception is broader than lying and encompasses many acts that are committed with the intention of misleading. The giving of a placebo medication is an example of deception. The nurse can give the placebo instead of a medication and avoid telling the patient what is being administered. The therapeutic benefit of this intervention is predicated on the deception.

All ethical frameworks contain strong precepts against deception. For all ethicists, deception requires justification, with the burden of proof resting on those who wish to initiate or maintain the deception.

Bok[4] equates deceit with violence and claims they are the two forms of deliberate assault on humans. Deceit is sneaky because it exerts control very subtly by working on beliefs and actions and shutting off alternative options. Bok emphasizes the psychological differences between the perspective of the liar and the perspective of the deceived. There is a tendency for the liar to overestimate the beneficial effects of the lie, to underestimate the damage the lie will do, to believe the lie is told for benevolent motives only, and to fail to see alternative courses of action that do not involve lying or deceit. When the lie is looked at from the viewpoint of the deceived, these characteristics become clear. When learning of the deception the deceived responds with resentment, disappointment, and suspicion. The perspective of the deceived supports Aristotle's position that falsehood is in itself mean and culpable, and truth is noble and full of praise.[4]

Veracity is the ethical principle that addresses the duty to tell the truth. Bok[4] presents veracity as a principle developed from Aristotle's premise that lying is mean and culpable and that truthful statements are preferred to lies, except in special situations. This premise gives negative weight to lies by requiring explanation and justification, and not requiring such qualifications for the truth. The veracity principle leads to the rule that truthfulness must be considered first in any situation and that lying must be ruled out if the truth can achieve a desirable result. This rule would negate a policy of not disclosing their medical conditions to patients, because this rule precludes looking at what telling the truth would do in a given situation. Like other duties, truth telling is prima facie, not absolute, so deception can sometimes be justified when veracity conflicts with other duties.

There are six major reasons that support the position that the nurse should tell patients the truth: it is essential to trust in the nurse-patient relationship, patients have the right to know, it is the moral thing to do, it alleviates anxiety and suffering, it is necessary to achieve patient and family cooperation, and it can meet the need of the nurse.

The trust relationship

Truthfulness is essential to a trust relationship. Several arguments can be made for the duty to tell the truth in a health care relationship. One argument is that nurses tell the truth and refrain from deceiving or lying because of the respect owed to people. We respect patients because they are self-determining, autonomous individuals with all the rights of autonomy, including the right to be told the truth and not to be lied to or deceived. A second argument makes a claim that a duty of veracity is derived from or is a way of expressing the duty of fidelity or promise keeping. There is no question that, in order to deliver their services, health care professionals must establish an implicit contract, a promise, with the patient that involves a trusting relationship. A helping relationship engenders a duty to tell the truth and not to deceive. The nurse-patient relationship creates the expectation that nurses will interact with a patient in a truthful manner. This trust is often needed by patients to cope with their illnesses. A third argument claims that relationships of trust, or the dependence on honesty, is necessary for cooperation between patients and health care providers.

The right to know

Patients have a legal right to information about their medical condition depending on where they reside and whether the information is related to an offered treatment. In all situations the patient has a legal right to information needed to make an informed consent regarding treatment decisions. However, states vary in regard to whether a patient has a legal right to personal medical records or medical information. In Massachusetts patients have the legal right of inspection and the right to a copy of their medical records. In 41 other states that allow access to medical records, this access can occur only when the records are subpoenaed for evidence in a lawsuit.[1] In general patients do not have a legal right to information regarding their diagnosis and prognosis except where this is pertinent to the giving of informed consent.

The legal and ethical status of a right are not the same. A moral right can exist in the absence of legal support for that right, as is the case with a patient's right to information. Patients do have a moral right to information about their health status and health care, and if they exercise this right by asking questions or asking for information, there is a duty to provide that information. When a patient asks questions about his or her condition, the nurse has a moral duty to answer honestly. The justification for this position is based on the principle of autonomy. When a patient is treated as an object, as a nonentity, or as merely a diseased body, that person is being denied identity. Failure to provide information to patients about their conditions is an effective way of denying their identity regardless of one's intent. Patients must have information about their conditions to exercise rational choice. Ramsey[19] takes the position that no one is good enough to cure or treat another without that person's consent. Patients have the right to be told the truth if for no other reason than they have a moral right to know.

In addition to the patient's moral right to know, research indicates that people want to know the truth about their conditions.[5,13,21] Knowledge of the true state of affairs helps people to gather the motivation and strength to do what is necessary to put their lives in order. Patients often want a nurse or doctor to decide when and how information is disclosed to them, but not to use a general policy to decide if disclosure should occur. A disclosure decision should be made based on individual needs. Norman Cousins, who cured himself with laughter, also advanced this position regarding truth telling.[6] Patients want to hear the truth, but they believe it is a professional responsibility to determine the most palatable and humane way of doing so.

The moral thing to do

There are at least three major ethical principles that support telling the truth as the moral thing to do: autonomy, beneficence, and justice. Although there is no controversy over whether truth telling is a moral act, differing opinions or choices of action regarding truth telling evolve from the interpretation of the duty to do no harm. This moral judgment is based on the decision that the duty to do no harm overrides the duty of veracity in the particular situation. Differing interpretations result from differing theoretical perspectives. A deontological viewpoint is less likely to obligate truth telling than a teleological viewpoint. Teleologically the nurse has a strong moral duty to tell patients the truth, and this duty should rarely if ever be overriden by a higher duty or a prior claim.

Alleviation of anxiety and fear

A main goal of nursing care is comfort, which includes the alleviation of anxiety and suffering. In fact, this is perceived internationally as the duty of a nurse. The International Code of Nursing states that one of the fundamental responsibilities of the nurse is to alleviate suffering. The American Nurses' Association Code also supports this position.

Fear of the unknown is a major source of anxiety. Telling the patient the truth about his or her condition and helping that individual understand what to expect should eliminate needless fears and anxiety. The patient needs truthful information to be able to begin the process of adapting and coping with illness. When the true condition is known, the nurse is able to use the intervention of anticipatory guidance to help the patient and the family to cope. When there is open communication among the nurse, patient, and family members, trust develops and needless anxiety is alleviated.

Gaining cooperation

It is essential to have the patient's cooperation in a health care situation. The care giver and patient are partners and need to establish mutual goals. If the patient does not receive truthful information, mutual goals are impossible.

Statutory laws regarding informed consent identify that the obligation, the duty of the health care provider, is to warn a patient of the hazards of experimental or unusual treatment and the possible complications of standard treatment. For consent to be truly informed and valid, the patient must be told the diagnosis, nature of the proposed treatment, prognosis with and without the treatment, and any alternative treatments that are available. Legally one must have consent and cooperation of the patient for treatment. It is extremely difficult to achieve this through deception.

Nurse's need

A nurse is human and has certain expectations and rights. The participation in deception compromises integrity and thus assaults the nurse's personhood. To fulfill many of a nurse's duties a trusting relationship must be developed with the patient. Deception puts the nurse in a negative position in developing a sound working relationship. To participate in deception is to do oneself a moral injustice.

WHEN DECEPTION IS RIGHT—THE CON POSITION

A teleological or utilitarian point of view holds that there are times when deception can be ethically justified. The principle of paternalism supports the use of the benevolent or therapeutic lie. The four major reasons that ethically allow altering the truth and deceiving a patient are that truthfulness is impossible to achieve, patients may not want to know the truth if it is unpleasant, professionals have a duty to do no harm, and deception may be a means of gaining cooperation to facilitate a therapeutic situation.

Incomplete knowledge

Nurses and doctors may be unable to tell patients the truth in regard to the patients' exact conditions, the meaning of their symptoms, or their prognosis if the health care professionals themselves do not know this information. If incomplete information is disclosed the patient may become confused as to the true situation. In this case withholding information is not a lie and is justified because the professional does not have certain or complete information.

Henderson[11] advances that there is no clear distinction between true and false information in medicine. Because in health care situations the outcome is not known with certainty, disclosure of what is thought to be true may unnecessarily confuse an ill person. Health statistics are meaningless to a specific case and their disclosure most likely will not be a presentation of the truth for an individual situation.

Patients do not want to know the truth

Most practitioners have had experience with persons who do not want to know information that is unfavorable in nature. When such information is presented they resist it, repress it, deny it, fail to understand it, and even claim never to have been informed. These patients do not want the truth and are unable to cope with it. The ethical duty of respecting others' wishes entails not forcing the truth on persons who indicate they do not want to hear it. When professionals read the clues or signals that indicate a patient does not want to hear the truth, and decide to respect these wishes, they are acting in accordance with the principle of paternalism.

The duty to do no harm

Two ethical principles, beneficence and nonmaleficence, call for doing good and not doing harm. If disclosure produces anxiety and fear it may cause the person to take harmful action, such as committing suicide or fulfilling the expectation of the prognosis. Because medical and nursing ethical codes make no mention of a truth-telling duty, it can be inferred that the duty to above all do no harm must be used as the

overriding duty. Meyer[5] has noted that traditionally medicine has been guided by a precept that transcends the virtue of uttering the truth for truth's sake, which is to as far as possible do no harm.

Responding to the duty to do no harm by not disclosing or lying is benevolent deception, where the care giver acts in a paternalistic manner by deciding what is best for the patient. All arguments used to justify nondisclosure have an element of paternalism. The traditional physician role has been one of authority, dominance, and respect. Patients believe that physicians will make the right decision for them simply because they are doctors. The ordering of principles for physicians is to first do no harm and then to do good. This ordering emphasizes the end rather than the means.

Ethically, paternalism requires justification in each situation because it sets aside respect for the individual's choices or wishes. When paternalistic intervention is used, the presumption of autonomy or self-determination no longer holds. The following three conditions ethically justify acts of paternalism: ignorance or impaired capacity for rational reflection by the patient, a high probability that patients will harm themselves without paternalistic intervention, and when it is reasonable to expect that patients would consent or recover the capacity for rational reflection with more knowledge.[3] Paternalistic acts are justified if they are truly in accord with the wishes and decisions of individuals able to make beneficial decisions.

Cooperation

Lying or deceiving may be exercised in critical situations as means of gaining consent and cooperation. The benefits of the necessary short-term cooperation must, however, be balanced with the risk of the trust that might be lost in the long run.

CONCLUSION

It is apparent that the principles and rules regarding truth telling do not produce a formula for the practicing nurse that states whether or not to tell the truth. To make a good ethical decision and provide quality care for patients a nurse needs to know how to avoid dilemmas and to set up win-win situations. A win-win situation has all individuals in the situation respected as persons. Once a specific situation progresses to the point that it meets the criteria of an ethical dilemma, the only outcome possible is a win-lose or lose-lose situation. Either one party maintains respect and the other parties lose, or all parties lose respect.

The nurse also needs to recognize how and why individuals can differ on a particular information-disclosure decision. The sharing of beliefs, feelings, and attitudes about disclosure with other members of the health care team can enhance such understanding. Nurses should clarify the ethical frameworks from which they are operating and place more emphasis on the principles for guidance rather than on rules or duties. This should help facilitate adaptation to various relationships and situations, because principles allow for more flexibility. Also, the emphasis on principles is needed because rules and duties are ordered or given different values according to the value assigned to principles in a given situation.

The truth-telling issue is embedded in broader practice issues that need clarification, verification, and illumination so that the nurse can become better equipped to deal with the how, what, and why of information disclosure. Two of these issues that have particular bearing on truth telling are the scope of nursing practice and professional dominance. Does the scope of nursing practice include providing diagnostic and prognostic information to patients? Does one professional group have the authority to tell another how to act when the action depends on a moral choice where there is no absolute right action?

A mechanism is needed that will affect medical ethics in a manner similar to the AHA's Patient Bill of Rights. Because these issues involve more than one professional group, the agency offering the health care must be involved in the establishment of a mechanism to help avoid the precipitation of ethical dilemmas regarding disclosure. The agency could establish policies or procedures that address ethical problems. For example, the agency could establish an ethical committee to address specific case situations. If the agency has a base policy of open disclosure then a decision not to disclose should be a committee decision. This decision would be based on whether an act of paternalism could be justified. The decision would also have to address whether justice would be rendered to all involved parties, the patient and the care givers. This type of policy would not allow one professional to impose a moral choice on another. It would also assure that truth telling would be considered the usual course of action and that an act of deception would have to be justified to a neutral party before it could be implemented.

REFERENCES

1. Anna G: The rights of hospital patients, New York, 1975, Avon.
2. Beauchamp TL and Childress JF: Principles of biomedical ethics, New York, 1979, Oxford University Press.
3. Benjamin M and Curtis J: Ethics in nursing, New York, 1981, Oxford University Press.
4. Bok S: Lying: moral choice in public and private life, New York, 1978, Pantheon Books.
5. Branch CH: Psychiatric aspects of malignant disease, CA 6(3):102, 1956.
6. Cousins N: A layman looks at truth telling in medicine, JAMA 244(17):1929, 1980.
7. Curtin L and Flaherty M: Nursing ethics: theories and pragmatics, Bowie, Md, 1982, Prentice-Hall Publications and Communications Co.
8. Fitts WT Jr and Raupin IS: What Philadelphia physicians tell patients with cancer, JAMA 153:901, 1953.
9. Frankena WK: Ethics, Englewood Cliffs, NJ, 1973, Prentice-Hall.
10. Friedman HS: Physician management of dying patients: an exploration, Psychiatr. Med. 1:295, 1970.
11. Henderson L: Physician and patient as a social system, N Engl J Med 212:819, 1935.
12. Kant I: Foundations of the metaphysics of morals, New York, 1959, The Liberal Arts Press, (translated by LW Beck).
13. Kelly WD and Friesen SR: Do cancer patients want to be told? Surgery 27:822, 1950.
14. Ladd J: The task of ethics. In Reich WT, editor: Encyclopedia of Bioethics, vol 1, New York, 1978, The Free Press.
15. Meyer BC: Truth and the physician, Bull NY Acad Med 45:59, 1969.
16. Novak D and others: Changes in physicians' attitudes toward telling the cancer patient, JAMA 241(9):897, 1979.
17. Oken D: What to tell cancer patients, JAMA 175:1120, 1961.
18. Popoff D: What are your feelings about death and dying? part I, Nurs. 75 5(8):15, 1975.
19. Ramsey P: Ethics at the edges of life: medical and legal intersections, New Haven, Conn, 1978, Yale University Press.
20. Rea MP, Greenspoon S, and Bernard S: Physicians and the terminal patient: some selected attitudes and behavior, Omega 6:291, 1975.
21. Samp RJ and Curreri AR: a questionnaire survey on public cancer education obtained from cancer patients and their families, Cancer 10:382, 1957.

CHAPTER 81

Viewpoints

The tyranny of ethics

M. PATRICIA DONAHUE

What we are is, in part only of our own making, the greater part has come down to us from the past. What we know and what we think is not a new fountain gushing fresh from the barren rocks of the unknown, at the stroke of our own intellect, it is a stream which flows by us and through us, fed by the far off rivulets of long ago. As what we think and say today will mingle with and shape the thoughts of men in the years to come, so, in the opinions and views which we are proud to hold today, we may, by looking back, trace the influence of those who have gone before.

SIR MICHAEL FOSTER
British Physiologist

The price of progress has been a health care delivery system that is beset with controversy, distrust, uncertainty, turmoil, complexity, and scarce resources. Nurses and other health care personnel function in an environment that is shaped by technology, malpractice suits, and cost containment. Machinery and money reign supreme in this setting at a time when consumers cry out for justice and equity in decisions related to health care, cry out for quality care that is based on humane treatment for all. These circumstances have provided a ripe arena for the entry of ethics as a powerful and potentially deciding force in health care.

No one can deny that ethics has been attended to in the past in a variety of ways for a variety of reasons. In addition, few people would be able to deny the fact that ethics currently has come to be regarded as a method of "immunotherapy," a way to attempt to resolve those crises in health care concerned with the ethics of caring. These crises are generated by the intricate interrelationships created by scientific and technological developments, institutional and professional problems, and societal, legal, and governmental constraints. The ethical problems that arise from these interrelationships are

an immunodeficiency problem in a social institution, a condition in which the values that defend the institution's existence and structure fall prey to some inner malaise. Ethical reflection is the first step in immunotherapy.[10]

According to Jonsen,[10] the appeal to ethics is heard when people, consciously or unconsciously, recognize that their familiar institutions are under stress and liable to crack."

The tyranny of ethics is rapidly becoming a reality, in the sense of ethics becoming an absolute power that may ultimately oppress. Public debates of ethical issues suffer from excess generalities in which oscillation occurs between narrow dogmatism limited to general assertions deemed "matters of principle" and shallow relativism that suggests value systems are chosen as freely as food is eaten. What is lacking is the translation to real-life situations in which a balance must be achieved between moral principles and individual, social, and cultural differences.

The rise of anthropology and the other human sciences in the early twentieth century encouraged a healthy sense of social and cultural differences; but this was uncritically taken as implying an end to all objectivity in practical ethics. The subsequent reassertion of ethical objectivity has led, in turn, to an insistence on the absoluteness of moral principles that is not balanced by a feeling for the complex problems of discrimination that arise when such principles are applied to particular real-life cases. So, the relativists have tended to overinterpret the need for discrimination in ethics, discretion in public administration, and equity in law, as a license for general personal subjectivity. The absolutists have responded by denying all real scope for personal judgment in ethics, insisting instead on strict construction in the law, on unfeeling consistency in public administration, and—above all—on the "inerrancy" of moral principles.[18]

Indeed, the subject of ethics has proved a battleground for debates between objectivity and subjectivity, theory and practice, rigidity and flexibility, justice and injustice. Unfortunately, the result is public distrust and the creation of absolute laws and public policies that are to be uniformly applied. The deeper demands within an ethic of caring ascribed to by nursing cannot survive in such a climate in which general rules and principles and absolute laws overshadow a consideration for individual differences and needs. Only with the analyses of actual practice situations will the answer(s) to ethical nursing care be found.

THE PROBLEM OF LANGUAGE

Ethics, medical ethics, social ethics, metaethics, normative ethics, descriptive ethics, biomedical ethics, nursing ethics. The list is endless and serves at times to create chaos and confusion. It is estimated that over 2000 books and articles on biomedical ethics alone appear in the English language annually.[14] Publications in the area of nursing ethics have also rapidly escalated during the last 12 years, with an emphasis originally on legal aspects rather than on moral principles and ethical dilemmas. In addition, a misleading idea surfaced in early publications—that the way to resolve an "ought" question is to decide upon a course of action and then choose the ethical theory that best supports the decision.[5] However, writings in the area of nursing ethics have demonstrated a consistent growth in sophistication and now focus on the entire realm of information necessary for ethical decision making. Yet the term *nursing ethics* itself is controversial. Some believe that the term is necessary because it signifies the uniqueness of moral problems that nurses face; others argue that there is little that is morally unique to nurses.[19]

Aside from the numerous categories and subcategories that classify the field of ethics, other difficulties are evident that may interfere with an adequate understanding of ethics and its role in health care. The term *ethics* has a variety of meanings, some of which have been outgrown by current society. As changes in society occur, different meanings are attached to specific phenomena. It is important, therefore, that nursing have ethical guidelines that are socially relevant, broad enough to be interpreted in various situations, and drawn from real-life situations. Essentially, nursing must start with the practice arena and must move from theory to practice. Only then will ethical theory for nursing be sound.

"To be sound, ethical theory, like all other kinds of theory, must be born out of experiences with actual problems. It is experimental, empirical, and data based; a posteriori, not a priori. Moral rules and principles ought to be empirical generalizations, changeable when experience changes. . . . In short, the process of ethics runs from practice to theory and then back to practice again."[6]

Even beyond the numerous definitions of *ethics* itself, other words associated with the realm of ethics have been burdensome. For example, attempts to adequately define such polarizing terms as ordinary-extraordinary, withholding-withdrawing, vegetative-nonvegetative state, medical-nonmedical treatments, dead-alive, passive-active euthanasia have become a challenge to all involved in the resolution of ethical issues in health care. At times, even the experts are unable to agree on definitions that are vital to legal determinations. Such was the case in *Brophy vs New England Sinai Hospital,* in which a judge had to choose among the differing opinions of seven ethicists who testified regarding whether a gastrostomy tube should be removed.[13] In the Matter of Nancy Ellen Jobes, five neurologists disagreed about whether a severely brain-damaged young woman was in a persistent vegetative state.[9] Three judged her to be so; two did not. These cases of course raise other questions, particularly those dealing with what criteria are valid in deciding between opposing viewpoints. Finally, our ethical language of today differs enormously from that used in the past. Certainly, the discretionary freedoms of physicians and nurses, as well as those of patients, are currently defended by concern for individual civil rights and autonomy.[21] Professional ethics can thus no longer be grounded on the historical models of professional duty but must be based on models consistent with the times. They must address the complex issues presented by a vastly different world of scientific advancement.

The language of nursing must be reflected in nursing ethics. Consequently, a theory of ethical practice must be carefully selected to avoid the male bias contained in many developmental theories and carefully developed by using necessary qualitative methods of discovery prior to quantitative validation.[11] Nurses should heed the work of Gilligan,[7] who suggests a female ethic of caring that occurs within the context of relationships. She states that the "activity of care is an activity of relationship, of seeing and responding to need, taking care of the world by sustaining the web of connections so that no one is left alone."[7] Huggins and Scalzi,[8] although cautious, recognize that such an ethic of care seems to intuitively suit the "reality of nursing." They emphasize that a theory for ethical practice should reflect the nurse's life experiences; that "nurses must be sure that when they speak of ethical issues, they speak with their own voices."[8] Ultimately, however, a crucial question must first be addressed: can nurses be ethical within the health care structure that presently exists?[1,17]

A LURKING FORCE IN HISTORY

The course of history has been shaped in numerous instances by the profound consequences of disease that has ravaged civilizations. The most powerful individuals and societies have not escaped its destructive effects. One need only read of the plagues that depleted the strength of ancient Rome and Athens, the Black Death that wiped out one fourth of the population of Europe and brought about the end of feudalism, the smallpox epidemic that became Cortez's ally against the Aztecs, and the yellow fever scourge of 1793 in Philadelphia (when most people who could, fled without regard for the health and safety of loved ones) to comprehend the scope of tragedies produced by disease.[3,20]

So, too, has the moral mission of health care been constantly tested by the impact of disease, with resulting ethical implications. The fear of contagious disease, however, in all probability has had the greatest effect on professional duty and professional ethics over time. Yet no consistent professional response to contagion has emerged. A review of medical responses to historic plagues revealed that many physicians "fled from patients with contagious epidemic diseases. Many of their colleagues, at considerable personal risk, remained behind to care for plague victims."[21] This clearly demonstrates that obligations to contagious patients have complex ethical overtones that cannot easily be resolved. Consequently, the issue of care for patients with acquired immunodeficiency syndrome (AIDS) currently occupies a primary position in ethical discussions. The traditional precedent related to professional duties in such cases is clearly inconsistent and inappropriate. A new professional ethic is thus needed to guide health care practitioners as they face a modern contagious disease and reflect on how the course of history will be influenced or altered by that disease.

Historically, physicians were not alone in their flight from contagious diseases. Nurses, too, lacked a consistent approach when faced with transmissible diseases. Many nurses fled from patients with contagious epidemic diseases; many remained behind in full recognition of the risks they faced. Isabel Hampton Robb lamented this dilemma in 1900:

A good deal might be said about the duty of nurses as regards contagious diseases. In the past, I fear that this has not been clearly understood, and I can call to mind not a few instances in which members of the profession have repeatedly refused to take care of such patients. The existence of this attitude among so many nurses is one of the strong evidences of the absence of an accepted code of ethics and a consequent lack of a proper comprehension of their moral duties as members of a profession. One hears sometimes of physicians who have spent valuable hours in vainly trying to find a disengaged nurse who was willing to take a case of scarlet fever or diphtheria, and yet have met with a firm refusal at every turn.[16]

Mrs. Robb devoted four pages to this narrative and was most explicit in her opinion of nurses who refused these cases. She stressed that there would be few instances in which a given reason for refusal would be justified, that a nurse was bound to take whatever case might come to her. She stressed further that nurses, like physicians, must aid the suffering whenever called upon; nurses do not have the moral right to pick and choose patients. Finally, Mrs. Robb strongly emphasized her position on professional duty:

If a nurse declines to go through fear of her own personal

safety, there is no excuse for her. She should have settled that question before she ever entered a hospital, for she must have known that there she would be expected to take any case assigned to her, and that any day she might be exposed to risks of various kinds. Such a position is very much on par with that of a man who has enlisted as a soldier and then later on wishes to make the provison that he shall always have the privilege of fighting in the rear, well protected against any chance of being shot.[16]

Although nursing now has a code of ethics, an inconsistent ethic still is apparent with respect to AIDS. Nurses have refused to care for patients afflicted with AIDS, even though they can be more secure in their knowledge of contagion and transmissibility than in the past, can be more secure that there is less probability of personal risk. Kim and Perfect[12] addressed this issue from the standpoint of physicians and elaborated on these pertinent issues. Their conclusion is an important one—that the answers to questions regarding physician involvement in the care of patients with AIDS will be difficult "in that they are more ethical than practical, more an issue of responsibility than of aseptic technique, and more a matter of conscience than of legal or professional liability." A similar statement can be made about nurse involvement.

The U.S. health care system is being seriously strained by the medical needs of HIV-infected persons, as it has been in the past from other high-risk diseases. Ethical issues raised by AIDS now occupy as prominent a position in discussions and decision making as those ethical issues concerned with technology, death, dying, and the prolongation of life. Eventually all nurses will be faced with caring for patients with this disease. To this end, the ethics that guide nurses need to be based on nursing's historical *aspirations* rather than on nurses' historical actions. Such ethics would commit nurses to obligations beyond those required by law and would include such attributes as compassion, courage, and integrity.

PAST REFLECTIONS, CURRENT PERSPECTIVES

It is interesting to note that both medicine and nursing have followed a similar course in their quests for relevant and effective codes of ethics. Both have a long, honorable, and at times difficult history regarding concern for the ethics of their respective professions. Both very early recognized that a code of ethics was a vehicle whereby respectability and a reputable image could be achieved through stated standards of conduct. Ulti-

mately, the code could and would legitimize their occupational groups as true professions.

The evolution of a medical code of ethics had its roots in the ancient world. For example, descriptions of the manner in which physicians should deal with patients and their problems, how they should deal with one another, and how early states tried to control the actions of physicians are recorded in ancient writings such as the Egyptian medical papyruses and the Babylonian Code of Hammurabi. The Hippocratic oath, however, was regarded for many centuries as the model of medical ethics. Paradoxically, this oath was probably not written by Hippocrates but by the philosophical Pythagorean sect, active in the latter part of the fourth century BC. The longevity of the oath, at least in the Western world, is perhaps due to "the approximation of the moral ideals expressed in the Hippocratic Oath with those of the early Christians."[15]

The primary focus of the majority of these writings, however, was on the conduct of the physician, with relatively little regard for the rights or the physical and mental welfare of patients. This was also true of the later medieval and more contemporary writers as they addressed the area of ethics. Percival, a well-known English physician, believed that good moral conduct would benefit not only the practitioner but also the patient and the profession. His treatise on medical ethics became the model for a number of codes of medical ethics, including the American Medical Association Code adopted in 1847. Thus for a long time medical ethics was concerned with conduct, or the deportment of physicians. This emphasis on etiquette and deportment finally began to shift to the current interpretation of medical ethics. According to Fletcher:

Until fairly recently, what physicians called medical ethics was little more than a body of moralistic advice about (a) medical manners and (b) the physician's guild or association rules. It consisted of paternalistic advice about not sitting on the patient's bed; not smelling of tobacco or pungent beverages such as Madeira (or maybe something even stronger); how to practice the art of touching—which is what medicine is—with Victorian propriety; and what one owed to one's professional brothers in the way of respect and discretion.[6]

Fletcher further commented that medical ethics was converted "into quite a serious value analysis of significant practices and innovation—at both research and clinical levels."[6] This progression in medical ethics was paralleled by a trend toward a more sophisticated and relevant code in which both practitioner and patient concerns would be addressed. Consequently, several revisions of the medical code of ethics occurred—in 1903, 1912, 1947, and 1955.

The evolution of nursing ethics is less clear, since it is difficult to ascertain just how far ethical considerations were considered in the early stages of modern nursing education. What is clear, however, is the attempt by nineteenth-century nurses to overcome a negative image and dubious reputation left from an era in which bedside nursing had been relegated to the servant class, or lower.[4] Florence Nightingale is credited as the founder of modern nursing because she fought this negative image and established the first formal school of nursing. In honor of her high ideals, American probationers memorized and repeated the "Florence Nightingale pledge." This pledge, distinctly similar to the Hippocratic oath, was written in 1893 by a committee headed by Lystra Gretter, who believed that nursing needed a code of ethics.

This was the beginning of a long struggle that led to the adoption by the American Nurses' Association of the first code of ethics for nurses in 1950. This occurred 77 years after the opening of the first U.S. school of nursing and after much argument, deliberation, and effort. Throughout this time the primary thrust of nursing ethics was on manners and morals, on etiquette and deportment. Eventually the focus of nursing ethics began to slowly change; the change resulted in the revised 1968 Code of Ethics, almost entirely free of an emphasis on etiquette but still concerned primarily with the practitioner. The most recent revision (1976) has broadened to include emphasis on the patient as well as on the practitioner. Other nursing codes were subsequently developed, such as the Code of Ethics adopted in 1953 by the International Council of Nurses (revised in 1965 and 1973) and used by many nursing associations throughout the world.

The development of codes of ethics has been an integral part of medical and nursing history. These codes have undergone numerous revisions in line with changes in society, health care, technological advances, and the professions themselves. They are, however, merely general guidelines that do not address the more troublesome issues inherent in the ethical dimensions of practice and education. Ethical situations are becoming increasingly complex, with resultant government and legislative involvement. Thus nurses cannot rely on codes of ethics to provide them with solutions or to prescribe "correct" actions to take when faced with ethical issues and dilemmas. In the final analysis legal decisions, history, and ethical codes can only indicate the direction being taken. "The most important thing they emphasize is that nurses should know where they stand as individuals, and then within their own belief patterns act as ethically as possible."[2]

The surging interest in health care ethics has led to increasing activities in nursing ethics at local, national, and international levels. Conferences, consultant activities, continuing education programs, ethics courses, interdisciplinary ethics seminars, and the establishment of ethics fellowships and centers such as the National Center for Nursing Ethics attest to the fact that the subject of ethics has become everyone's concern. But after all is said and done, the most crucial aspect of this scenario is how nursing will prepare its practitioners to cope with ethical issues and ethical dilemmas. It is not enough to raise the ethical consciousnesses of students or their sensitivities to ethical issues. Nor is it enough to emphasize ethical theory and analysis. Students must be taught how to think critically in order that they may develop confidence to act on their analyses.

In the present relatively narrow focus of professional education, nurses are trained, as William May put it, 'to use operational intelligence'; they also need to learn how to exercise their critical intelligence.[17]

REFERENCES

1. Aroskar MA: Are nurses' mind sets compatible with ethical practice? Topics in Clinical Nursing 4(1):22, 1982.
2. Bullough VL and Bullough B: History, trends, and politics of nursing, Norwalk, Conn, 1984, Appleton-Century-Crofts.
3. Cartwright FF (in collaboration with Biddiss MD): Disease and history, New York, 1972, Thomas Y Crowell Co.
4. Crowder E: Manners, morals, and nurses: an historical overview of nursing ethics, Texas Reports on Biology and Medicine, Spring, 1974, 32(1):173, 1974.
5. Donahue MP: Tough decisions, Intercom (Des Moines) 87(3):2, May-June 1987.
6. Fletcher J: Humanism and theism in biomedical ethics, Perspect Biol Med 31(1):106, 1987.
7. Gilligan C: In a different voice, Cambridge, Mass, 1982, Harvard University Press.
8. Huggins EA and Scalzi GC: Limitations and alternatives: ethical practice theory in nursing, Advances in Nursing Science 10(4):43, 1988.
9. *In the Matter of Nancy Ellen Jobes.* Docket C-4971-85E, Superior Court of New Jersey, Chancery Division, Morris County, April 23, 1986.
10. Jonsen AR: Ethics as immunotherapy, Forum on Medicine 1(7):50, 1978.
11. Ketefian S: A case study of theory development: moral behavior in nursing, Advances in Nursing Science 9(2):10, 1987.

12. Kim JH and Perfect JR: To help the sick: an historical and ethical essay concerning the refusal to care for patients with AIDS, Am J Med 84(1):135, 1988.
13. *Patricia E. Brophy, Guardian of Paul E. Brophy, v. New England Sinai Hospital.* Docket 85E0009-G1, Commonwealth of Massachusetts, Trial Court, Probate and Family Court Department, Norfolk Division, Oct 21, 1985.
14. Pellegrino ED: Medical ethics, JAMA 256(15):2122, 1986.
15. Reiser SJ, Dyck AJ, and Curran WJ, editors: Ethics in medicine: historical perspectives and contemporary concerns, Cambridge, Mass, 1977, MIT Press.
16. Robb IH: Nursing ethics: for hospital and private use, Cleveland, 1900, CC Koeckert.
17. Steinfels MO: Ethics, education, and nursing practice, Hastings Cent Rep 7(4):20, 1977.
18. Toulin S: The tyranny of principles, Hastings Cent Rep 2(6):31, 1981.
19. Veatch RM and Fry ST: Case studies in nursing ethics, Philadelphia, 1987, JB Lippincott Co.
20. Zinsser H: Rats, lice, and history, Boston, 1963, Little, Brown & Co.
21. Zuger A and Miles SH: Physicians, AIDS, and occupational risk: historical traditions and ethical obligations, JAMA 258(14):1924, 1987.

CHAPTER 82

Rationing health care services

Ethical issues for nursing

SARA T. FRY

It is not surprising that health care costs have risen sharply in recent years. The growth of medical knowledge, development of new technologies, public demands and expectations concerning health issues, and other matters have helped create a spiraling escalation of private and public costs for available health care services. With the United States currently spending 11% of its gross national product (GNP) on health care,[20] and about 1% of the GNP on health care for the elderly in their last year of life,[9] questions are now being raised about the benefits of such care in relation to its costs. These questions are being asked by economists, legislators, the consumer, and ethicists. At issue are the appropriate amounts of government spending for health care, restrictions that should be made to genuinely reflect the health priorities of the American people, and the ethical implications of various rationing strategies.

It is generally believed that the ethical implications of various actions and their alternatives should be considered before choosing a course of action and putting it into practice.[2] Therefore it is appropriate, if not prudent, that the ethical implications of various cost-containment measures in health care be considered before the amount of government spending for health care is decided and potential limitations of resources are created. A cautious approach to these matters is very important because rationing strategies often have serious implications for the health professions. The implications of various health care rationing strategies for the practice of nursing is the subject of this chapter.

First, I describe several well-known methods of rationing that are currently used in the allocation of health care. Second, I analyze the relatively new attempt at rationing that focuses on limiting costly health care services to the elderly. Throughout these discussions, the ethical implications of these rationing strategies and their particular implications for the practice of nursing will be explored. Finally, a brief proposal for the provision of nursing care under conditions of rationing is considered.

My goal in this chapter is to emphasize how rationing strategies in general, and the rationing of health care resources to the elderly in particular, pose a significant challenge to professional ethics. Current rationing strategies are creating some troublesome ethical problems in the provision of health care and have the potential to dramatically affect the ethical foundations of the health professions, particularly the practice of nursing and medicine.

CURRENT RATIONING STRATEGIES

It is widely understood that current cost-containment measures in health care use a mixture of rationing methods that affect access to health care.[14] These methods influence either the behavior of the consumer (market rationing), the behavior of the health professional (implicit rationing), or the administration of health care services (explicit rationing).

Market rationing

In the market system prior to the 1950s, health care was rationed by the consumer's ability to pay for services, the availability and distribution of medical personnel and services, and professional decisions about the allocation of professional services.[15] This was essentially a fee-for-service system that was gradually eroded by social forces resulting from the rapid rise in medical knowledge and technology and government subsidy of health care. The market system then slowly shifted to a system dominated by a variety of third-party payments for health care services. As the new system grew, however, availability of health resources everyone and to choose the alternative that maximizes the benefit or good for all.

Ethical formalism, or deontological ethics, which is often philosophically in opposition to utilitarianism, considers individual rights as unconditional and absolute. Individual rights are not to be compromised in the interest of the larger group. Deontologists view human rights as ends in themselves without recognition of consequences. To compromise an individual's rights in the interests of other human beings is to violate Immanuel Kant's well-known maxim, treat people as ends in themselves and never as means only. If one fails to recognize and act on the right of an individual, one is then treating that person as a means to ones own end. Deontology stresses individual rights, not the rights of the majority. It is concerned with self-determination, keeping promises, privacy, personal responsibility, dignity, individual worth, and the sanctity of life.

Given the increasing ability to preserve and maintain human life via technological intervention, the questions dealing with life become complex conceptually as well as ethically. From a conceptual perspective it becomes more and more difficult to define terms such as "extraordinary treatment" and "human life" because our concepts of living and dying have changed dramatically as a consequence of technology. Because we have such an increasingly difficult time achieving consensus on such concepts, it becomes proportionately difficult to achieve consensus on the ethical issues of how to interpret and apply universal ethical principles in resolving technological dilemmas. The ethical problem becomes which principles should be applied and which ones should take precedence over others when there is a conflict between principles relevant to the solution of a particular ethical dilemma.

For example, use of chemotherapeutic agents in the control of pain presents the dilemma of how to relieve pain and suffering without hastening death. Often the beneficent act of medicating violates the principles of preservation of life (sancity of life) and avoiding harm (nonmaleficence) because the side effects of medicating the patient can cause central nervous system depression and decreased physical activity, subjecting the patient to the hazards of immobility and respiratory arrest. The question for nurses then becomes, which is the greater harm—hastening death as a side effect of treatment or failing to adequately relieve human suffering?

Another instance is when patients refuse treatment and make decisions concerning their bodies, their lives, and their desires to control events related to both. Does the principle of autonomy and self-determination always and absolutely take precedence over all other principles, or is it relative to the other ethical principles of beneficence, nonmaleficence, and sanctity of life? Most members of American society would agree that freedom and self-determination are the most important things we can enjoy, but we cannot have unlimited rights and freedoms when living in a group. No person is an island unto themselves. We are all members of the moral community and have obligations to family, friends, and society.

When patients enter the health-care system, we as nurses are obligated to help them under the principle of beneficence and sanctity of life, which is the source of the right to health care. How can we stand by and allow harm to come to an individual? When patients refuse treatment, the health care provider, family members, and society at large are affected by the decision. If a patient is a viable member of a family with responsibilities to others, does the nurse, family, or community have a right to oppose the decision?

Philosophers tell us that rights and duties are correlative among as well as within individuals. If I have a certain right to something, someone else has a correlative duty to give it to me. Likewise, if I have a right to something, I have a corresponding duty, obligation, or responsibility to maintain and support that right. Some would argue that each patient has the basic right to life as a human being and that health care professionals, as the guardians of life for society, are obligated to see that patients are accorded that right when they are unable or unwilling to assume responsibility for their own right to life.

A counterargument in the resolution of this dilemma is that nurses are mere technicians who implement third-party decisions regardless of whether the decisions are consistent with their personal or professional beliefs and code of ethics. What do nurses do about their duties as professionals and their rights as individuals with certain value systems? If patients have a right to die, does the nurse have the duty at all times to see that patients have that right met?

If one allows patients to die by allowing them to refuse treatment, one is respecting their autonomy and self-determination. One avoids dehumanizing patients through the use of paternalistic practices that may prolong life. But is one recognizing and preserving the patient's autonomy by doing so? By refusing treatment the patient dies more quickly. Some would argue that once one is dead one has no more autonomy or freedom to make or act on one's own decisions because one no longer exists. Therefore it would follow that if we really want to preserve the patient's autonomy, should we not keep that person alive as long as possible so that the patient at least possesses the potential for being an autonomous person?

Nurses as health care providers continually hear that patients want to die a dignified death. What really is death with dignity? Can death ever really be dignified? Dempsey[1] notes that withholding treatment does not mean that a patient will necessarily die with dignity, it simply means that the patient will die sooner. Nurses who have witnessed patients dying of malnutrition and dehydration in cancer-related deaths, for example, can attest to this fact. The pain, discomfort, and debility of anemia, the development of decubitus ulcers, and the edema of protein deficiency are not consistent with what many would consider death with dignity.

When death is inevitable despite treatment, life is immediately threatened, the treatment is particularly hazardous, or if treatment will either be temporarily or permanently mutilate or incapacitate the patient, we do not feel so uncomfortable if the competent patient refuses treatment. But what do we do as nurses when the patient is not competent and when the prognosis may improve with painful or mutilating treatment? A frequent source of ethical dilemmas is the use of invasive technological treatment to prolong life for patients with limited or no decision-making capacities. Nurses continue to be faced with complex quality-of-life and treatment decisions with incompetent patients. By what criteria should mental competency be determined? Is mental competency a static, all-or-nothing phenomena? Just because a patient is confused or depressed some or most of the time does that mean the person has nothing to say in the decision-making process? Is there such a thing as partial mental competency? Is an incompetent person a full human being or less than human and hence not accorded full human rights, among them the right to make decisions and the right to life? Because we traditionally accord the right to life and the right to treatment to human beings only, how do we define humanness or personhood?

Should decisions about incompetents be based on social consideration—the best interest of loved ones or the state—or on their own best interests? In the harm-benefit, cost-benefit analysis should economic factors as well as human suffering enter into the calculation? Should the senile, confused, retarded, or "unproductive" incompetent be less entitled to expensive, exotic life-saving treatment than the "productive" competent citizen?

Do we have the right to make a judgment about the quality of someone else's life? How do we determine the criteria by which we judge the quality of life for another human being? My idea of the good life may not be the same as those closest to me, much less the same as my patient.

These are but a few of the very serious ethical dilemmas facing nurses in a technological health system that at times presents seemingly unlimited choices in determining who shall live and who shall be permitted to die. Ethical decisions are social decisions because they take place in a highly complex social environment consisting of different health team members who may have widely different value systems.[6] In addition, the prevalent philosophy of society at large and the particular health care institution also add to the dynamics of the social component of the decision-making process. No matter how much the decision maker may attempt to remain objective, there is a large subjective element present in the ethical decisions of health care providers.

Technological health care institutions strive foremost for efficiency and cost-effectiveness. Physicians as scientists often perceive their goal of treatment as the cure of diseases and the extinction or control of pathological bodily functioning. In determining the cost-benefit ratio, the technological, bureaucratic institution perceives its ethical mandate to be utilitarian in nature—the greatest good for the greatest number. Consequently, self-preservation of the bureaucracy is foremost. In this cost-benefit decision-making process, quality patient care can easily be traded off in the interest of financial cost savings.

In the case of ethical decision making on the part of physician-scientists, the reductionist orientation of science socializes physicians to look at bodily systems and disease entities—not at the patient as a person.[5] Factors considered in the cost-benefit ratio for physicians are often limited to physiological harms and benefits because physicians perceive their ethical mandate of "doing no harm" or "doing good" to be an all-out attack on the disease process.

The nursing profession holds a more holistic orientation and has as its goals the treatment of the patient's response to the particular health problem. For nurses the ethical mandate in the cost-benefit decision-making process is to consider the costs and benefits of treatment in terms of preserving the patient's human dignity and ability to function at the highest level of potential. Nurses, therefore, are far more concerned with individual patient welfare and the impact of technological intervention as it affects the immediate and long-term quality of life of the patient and family. Herein lies the ever-increasing source of tension and conflict between nurse, institution, and physician. The development of science and technology appears to be a necessity and no doubt will continue to have high priority in our society. Science and technology give us means but not ends and therefore must be directed toward ends determined by society. Nurses are the key personnel in the health care system to mediate the interaction among science, technology, and the patient because of their unique role as care givers who preserve the patient's humanity. The challenge for the nursing profession is how to continue to render humane and moral care that gives life, health, and death its meaning when nurses have to function in technological orga-

nizations that strive foremost for technological efficiency and cost-effectiveness.

REFERENCES

1. Dempsey P: The way we die: an investigation of death and dying in America today, New York, editors: 1975, McGraw-Hill Book Co.
2. Eden HS and Eden, M. editors: Microprocessor-based "intelligent" machines in patient care, US Department of Health, Education and Welfare, National Institute of Health Pub No 79-1852, Sept 1979.
3. Frost SB, Fearon Z, and Hyman HH: A consumer's guide to evaluating medical technology, New York, Consumer Commission on the Accreditation of Health Services.
4. Gordon G and Fisher GL, editors: The diffusion of medical technology, Cambridge, Mass, 1975, Ballinger Publishing Co.
5. Murphy CP: Nurses' views important on ethical decision team, American p12, Nov-Dec 1983.
6. Murphy CP and Hunter H, editors: Ethical problems in the nurse-patient relationship, Boston, 1983, Allyn and Bacon.
7. Pollack A: A new automation to bring vast changes, Supplement on Employment in High Technology, section 12, March 28, 1982.
8. Taylor P: Principles of ethics, Encino, Calif, 1975, Dickenson Publishing Co.
9. Walters, LR: Technology assessment. In Reich W, editor: Encyclopedia of Bioethics, New York, 1978, The Free Press.

CHAPTER 84

Knowledge technology

Costs, benefits, ethical considerations

LINDA K. AMOS
JUDITH R. GRAVES

Advances in technology over the last 50 years have been cited as the primary factor in the movement of the economy of the United States and the world. Nationwide in 1986 a total of $458 billion was spent for health, an amount equal to 10.9% of the gross national product.[4] Health care expenditures are projected to reach $1.5 trillion by the year 2000—15% of the gross national product. Technology in health care has revolutionized the nature of care delivery and has significantly influenced costs, mechanisms of care delivery, and the nature of health care benefits and outputs. Consumers of health care are demanding and expecting the highest quality of health care and technology. That demand is expected to continue at an ever-accelerating rate.

The issues of quality of care, access to care, cost of health services, and allocation of scarce resources have been paramount for the past few years and remain the priority issues for consumers and health care policymakers. Technological advances have created more complex dilemmas in each of the policy priority areas. In health care, the advances in biomedical and information technology have had a significant influence on the ability to address the major problems confronting health care providers today. In nursing, new and complex challenges are confronted in the implementation, utilization, evaluation, and development of new technologies while nurses at the same time strive to maintain and advance the basic core of nursing practice—humane approaches to the care and treatment of clients and their families.

The focus of this chapter is a relatively new technology on the health care scene, knowledge technology. The purposes of this chapter are (1) to define and describe knowledge technology, contrasting it to the other two main types of health care technology; (2) to describe the influence of this new technology on nursing practice and research and suggest a future based on such knowledge technology; (3) to examine the ethical implications involved in knowledge technology; and (4) to examine the costs and benefits of a future with knowledge technology.

TYPES OF HEALTH CARE TECHNOLOGY
Biomedical technology

Health care technology can be grouped into three major categories: biomedical technology, information technology, and knowledge technology. Biomedical technology conjures up the image of complex machines and implantable devices for use in the patient care setting. Artificial organs (hearts, arms, and ears), gene therapy to identify and correct faulty genes, diagnostic tests that spot early indications of disease or determine the exact site of tissue damage, transplantation of brain tissue to treat Parkinson's and other diseases, robot servants for people who are disabled, and the use of electrical currents in the body to stimulate repair of damaged tissue are all examples of biomedical technology that is currently available or in the development process.

The trend in this area is toward less invasive technology. Lithotriptos, micropumps, and lasers are good examples. On a larger scale, the CT (computed tomography) scanner and magnetic resonance imager have provided a greater ability to look inside the body and have decreased the need for exploratory surgery. Although biomedical technology is largely grounded in hardware and appliances, it may be combined with information technologies such as those used to assist paralyzed persons walk. Here a computer using information and even knowledge technology is used to transmit signals to muscles, enabling persons who are paralyzed to walk.

Biomedical technology has had a significant impact on nursing practice. Nurses have often been the ones to assume responsibility for monitoring the data generated by these devices, and they have frequently taken responsibility for assessing the effectiveness of such equipment.

Information technology

Information technology is used here to refer to the electromechanical matrix, that is, the hardware and software used to manage and process information. Used collectively and generically, *data, information,* and *knowledge* are referred to as information. It is helpful for the purposes of this chapter, however, to define these concepts more precisely so the differences in technological base can be grasped more clearly.

Using conventions described by Blum,[2] *data* is defined as uninterpreted but measured objects or elements. *Information* is interpreted sets of data, and *knowledge* refers to the rules, relationships, and experience by which data become information. Data applications such as signal processing, imaging, and modeling rely on computational processing and fit largely into the realm of biomedical technology. They produce information by computationally processing limited amounts of data. Information applications, in contrast, combine data so that meaning is emphasized. Here the emphasis is on organization, storage, retrieval, and communication management. These applications imply a database. In the health care field, information systems are the primary information application. These information systems are usually named to indicate the discipline or function they serve. For example, hospital information systems support hospital functioning and manage information for accounting and other tasks; nursing and medical information systems manage clinical information required for the practice of nursing and medicine; and nursing management-information systems support nursing administration functions such as staffing. This technology, at its best, stores information needed to support a type of practice or decision making and can restructure and re-present the information in ways requested by and useful to the decision maker.

Knowledge technology

Although there is a lot more electronic and mechanical gadgetry interposed between patient and nurse that has greatly influenced the technical practice of nursing, technology has had little influence on the core of nursing practice, which is caring for and nurturing persons in health and in illness. Computers, however, bring a technology that promises to be more than another electromechanical contrivance interposed between nurse and patient or client. The technology that computers enable is broader than the mechanical and electronic properties by which they operate. Because computers process symbols, they bring a technology of mind, a knowledge technology. Knowledge technology is defined here as computer systems that generate or process knowledge. The generating component is the transformation of information into knowledge. The processing component of knowledge technology is analogous to the processing of information by practitioners of the discipline to make clinical decisions.

The study of the use of the computer as a knowledge technology for the practitioner of nursing is part of *nursing informatics.* Informatics is an emerging academic discipline within nursing in which the processing and management of nursing data, information, and knowledge are the central focus of study. The term *informatics* originated in Europe, where it refers to computer science. The term has broadened to mean computer science and information science. It is used in conjunction with the names of disciplines or domains of knowledge to denote an application of computer science and information science to the management and processing of data, information, and knowledge in a particular domain. Nursing informatics combines computer science and information science with nursing science to assist in the management and processing of data, information, and knowledge to support the practice of nursing—the care of clients or patients. It is the commodity that computers process (i.e., nursing data, information, and knowledge), not the computer itself that is important to the science of informatics.[1]

The management component of informatics speaks to the functional capacity to collect, aggregate, organize, and move information between point of origin and point of use in a way that is economical, efficient, and useful to the clinician. This component generates most of the ethical difficulties posed by any electronic information system, including the privacy and security of data. These dilemmas have been the focus of most critiques to date.

The processing component of informatics stems from the recognition that data and information are processed by practitioners of the discipline to make clinical decisions, by researchers to build knowledge strategies, and by theorists to develop nursing theory. Processing can be considered a transformation of data or information from one form to another, usually at a higher level of complexity and organization. The automation of processing thus requires an understanding of the nature and structure of the information to be processed, of the potential for transformations useful in the domain, and of the algorithms (i.e., rules, knowledge) used by experts in the field to transform information from one level of complexity to another for use in practice, research, and theory building.

Data are discrete entities that are objectively described without interpretation. The number 7 is data. Unless more is known, the number is meaningless and largely useless. Data processing implies the transformation of data in raw form to data that are organized and structurally meaningful. Because information refers to data that are interpreted and organized or structured, the processing of data generates information as a product. Thus, individual data groupings such as hourly fluid intake and output values are transformed into 8-hour, 24-hour, and even weekly values. To automate this processing, the necessary data elements must be identified and rules for combining the data established. The critical assumption underlying this processing is that the same data elements are always required and the same formula or rule is always applied in the same way to the data.

The next level of processing, the processing of information, is much more complex. The term *information* denotes data to which meaning has been attached by virtue of context or by virtue of having been organized into a structure that carries meaning. Processing, then, must somehow deal with meaning. The processing of information may result in the development of new or different information or, more to the point, the product, knowledge. Knowledge is information that has been synthesized so that interrelationships are identified and formalized. The research process is a familiar example of processing data or information into knowledge. In what might be called research processing, a structured set of rules and procedures is applied to transform raw data into knowledge about relationships between the variables of interest. This processing is sufficiently structured and algorithmic to allow computer programs to design research studies and test of interesting hypotheses in some situations.[22]

The same idea can be taken one step further, to the processing of knowledge to produce decisions. This, in effect, is what expert system technology does. An expert system is a computer program that mimics the deductive or inductive reasoning of a human expert or the outcome of that reasoning process by making inferences from internalized facts and rules.[17] To wit, the expert system processes knowledge to produce decisions. The system is composed of two main sections: (a) a knowledge base (as opposed to a database) containing the knowledge (rules, heuristics) that an expert applies to data and information in order to solve a problem; and (b) an inference engine, that is, a computer program that controls the use of the knowledge.

The creation of expert systems is one implementation of knowledge technology that shows considerable promise in assisting nurses with clinical management problems. Computer processing of the expert and research knowledge captured in domain-specific knowledge bases can suggest how to apply and interpret nursing data and information in such a way as to make better clinical nursing decisions.

Because expert knowledge is a key component of such systems, it is important to ask, What is an expert? The question of what distinguishes the expert from the nonexpert was posed by Socrates, who attempted to pry the secrets of expertise from the known experts of his day.[5] Socrates found that the experts he questioned did not reply with a generalizable process or even a specific set of rules and principles as anticipated, but instead gave numerous different case examples from experience to illustrate given points. Knowledge gained in building and testing expert systems in medicine and in the physical sciences has confirmed the domain-specific nature of expertise. Thus expertise is defined as knowledge about a particular domain, understanding of domain problems, and skill in solving some important subset of these problems.[15] The domain knowledge captured in the expert system involves specialty knowledge. Specialty knowledge encompasses the public or published definitions, facts, and theories contained in the references and texts of a field. Specialty knowledge also includes the private knowledge of the expert, which is not published and seems to consist largely of rules of thumb or heuristics about how to combine the facts to make correct decisions under varying conditions.[15] These heuristics are developed by the expert as experience and expertise in the domain is developed. To reproduce, clarify, and represent the private as well as public knowledge of the specialty expert is the central problem of expert system development.

The expert system, like the expert, must have great knowledge of the domain and skill at solving the given problems. Despite the observation that computer programs can be written to discover scientific laws from data, the representation of problems and the associated operations that permit experts to extract information from situations is thought to be associated with the field of expertise, not with expertise generally.[14]

Case study of an expert system

Consider a specific expert system, the issues it raises, and how those issues are being explored. In collaboration with clinical nurses from local hospitals and colleagues from the medical informatics department, the faculty of the College of Nursing at the University of Utah are developing an expert consultation system for nursing management of acute pain in patients who have had total hip arthroplasty.[11] The system, begun in 1986, now contains the knowledge that clinical nurse experts in pain management use in making some 58 decisions to (a) define the current pain state, (b) determine the need for, appropriateness of, effectiveness of, and need for change in pharmacological and nonpharmacological nursing therapies, (c) alert the nurse for treatment-specific nursing measures, and (d) assess and plan patient education.

The system uses a frame-based model in which a number of items and conditions may be used to make a single decision. The system then uses Boolean reasoning to combine the facts into a correct decision. A simple decision is modelled in the box above.

The logic of the frame indicates that a maximum dose of the prescribed opiate—in this case, morphine sulfate—is given on schedule every 4 hours in the first 48 hours after surgery as long as there are no contraindications, even though the patient may not be in severe pain or a painful procedure is not planned. If the patient is in severe pain, or if a painful procedure is planned, and there are no contradictions, the morphine may be given three hours after the last dose.

Case study of a literature-based knowledge-building system

A second type of knowledge system is under development at the University of Utah by Graves.[9] ARKS, an acronym for "a research knowledge sys-

---

> **DECISION FRAME FOR "GIVE MAXIMUM DOSE OF MORPHINE SULFATE"**
>
> A   @Pain is severe
> B   @Painful procedure is planned
> C   There is an existing order for morphine sulfate
> D   @Contraindications to morphine sulfate
> E   @History of allergic reaction to opiate analgesic
> F   @Contraindication to maximum dose of opiate analgesic
> G   Time since last dose of morphine sulfate
> H   Time since surgery
>
> *Logic: Give the maximum dose of morphine sulfate IF:*
> (A OR B) AND (C AND H < 48 hours AND G > 3 hours) AND NOT (D OR E OR F)
> OR
> (C AND H < 48 hours AND G ≥ 4 hours) AND NOT (D OR E OR F)

The @ sign indicates that another decision frame exists to fully define that item or condition.

tem," is a program designed to build literature-based knowledge bases in a domain. Development has been based on the opinion that it is both possible and desirable to turn health-relevant libraries into databases of findings instead of databases of document information provided by the current generation of bibliographic databases. By aggregating variables linked together in (quantitative) research in a field of study with the nature and direction of the relationship demonstrated, its stochastic significance, and the findings, and representing them as causal or directional maps, ARKS can assist clinicians in designing treatment strategies, researchers in designing research protocols, and nurse theorists and students in understanding the definition and structure of nursing concepts. The domain-specific databases that result from the use of ARKS are considered knowledge bases, because they store related variables and describe the knowledge that describes the relationship. In addition, ARKS processes the knowledge contained within the knowledge base by restructuring it into concept structures that can represent new knowledge in a field.

Ethical considerations

Knowledge technology brings with it important ethical considerations. In the context of expert systems, how expert is the expert system? If it is in fact expert, are there normative effects? Will use of the system become prescriptive for the average practitioner? Will some systems become so expert and accepted that it will be considered inappropriate or evidence of malpractice to reach decisions without consulting them? Will use of the system diminish the performance level of the human domain expert?

Currently only the first question can be answered. Until actual systems can be tested in clinical situations, answers to the remaining questions must wait or rest on theory and philosophy.

How expert is an expert system? The answer to this question resides largely in the quality of the system's decisions and advice and the correctness of the reasoning techniques used.[10,19] Regardless of the type of system, the decision or recommendation may be correct or incorrect. Error can occur in the facts, in the logic, or perhaps in the method for dealing with uncertainty. In systems that model the reasoning process (not just the outcome), a particularly worrisome possibility is the fact that the program may come up with the right answer, so to speak, for the wrong reasons. Should the right answer be accepted? In systems that do not model the reasoning process, should right answers be accepted if it is not understood how the computer arrived at an answer?

Factual items must be verified from the research literature if at all possible. In addition, research documentation of the logic is obtained. Because most research in nursing deals with simple relationships rather than decisions, this latter requirement is not always met. In the decision example given on p. 595, research has been found to substantiate that longer periods of satisfactory pain relief are obtained when opiate analgesic is administered on schedule rather than on demand. The research sample, however, and the population for whom the expert system is built, are sufficiently different to require expert confirmation of standards of practice. A system such as ARKS may help to document decision logic by producing maps of related variables, thus documenting necessary relationships.

One potentially major source of unreliability of the decision frame on p. 595 is the limitation of the logic form itself. When representing knowledge as rules and using Boolean combinations, it is very difficult except in the simplest of situations to represent all the items of information that the expert actually considers in making a decision. Further, all data items must be

"known" in the decision to be recommended, yet clinical decisions are rarely made on complete information. Thus, even when all conditions are met, the most important conditions represented, and the logic correct, the decision frame must be demonstrated in clinical practice to work reliably with different patients. This requires clinical testing with real patients against an expert decision standard. Such systems are labor intensive to build and labor intensive to test. The more rapidly the knowledge of a domain is changing, the greater the demand for updating and reevaluating the knowledge base. Because they operate in real time, clinical management systems are far more difficult to build than diagnostic systems, which can assume that time is unimportant.

The rule-based decision system illustrated on p. 595 mimics nonexpert processes, not the case-example reasoning process of the experts.[5] For this reason, the model for the pain management system is due to be transformed to Bayesian reasoning, a statistical model. Taking as an example the decision of what defines severe pain, as expert would be asked to estimate the probability with which a finding such as "verbal report of severe pain from the patient" occurs in patients who indeed have severe pain and another probability in which the same finding occurs in patients who do not have severe pain. This type of probability estimate is obtained for each condition that is believed to contribute to a discrimination of the level of pain. To estimate the likelihood of severe pain in any one patient, the probabilities are then combined using the Bayes formula and, given an a priori probability of severe pain in the population of persons having undergone total hip arthroplasty, the computer can calculate the probability that a given patient is in severe pain, given the signs and symptoms expressed by that patient. When experts are asked to estimate the probabilities, in essence they are asked to sift through their experiences with patients (case experiences) having pain for the same reason. Thus a more realistic model for deciding that severe pain is present is obtained, at least in theory. This type of reasoning works well in medical diagnostic systems such as HELP.[3] Whether or not the same model will be reliable for decisions that do not have the same degree of discreteness in the real world as diseases is impossible to determine until the reasoning is transformed and tested. In the meantime, what is learned about novice and expert decision making, about expert domain problem structuring, and about the domain of pain management, is invaluable to the discipline of nursing. The knowledge base alone (containing the facts and conditions and the rules for combining them to make a decision), even when unaccompanied by an inference engine, is a completely new offering to the discipline.

The pain management system has undergone several levels of formative evaluation already. In addition to expert help in formulating the decisions and validating the knowledge or fact in the literature, another outside clinical expert has reviewed the decisions for factual content, accuracy of logic, comprehensiveness, and practicality for clinical practice. The system currently is being readied for clinical testing of the rule-based version.

What is an acceptable level of performance of this system and of the individual decisions within the system? Medical diagnostic systems can be expected to outperform experts. At that, accuracy is considerably under 100%. Accuracy of a clinical management decision is much more difficult to measure than accuracy of a diagnosis of a disease. Unlike a disease, a clinical management decision is highly context dependent. That context includes at least the patient and the surrounding environment, the patient's past experience with pain, and pain treatments. Is clinical management of acute pain too difficult a problem to model at all under these circumstances? Obviously we do not think so; however, we are aware of our obligations as domain experts and informaticists building the system to ask the hard questions, to find the boundaries of the problem, to explore the limits and benefits and consequences to use of such systems.

BENEFITS AND COSTS

The costs of technology can be divided into the categories of development, capital acquisitions, maintenance, operation, and equipment replacement. These categories of costs of technology vary considerably among the different types of biomedical, information, and knowledge technology, especially in the development phase. Equipment replacement was cited as accounting for only 5% of the annual cost of technology in hospitals in 1986, and the deployment of staff for maintenance and operation as the most expensive component of technology after the initial capital purchase. The marginal costs of repeated or additional use of some technology offsets the initial outlay of the capital purchase.[12] Thus the cost of high technology can be cut—without losing benefits—by

increasing use or enhancing productivity, abandoning unnecessary and ineffective technology, and working to avoid duplicative acquisitions of high-cost equipment in settings or geographical areas where it can be shared.

There are additional cost considerations after the initial investment in information or knowledge systems for a health care system, such as the needs for space, security, and special furniture. Also, continuing costs for maintenance contracts, supplies, personnel, and upgrading need to be considered. The costs for repair and upgrading sometimes can be major. There may be hidden costs that are difficult to assess on initial investment in a system. The competitive market in computer technology presently is to the advantage of the purchaser. Opportunities to gain access to hardware and software with multiple capabilities, along with staff trained to develop unique software packages, will be important developments. The potential for distributing software packages to other settings throughout the country makes it advantageous for institutions to give serious consideration to the need to invest in computer technology.

The ease with which an individual can use computers is another cost factor. Expensive training and availability of sophisticated programmers and technicians add considerably to the cost of computer use and any management information system. The cost of building expert systems is very costly right now because of the length of time required to harvest the knowledge of the expert. This is changing as tools such as development shells and tools for converting the logic that is originally written in English text form into programming language become available. Microcomputers are now being produced in a manner that encourages friendly interaction through use of common language. At the same time, administrators must consider the cost of training staff so they can use the computers. A careful approach to the introduction of development programs for staff is key to a major investment in computer technology. The lag time in preparing personnel and developing suitable programs interjects the costs of personnel time and preparation needed to move programs forward without delays.

Implications

The question of how much technology we can afford can be partially answered through a cost-benefit analysis.[13] This is an analytic approach in which the major consequences of technology versus other methods are measured in dollars. Because the major consequences of technology in health care delivery cannot be measured meaningfully in only monetary terms, it is essential that some qualitative indication of the impact of technology be assessed. This impact relates mainly to the intangible benefits discussed earlier. Examples include quality of information, speed of decision making, personnel satisfaction, improved services, impact on the quality of life for clients, advances through discovery of new knowledge, improved efficiencies in management and financial operations, and greater fiscal control as a result of more precise accounting methods. The costs of technology are high and the question of how much technology can be afforded must be answered based on an analysis of the cost-benefit ratio and the marginal rates of return from the purchase and use of technology. Marginal effects refer to a measure of the changes in costs or effectiveness associated with the next activity or unit of output. This means that the cost for an information and decision support system will be high for the first several months of operation, but will decrease with continued use.

If it is determined that the technology's real or perceived value approximates its costs, the next question is whether it is possible to have the same benefits at a lower cost; or whether for the same cost it is possible to have more benefits. The first question relates to technical efficiency, where it must be determined if the resources currently in use achieve their maximum outputs while maintaining quality and consumer satisfaction.

The discussion thus far has focused on cost-benefit analyses of physical rather than human issues. It is far more difficult to analyze the costs and benefits of saving or prolonging human lives through technology. The real question is, at what point is the cost of extensive information or human life too high? Commercial insurers already face the dilemma of how much they will pay for organ transplants that save lives. If the cost remains as high as at present, the time may come when organs are available only to the rich. Small or rural hospitals may find the costs of installing and maintaining an information and clinical decision support system for clinicians prohibitive. Technological discrimination against the poor already exists, because the poor have not had the opportunities enabling them to fully benefit from present technology.

A benefit usually is defined as some measure of the ultimate worth or value of a desired outcome. Benefits can also be defined as the effects expected or achieved as a result of using technology. Tangible benefits are frequently specified in dollar equivalents, whereas intangible benefits refer to aspects of quality or effectiveness. Tangible benefits from technology in health care delivery can be viewed in a number of ways. An obvious tangible benefit of technology is the reduction in cost resulting from shorter hospital stays than would have been possible otherwise. The number of days someone with a chronic illness or disability is kept from work can be decreased by technology and measured in dollars. Another fiscal benefit is the savings created by technology freeing professional personnel from tedious and time-consuming administrative tasks. A more difficult issue to address is the value placed on the lives that are prolonged through modern technology.

At the same time, society is acutely aware of the crisis in health care financing. Consumers, providers, and policymakers are all concerned about cost-effectiveness, efficiency, and new alternatives for health care delivery because health care costs are growing at an unacceptable rate. Evidence of overuse and abuse of health care technology is abundant. It is incumbent on nurses and computer companies to develop approaches to the use of informatics that cost less and increase productivity while maintaining a high-quality product.[7] Information management technology has been described as saving costs, but no documentation has yet been published. Several authors, however, describe the use of information systems and decision-supported assistance in the clinical area as having the potential to help nurses improve their productivity.[6,16,18]

The intangible benefits of technology often have greater appeal for most health professionals and consumers than its tangible benefits. In the practice area, technology can improve client services. At the very least there should be an improvement in the quantity and quality of services and information, resulting in faster and better decision making. For nurses, it is possible that job satisfaction will increase because informatics will provide opportunities for greater knowledge and control over data and its uses.

Time is a variable that will have to be taken into consideration as either a cost or a benefit of technology. Large amounts of time will be expended as personnel learn to use the technology and to develop programs suitable for saving time in the long run. It is likely that one of the greatest benefits of computer applications in the practice setting will be the amount of time saved and increased accuracy and efficiency. The crucial decision will be how to use the time saved. Given severe nursing shortages throughout the country and the likelihood that they will continue in the future, the time savings factor could have important ramifications for nursing practice.

What are the benefits of expert knowledge technology that make the extensive development effort worthwhile? First of all, expert systems outperform nonexpert human clinicians, at least in the medical domain. If this relationship holds true in nursing, a beneficial effect on decision-making might be expected for novices, and nurses working outside of their usual area of expertise, a useful effect for orientation and in-service education. A major benefit exists when this expert system is used with a clinical nursing information system (CNIS) and gets its data directly from the electronic charting of the nurses. Not needing time off for lunch and breaks, not tied up unexpectedly with another patient, the computer never forgets when the patient needs to be treated for pain or checked for effectiveness of the last treatment. Thus even trivial and obvious decisions in such an on-line system can help improve the quality of care. Also if the expert system is used with a CNIS, the documentation of observations, care, and patient outcomes can be expected to improve significantly. More important, perhaps, is that the information system can be used to gather the data needed to measure the incidence of findings associated with pain states and treatment outcomes under varying conditions, thus allowing the problem to be modeled in a statistical rather than a Boolean mode.

The Nursing Pain Management System is built on the premise that it must be self-explaining. If the nurse questions the computer's recommendation, the computer must explain how it arrived at the decision. It must show all the conditions used and how it applied the rules (logic) to arrive at the condition. In addition, the pain management system is designed to display research knowledge or (in the absence of research) declarative knowledge or expert opinion. Eventually, actual clinical data taken from the local CNIS will be used to document the reasoning used. This provides the potential for more timely implementation of new knowledge into practice, that is, it constitutes a direct use of research. Because the research used to document the system is filtered by a domain expert, some of the major obstacles to research utilization are overcome.[8] The linking of the research to the decision ensures relevance. The expert filters out research reports of poor quality or weak design and methodology and knows enough about the existing research in the domain to know which studies present conflicting results and which have be replicated sufficiently for enactment into practice.

Expert system development, like other knowledge technology development, is costly. Knowledge acquisition—that is, obtaining the knowledge from the source and getting the knowledge into the computer system—is extremely time consuming. For example, the Nursing Pain Management System took 3 years to develop a 58-frame prototype, and development involved 2 to 3 experts (domain and informatics) and 2 knowledge engineers on an ongoing basis. All told, an estimated 12½ full person-months plus another month of programming time were spent. This was the first system of its type built in nursing, and there were no guidelines for the development process. The first two years of development used an approach that depended largely on a domain expert identifying the decision set and logic and working with knowledge engineers to represent that knowledge in the HELP system language. In the third year, we moved to a method of development that was largely literature based. Instead of a clinical domain expert, we used a doctoral student who had a background in chronic pain management and was generally familiar with the literature. Within six months the decision set was nearly quadrupled in size and the logic polished. As the set neared completion, we were able to determine a structure for the decision set. Because we can now predict the overall structure of needed decisions and build the initial logic from the literature prior to requiring a clinical expert, we expect to reduce our production time for development of new clinical management systems to one third or perhaps one fourth of this initial time.

A second breakthrough promises to reduce the time and therefore the cost of expert system production. Homer Warner and his colleagues in the medical informatics department at the University of Utah have developed a set of automated knowledge engineering tools that can take the near-English text logic written by domain experts and engineers and translate it into the programming language required to run the system.[21] The programming and debugging time can therefore be significantly reduced. This also reduces the number of people that need to be involved in the development process, thus significantly reducing cost.

CONCLUSION

There have been many criticisms of the possible dangers of a technological society, particularly with regard to the loss of the human element, but it is important to recognize that human beings can assess information technology in the same way progress has always been assessed in society; namely, through careful, critical, and imaginative analysis. "The dichotomy between caring and technology reflects a fear of technology. Nurses must view technology and humanism as complementary in their contribution to human welfare, and we must see ourselves as the agents capable of melding the two as we help drive the changes for the future."[20]

Technological and computer advances cannot be thought to provide answers to all things. No matter how sophisticated computer technology becomes, the question of individual use or abuse of the system will be the true limiting factor in its ability to provide efficiency and quality of care. Inappropriate use of technology cannot be afforded either in humanitarian or economic terms. When the full range of implications of modern technologies is considered, one begins to realize the possible consequences of misuse or misinterpretation as well as the vast potential for good.

The information revolution in nursing and health care will provide an opportunity to better control practice and activities in ways previously unknown. Nurses should view the advent of inexpensive and sophisticated microcomputers with complex capabilities as a major opportunity for nursing to advance its knowledge base at a pace faster than ever thought possible. Without investing in the costs of technology, an institution is likely to become outdated in a short time. Although the costs of initial investment in hardware and software, personnel, instruction, supplies, space, and ongoing maintenance may be considerable, we cannot afford not to take advantage of this significant opportunity to mainstream nursing so that significant strides can be made in the quality of care delivered and the expansion of the profession's knowledge base.

REFERENCES

1. Blois MS: What is it that computers compute? Clinical Computing 4(3):31, 1987.
2. Blum BI: Computers in medicine: information systems for patient care, New York, 1984, Springer-Verlag, Inc.
3. Bouhaddou O, Haug PJ, and Warner HR: Use of the HELP clinical database to build and test medical knowledge. In Stead WW, editors: Proceedings of the eleventh annual symposium on computer applications in medical care, 1987, Computer Society Press.
4. Division of National Cost Estimates 1986-2000, Office of the Actuary, Health Care Financing Administration: National health expenditures, Health Care Financing Review 8(4), 1987.
5. Dreyfus H and Dreyfus S: Mindless machines, The Sciences 24:18, 1984.
6. Edmunds L: Computers for inpatient nursing care, Comput in Nurs 2:102, 1984.
7. Edwardson SR: Measuring nursing productivity, Nursing Economics 3(1):9, 1985.
8. Graves JR: ARKS: a research knowledge system, in process.
9. Graves JR and Cocoran S: Design of nursing information systems: conceptual and practice elements, J Prof Nurs 4(3):168, 1988.
10. Hayes-Roth F, Waterman D, and Lenat D, editors: Building expert systems, New York, 1983, Addison-Wesley Publish Co, Inc.
11. Heriot C, Graves J, Bouhaddou O, Armstrong M, Wigertz G and Ben Said M: A pain management decision support system for nurses: Proceedings of the twelfth annual symposium on computer applications in medical care, Los Angeles, 1988, Computer Society Press.
12. Jennett B, editor: High technology medicine: benefits and burdens, New York, 1986, Oxford University Press.
13. Keller J, editor: Making resource allocation decisions based on policy analysis and program review, Boulder, Colo, 1983, National Center for Higher Education Management Systems.
14. Langley P and others, editors: Scientific discovery: computational explorations of the creative process, Cambridge, Mass, 1987, MIT Press.
15. McGraw-Hill expert system. In the McGraw-Hill encyclopedia of electronics & computers, New York, 1984, McGraw-Hill Book Co.
16. McHugh ML: Information access: a basis for strategic planning and control of operations, Nursing Administration Quarterly 10(2):10, 1986.
17. Negoita CV: Expert systems and fuzzy systems, Menlo Park, Calif, 1985, The Benjamin/Cummins Publishing Co, Inc.
18. Saba VK: The computer in public health: today and tomorrow. Nurs Outlook 30(9):510, 1982.
19. Shortliffe EH, editor: Rule-based expert systems, Reading, Mass, 1984, Addison-Wesley Publishing Co, Inc.
20. Smith GR: The evolution of alternative delivery systems: what will be nursing's role? In Nursing practice in the 21st century, Kansas City, Mo, 1988, American Nurses' Foundation, Pershing Road, Kansas City, Mo.
21. Sorenson O, Bouhaddou O, Wang W, Canfield G, Fu L, and Warner HR: Generation and maintenance of Illiad™ medical knowledge in a Hypercard™ environment. In Greenos RA, editor: Proceedings of the twelfth annual symposium on computer applications in medical care, Los Angeles: Computer Society Press, 1988.
22. Walker MG and Blum RL: Towards automated discovery from clinical databases: the RADIX project. Medinfo 86: Proceedings of the fifth Conference on Medical Informatics, part I, Washington, D.C., October 26-30, 1986.

CHAPTER 85

Computer technology

Endangering the essence of nursing?

CONNIE DELANEY

The question for [our] era, stated broadly, is whether technology will be the master or servant—a tool of oppression or an instrument for the general welfare.[16]

The first response of society to scientific, technological innovations is to marvel at their capabilities. Technology in general and computer technology in particular have made significant contributions to nursing practice, administration, research, and education. Nurses functioning as care givers, advocates, leaders or managers, teachers, and collaborators have felt the impact of computers and have identified numerous advantages to incorporating this technology into their roles.

However, technological revolution indelibly transforms society at large, the profession that utilizes the technology, and the individuals at whom the technology is directed. Because scientific and technological advances can shatter personal and professional beliefs, it becomes equally important to recognize the disadvantages and limitations of the technology. It is essential that nursing reexamine its practice and the values, beliefs, and knowledge base on which that practice is built. The fundamental issue surrounding computer technology is how to integrate computers into nursing practice while preserving and enhancing human dignity, respecting the uniqueness and freedom of the individual, and sustaining a common humanness.

This chapter explores technological change brought about by computers within the framework of nursing's commitment to caring.[28] The discussion examines the adoption of technology by society and nursing, caring in a technological society, and nursing practice strategies for balancing computer technology and the profession's commitment to caring.

THE ADOPTION OF TECHNOLOGY BY SOCIETY AND NURSING

Historically, technology has released people from the dull and routine, enabling them to reduce the dehumanizing elements of their jobs and expand their intrapersonal and creative lives. Technology also has challenged the limitations of being human, extending and amplifying the human body. The development of computer technology has paralleled this evolution from performing the dull and routine to challenging the entire range of human abilities. Early computing machines facilitated basic arithmetic activities. The advent of electronic devices made possible data storage and programming languages. Transistorized computers promoted reliability and interactive time-sharing. Integrated circuits made large computers commonplace and personal computers a reality. And the newest innovations allow for the development of knowledge-based expert systems that can simulate certain human thought processes.[22] Indeed, computers will be able to extend and amplify human capabilities to levels never before reached with other industrial technologies.[3,6,19]

Technology is adopted by society in stages. Initially, technology does work previously performed by people. That is, technology simply replaces a manual method of doing some activity. As technology allows work to be accomplished that previously was not possible, true innovation occurs. Finally, adoption becomes so complete that all dimensions of society itself are transformed by the technology. Currently many parts of our society—communications, financial and health care systems—have moved to the third stage and have "accepted computer technology as a means to enhance life."[14]

The widespread use of computers in nursing practice, research, education, and administration reflects professional acceptance. Nurses in both acute care and community health settings have used computers for physiological monitoring, diagnostic testing, drug administration, and therapeutic treatments such as dialysis and mechanical ventilation. Extensive computerized monitoring systems, particularly in critical care environments, collect and manage a wealth of data. Access to these data can facilitate prompt recognition of trends in patient status and promote rapid decision making. Evaluation of data through a decision-support system can improve rational decision making even more. Monitoring systems can accommodate patient assessment from remote locations, and automated patient care data systems can provide several clinicians with simultaneous access to data.

Computerized patient care planning and documentation exist in many institutions. Computer technology can enhance nursing diagnoses, treatment selection, and outcome evaluation. Improvements in the accuracy and completeness of documentation and in the availability of current information inevitably will enhance professional practice. Computers have been credited with making nursing practice more visible and placing the nurse in control of information.

Bibliographic searches, data gathering and analysis, and report preparation, revision, and communication capabilities enhance nursing research. Patient education and staff development activities are facilitated through computer-assisted instruction and educational resource databases. Computer-assisted and computer-managed instruction also are used in nursing education and continuing nursing education.

Automated nursing administrative and management information systems support personnel, scheduling, staffing, budget and payroll, costing out of nursing services, patient census, standards of care, quality assurance, forecasting and planning, and communication networks. Computers have been credited with

saving time, money, and energy, decreasing repetitious tasks and duplicative charting, increasing nursing's thoroughness, accuracy, efficiency, and reliability, and ultimately increasing nursing time for the patient.[14,9,17]

Computer technology has clearly replaced some of the work traditionally done by nurses and made it possible for nurses to do other new kinds of work. Nurses are well into the second stage of adoption. If nursing, like other components of society, follows the usual pattern of adoption, the profession itself will eventually be transformed by its technology.

CARING IN A TECHNOLOGICAL SOCIETY

Modern technological society values autonomy, individualism, and competitiveness. Our society's view of what it means to be a person, to be a human, has roots in the mechanistic model that grew out of the causal-mechanistic framework of the seventeenth and eighteenth centuries. This framework supports the following philosophical conclusions: the mind and body are separate; rationality is all-important; understanding comes from being able to represent things clearly; cost-benefit analysis underlies decision-making; the world and people are simply material to be used to reach goals; and behavior results from cognitive choice or intentionality only. Although this view is effective for understanding inanimate objects, it falls short when used for studying people. It ignores humans' connectedness within a given situation, and does not relate individuals' behavior to their skilled practices, habits, or languages.[4] Ultimately, technical-purposive rationality thrives at the expense of human interest and prevails over newer twentieth-century philosophies supportive of our common humanness.[13]

Moreover, the assimilation of technology itself promotes several value changes, further subverting many "basic human qualities on which society is built."[1] Nature tends to be viewed as simply an object to be exploited for satisfaction of human wants. Emphasis is placed on quantity (rather than quality) as a measure of good. And knowledge becomes viewed solely as a source of power.[11] In addition, the individual becomes assimilated into the machinery of society. Absorption occurs, with the individual becoming a number, and freedom and identity being distorted. Such changes in values and perspectives culminate to produce a society composed of standardized moving parts acting on each other to produce standardized products.

Society has reached a fault line, a point at which the traditions and culture steeped in the mechanistic philosophy and technological advances that have shaped contemporary life can neither sustain nor nurture people or their civilizations.[18] Yet an alternative path exists. By choosing to value people, human concerns, human worth, and individual decision-making, a new way of living can be effected. Indeed, Ray[23] has asserted that the future of health care delivery depends not only on technological abilities to generate computer-assisted costing and monitoring systems but also on abilities to interact, communicate, and understand what it means to be human. Herein lies the nursing profession's central dilemma: "being [committed] to care in a society that refuses to value caring."[24]

Caring has been defined as the essence, the "moral ideal of nursing whereby the end is protection, enhancement, and preservation of human dignity."[28] Encompassed in caring is a commitment to the preservation of common humanness and an unrelenting respect for the uniqueness and human dignity of each individual. Experiencing this duality of common humanness as well as separateness is accomplished by maintaining a holistic focus. Caring is situation specific, occurring in a relationship between the caring and the cared for. The sense of obligation inherent in the caring relationship is limited and delimited by the relationship.

For caring to be a true moral imperative and serve as the basis for nursing practice, it must be prescriptive, other regarding, and the ultimate overriding value that guides actions in relation to all persons.[12] Caring must encompass knowledge and skill in the ability to identify care needs and nursing actions that will bring about positive change; that is, movement toward the protection, enhancement, and preservation of human dignity. Consequently, care givers' activities should create and maintain an environment that allows caring to flourish.

If caring serves as an ethical standard of practice, the meaning of caring for things and ideas takes on an interpretation different from that generated by the mechanistic framework. An awareness surfaces that moral behavior occurs only through things and ideas, not toward them.[20] Examples of verbalisms commonly used in nursing literature—"the caring computer," "self-regulating machines"—raise the question as to whether this awareness currently exists in nursing. Indeed, the computer is changing the way people think, especially about themselves,. Turkle[27] notes that the question is not what the computer will be like in the future, but what will people be like.

BALANCING COMPUTER TECHNOLOGY AND CARING
Strategies for nurses

The widespread adoption of computer technology creates a serious challenge for the nursing profession. As a result of technology, dehumanization, loss of privacy, and breaches of confidentiality and security emerge as real threats to the outcomes of nursing practice. The use of expert systems and artificial intelligence, the impact of technology on organizational structure and processes, and the cost and resource consumption needed to support the technology create further concerns for nursing. Yet nursing can develop proactive strategies for addressing each of these issues and concerns as long as those strategies reflect nursing's commitment to caring.

Increased use of machines may lead to decreased human contact and interaction.[14,15] Lack of reliance on human skill and perception, overreliance on computer printouts and the products of machines, and more authority being invested in the machine are possible specific outcomes of computer technology.[17]

Weizenbaum[29] harshly judges: "All projects which substitute a computer for a human function that involves interpersonal respect are obscene and a fraud." Nursing indeed can maintain some control over the dehumanization process. Unfortunately, nurses can also accelerate the process. The question one must ask is, "Does in fact the computer remove the interpersonal aspect of nursing or do nurses diminish this aspect of their role as they become involved in managing the technology?"[10]

The relationship between one's level of computer literacy and one's ability to act on caring has been substantiated in the nursing literature. For example, in a qualitative study of technological caring, Ray[23] found that a comfortable level of technical competence preceded both nurses' skill at concentrating on the needs of the patient and the family, and their ability to perceive the impact of the technology on the patient. In short, the nurse's ability to function as an advocate, protecting the patient and preserving human dignity, is preceded by a belief in the power of technology to change or reverse the patient's condition. The nurse then develops compassion and a close sense of interconnectedness with the patient and is better able to balance the technology with caring. The main strategy that nurses can adopt to counter the potential dehumanizing effects of computers is to improve their own computer literacy. Increased knowledge and skill will enable nurses to use computer technology more efficiently and more appropriately and to incorporate technology into a caring-based practice.

Computer literacy, therefore, represents a proactive response to technology that ultimately supports caring in nursing. Sources are available to help nurses gain competency at a variety of levels ranging from informed user to developer.[25] It is also essential that some nurse professionals advance beyond computer literacy and attain competency in the field of nursing informatics. Nurses in this field of specialization explore the relationships among nursing data, information and knowledge, nursing reasoning, and information science. Understanding these relationships will enable nurses to more effectively develop and use nursing's knowledge base, thereby enhancing the quality of practice. Here too levels of competency range from the user to the innovator.

Client privacy, confidentiality of client information, and security of patient data are all threatened by computer technology. Privacy issues concern who should control overexposure of self and information about oneself, ensure freedom from intrusion and the ownership of information, and counter the misuse of information.

Confidentiality issues involve the relationship between one individual disclosing information and another receiving that information. Redisclosure of shared information is the major concern in discussions of confidentiality. A health professional's duty has traditionally included an obligation to safeguard the secrecy of information collected, stored, transmitted, and retrieved in the health care system. Security issues arise over the protection of client data and information from accidental or intentional disclosure to unauthorized people, from unauthorized modifications, or from destruction.

The impact of the computer on privacy, confidentiality, and privacy concerns in health care was investigated in a national, government funded study. Westin[30] reported that patient information from the medical record flowed regularly out of the primary care setting in ways that allowed the patient little control over the disclosures. In addition, the study found considerable disagreement between health care professionals and third-party payers regarding just how much personal data from medical records needed to

be disclosed for the payment-review process. Existing practices did not prevent leakage of personal information to persons the patient did not consent to allow access to such facts. This study also documented the multiple social uses of health data, ranging from employment and life insurance uses to law enforcement to social research. Westin noted that traditional laws and organizational policies have not kept pace with the new flows and uses of information.

One of the biggest events in health care delivery, which revolutionized the client-health care professional relationship, was the computerization of the health record. The ability of the computer to provide storage, analysis and retrieval of enormous amounts of accurate, comprehensive, selective, sensitive, and readily identifiable client information greatly contributed to the need for ethical and legal clarification regarding clients' rights to privacy and confidentiality.[8]

Nurses who are computer literate will be better able to safeguard clients' rights to privacy, confidentiality, and security. Nurse advocates can support adoption and enforcement of guidelines advanced by an international study group on privacy, confidentiality, and security of computer systems.[7] These guidelines include lawful collection of data with the knowledge and consent of the client; assuring that the data are relevant, accurate, complete, and up-to-date; disclosure of the purpose of data collection at the time of collection; limitation of subsequent use to the stated purpose; safeguarding the security of client data; informing the client what is being collected and stored and where it is stored; allowing clients to participate in review of the data; and placing accountability with the organizations and persons collecting the data. Confidentiality can be promoted through implementation of the American Nurses' Association (ANA) Code for Nurses. Nurses can also work to establish privacy, confidentiality, and security guidelines in policy development. Policy development should involve persons representing citizens' rights. A full-scale privacy audit conducted by each organization operating health information systems is also advocated.

Expert systems are computerized systems

in which the expertise of an expert or panel of experts, in a relatively narrow area of knowledge, has been modeled and stored in a manner that allows this expert knowledge to be accessed and used by others to assist in making decisions and solving problems.[26]

However, can expert systems be truly expert when their development depends on the ability of humans to express what they know, or, in other words, on reconstructed methods of reasoning? Because human experts are seldom able to make explicit what they know, expert systems do not often reflect the heuristics and processing constraints of the system user. Ackoff[2] acknowledges the problem of integrating the "breadth" of people's lives into the order of the expert system. Integrating breadth requires intuitive, holistic thinking: it is a problem not solved by taking knowledge apart but rather by viewing it as part of the larger arena. Although expert systems provide consistent performance, increase productivity, preserve expertise, promote a better understanding of problems, and promote staff development, they will not replace the decision maker.[26]

Computer technology can also negatively affect organizational structure. Incorporating computers into the organization promotes increased formalization of rules and procedures, greater centralization of decision making, and greater numbers of specialists. Incorporation of computers has been associated with an increased need for clarification of status differences, which, in turn, has promoted rigidity and decreased communication among computer levels and organizational units. These concerns are especially weighty when one remembers that low formalization, low centralization, and low stratification all contribute to employee acceptance of computer technology.[15] Nurses, therefore, need to counteract the effects of computer technology on organizational structure so that a caring environment for their coworkers and clients can be maintained.

Several factors will make this goal difficult to attain.[5] First, corporations tend to focus their energies on insuring corporate survival and corporate profits, not on the needs of individuals. Therefore computer technology, which is largely funded by organizations or corporations, often is used primarily to satisfy the profit motive of the corporation rather than the interests of individual patients. Nurses, who traditionally have not participated in corporate-level decision making, may find it difficult to change this. The potential exists for conflicts of interest between health care institutions as corporations concerned with profits and patients as individuals served by the corporation. The advocacy role of the nurse in protecting patients' rights assumes critical importance as nursing struggles with questions of patients' rights versus corporate rights. Second, unconditional positive acceptance of new technology can have several negative consequences. Nurses may have trouble identifying when the profession begins accommodating the machine, rather than the machine serving nursing and nursing's clients. Mastery of technology can induce a sense of power and control that allows individual nurses' commitments to caring to be subjugated to the technology. Patients who perceive that a machine is in control may become passive and cease to view themselves as valuable sources of input regarding their own health status.[5]

Questions have been raised related to the cost justifications of computer technology. This includes not only cost-benefit analysis, which measures in dollars the value of all resources used, but also cost-effectiveness, the qualitative, subjective effects of adopting computer technology. Affordability must include consideration of hardware and software outlays, staffing needs, supplies, environmental modifications, and maintenance. The initial outlay for computerization, whether for a hospital information system, nursing information system, or expert system, is great. At this point, unsubstantiated claims regarding the costs and benefits and cost-effectiveness of computer technology are prevalent. Attention to accurate forecasting, in which nursing should have consistent input, will play a major part in determining the survivability and success of computer applications.

CONCLUSION

The impact of computer technology on current and future nursing practice must be carefully evaluated. Professional nursing's dedication to caring provides a means for balancing the art and science of the profession. Nurses will need varying levels of computer literacy, with some attaining competency in nursing informatics. It is essential that this expertise, however, not occur in a vacuum. Ferkiss[11] warned that the nurse, on becoming literate and sensing the power, sense of control, and concomitant satisfaction that comes from working with machinery, may not move onward to the goals of nursing, to preserving the essence of nursing. As Baumer[21] noted, "It is not the technology here that is the problem; it is the uses to which it is put."

Consequently, teaching and learning must occur within the context of a philosophy of caring. The needs of clients and their families can be addressed by nurses who have attained understanding and proficiency in computer use. If this understanding and skill is based on a foundation in ethics with a commitment to the essence of nursing, nurses can meet the responsibilities of their advocacy role. Nurses' abilities to achieve a balance between the technology and the humanness of nursing practice will be measured by the degree to which human dignity is protected, preserved, and enhanced.

REFERENCES

1. Adams G: Computer technology: its impact on nursing practice, Nursing Administration Quarterly 10(2):21, 1986.
2. Ackoff R: Redesigning the future: a systems approach to societal problems, New York, 1974, John Wiley & Sons, Inc.
3. Banta D: Technology: review of medical technology policies show need, opportunities for change, Hospitals 56:87, 1982.
4. Benner P and Wrubel J: The primacy of caring, Menlo Park, Calif, 1989, Addison-Wesley Publishing Co, Inc.
5. Birckhead I: The need for nurse support systems in affecting computer systems, Journal of Nursing Administration 8(3):51, 1978.
6. Bolter J: Turing's man: Western culture in the computer age, Chapel Hill, 1984, The University of North Carolina Press.
7. Burton R: Transnational data flow, Data Management 18(6):68, 1980.
8. Cox HC, Harsanyi B, and Dean LC: Computers and nursing, Norwalk, Conn, 1987, Appleton & Lange.
9. Davenport D: Computerized monitoring systems, Nurs Clin North Am 22(2):495, 1987.
10. Fagerhaugh S and others: The impact of technology on patients, providers, and care patterns, Nurs Outlook 28(11):666, 1980.
11. Ferkiss V: Technological man: the myth and the reality, New York, 1969, Braziller.
12. Fry S: The ethic of caring: can it survive in nursing? Nurs Outlook 36(1):48, 1988.
13. Habermus J: Toward a rational society, Boston, 1970, Beacon Press.
14. Happ B: Should computers be used in the nursing care of patients? Nursing Management 14(7):31,34, 1983.
15. Kelly L: Dimensions of professional nursing, ed 5, New York, 1985, Macmillan Publishing Co.
16. Mackey C: Address to University of Michigan graduates, MSU Today, p 2, Winter 1987.
17. McMullen E: Diagnosis by computer, J Med Philos 8:5, 1983.
18. Moccia P: At the faultline: social activism and caring, Nurs Outlook 36(1):30, 1988.
19. Naisbett J: Megatrends, New York, 1982, Random House, Inc.
20. Nodding N: Caring: a feminine approach to ethics and moral education; Berkeley, 1984, University of California Press.
21. Opp M: The confidentiality dilemma, Modern Health Care 3:49, March 1975.
22. Protti D: The impact of informatics on nursing. In Ball MJ and others, editors: Nursing informatics: where caring and technology meet, New York, 1988, Springer-Verlag New York, Inc.
23. Ray MA: Technological caring: a new model in critical care, Dimensions of Critical Care Nursing 6(3): 166, 1987.
24. Reverby S: A caring dilemma: womanhood and nursing in historical perspective, Nurs Res 36(1):5, 1987.
25. Ronald J and Skiba D: Guidelines for basic computer education in nursing, New York, 1987, National League for Nursing.
26. Schank MJ, Doney LD, and Seizyk J: The potential of expert systems in nursing, Journal of Nursing Administration 18(6):26, 1988.
27. Turkle S: The second self: computers and the human spirit, New York, 1984, Simon & Schuster.
28. Watson J: Nursing: human science and human care, Norwalk, Conn, 1985, Appleton-Century-Crofts.
29. Weizenbaum J: Computer power and human reason: from judgment to calculation, San Francisco, 1976, WH Freeman, 1976.
30. Westin A: Computers, health records, and citizens' rights, Washington, DC, 1976, US Government Printing Office.

CHAPTER 86

Indigent care

CATHERINE MALLOY

The 1987 American Public Health Association annual meeting theme was "Health Care: For People or Profit?" How does American society balance humanitarian values with cost containment in creating a just health care policy? How are questions of equitable access and quality considered in a fiscally conservative environment? Can a just society permit the creation of a two-tiered system of health care: one for the "haves" and one for the "have-nots"?

Ethical questions of care for the medically indigent are embedded in the social-political system and the organization of health care delivery in the United States. Although it is generally agreed that the U.S. health care system was founded on the premise that quality care should be available to all without discrimination or rationing, actual practice is often at odds with this belief. Because a society is judged by how it cares for its most vulnerable members, the principle of social justice is particularly relevant in considering the problem of indigent care.

Providing health care for indigent patients has been a persistent problem throughout the history of U.S. health care. However, "the obligation to aid the sick and afflicted is ubiquitous in the code of ethics. The medical profession is appropriately pledged to promote high quality health care for all people. Likewise, the mission statement of most hospitals contain similar commitments."[20] Access to health care as a basic right of the citizen is an assumption supported by professional nurses. In fact, access to health care is viewed as a social contract, as illustrated in the American Nurses' Association Social Policy Statement.[2] Why is it, then, that there are more and more reports of people being turned away from hospitals due to inability to pay, the new "dumping syndrome"? Why is it that some physicians refuse to treat Medicaid and even Medicare patients?[7] How can a society built on humanitarian values shun those in need? Indigent care, with its inherent questions of access and financing, has become a serious social problem and ethical dilemma. Aydelotte[3] noted that an ethical dilemma emerges when a society perceives its resources to be limited. In the case of indigent care, the dilemma emerges from the competing pressures of the need to provide care and the need to control costs. Nurses need to understand the social, political, economic, and practice issues involved in the problem in order to become part of the solution.

FROM THE GREAT SOCIETY TO CORPORATISM

During the Great Society of the 1960s, health care policy focused on providing accessible, quality health care for all. The passage of Medicare and Medicaid legislation in 1966, and programs for mothers, infants, and children, as well as for other categorical populations, reflected the social value for ensuring adequate health care to all.[11]

Ironically, the passage of Medicare and Medicaid opened up a Pandora's box. For those clever enough to see that public financing could be profitable, a revolutionary era was born: the corporate transformation of American health care delivery. Thus, Medicare and Medicaid, which were enacted to increase access to health care, paradoxically have led to the penetration of health care markets by corporate conglomerates.[16]

The implications of corporatism are particularly ominous for indigent health care. Corporations will not locate their hospitals in areas with large Medicare and Medicaid populations. Also, decreasing reimbursement for Medicare and Medicaid recipients have serious consequences for those hospitals serving large numbers of poor and uninsured.

Moreover, the shift from retrospective to prospective payment combined with federal budget cutbacks has further eroded indigent accessibility to health care. Yet the United States has seen increased federal expenditures in health care from \$4 billion in 1975 to an estimated \$65.7 billion in 1980.[5] Continuing increases in the national debt and ominous predictions of a depleted Medicare fund by 1990 make cost containment a matter of the highest concern. Cost containment has led to serious cutbacks in federal and state programs for the indigent. Further, policies of the Reagan administration promoted antiregulatory approaches to a free market in health care and lessened responsibility of the government for people's health.[15] A national health care policy of competition as key to cost containment has emerged.[13]

FALLING BETWEEN THE CRACKS: A WIDENING CHASM

Medically indigent people are those who have no public or private insurance and who cannot afford to pay for health care out of pocket. "The number of uncompensated care patients—the medically indigent—has almost doubled from an estimated 25 million to 40 million in the past 10 years."[21] According to the American Hospital Association Report on Care for the Indigent,[1] the best indicator of medical indigence is whether or not a person is insured. Medically indigent patients are composed of three groups: the nonworking uninsured, the medically uninsurable, and the employed uninsured.[22] In 1983 approximately 15% of Americans, 35 million people, lacked health insurance coverage.[6] Whitman and colleagues[23] reported that the "common thread that binds the working poor together most tightly is the absence of health insurance. . . . two out of three poor workers, representing more than 9 million Americans and their dependents, have no employer or union subsidized health insurance." Almost 65% of the uninsured are working adults or their dependents, including 4.1 million uninsured dependents of insured working adults.[1] According to Moccia and Mason,[12] 15.2% of the population is struggling financially. A dramatic increase in the numbers of poor families headed by women has given rise to the concept of the "feminization of poverty." Almost 40% of all poor are children; in fact, poverty affects blacks, Hispanics, other minorities, and women disproportionately.[12] Tragically, reports abound of elderly individuals who have their life savings depleted because of an illness requiring long-term care. The spouse and patient often end up indigent, having to choose between food, heat, and medicines.[19]

Many Americans hold distorted perceptions of the medically indigent. Inner-city welfare poor represent only a small fraction of America's poor. The working poor tend to be low wage, semieducated people who work in agriculture and the private sector. The public can identify with the working poor, and their numbers have swollen tremendously. Surprisingly, the number of poor adults who work has increased by 52% in the last decade, to include 7 million Americans.[23]

Other uninsured are newly unemployed workers and their families who have lost insurance benefits. Health insurance loss due to job layoff has become a more serious problem than anticipated. Those already ill or disabled for whom finding insurance at an affordable rate is impossible are also included in the indigent group.[5]

A QUESTION OF PRIORITIES

The major barriers to accessing health care are lack of insurance, inadequate insurance, or a longstanding or catastrophic illness, all having financial implications. Corporate restructuring of health care has further excluded the underinsured from care. McCarthy[10] reported that the competitive market produced many desirable results but cautioned that competition and cost-containment measures were placing "increasing numbers of uninsured in serious jeopardy." It seems clear that the trend toward corporatism is unlikely to benefit the medically indigent. For-profit organizations find little incentive to assume responsibility for care of the uninsured. In assessing the competitive environment, Kuder[8] reported that because Medicaid rates were below the usual physician fees, there was a "disincentive for physicians to treat the poor with the same standard of care as for patients who pay higher fees."

All traditional ways of financing care for indigents have been eroded as competition among providers has increased. In the past, care may have been subsidized by taxes, by governmental health insurance or welfare programs (Medicare and Medicaid), by cost shifting from insured patients, or by charitable donations. The prospective payment system eliminated cost shifting, the Reagan administration reduced programs, Medicare and Medicaid recipients cannot always access care because of inadequate coverage or the refusal of some providers to treat patients on the Medicare or Medicaid programs. It is easy to see that current policy does not address continuity or comprehensiveness of care.

HEALTH AND POVERTY

The relationship between poverty and health status has been well documented. Due to lack of insurance or lack of funds for medical care, people do not seek care until it is "too late, leading to complications that require more and longer care."[6] The poor or near poor have a higher prevalence of infant mortality, chronic diseases, and disability.[11] Throughout life, poverty exposes the poor to more health risks. Poor people get sick more often, have more serious complications, take longer to recover, and are less likely to regain their full level of functioning.[12]

Often the magnitude of social disability is as much a result of social definitions, inadequate coping skills in dealing with the illness and the treatment regimen, and deficient problem-solving capacities as it is a result of the illness as such.[11]

Indigent patients often feel powerless in the system. Preoccupation with securing the basic necessities of life (food, shelter) precludes a future-oriented approach to their health. Consequently, they tend to seek help only when in pain or acutely ill.

THE ETHICAL DILEMMA: WHO PAYS?

The Medicaid program is often misunderstood. Although people generally believe that Medicaid is the major source of financing of medical care for the poor, in reality it covers less than 40% of the poverty population. In fact, Medicaid has become more of a supplemental insurance for individuals receiving Medicare. Only one quarter of Medicaid's expenditures paid for medical care to the poor in 1984.[1] In 1982 more than one third of the uninsured, 11.6 million people, were below the poverty line but still did not qualify for Medicaid. Two thirds of the uninsured population had incomes below 200% of the poverty levels.[11]

Responsibility: public or private

Barriers to public action are many. A Gallup poll reported that 62% of adults felt it was the government's responsibility to pay for the health care of the poor. When asked to specify the level of government that was responsible, 37% indicated it was the federal government's responsibility, 15% judged it to be a state governmental responsibility, and 6% indicated it was a local government responsibility. Of those responding, 69% reported they would be willing to pay higher taxes for indigent care.[17] However, many people with adequate health care insurance fear that more taxes will result if indigent care is addressed. Some analysts believe the public cannot afford additional taxes or increased insurance premiums and will not support measures likely to have those consequences. Basically the debate comes down to two questions. Who receives care? Who pays?

The dilemma

In a culture of contradictions and competing values, an ethical dilemma emerges. The American ideal of self-reliance and rugged individualism is in opposition to the realities of the indigence problem. Perhaps the dilemma is best expressed in the context of social responsibility versus individual responsibility or, stated another way, access and quality versus rationing.

Veatch[18] holds that defining health care as a product in typical economic terms is unacceptable if a society affirms health care to be a right. A society professing humanitarian values should not treat health care as a market commodity to be regarded as any other product in a competitive arena. This would not be consistent with the ethical codes of nursing and medicine that have always included the patient's right to care.

Should a society offer its citizens equal opportunity in the pursuit of personal-social goals, and equitable access in an increasingly complex society? Should a just society tolerate escalating levels of poverty and hunger and increasing numbers of persons without adequate care? People hold to the belief that a middle-class lifestyle is available for anyone who works hard enough to get it. The indigence problem suggests that conviction simply is not true.

ACCESSIBLE AND EQUITABLE CARE: NURSING STRATEGIES

Current approaches in health care are failing to provide access and quality care for all. Perhaps the strategies implemented to restructure the health care system rely too heavily on high technology and on the illness model with the physician as provider. A radical departure from the medical model may provide alternative solutions to some of the indigent care problems. Nurses are strategically positioned to create such a change. From the early days of nursing to the present, nurses have been the architects of creative practice arrangements to meet the health care needs of the poor and the vulnerable, while promoting their well-being. What is needed is a modern-day Lillian Wald, a mover and shaker of society's purse strings and conscience.

Nurses as a collective force can create a Waldian composite to expand their contribution to the pressing problem of indigent care. Two major approaches for nursing intervention are suggested: (1) developing a role in policy formulation, and (2) designing innovative indigent care projects.

Policy formulation

Attention needs to be centered on shaping public policy and increasing public knowledge about the indigent care issue. Nursing's contribution to health policy can be made through research and practice. Nurses should document issues related to access, services provided, advantages of health promotion services as cost containment. Research should be conducted regarding the health needs, practices, coping mechanisms, and environment of the poor.[12] Nurses can serve as advocates for the medically indigent by presenting this research to legislators and the public.

The socialization of nurses should emphasize the nurse's role in policy formulation. Nursing skills must include assertive decision making, political skills, and advocacy. Nurses should be actively involved in policy formulation at every level: local, regional, state, national.

Designing innovative projects

It is time for nurses to take a bold step in creating nurse models for indigent care. Nurses can develop comprehensive care projects as demonstrations of compassionate and dignified care. Such projects can integrate preventive and therapeutic services and coordinate resource management. Nurse-managed clinics can serve as models of case management demonstrating the effectiveness, cost-efficiency, and continuity of service.[9] These projects, which are targeted to the homeless, the elderly, and other underserved groups, need to be showcased to illustrate to the public what nurses can do as part of the solution.

Weis[4] reported on the common risk factors of the indigent. The most frequently recorded risk factors are smoking, alcohol, obesity, lack of prenatal care, and street drug use. Clearly these risk factors call for lifestyle modification. The nurse has a role in assisting indigent patients to decrease risk factors through health promotion activities. Improving self-care practices, developing more effective ways of coping, maintaining functioning, and preventing disability will positively affect the ultimate cost of health care for indigents. Currently, the federal government spends only 3% of the budget on health promotion. Perhaps a policy shift from illness care to prevention would be more cost effective in the long term.

The crisis in indigent health care presents an opportunity for nurses to take adversity and turn it into advantage. At a time when the health care system is strained, when predictions of economic disaster loom everywhere, nurses can improve access, promote quality, and demonstrate cost savings. An excellent opportunity awaits nurses in the competitive arena. By establishing partnerships with indigents, nurses can take an active part in changing community use of resources. Efforts toward self-care will empower indigents to reframe their own definitions of health care.

A sterling example of what nurses can do to address the indigent care dilemma is the community nursing model in Lubbock County, Texas. The project was specifically designed by Ridenour[14] to meet the health care needs of the uninsured. By developing a health care delivery approach as the basis for a cost-effective prepaid system, services can be marketed directly to the uninsured, to employers, and to the responsible units of federal and state government. The goal of the project is to demonstrate cost-effective, quality health and medical care for the uninsured. The project is using a case management approach to provide care for targeted uninsured groups.[14]

In regard to the question posed above about access versus competition, the nursing profession has the opportunity to show how nurses can make a difference. To do less would not be in keeping with the profession's heritage.

REFERENCES

1. American Hospital Association: Cost and compassion: recommendations for avoiding a crisis in care for the medically indigent. Report of the Special Committee on Care for the Indigent, Chicago, 1986, The Association.
2. American Nurses' Association: Nursing: a social policy statement, Kansas City, Mo, 1980, The Association.
3. Aydelotte MK: Catastrophic, long term, and indigent care. In McCloskey JC and Grace HK, editors: Current issues in nursing, ed 2, Boston, 1985, Blackwell Scientific Publications.
4. Weis D: Health care for low income, Journal of Nursing Administration 17(12):18, 1987.
5. Davis K and Rowland D: Medicare financing reform: a new medicare premium, Milbank Quarterly 62(2):300, 1984.
6. Jones K and Kilpatrick K: State strategies for financing indigent care, Nursing Economics 4(2):61, 1986.
7. Kirkman-Liff BL: Refusal of care: evidence from Arizona, Health Aff 4(4):15, 1985.
8. Kuder JM: No miracle remedies in sight for financing health care for the poor, Henry Ford Hosp Med J 34(4):252, 1986.

9. Malloy C: Nurse-managed clinic for the homeless. Paper presented at the fifth annual nursing practice symposium, meeting of the American Academy of Nursing, Atlanta, Georgia, January 29, 1988.

10. McCarthy CM: Financing indigent care: short- and long-term strategies, JAMA 259(1):75, 1988.

11. Mechanic D: Health care for the poor: some policy alternatives, J Fam Pract 22(3):283, 1986.

12. Moccia P and Mason DJ: Poverty trends: implications for nursing, Nurs Outlook 34(1):20, 1986.

13. Nutter DO: Access to care and the evolution of corporate, for profit medicine, N Engl J Med 311(14):917, 1984.

14. Ridenour N: A community approach to providing quality health care for the uninsured. Paper presented at the fifth annual nursing practice symposium meeting of the American Academy of Nursing, Atlanta, Georgia, January 29, 1988.

15. Roemer R: The right to health care—gains and gaps, American Journal of Public Health 78(3):241, 1988.

16. Starr P: The transformation of American medicine, New York, 1982, Basic Books, Inc.

17. Steiber S: Indigent care: public wants government to pay, Hospitals, p 152, Oct 5, 1987.

18. Veatch RM: Ethical dilemmas of for-profit enterprise in health care. In Gray BH, editor: The new health care for profit, Washington, DC, 1983, National Academy Press.

19. Vehara ES, Geron S, and Beeman SK: Gerontologist 26(1):48, 1986.

20. Weems WL: Medical care for the indigent, J Miss State Med Assoc 28(8):218, 1987.

21. Weis D: Speaking out: who are the working poor? Am J Nurs 87(11):1451, 1987.

22. Wilensky GR: Viable strategies for dealing with the uninsured, Health Aff 6(1):33, 1987.

23. Whitman D and others: America's hidden poor, US News and World Report, p 18, Jan 11, 1988.

CHAPTER 87

AIDS in the 1990s

An ethical challenge

DAVID ANTHONY FORRESTER

The need for nursing is universal. Inherent in nursing is respect for life, dignity, and the rights of humans. It is unrestricted by considerations of nationality, race, creed, color, age, sex, politics, or social status.[3]

Since the first cases of acquired immunodeficiency syndrome (AIDS) were reported among members of the gay community in the United States in 1981, the human immunodeficiency virus (HIV) that causes AIDS and AIDS-related complex (ARC) has precipitated a global pandemic unprecedented in modern history. In the United States it is currently estimated that about 175,000 Americans will be persons with AIDS or ARC (PWAs) by 1991, and about 1.5 million people in the United States are already infected with HIV.[19] Over 130 countries throughout the world have reported cases of AIDS[7] and it is anticipated that in the next five years there will be as many as 1 million new cases of AIDS worldwide.[19] Thus AIDS is a vastly complex, global phenomenon with extraordinary social, cultural, economic and political dimensions and impact.

The worldwide fear and hysteria AIDS has engendered is unprecedented in contemporary society. The profound scope of the AIDS pandemic forces all segments of society to reexamine their values and address many troublesome ethical issues. Nurses are no exception. Many of these issues are born out of the unique epidemiological features of AIDS and the pervasive social stigma associated with those afflicted with it. From a nursing perspective, this stigma is as much a part of the pathology of AIDS as the virus itself.

Exploring some of the factors contributing to the stigmatization of PWAs may be helpful in formulating an understanding of the challenges nurses must address during this pandemic. After a brief etiological exploration of the stigmatization of PWAs, this chapter focuses on some of the ethical challenges AIDS poses for nurses in the 1990s.

STIGMATIZATION OF PWAs

It may be considered an accident of history that AIDS was discovered in the gay community of the United States. In 1980 or 1981, it could just as easily have been discovered in a number of countries. Had it been discovered in Africa, for example, it might have been known as a heterosexual syndrome, which, because sexually transmitted, also affects gay men. Thus the unfortunate, worldwide and false impression that AIDS is a "gay disease" might not have come about.[19] Unfortunately, the history of this syndrome cannot be rewritten and the social and cultural meanings of AIDS continue to contribute to widespread stigmatization of PWAs, frequently resulting in unfair AIDS discrimination.

Undoubtedly, one of the most serious threats PWAs face is the powerful social stigma associated with AIDS. AIDS has so far had its greatest impact on already stigmatized socially "deviant" groups including gay and bisexual men, intravenous (IV) drug users and prostitutes.[6] The indigent and black and Hispanic racial minorities are also disproportionately affected.[13] PWAs and HIV-positive individuals have lost jobs and insurance benefits and have even occasionally been denied educational opportunities and medical care.[20]

During the social crisis of a pandemic, further stigmatization of already disenfranchised groups serves to project that which is feared (e.g., contagion, immorality, mortality) outside the normative social group. This, of course, occurs at great expense to the non-normative groups and results for them in the double bind of being stigmatized individuals with a stigmatized life-threatening illness.

As a result of the stigma associated with AIDS, PWAs frequently encounter unfair discrimination. Like other forms of discriminations, AIDS discrimination is "the unfair treatment of individuals based upon irrational fears and prejudices about groups."[22] The resulting "us" versus "them" mentality is potentially very costly to society as a whole. Because they fear unfair discrimination, stigmatized groups, whether HIV infected or not, may naturally be less willing to come forward and participate voluntarily in efforts to control the spread of AIDS.

AIDS engenders much fear and apprehension. For many people, including some health care providers, "AIDS carries with it all the connotations of sin"[18] and images of an illicit disease associated with illicit behavior. Two important aspects of "AIDS fear" are the fear of disease and the fear of social disorder.[22]

Far more complex than the obvious and possibly realistic fear of contagion, fear of AIDS as a "disease" is compounded by a number of factors. First, human sexuality, and more specifically, homosexuality and bisexuality, are issues about which many members of society are uncomfortable and uninformed. A second factor is widespread ambivalence toward mental illness. As treatment modalities improve and life expectancy lengthens for PWAs, it is likely that there will be greatly increased numbers of HIV-demented people. These individuals will make increased physical and fiscal demands on mental health care systems and on other social resources. Finally, a third factor contributing to the fear of AIDS is its incurable and invariably fatal prognosis. The fear of death is primal and pervasive, even among health care providers. In fact, health practitioners' personal fears regarding mortality may be particularly exacerbated by a fatal illness affecting large numbers of young, previously healthy people—in other words, people very much like themselves.

The fear of social disorder relative to the AIDS pandemic stems from the attrition of PWAs from the work force, thus removing their economic contributions from society. This is further compounded by their acutely increased needs for public support for medical care, food and housing.

Historically, making such stigmatized groups the focus of social panic has resulted in scapegoating and isolation. For example, in an effort to control the spread of sexually transmitted diseases (STDs) during World War I, 30,000 prostitutes were isolated. Despite the restriction of these individuals' civil liberties, the incidence of STDs increased dramatically during this period.[4] Similarly, as a result of fear during World War II, the U.S. Supreme Court upheld the incarceration of Japanese-Americans.[22]

More recently, in 1986 California voters defeated a Lyndon LaRouche-supported referendum that would have declared AIDS an infectious, contagious and easily communicable disease. This legislation would have mandated the quarantine of HIV-infected persons in camps and would have resulted in all infected food handlers and teachers losing their jobs. In 1988 California voters were asked to vote on the Dannemeyer AIDS initiative, which would have among other things eliminated all anonymous screening for HIV in California and would have allowed employers and insurers to require applicants be tested for HIV as a condition of employment and insurance coverage. Such extreme measures would clearly be counterproductive, because few who believed they had been exposed to HIV through risk-taking behavior would voluntarily come forward. In effect, such measures would simply serve to drive AIDS "underground" and would surely thwart public health efforts such as screening, counseling and education to prevent the further spread of this deadly syndrome.

ETHICAL CHALLENGES TO NURSES

As members of society, health care professionals also participate in the stigmatization of PWAs. A number of research studies have documented negative attitudes of physicians and nurses toward gay men, IV drug users and PWAs in general.[14,15,24] Such attitudes may be based on practitioners' opinions about patients' personal attributes, lifestyles or personal worth. Whatever their origins, such attitudes engender social prejudice from which discrimination emerges.

The complex phenomenon of AIDS stigma in itself poses major personal and professional challenges to nurses who wish to provide PWAs with optimal, sensitive health care. Understanding the social etiology of AIDS stigma should assist nurses in (1) rejecting and counteracting social stereotypes, (2) assessing personal values and risks more accurately, and (3) identifying their professional responsibilities in providing health care that demonstrates value for the personal autonomy of PWAs.

Personal safety

The nursing profession has a long and distinguished history replete with examples of nurses who have knowingly risked their personal safety in order to benefit others. Providing care for PWAs holds at least some degree of risk to nurses' personal safety. For example, current estimates place the risk of becoming HIV infected as a result of an accidental needlestick injury at approximately 0.13 to 0.39%.[12] Thus nurses are at far greater risk of contracting other serious infectious diseases (such as hepatitis B) in the health care setting than of contracting AIDS.[16] Although the risk of becoming HIV infected while providing patient care is minimal, it still must be factored into nurses' calculation of personal risk incurred by providing care for PWAs.

In 1986 the Committee on Ethics of the American Nurses' Association (ANA)[2] published a position paper entitled "Statement Regarding Risk Versus Responsibility in Providing Nursing Care." This document offers nurses four fundamental criteria to consider when differentiating between a *moral duty* and a *moral option* to provide care for patients with communicable or infectious diseases.

1. The patient is at risk of harm, loss, or damage if the nurse does not assist.
2. The nurse's intervention or care is directly relevant to preventing harm.
3. The nurse's care will probably prevent harm, loss, or damage to the patient.
4. The benefit the patient will gain outweighs any harm the nurse might incur and does not present more than minimal risk to the health care provider.[2]

If *all* of the above criteria are satisfied, nurses are morally obligated to provide care. Therefore nurses would be morally obligated to provide care to PWAs in most instances. If, however, one of these criteria is not met, nurses have a moral option to provide care. Nurses must arrive at ethically defensible decisions by weighing their personal risk against their moral responsibility to provide care. For example, nurses who

are pregnant or receiving immunosuppressant therapy may choose to exercise their moral option by not providing care for PWAs.[2,5]

Another instance in which nurses may ethically exercise choice is if the employing agency is in compliance with currently accepted guidelines to prevent transmission of HIV in the health care environment. Clearly, it is an ethical obligation for employers to comply with such guidelines as the Centers for Disease Control's "universal blood and body fluid precautions."[8] This requires employers to provide resources necessary for proper infection control including appropriate equipment, education, enforcement and evaluation on an ongoing basis.[21] However, it should be pointed out that even in situations of significant employer failure to comply responsibly with such guidelines, there are no "cookbook" solutions. Ultimately, nurses are responsible for their own ethical decisions, even when others act irresponsibly.

Personal and professional values

Holistic health care for PWAs requires that nurses gain insight into their own opinions, attitudes and values. For example, nurses typically place a high value on health and health-seeking behaviors in patients. PWAs who continue to use IV drugs or to engage in high-risk sexual activity are often perceived as nonhealth seeking and therefore pose a substantial challenge to nurses attempting to provide nonjudgmental care. Such conflicting values are almost sure to result in an ineffective nurse-patient relationship. To counter this, nurses must engage in a process of clarification. This process fosters personal and professional growth and takes place through frank discussions of value conflict and activities such as participation in ethics committees and organized educational programs regarding PWAs.[10]

Excellent health care for PWAs is characterized by open interpersonal communication and social support. Effective care for PWAs, as with *all* patients, requires an accepting, nonjudgmental approach by competent health professionals. Such practitioners are unencumbered by unrealistic fears of contagion or unfair personal prejudice.

Again, the ANA offers guidance regarding personal risk, social prejudice and moral responsibility.

Nursing is resolute in its perspective that care should be delivered without prejudice, and it makes no allowance for the use of the patient's personal attributes or socioeconomic status or the nature of the health problem as grounds for discrimination.

Nursing's code of professional ethics insists,

The need for health care is universal, transcending all national, ethnic, racial, religious, cultural, political, educational, economic, developmental, personality, role, and sexual differences. Nursing care is delivered without prejudicial behavior.[1]

At least two conclusions can be drawn from these statements with regard to PWAs. First, although it is true that nurses may exercise a moral option (that is, refuse to provide care) in certain instances where there exists an irreducible risk to personal safety that is perceived as insurmountable, there is no circumstance in which nurses can ethically refuse to provide care based on personal prejudice.[11] Second, personal attributes of patients and the social aspects of their illness are to be used only for their benefit in individualizing their care, not to their detriment.[11]

Patient autonomy

Decision making regarding what constitutes appropriate medical treatment is the right of the patient.[16] However, the ethical challenge of respecting the autonomy of PWAs' in decision making is complicated by many factors. For example, AIDS raises special considerations regarding autonomy due to the high incidence of either primary HIV infection of the brain or secondary opportunistic infections resulting in dementia or other mental impairment. PWAs are often unable to participate in decision making when decisions need to be made.

Nurses have an ethical obligation to assist PWAs in making health care decisions early in course of the illness. Advance directives such as a "durable power of attorney for health care" (DPAHC) should be discussed with patients in a frank and thoughtful way. These documents allow patients to indicate treatment preferences and to designate a surrogate decision maker prior to becoming incapacitated. Proxy decision makers are particularly helpful in planning care for many gay men who wish to have their life partners rather than legally sanctioned family members make decisions on their behalf. As knowledgeable practitioners, nurses have a responsibility to anticipate the need for advance directives and to initiate discussion of such documents with PWAs.

Other ethical challenges confront health practitioners when the expectations and treatment preferences of PWAs or their proxy decision makers are inconsistent with those of the health team. For example, in one study of PWAs a sample of gay men, although generally well educated about AIDS, significantly overestimated their chances of surviving intensive care treatment for *Pneumocystis carinii* pneumonia (PCP). Of this group of 118 men, 55% wanted mechanical ventilation and 46% wanted cardiopulmonary resuscitation.[23] Such unrealistic expectations seriously impair patients' abilities to accurately evaluate risk-benefit ratios in care planning and, thus, their abilities to give truly informed consent.[16]

Medical and nursing paternalism is very tempting in such instances. However, paternalism by definition, even though altruistically motivated, negates the ethical principle of patient autonomy. Nurses are ethically obliged to be knowledgeable regarding currently available therapies as well as their potential risks and benefits for PWAs. Furthermore, nurses have a moral responsibility to share this information in a way that is sensitive, supportive and truthful.

AIDS treatment

As has been previously established, nursing recognizes an ethical obligation to provide care for PWAs. To meet this obligation nurse faculty and practicing nurses have an ethical responsibility to be sufficiently knowledgeable of the disease in order to (1) overcome their fears and personal prejudices, (2) prevent transmission of HIV through occupational exposure, and (3) provide competent, safe, quality care. The nursing profession, therefore, has a responsibility to assist nurses in meeting these objectives.

This decade should see a marked increase in efforts to further educate nurses and the public about AIDS. These efforts may best be carried out through nursing's various academic curricula and professional associations. Just as there is no segment of society unaffected by AIDS, there is no area of specialization in nursing not directly affected by AIDS. Nurses have a responsibility to seek out educational opportunities regarding AIDS. It is incumbent on all of nursing's academic programs and speciality associations to develop, implement and evaluate AIDS educational programing for nursing students, practicing nurses and consumers of nursing services.

AIDS research

Nurse researchers have an obligation to consider the importance of AIDS to national and international health. Furthermore, nurses should identify areas in which they might contribute individual or collaborative research efforts. Interdisciplinary studies should be undertaken that will result in valuable nursing contributions to the growing body of knowledge about AIDS.[17]

As nurses become increasingly involved in scientific study regarding AIDS and PWAs, many ethical dilemmas emerge. Research involving highly stigmatized groups at risk of unfair discrimination brings into view ethical issues involving PWAs' rights to privacy, anonymity and confidentiality. For example, how heavily does the individual's right to privacy weigh in the balance against the potential social good of health research? And, given the communal nature of in-patient care facilities and the age of computerized (and therefore easily accessible) patient records, how can research participants be *guaranteed* anonymity or confidentiality? Also, because it is generally agreed that intrusions into privacy in clinical care and research require informed consent from participants, how can the ethical participation of HIV-demented individuals be obtained? Finally, do the findings of scientific inquiry hold potential threats of harm either to PWAs directly or to future public policy regarding AIDS?

The personal and social risks to PWAs agreeing to participate in AIDS research are obviously quite high. Study participants must be fully informed about how research data are to be collected, used and stored, and who will have access to these data.[9] Researchers and clinicians must (1) faithfully adhere to published guidelines for research involving PWAs, (2) minimize intrusions into PWAs' privacy, (3) assure anonymity whenever possible, (4) take necessary precautions to ensure confidentiality, and (5) carefully consider the potential influence of study findings on the lives of PWAs and the course of public policy.[9]

CONCLUSION

As nurses we must be active participants in an organized response to the profound ethical challenges that AIDS poses in the 1990s. An appropriate nursing response to the AIDS pandemic in this decade should have three main objectives: (1) to prevent HIV infection, (2) to provide care for those already HIV infected, and (3) to participate in national and international efforts to fight AIDS and its associated stigma.

First, in order to prevent HIV infection, we must base our actions on a sound epidemiological under-standing of AIDS. From this knowledge is derived the concept that the proper focus of prevention is *behavior,* not "risk"-group membership or HIV antibody status. Information and education are essential but not sufficient. Only if we as nurses make ourselves available in a supportive social environment will prevention truly have a fair chance of success.

The second objective is to ensure that all PWAs receive humane care of a quality at least equal to that provided to people suffering from other illnesses, and to provide comprehensive support and services to all who are HIV infected. Implicit in this goal are the responsibilities that all nurses share to (1) avail ourselves of accurate, up-to-date information pertaining to the occupational risks, epidemiology and treatment of AIDS, (2) act in accordance with this knowledge both in our personal and professional lives, and (3) model appropriate behaviors to educate professional colleagues and the public about AIDS.

The third objective is nurse participation in national and international efforts to fight AIDS and its associated stigma. As litigation in the courts and debate in legislative bodies proliferates regarding the civil liberties of PWAs, nurses must be active participants providing their peers and the public with appropriate education and leadership. "Nurses, as health professionals, have an obligation to engage in the ensuing national [and international] debate about AIDS health policy issues in an informed manner.[16] We must be a knowledgeable and vocal force in future decision making regarding such issues as international travel, AIDS in prisons, the neuropsychiatric aspects of HIV infection and AIDS in the workplace.

The AIDS pandemic clearly poses some of the most compelling ethical challenges for nurses imaginable. Some of these challenges are unique to AIDS; some are common to other serious illnesses as well. The ethical issues raised by AIDS are amplified by the urgency associated with the pandemic and the complex psychological, political, legal and social problems it engenders. For this generation and future generations of nurses, the ultimate challenge of AIDS will be to provide sensitive, compassionate care while balancing individual rights and liberties against the duty to protect the health of the general public.

REFERENCES

1. American Nurses' Association: Code for nurses with interpretive statements, Kansas City, Mo, 1985, The Association.
2. American Nurses' Association Committee on Ethics: Statement

regarding risk versus responsibility in providing nursing care, Kansas City, Mo, 1986, The Association.

3. Bandman E and Bandman B: Nursing ethics in the life span, Norwalk, Conn, 1985, Appleton-Century-Crofts.

4. Brandt AM: AIDS: from social history to social policy, Law, Medicine, and Health Care 14:231, 1986.

5. Bremner MN and Brown LB: Learning to care for clients with AIDS—the practicum controversy, Nursing and Health Care, p 251, May 1988.

6. Centers for Disease Control: Quarterly report to the domestic policy council on the prevalence and rate of spread of HIV and AIDS in the United States, MMWR 37(14):223, 1988.

7. Centers for Disease Control: Update: acquired immunodeficiency syndrome (AIDS)—worldwide, MMWR 37(18):286, 1988.

8. Centers for Disease Control: Update: universal precautions for prevention of transmission of human immunodeficiency virus, hepatitis B virus, and other bloodborne pathogens in healthcare settings, MMWR 37(24):377, 1988.

9. Durham JD: The ethical dimensions of AIDS. In Durham JD and Cohen FL, editors: The person with AIDS: nursing perspectives, New York, 1987, Springer Publishing Co.

10. Farrell B: AIDS patients: values in conflict, Critical Care Nursing Quarterly 10(2):74, 1987.

11. Fowler MDM: Acquired immunodeficiency syndrome and refusal to provide care, Heart Lung 17(2):213, 1988.

12. Friedland GH and Klein RS: Transmission of the human immunodeficiency virus, N Engl J Med 317(18):1125, 1987.

13. Jakush J: AIDS: the disease and its implications for dentistry, J Am Dent Assoc 115:395, 1987.

14. Kelly JA and others: Nurses' attitudes toward AIDS, Journal of Continuing Education in Nursing 19(2):78, 1988.

15. Kelly JA and others: Stigmatization of AIDS patients by physicians, Am J Public Health 77(7):789, 1987.

16. Koenig BA: Ethical and legal issues in the AIDS epidemic. In Lewis A, editor: Nursing care of the person with AIDS/ARC, Rockville, Md, 1988, Aspen Publishers, Inc.

17. Larson E: Nursing research and AIDS, Nurs Res 37(1):60, 1988.

18. Loewy EH and Smith SJ: Duty to treat AIDS patients clouded by fears, Medical Ethics Advisor 2(3):29, 1986.

19. Mann J: Global aspect of AIDS. Paper presented at AIDS/ARC Update, University of California at San Francisco, July 15, 1988.

20. New York City Commission on Human Rights: Report on discrimination against people with AIDS, New York, Nov 1983 to April 1986.

21. Schobel DA: Management's responsibility to deal effectively with the risk of HIV exposure for health care workers, Nursing Management 19(3):38, 1988.

22. Schulman DI: AIDS discrimination: its nature, meaning and function. AIDS and the Law Symposium, Nova Law Review 12:1113, 1988.

23. Steinbrook R and others: Preferences of homosexual men with AIDS for life-sustaining treatment, N Engl J Med 314:457, 1986.

24. Wachter RM and others: Attitudes of medical residents regarding intensive care for patients with the acquired immunodeficiency syndrome, Arch Intern Med 148:149, 1988.

CHAPTER 88

In vitro fertilization, artificial insemination, and reproductive controls

ELLEN FRANCES OLSHANSKY

In vitro fertilization (IVF) and artificial insemination are but two among many new technologies used to achieve reproductive control. Other techniques are gamete intra-fallopian transfer (GIFT), oocyte donation, and frozen embryo transfer, with newer technologies being developed. Surrogate mothering, too, is a technique used for reproductive control. These treatments offer hope for many infertile persons, while at the same time they pose many ethical dilemmas and conflicts not only for infertile persons but also for the larger society. For those who keenly feel the aching pain associated with infertility, this technology offers hope and the possibility of control over one's reproductive function. For others, however, this technology represents exploitation, immorality, and the possibility of loss of control over one's reproductive function. The use of this technology raises important feminist issues. This chapter examines these issues in terms of three concepts: (1) choice, (2) control, and (3) the meaning of parenthood. A section on nursing practice and research is included as a means of suggesting how nurses can integrate humanism and caring in a world of high technology.

OVERVIEW OF REPRODUCTIVE TECHNOLOGIES

A brief overview of the various current technological procedures used in the control of reproduction will assist in the discussion that follows.

IVF represents a method of conception in which the woman's fallopian tubes are bypassed. This procedure consists of medical hyperstimulation of the ovaries to achieve several mature eggs, or follicles; the subsequent surgical retrieval of these eggs; and the fertilization of the retrieved eggs, in a test tube by mixing the eggs and masturbated sperm from the woman's partner or from a donor. The resulting fertilized eggs, after undergoing a series of cell divisions, become embryos and are then transferred to the woman's uterus in the hope that a pregnancy will result.

Artificial insemination consists of collecting sperm from the male and inserting it into the woman's vagina, cervix, or uterus at the presumed time of ovulation. Sperm can be collected from the woman's husband or partner or from a known or anonymous donor. Various methods of artificial insemination exist.[13] Recently a more technologically sophisticated form of artificial insemination has become popular, involving the use of ultrasound and medical stimulation of the ovaries so that ovulation can be precisely timed and chances are greater that the woman will, in fact, ovulate. Sperm are washed in a special solution to improve motility and are inseminated into the woman's uterus.

GIFT involves surgical retrieval of the egg or eggs as well as retrieval by masturbation of the partner's sperm. Both the sperm and the egg(s) are placed into the fallopian tube via laparoscopy in the hope that fertilization will occur in the tube and the resulting embryo will implant normally into the wall of the uterus.

The use of donor oocytes involves retrieving an egg or eggs from a known or anonymous donor, who must undergo medical hyperstimulation of her ovaries. The recipient, too, must undergo hormonal therapy to ensure correct timing of her menstrual cycle so that her uterus is ready to accept a fertilized egg (fertilized by her partner's sperm or by donor sperm). In addition, the recipient must continue hormonal therapy for several weeks to ensure that her uterus can maintain the embryo until the placenta takes over this functioning. Frozen embryo transfer involves the freezing of embryos that have been created in a test tube, as described for IVF. These embryos can be frozen for an indefinite period of time, although the procedure is so new that no long-term studies exist regarding the efficacy of length of time of freezing. The embryos can then be transferred to the uterus of the woman (most likely the woman from whom the egg has been retrieved for fertilization and subsequent freezing).

Surrogate mothering is the process of artificially inseminating a woman, with the intent that she will carry the resulting conceptus to term and then, under contract, give up the baby for adoption by a couple with whom she has contracted. The couple usually consists of the sperm donor and his wife.

GENERAL ETHICAL CONSIDERATIONS
Greater good versus individual good

Several ethical dilemmas are posed by the technologies described above.[4] Religious concerns verbalized most strongly by the Catholic church address the issue of the sanctity of life and the question of when, in fact, life begins. Societal concerns related to the preservation of family values are manifested in debates over such questions as: What constitutes a family? Are single men and women or homosexual men and women considered a family? Where do third parties—such as surrogate mothers, egg donors, or sperm donors—fit? Many legal and ethical dilemmas are posed by the use of high-technology reproductive controls.[1,17]

Many authors describe these technologies as providing alternatives and options for infertile persons. They tend to see the value in these technologies but are cautious regarding the potential human price. Menning[10] and Lasker and Borg[6] have sensitively detailed the conflicting nature of hope and despair with which infertile persons are confronted in choosing such technologies. Olshansky[12] describes the complex human responses to the possibility of pursuing such technologies. The psychological responses to IVF have been outlined by Mahlstedt, MacDuff, and Bernstein[7] as well as by Seibel and Levin.[16]

Although these controversial issues often are discussed only in terms of infertile persons, several authors address the dilemmas posed by these technologies in terms of society in general. Corea,[3] Arditti, Klein, and Minden,[2] and Rowland[15] raise many thought-provoking issues in discussing the implications of such technologies. They note the potential of women being subjugated and controlled by a medical system run predominantly by men. The exploitation of women is a central focus of Corea's account of how

women would be used purely for reproductive purposes and is particularly evident in her description of "breeding brothels." A strong argument against the use of surrogate mothers, in fact, is that surrogates tend to be of a lower socioeconomic status and the potential adoptive parents of a much higher socioeconomic status. The potential for exploiting poor women is evident.

A difficult dilemma is noted in the literature, posed by the question of the greater good versus the individual good.[2,13,15,18] In more concrete terms, the questions addressed are as follows: Is there a conflict between the good of society and the good of individuals, such as infertile persons? Although infertile persons may benefit from technologies such as IVF by achieving a much-wanted pregnancy, is this at the expense of the larger society, particularly in relation to women?

This is an extremely complicated issue, and it is clear that the potential exists for harm to be done to society in general and women in particular. At the same time, however, opportunities and choices that can be available to infertile persons should not be denied them. With proper regulation of the providers of the technology and with sensitive counseling and care of the recipients of such technology, perhaps the serious negative consequences can be averted. The issues are quite complex and deserve a thorough analysis. A more detailed examination of the concepts of choice, control, and the meaning of parenthood will help to elucidate some of these issues.

The concept of choice

The women's movement and feminism have addressed the importance of choice, especially in relation to reproduction. The right of women to choose abortion is a prime example and the potential loss of this choice in the current political climate poses a clear threat to a very basic right of women—the right to choose whether or not to bear a child. This concept also can be applied to infertile women, who represent the other end of the reproductive continuum in that they desperately want to bear a child but are unable to do so. These women also would like the right to choose. For them, techniques such as IVF represent the right to choose to bear a child, just as abortion represents the right of other women to choose not to bear a child.

The concept of choice related to high-technology infertility treatments is not quite so simple, however. Rothman[14] aptly addresses the issue of "choice" that actually becomes "lack of choice" in particular situations. She advances the view that technology does permit choice, but questions whose choice this is, arguing that the medical practitioners rather then the patients are making those choices. She cites the example of physicians choosing to perform cesarean sections on women because of mild fetal distress apparent on the fetal heart monitor, and asks whether this choice is actually appropriate.

One can raise the question as to whether women truly are gaining more choice in the matter of fertility. When IVF and other techniques are prohibitively expensive, this choice may only be available to upper-middle-class women. Access to infertility treatment and specifically high-technology treatment is rarely available to poor women, although infertility does not limit itself to a particular socioeconomic status.

One can also question whether choice truly exists for all women when the medical profession often limits the criteria for eligibility for such choices, particularly with respect to certain high-technology procedures. Many IVF clinics have used 35 years as an age limit, although some are raising this limit to 40 and even 42 years. Single women or homosexual women are often excluded from the criteria, raising ethical and moral issues having to do with family values. The concept of choice, then, becomes intertwined with the concept of control.

The concept of control

Who controls women's bodies has long been a concern of the feminist and women's health movements. The area of reproductive control reflects this concern. With the advent of newer methods of contraception, particularly with oral contraceptives, women have gained a degree of control over their reproductive lives. However, issues of control over women's reproduction remain a central issue. Important questions include: Who has control over reproduction, the providers or the recipients of such control? What are the consequences of such control (e.g., the side effects of oral contraceptives)? Under what conditions does such control exist (for example, pharmaceutical experimentation with various contraceptive methods on women in Third World countries)?

It is clear that many infertile women view the new technologies as means of gaining more control over their reproductive functions, because they now feel that the possibility exists to achieve a pregnancy. This is crucial, since a common feeling verbalized among those experiencing infertility is that of being "out of control."[8]

Hubbard,[5] however, views the new technologies as means for the medical profession to gain more control over women's bodies. She views this as a greater threat than the benefit to a few individual infertile persons. Menning,[9] taking an opposing stance, clearly notes the value for infertile persons in terms of assisting them to gain more control over their own bodies. This debate elucidates the complexity of the issues surrounding reproductive controls.

The meaning of parenthood

The two concepts of choice and control are intimately related to the meaning of parenthood. In Western society, parenthood has come to connote aspects of choice and control. The decision or choice to have children is evident; much is written and spoken about the decisions women must make as they confront their "biological clocks." Choosing to use or not use contraception—"family planning"—is evidence of the importance of controlling childbearing by either delaying it or avoiding it completely. The underlying connotation is that people have a choice in and control over decisions about parenthood. It is important to note, however, that this is not necessarily the case for all, as witnessed in the soaring adolescent pregnancy rate and large family sizes among those in whom contraception is not readily available.

Lasker and Borg[6] aptly title their recent book *In Search of Parenthood*, which addresses the exhausting search infertile couples endure as they attempt to achieve the ability to "choose" to become parents and to have "control" over their choice. In many ways the new technologies assist them in gaining such choice and control.

Of course it can be argued that the new technologies remove choice and control from parenthood. Corea[3] certainly makes that argument as she discusses how women may simply become "breeders" for those in control; she foresees that women's choices and their control over their lives will become nonexistent. Again, the philosophical and ethical question is raised regarding the greater good versus the individual good.

FUTURE DIRECTIONS

It is clear that these new reproductive technologies can lead to many adverse consequences if not regulated. The benefits of such technologies, however, cannot be discounted. Many infertile couples have achieved parenthood as a direct result of these technologies. In taking this position, though, it is essential to point out that it is far from simplistic or clear-cut. The human pain and suffering that accompany the decision to pursue something like IVF, which has at the most a 25% success rate, is not a trivial matter. The very real and painful human responses to subjecting one's body and one's emotional self to such invasion for the purpose of achieving what most achieve without comparable effort cannot be ignored. The very real and painful human responses to the inability to conceive and bear a child, however, also cannot be ignored.

The need for these technologies within a context of regulation is apparent. Corea,[3] in fact, proposes one method of regulation. She draws her ideas from an environmental engineer, Patricia Hynes, who suggests a regulatory model based on one currently in use to deal with hazardous waste. This model is analogous to the function of the Environmental Protection Agency. Through such a model, the use of reproductive technologies would be regulated. Much detailed planning is needed to develop and implement such a model, but the idea holds great promise.[3]

In addition, nursing can play a key role in counseling persons who are considering using such technologies, to ensure that they are informed and knowledgeable and are making decisions that are right for them. The following section describes the role of nurses in both practice and research in the area of high-technology infertility treatments.

NURSING'S ROLE IN PRACTICE AND RESEARCH

The experience of infertility, whether or not one chooses an option like IVF, is very distressing and often affects one's self-concept.[11] The stresses and demands of pursuing expensive technologies with uncertain results clearly add to the distress of infertility. Nursing plays a key role in caring for patients who are considering or are currently involved in using high technology to enable them to become parents.

One important area for nursing practice is assisting patients in the decision-making process. Nurses can help individuals or couples examine the options available to them and, in so doing, aid them in making decisions that are best for them. The decisions can include ending treatment and either adopting a child

or choosing a childfree lifestyle, or aggressively pursuing any and all treatments available that provide even the slightest hope of conception. A very important aspect of counseling is helping patients make decisions as they proceed with their infertility treatment(s). There may be a time when some patients want to stop treatment and "get on with their lives," a phrase commonly used by infertile persons in describing the desire to complete the very disruptive and stressful infertility treatments. The nurse-counselor plays a key role in validating this desire and in assisting patients to realize their wish to stop treatment. It is often the case that patients do not receive validation for stopping treatment, but instead see themselves as failures for not continuing with everything possible to try to conceive. An important role of the nurse-counselor is to help patients achieve good self-images and to view themselves as successful if they can come to some resolution regarding their infertility treatment.[12] For some this resolution means stopping treatment, whereas for others it means attempting every possible treatment available to them, even if experimental. A sensitive, insightful counselor can help tremendously in this area.

Another important nursing function is to educate patients by making sure they understand the procedure(s) they are choosing and by answering their questions. This will result in more informed consumers, possibly leading to increased consumer or patient control over their own decisions.

The counseling function of nursing is most apparent, because patients clearly are facing important, stressful, and difficult decisions with potentially significant consequences. Helping individuals or couples to understand the issues they are confronting and to put these issues into perspective is an essential role of counseling. The nurse can help couples assess their marital relationships, motivations for parenthood, and responses to infertility and its treatment.

Nursing research can contribute important data to the humanistic aspects of the use of reproductive technologies. More research is needed to investigate the human responses to high technology, the consequences of not conceiving despite the use of technology, and the experience of pregnancy that may result from such technology. In addition, research into the therapeutic aspect of nursing practice in relation to patients who choose high technology would provide important data for effective nursing interventions. With well-designed research studies nurses may be better able to provide caring, humanistic health care within a context of high technology.

SUMMARY

The intent of this chapter has been to convey the very complex nature of the issues raised by the new technological reproductive-control mechanisms. Although the potential dangers of such mechanisms were addressed and a cautious approach to their use advocated, the benefits to infertile persons were highlighted. The technologies were discussed in terms of the concepts of choice, control, and the meaning of parenthood.

The viewpoint taken in this chapter is that reproductive technologies, while posing potentially serious problems for society, also provide many persons with hope and the opportunity for parenthood. Although these technologies may not be chosen by all infertile persons, a significant number do choose them and should not be denied access to them. Much caution is advocated in the use of such technologies, in the form of more stringent controls over the providers of the technologies and careful, sensitive counseling of the recipients.

REFERENCES

1. Andrews LB: Legal and ethical aspects of new reproductive technologies, Clin Obstet Gynecol 29(1):190, 1986.
2. Arditti R, Klein RD, and Minden S, editors: Test-tube women, London, 1984, Pandora Press.
3. Corea G: The mother machine, New York, 1985, Harper & Row Publishers, Inc.
4. Grobstein C and Flower M: Current ethical issues in IVF, Clin Obstet Gynaecol 12(4):877, 1985.
5. Hubbard R: The case against in vitro fertilization. In Holmes H, Hoskins B, and Gross M, editors: The custom-made child? Clifton, NJ, 1981, Humana Press.
6. Lasker JN and Borg S: In search of parenthood, Boston, 1987, Beacon Press.
7. Mahlstedt PP, MacDuff S, and Bernstein J: Emotional factors and the in vitro fertilization and embryo transfer process, J In Vitro Fert Embryo Transfer 4(4):232, 1987.
8. McCormick TM: Out of control: one aspect of infertility, J Obstet Gynecol Neonatal Nurs 9(4):205, 1980.
9. Menning BE: In defense of in vitro fertilization. In Holmes H, Hoskins B, and Gross M, editors: The Child?custom-made child? Clifton, NJ, 1981, Humana Press.
10. Menning BE: Infertility: a guide for the childless couple, ed 2, New York, 1988, Prentice-Hall, Inc.
11. Olshansky EF: Identity of self as infertile: an example of theory-generating research, Advances in Nursing Science 9(2):54, 1987.
12. Olshansky EF: Human responses to high technology infertility treatment: a grounded theory analysis, Image 1988 20(3):128, 1988.
13. Olshansky EF and Sammons LN: Artificial insemination: an overview, J Obstet Gynecol Neonatal Nurs 14(6s):49, 1985.
14. Rothman BK: The meanings of choice in reproductive technology. In Arditti R, Klein RD, and Minden S, editors: Test-tube women, London, 1984, Pandora Press.
15. Rowland R: Reproductive technologies: the final solution to the woman question? In Arditti R, Klein RD, Minden S, editors: Test-tube women, London, 1984, Pandora Press.
16. Seibel MM and Levin S: A new era in reproductive technologies: the emotional stages of in vitro fertilization, J In Vitro Fert Embryo Transfer 4(3):135, 1987.
17. Singer P and Wells D: Making babies: the new science and ethics of conception, ed 2, New York, 1985, Charles Scribner's Sons.
18. Strickland OL: In vitro fertilization: dilemma or opportunity? Advances in Nursing Science 3(2):41, 1981.

CHAPTER 89

What are the ethical issues from a worldwide viewpoint?

CONSTANCE A. HOLLERAN

Should ethical standards vary throughout the world? This is a controversial question that can be debated from a variety of perspectives. From a truly moral absolutist viewpoint, ethical standards should be the same everywhere, no matter which culture one is born into. From a cultural relativist viewpoint, there can be no one standard because philosophical traditions in different parts of the world have come to different conclusions regarding ethical conduct. In some Western Pacific cultures it was ethically acceptable up to 100 years ago to eat human flesh. In 1988 one still reads of female circumcision, a culturally accepted practice that must be considered ethical in societies in which it is practiced openly. Many people know about the ancient custom of allowing or even assisting the elderly to go to an isolated area to die a quiet death. They also may know of Americans in their nineties who have been kept alive even though unconscious through the use of sophisticated equipment and drugs. Is one practice ethical and the other not, or do technology and resources make a difference?

RAPID CHANGES AHEAD

"A few days ago, a team of researchers took the first steps towards the creation of a radical new medical treatment, one that has profound implications for society. The group asked for permission to carry out the genetic alteration of a human being."[7] So begins an article on the editorial page of a London newspaper. The report discussed an actual event, not, as one might guess, a science fiction story.

Changes brought about by scientific advancement are having profound effects on the health field and on nursing. Developments that in the past were not seriously even dreamed about are today a reality. So much of a reality that in several developed or indus-

trialized countries the citizens feel they must put limits on some types of scientific research to provide safeguards for the public. In some countries that means a requirement of extensive peer review. In another, the government may start requiring researchers to obtain a government license before even beginning certain kinds of projects.[7]

Aroskar states: "Dealing with ethical concerns in the world of nursing practice and service requires dealing with the political dimension as well. Ethics and politics interface and overlap. . . . Isn't ethics about right or good action and politics about power and manipulation?"[1] From an international perspective that is true, not that current politics changes the ethics of an issue, but political changes can change the way a society sees things. Take attitudes on abortion in the United States in 1950 compared to those in 1980, for example. Although many groups in that society have not changed their views, the court rulings and laws have changed dramatically.

ARE INTERNATIONAL ETHICAL ISSUES OF CONCERN TO AMERICAN NURSES?

Nurses need to raise this question in many settings. I personally feel very strongly that U.S. nurses have a responsibility to speak out on several types of issues of concern to nurses worldwide, and I will discuss just a few of those.

Drugs—usefulness and need

The availability of drugs in developing countries leads to headlines that for a day or two spark heated discussions. Otherwise things seem to go on as usual. Three major controversial topics in the 1980s are the export of outdated drugs, the export of drugs not yet certified as safe and effective for American distribution, and the promotion and aggressive sale of nonessential drugs. In countries facing grave financial crises this expenditure on drugs can restrict the availability of needed health services. These are all issues that are decided by those with more power than hospital nurses. Yet hospital and community nurses see the results of decisions about such drugs, and they can have some influence on policies regarding them.

Diplomatic pressure from the United States was reported to have been applied quite recently to one of the poorest countries in the world when the government of that country decided it would import only the 200 essential drugs identified as essential by the World Health Organization (WHO). Is this appropriate action to be taken by **your** government? Outdated drugs, the efficacy of which must be in doubt, are still being sent to developing (nonindustrialized) countries either as contributions or for sale. Is it safe and ethical to give such a drug to a dying child in Uganda but not in New York? Yet another situation arises when drugs not cleared for use in the United States are tested, tried, or used regularly in other countries so the market can be developed. Is it ethically sound, for example, to export an experimental contraceptive when it has not yet been determined to be safe for use in one's own country?

How can and should nurses make their ethical concerns known? To me these are natural issues on which the state nurses' associations and the American Nurses' Association should speak out. To do so they need to hear from their members, after which they can approach the appropriate policymakers. Individual members should contact their own elected officials to make their wishes known on these issues, which are of international significance.

Infant formula and weaning foods

A few years ago the aggressive promotion of commercially prepared infant formula in poor countries made headlines in the United States, prompting congressional hearings, lobbying by health professional organizations and others, and the organization of boycotts. A WHO code was developed and agreed to by the World Health Assembly (WHA), which meets in Geneva each May to set policy and budget for WHO. The only country voting against that code was the United States.

Eventually the code was accepted by the companies involved, and the controversy quieted down. Yet quite recently many people have expressed concern that costly weaning foods are now being promoted among people who can barely afford subsistence diets. Commercial trade is important to every country. Yet it is also important, in terms of moral responsibility, to see that people are not made to feel they must buy costly imported foods when perfectly good and inexpensive local products are readily available. Wealthy people in all countries may wish to spend money on such things, but that is not the issue. The problem I see arises when parents feel their children must eat on a regular basis the food the hospital had given the parents as free samples. And to provide these samples where water may be unsafe, refrigeration unavailable, and the cost high can lead to health and other problems for a family. I have seen mothers give very diluted formula to babies that resulted in malnourishment, illness, and even death. Nurses are usually the ones responsible for patient education. Are they giving out those samples? These are not necessarily direct care or cure ethical issues, but I believe they are international ethical issues of nursing.

CULTURAL DIFFERENCES

Ethics evolve from the mores and values held by a society. Such values develop from religious, historical, and cultural traditions and these may vary from country to country. For example, the rights of the individual versus the rights of society at large, and the right to know (information about illness outcomes, etc.) versus the right to withhold information are perceived very differently in different cultures. In other words, what is generally felt to be "right" in the West may not be "right" in some Eastern or other cultures. Currently there is much discussion about rights of privacy because of the spread of AIDS. Some countries say the right to privacy requires that testing for the virus can be done only if a person requests it. Yet other countries require testing of all foreigners and may test without an individual's consent. The clash centers around the rights of the many versus the rights of the individual. If ethics are seen as being universal, such issues create dilemmas that are not easily resolved.

SOURCES OF ORGANS FOR TRANSPLANTS

The expansion of high technology in the health care system of the industrialized countries has raised many new issues for health care workers to consider. Some of the more controversial ones revolve around when death occurs, how long people should be kept alive, and the quality of life of patients who are being kept alive by artificial means. I will not deal with those issues here.

But, have you considered the ethical implications of where some organs for transplantation come from? Should you know? Should you raise the issue? In a newspaper report early in 1988[8] it was reported that children in Bangladesh were being kidnapped to make their organs available for transplants! Consider the implications. Do health professionals play a role in such situations? When transplants are done, do they ask about the source of the organs? Should poor children from poor countries lose their lives so that children in industrialized countries can live? There have been reports that this issue is being exploited for political reasons. Yet the article I quoted from was quoting a government official of the country involved. It is something to think about.

HEALTHWORKERS AT RISK

Few health professionals, it is hoped, will ever have to help the wounded and suffering during an armed conflict, guerrilla war or political or civil disturbance. But everyone should be prepared and know how to face such situations. The International Committee of the Red Cross (ICRC) constantly monitors the Geneva Conventions.[5] Not all countries that have recognized those conventions abide by them. Everyone should be familiar with them, however.

At the International Council of Nurses (ICN) I heard about several nurses and other healthworkers who still are jailed and some who were physically tortured for providing emergency care to wounded people who were in opposition to the government. Also nurses and other community workers have been jailed for helping to bring about social changes that would improve the health and well-being of the poor.

NURSE-CLIENT OR PRISONER-SECURITY WORKER'S ROLE

Nurses working in prisons are often asked to do body searches on prisoners to look for drugs or weapons. Does this raise ethical issues? Does such a dual role jeopardize the confidentiality rights of the prisoner in the nurse-client relationship?

Some nurses believe it does and that security personnel should be trained to do body searches. They

asked ICN to develop an official position on that issue.[6] However, nurses in some countries argue that nurses should do such searches, so there is not universal agreement among nurses on this matter.

In addition to the body search problem, nurses who work in prisons face other issues involving confidentiality. They may have access to confidential information about a prisoner that could be important for others to know. How should such situations be handled?

ETHICS IN NURSING AND OTHER PROFESSIONS

A recent text on ethics edited by Joan Callahan looks at similar ethical issues in a variety of professions.[3] Again, the ethical implications of many of those topics will be viewed differently in different parts of the world. The recognition that nurses, lawyers, social workers, and others confront similar problems should encourage nurses to open lines of communication to colleagues in other professions.

The Council for International Organizations of Medical Sciences (CIOMS), to which ICN belongs, has sponsored conferences on ethical issues. The most recent one was held in the Netherlands in 1987.[2] One of the topics discussed at that conference was euthanasia, a topic that has received considerable press attention in Europe recently. Cases of individual doctors and nurses taking active steps to bring about death in the terminally ill have been reported. Devaneson cites a specific case of a lethal dose of morphine being ordered for a dying patient.[4] Even when euthanasia is not actually legal, legal action against the persons involved is not always taken. The ethical implications of this issue are a long way from being resolved. It is one of the real ethical crisis nurses must deal with.

ICN developed its first Code of Ethics in 1953. It has been revised and updated periodically. Its current format offers broad guidelines rather than specific suggestions for resolving individual issues. This approach has proved to be advantageous when the national nurses' associations needed to adapt the code to meet their specific needs. In 1988 it was agreed, after considerable discussion and review, to keep the current code to guide nurses as they deal with ethical issues worldwide.

The pace of change is so rapid in these days of genetic engineering and technological advances that we all need to remind ourselves to stop to consider the ethics of some aspects of progress. No one chapter can deal with all ethical issues of a global or international nature—all we can hope to do is to broaden our awareness, recognize and respect our differences, and think together.

REFERENCES

1. Aroskar MA: The interface of ethics and politics in nursing, Nurs Outlook 35(6):268, 1987.
2. Bankowski Z and Bryant JH: Health policy, ethics and human values: European and North American perspectives, England, Geneva, 1988, The Council for International Organizations of Medical Sciences.
3. Callahan JC: Ethical issues in professional life, New York, 1988, Oxford Univ Press, Inc.
4. Chandaramani M and Devadas RP: Ethical values in a changing world. Coimbatore. Sri Ramakrishna Mission Vidyalaya Insutrial Institute, p 165, 1987.
5. International Committee of the Red Cross (ICRC): Basic rules of the Geneva conventions and their additional protocols, Geneva, 1983, ICRC.
6. International Council of Nurses (ICN): The nurses' role in the care of detainees and prisoners, Geneva, 1986, ICN.
7. McKie R: Designer baby ethics, Observer (London), p 14, August 7, 1988.
8. Slave trade. The Sunday Times (London), p A19, April 17, 1988.

Concluding notes and future directions

JOANNE COMI McCLOSKEY
HELEN KENNEDY GRACE

As we have said before in previous editions, there is no conclusion to a book on issues in nursing. Given the purpose of the book, "to provide a forum for knowledgeable debate on today's nursing issues so that intelligent decision making can occur," an ending is, in fact, inappropriate.

An issue is an issue for one of two reasons: either what is known is not well understood, or not enough is known. What is needed is debate on what is known to foster understanding and an ongoing search for knowledge about what is not known. Thoughtful debate and research are the keys to understanding a professional issue. Yet searching and debate are not enough for continued growth. Decision making also has to occur, and sometimes it has to occur in the absence of full knowledge. In this case, it is even more important to understand what is known and to be able to put this knowledge into a broader perspective.

The broader perspective requires that one keep current on the changes in the profession and health care field. Many things have changed since the 1985 edition of this book. Recent changes in nursing include a severe national nursing shortage, declining enrollments in schools of nursing, more employment opportunities for nurses outside of hospitals, more use of the computer and recognition of a standardized nursing language for documentation, more concern with costs and delivery of a quality product, more push by more nurses for participation in policy-making, a beginning effort to restructure hospitals to allow more nurses to have input into organizational decision making, more concern by all nurses with the care of the elderly and those with chronic illnesses, and more interest in nursing in other parts of the world.

Yet despite the many changes, the dilemmas faced by nursing remain the same as in the past. Stating them in the debate format, the dilemmas are

- unity versus diversity
- standards versus access
- quality versus cost
- independence versus dependence
- inside control versus outside control
- safety versus risk

The general recommendations to aid resolutions also are the same as in the past. In alphabetical order, they are

1. to clarify our mission
2. to get more involved professionally and politically
3. to produce more and better prepared leaders
4. to promote flexibility and diversity
5. to realign education and service
6. to support nursing research
7. to take control of our own destiny
8. to widen our horizons to include relevant issues outside the profession

Just looking over the list of recommendations, one can see that nursing as a profession is changing. We have made considerable progress on many of these recommendations in the past few years. Nurses are more involved and more influential in health care policy-making arenas, nursing research is alive and healthy, more nurses are preparing for leadership positions, and education and service have closer ties than in the recent past. This is not the time, though, to sit back and congratulate ourselves. The staff nurse and student nurse shortages threaten to undo some recent gains. The average staff nurse is still largely unaware of the broader issues, and most are not professionally committed. We need to push forward using the momentum that we have. Many old problems and issues still exist with new ones developing every day.

We believe that continual debate on important issues can lead to effective decision making and professional growth, both for the individual and the profession. This book, now in its third edition, has been our contribution to that process.

INDEX

ALSO AVAILABLE!

LEADERSHIP: THE KEY TO THE
PROFESSIONALIZATION OF NURSING
2nd Edition
Linda Ann Bernhard, Ph.D., R.N.; Michelle Walsh, Ph.D., R.N.
February 1990
ISBN 0-8016-0547-4

This concise, contemporary text provides a thorough background of leadership theories for future nurse leaders. A wide range of models and practical examples related directly to current nursing practice are presented to teach the nurse how to apply the most appropriate theory to a particular group and setting.

CASE STUDIES IN NURSING MANAGEMENT:
PRACTICE, THEORY, AND RESEARCH
Ann Marriner-Tomey, Ph.D., R.N., F.A.A.N.
February 1990
ISBN 0-8016-5848-9

This comprehensive new text, based on the management process of plan, organize, lead, motivate, and evaluate, helps nursing students and nurse managers apply nursing management theory to all levels of nursing management by analyzing case studies. Thirty-nine tested management theories from many different disciplines are related to real-life case studies in nursing.

NURSE'S LIABILITY FOR MALPRACTICE:
A PROGRAMMED APPROACH
5th Edition
Eli P. Bernzweig, J.D.
April 1990
ISBN 0-8016-6069-6

This authoritative resource helps students understand the meaning and relevance of nursing liability and malpractice through the exploration of numerous malpractice doctrines and statutes applicable to nurses. In this new edition, all cases, citations, examples, and legal guidelines have been updated to provide the most current legal information available.

To order, ask your bookstore manager or call toll-free 1-800-426-4545.
We look forward to hearing from you.

NMA-039